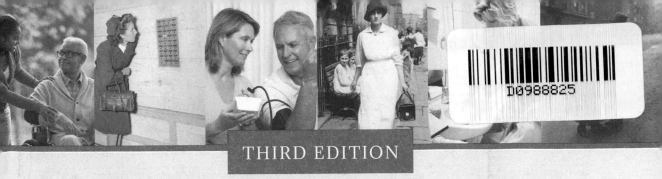

D0988825

THIRD EDITION

Public Health Nursing

Practicing Population-Based Care

Edited by

Marie Truglio-Londrigan, PhD, RN

Professor
Pace University, College of Health Professions
Lienhard School of Nursing
Pleasantville, New York

Sandra B. Lewenson, EdD, RN, FAAN

Professor
Pace University, College of Health Professions
Lienhard School of Nursing
Pleasantville, New York

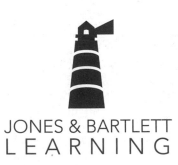

JONES & BARTLETT
LEARNING

World Headquarters
Jones & Bartlett Learning
5 Wall Street
Burlington, MA 01803
978-443-5000
info@jblearning.com
www.jblearning.com

Jones & Bartlett Learning books and products are available through most bookstores and online booksellers. To contact Jones & Bartlett Learning directly, call 800-832-0034, fax 978-443-8000, or visit our website, www.jblearning.com.

Substantial discounts on bulk quantities of Jones & Bartlett Learning publications are available to corporations, professional associations, and other qualified organizations. For details and specific discount information, contact the special sales department at Jones & Bartlett Learning via the above contact information or send an email to specialsales@jblearning.com.

Copyright © 2018 by Jones & Bartlett Learning, LLC, an Ascend Learning Company

All rights reserved. No part of the material protected by this copyright may be reproduced or utilized in any form, electronic or mechanical, including photocopying, recording, or by any information storage and retrieval system, without written permission from the copyright owner.

The content, statements, views, and opinions herein are the sole expression of the respective authors and not that of Jones & Bartlett Learning, LLC. Reference herein to any specific commercial product, process, or service by trade name, trademark, manufacturer, or otherwise does not constitute or imply its endorsement or recommendation by Jones & Bartlett Learning, LLC and such reference shall not be used for advertising or product endorsement purposes. All trademarks displayed are the trademarks of the parties noted herein. *Public Health Nursing: Practicing Population-Based Care, Third Edition* is an independent publication and has not been authorized, sponsored, or otherwise approved by the owners of the trademarks or service marks referenced in this product.

There may be images in this book that feature models; these models do not necessarily endorse, represent, or participate in the activities represented in the images. Any screenshots in this product are for educational and instructive purposes only. Any individuals and scenarios featured in the case studies throughout this product may be real or fictitious, but are used for instructional purposes only.

The authors, editor, and publisher have made every effort to provide accurate information. However, they are not responsible for errors, omissions, or for any outcomes related to the use of the contents of this book and take no responsibility for the use of the products and procedures described. Treatments and side effects described in this book may not be applicable to all people; likewise, some people may require a dose or experience a side effect that is not described herein. Drugs and medical devices are discussed that may have limited availability controlled by the Food and Drug Administration (FDA) for use only in a research study or clinical trial. Research, clinical practice, and government regulations often change the accepted standard in this field. When consideration is being given to use of any drug in the clinical setting, the health care provider or reader is responsible for determining FDA status of the drug, reading the package insert, and reviewing prescribing information for the most up-to-date recommendations on dose, precautions, and contraindications, and determining the appropriate usage for the product. This is especially important in the case of drugs that are new or seldom used.

Production Credits
VP, Executive Publisher: David D. Cella
Executive Editor: Amanda Martin
Editorial Assistant: Emma Huggard
Production Manager: Carolyn Rogers Pershouse
Production Assistant: Molly Hogue
Senior Marketing Manager: Jennifer Scherzay
Product Fulfillment Manager: Wendy Kilborn
Composition: S4Carlisle Publishing Services
Project Management: S4Carlisle Publishing Services
Cover Design: Kristin E. Parker

Rights & Media Specialist: Wes DeShano
Media Development Editor: Troy Liston
Cover Image (Title Page): (clockwise) Courtesy of the Visiting Nurse Service of New York; © SilviaJansen/iStock/Getty Images Plus/Getty; Courtesy of Visiting Nurse Service of New York; © Terry Vine/Blend Images/Getty; Courtesy of the Visiting Nurse Service of New York; © kurhan/Shutterstock
Printing and Binding: Edwards Brothers Malloy
Cover Printing: Edwards Brothers Malloy

To order this product, use ISBN: 978-1-284-12129-2

Library of Congress Cataloging-in-Publication Data
Names: Truglio-Londrigan, Marie, editor. | Lewenson, Sandra, editor.
Title: Public health nursing : practicing population-based care / editors, Marie Truglio-Londrigan, Sandra B. Lewenson.
Other titles: Public health nursing (Truglio-Londrigan)
Description: Third edition. | Burlington, MA : Jones & Bartlett Learning, [2018] | Includes bibliographical references and index.
Identifiers: LCCN 2017002918 | ISBN 9781284136500 (pbk.)
Subjects: | MESH: Public Health Nursing | Evidence-Based Nursing | Models, Organizational | United States
Classification: LCC RT42 | NLM WY 108 | DDC 610.73--dc23 LC record available at https://lccn.loc.gov/2017002918

6048

Printed in the United States of America
21 20 19 18 17   10 9 8 7 6 5 4 3 2 1

Contents

1   What Is Public Health and Public Health Nursing? 3

2   Public Health Nursing in the United States: A History 23

3   Assessment: Using the Public Health Nursing Assessment Tool 49

8 Considerations of Culture in the Health of the Public 173

9 Healthcare Policy and Politics: The Risk and Rewards for Public Health Nurses 197

10 Social Justice and the Ethics of Public Health Practice 217

11 Hitting the Pavement: Intervention of Case-Finding: Outreach, Screening, Surveillance, and Disease and Health Event Investigation 229

Foreword

Some things remain the same, but the context is different. In the preface to the second edition, I described public health nursing as the "linchpin" of America's health. Presciently, the 2010 National Academy of Medicine report *The Future of Nursing* highlighted the importance of public health nursing. In 2017, as it has across the last century, public health nursing remains critical to the health of our nation, and in particular, for our most vulnerable populations. Because of the uncertainties surrounding the payment and provision of health care and changes we will see in future healthcare legislation, public health nurses are indeed the line in the sand, the safety net for many people.

The third edition of *Public Health Nursing: Practicing Population-Based Care* refines the salient issues from the previous volume. There is a new chapter on social justice, a critical construct in our current environment of cost-cutting and marginalization of certain population groups. Throughout the last century, we have seen the rise and fall of particular social movements—the Civil Rights Movement, the Consumer Movement, the Women's Movement, just to name a few. Social justice has been a critical foundation for all of these. But it is wise for us to remember that social justice and social movements exist in particular forms at particular times and places. For this reason, the historical foundations in this volume are critical for understanding nurses' participation in these movements. It is also critical to recognize that nurses' frame of social justice is context dependent, another reason for understanding the historical underpinnings of constructs and ideas. For example, nurses participated in both the January 2017 Women's March on Washington, as well as the Right to Life March a week later. Understanding social justice from an historical frame helps us see the value of history as well as the importance of creating alliances that bridge divides across political beliefs, professional practice, and policy standpoints.

Public health nursing is based on these critical alliances, and the work of public health nurses relies on the ability to bridge diverse interests of individuals, families, communities, and populations in order to support the seamless movement of the public across healthcare settings and to access resources. Health for all is an implicit philosophy in public health nursing practice. But health for all cannot be actualized by reinforcing silos of all kinds. As this volume explicates, creating alliances through interdisciplinary care, a shared understanding of a culture of health, and a firm foundation of social justice can create a movement that supports public health and primary health care—for all.

The third edition of *Public Health Nursing: Practicing Population-Based Care* is more than a textbook. It is a rallying cry for health care for everyone, and it offers historical evidence for action and for advocacy.

The editors, an expert practitioner and a historian, use the concept of a quest—to search for something that may be undefined—and it is a well-chosen ideal. Public health nursing is in itself a quest. Each one of us must find that public health nurse that is in all of us. Our quest should also train laser-like on a search for the best strategies to care for individuals, families, and communities in uncertain times that may need to be reformatted, revised, and reimagined. Public health nurses will need partners on this quest as they form alliances to support the public. As the editors note, "It is only through the applying and doing of public health nursing that society may attain 'health for all'" as stipulated in the World Health Organization's 1978 Declaration of Alma-Ata. This should be nurses' rallying cry and call to action no matter their politics or their clinical focus, and the tools to support this "movement" can be found in this volume.

Julie Fairman, PhD, RN, FAAN
Nightingale Professor of Nursing in Honor of Military Veterans
Chair, Department of Biobehavioral Health Sciences
Director Emerita, Barbara Bates Center for the Study of the History of Nursing
School of Nursing
University of Pennsylvania
Philadelphia, PA

Preface

Lillian D. Wald (1913) wrote about the "prophets among the nurses and among the students of social movements who see the veil lifted, and who know that the great aray [sic] of nurses are educating the people, translating into simple terms the message of the expert and the scientist" (p. 2). We take Wald's early-20th-century message to heart as we revise our third edition of *Public Health Nursing: Practicing Population-Based Care*. To begin the process of revision, we turned to the nurses, the experts, the scientists, and to the people that we serve to help us educate new nurses in this extraordinary role. We asked our publisher, Jones & Bartlett Learning, to share feedback from those who used the book in their courses—what they liked and what they wanted to see added. Faculty liked the public health assessment tool; they liked the case studies and wanted to see more of them; and while some questioned the overabundance of history, some wanted even more to use as they integrated the past into the current and future role of the public health nurse. We also turned to the origin of this—our own evolutionary history as public health nurses and educators—to use and expand upon in this revision.

We first revisited our earlier exploration of what it means to practice population-based public health nursing. We continued to raise and refine the questions that we had asked previously about public health nursing. We considered the evolutionary nature of public health nursing and how one learned to become a public health nurse. We then considered how a "carry the bag" type of experience, usually found in visiting nurses service associations, and surveillance-type activities, like those found in publicly funded health departments, would develop a student's understanding of the scope of practice of the public health nurse. We finally reflected on ways in which we could integrate the ideas of evidence-based practice, technology, cultural competence, diversity, primary health care, social justice, environment, and history into the curriculum (and ultimately the work) of public health nurses.

This third edition of *Public Health Nursing: Practicing Population-Based Care* addresses these questions, and in so doing, offers a variety of perspectives on community and public health nursing from other texts already in use. Using the reader feedback, we continue to address the relevance of historical evidence in coming to know the meaning of the terms used to describe public health nursing, such as primary health care, primary care, disaster nursing, environmental nursing, and global perspectives. We updated each chapter and rewrote several chapters including the chapter on the use of technology in public health, the education chapter, the chapter on collaboration, coalition building, and community organizing, the chapter on contemporary emergency disaster management, as well as the chapter on advocacy, social marketing, policy development, and enforcement. We added two new chapters—one on social justice and the other on environmental health.

In this edition, we offer an innovatively designed and recently revised assessment tool that uses *Healthy People 2020* as its framework. Another highlight of this book (which we used previously and continue to use) is the focus on the 17 intervention strategies identified in the Population-Based Public Health Nursing Practice Intervention Wheel (Intervention Wheel), developed by the Minnesota Department of Health in the mid-1990s. In addition, these chapters examine how public health interventions may be applied throughout the three levels of practice: individual/family, community, and systems (Keller & Strohschein, 2016; Minnesota Department of Health, 2001). We included in each Intervention Wheel chapter a case study, contributed by our readers, that depicts how the particular strategies of that chapter are applied in public health nursing practice.

Each intervention strategy chapter also includes a box that highlights historical research about various aspects of the American Red Cross Town and Country, a little known rural public health nursing service that started in 1912 and ended in 1948. We used historical data to illustrate concepts of public health nursing within a primary health care framework such as collaboration, shared decision-making, evidence-based practice, and both interprofessional and intersectoral relationships.

At the end of each chapter, we also include an Additional Resources box to be used by the reader in a web quest. A *quest* is a journey in search of something, even though the destination is not clear. Those who embark on quests are explorers who are courageous, open, and willing to search and to take in information and learn from that information. We ask the reader to be that explorer and take some time using the websites in these boxes, and then consider what they learn and how to apply this information to their practice.

Another unique feature of this book is the opening quote in each chapter. In previous editions of the book, we used quotes from published materials in the literature. But this time, we wanted the futuristic words of Lillian D. Wald to resonate and lead us in our book. Therefore, we selected poignant excerpts from many of her unpublished papers (found in the New York City Public Library, Lillian D. Wald collection) to demonstrate the links between the past and current thinking about nurses, women, civic responsibility, the suffrage, and public health.

Other key concepts in public health, like social justice, health equity, health policies, and economics of care, appear in Wald's papers and still resonate today. As the American Association of Colleges of Nursing (AACN, 2008, 2011) calls for an integration of the liberal arts into nursing curricula at both the undergraduate and graduate levels, this book excels (we hope) in raising the interest of students, faculty, and professionals who will use this book going forward. It's what our readers called for, and what we believe that we have the expertise to offer.

Finally, one particularly unique feature of this book is the ongoing placement of nurses within a broad primary health care framework that calls for, among other things, health care for all. In our second edition, we began that conversation as an epilogue. This time, the final chapter on primary health care provides more than just a conversation. It shows how we, the editors and the contributing authors of this book, believe that public health nurses have an important role to play in helping individuals, families, communities, and populations move toward a culture of health (Hassmiller, 2017). Public health nurses have had and will continue to have a place in communities that demands clear decisions and leadership.

Neither nurses, nor any other professional groups or stakeholders, work in a vacuum. Yet, too often we work in our professional silos and rarely have an opportunity to fully understand the many roles and relationships that it requires to provide that culture of health we seek. To this end, we invited several professionals outside of nursing to participate in the development of an interprofessional perspective to be included in this third edition.

As a result, in this final chapter, we reached out to other professionals—dentistry, criminal justice, technology, law, occupational therapy, and political science—to ascertain their views on the vulnerable and on a particular public health issue. Furthermore, that dialogue begins a conversation on how we together may potentially collaborate to develop interventions with the population. We asked our contributors to consider an issue that they faced in practice and the population it focused on; we asked them to consider what collaboration with others meant to them, how they valued another discipline within a collaboration, and how they envisioned a collaborative effort with nurses. By doing so, we challenge faculty and students to begin a conversation about population engagement in the determination of priority initiatives and the corresponding public health interventions. It also encourages us to talk with other professionals in an attempt to facilitate collaboration. Collaborative interprofessional and intersectorial work is essential if the complex healthcare problems of our contemporary society are to be addressed. The ability to engage in collaborative work starts with a dialogue that broadens the worldview about oneself and collaborative relationships. To this end, we asked our new contributors and you, the reader, to begin this work.

Public Health Nursing: Practicing Population-Based Care aims to add greater clarity to the body of public health nursing literature, inclusive of primary health care, and serve as a useful tool for educators, students, and practitioners of public health nursing. Although the editors have revised many of the existing chapters and developed several new ones, they would like to include the caveat that knowledge evolves, and we urge the reader to continually support this work with additional sources as they become available.

Audience for This Book

This book can be used by nursing students in both baccalaureate and graduate degree programs. In addition, all nurses, whether practicing in public health, community health, or home care settings, can benefit from this book because it offers a way to understand how care of the individual, family, and population relates to larger systems and the care of communities. Nurses in all healthcare delivery systems should already practice population-based care; this book simply provides nurses with the information that they need to provide this care.

Organization and Pedagogical Features of the Book

Each chapter begins with a quotation and a photograph from nursing history that resonates with the content of the chapter. In this edition, as stated previously, we use excerpts from the noted early-20th-century public nursing leader Lillian D. Wald. Many have heard about her work, but few have read her unpublished ideas, which she frequently shared with the world during her lifetime. Objectives and key terms for each chapter offer direction to the reader as to what can be expected. Those chapters that address public health intervention strategies contain new case studies that reflect the geographical diversity of the United States.

The use of history as evidence is threaded throughout the chapters, where it illuminates the didactic content and case studies. Noted historians from around the world participated in the writing of several chapters that provide this evidence. We also included ongoing research in a separate box in each of the intervention chapters to illustrate how public health nurses historically may have applied these very same strategies. To aid the reader further, a glossary defining the various key terms used in the book can be found at the end of the book.

Although the editors wrote several chapters, they also turned to experts to write many of the chapters throughout the book. These contributing authors represent a cadre of outstanding nursing professionals who were willing to rethink the way that they practice and share their thoughts with the reader. Another unique feature of this book is that each contributor's "voice" can be heard in his or her own chapter. This means that the authors avoided consistency of style and pedagogy on purpose so they could showcase a diversity of ideas about how to approach public health nursing.

Chapter 1, "What Is Public Health and Public Health Nursing?" explores the ideas of health promotion and disease prevention and refers the reader to the evolutionary nature of nursing activities in primary, secondary, and tertiary prevention. Truglio-Londrigan and Lewenson point out that nursing care, especially public health nursing, is not a linear process. Using a nonlinear approach encourages us to think about providing care for diseases while simultaneously promoting health. The chapter includes definitions of public health and public health nursing, the three core functions of public health, 10 essential public health services, and an explanation of *Healthy People 2020*. The authors use these various documents and meanings of public health to help explain the work of public health nurses.

The reader finds an unusual approach to public health nursing history in Chapter 2, "Public Health Nursing in the United States: A History." Lewenson, a nurse historian, wrote this chapter from the standpoint of how changing definitions show the social, political, and economic influences that altered the work of nurses in the home setting. The author turns to past nursing leaders in public health nursing and examines how they defined public health nursing. Instead of writing a traditional history of public health nursing, she uses the past to explain the tensions that exist between and among the various titles that nurses have used to delineate care provided in the community, including district nurse, health visitor, public health nurse, community health nurse, and home care nurse. These changing definitions and titles show the evolutionary nature of public health nursing and the response of these nurses to the social, political, and economic environment. The use of historical evidence also offers insight into the questions that Truglio-Londrigan and Lewenson asked, including "What is public health nursing?" "How is public health nursing different from community health nursing or home care nursing?" and "How do we educate students about the role of public health nursing when the names and contextual meanings change over time?"

Chapter 3, "Assessment: Using the Public Health Nursing Assessment Tool," presents the innovative Public Health Nursing Assessment Tool (PHNAT) designed by Lewenson and Truglio-Londrigan. The PHNAT engages nurses, nursing students, and public health nurses in an assessment process that applies the newly published Process Model for *Healthy People 2020* (U.S. Department of Health and Human Services, 2010), with specific emphasis placed on the determinants of health and health status. In addition, the PHNAT directs the reader to use the Intervention Wheel strategies in their work. This chapter sees assessment as a fluid process, and the PHNAT offers the user a kaleidoscopic view of this process.

In Chapter 4, "Fundamentals of Epidemiology and Social Epidemiology," Moscou presents the science of epidemiology. She begins with a discussion of the history of epidemiology that highlights two revolutions in the field. The chapter covers the terms descriptive epidemiology, analytical epidemiology, the epidemiological triad, and the chain of infection. The author then introduces social epidemiology and the social determinants of health in the second part of the chapter. Comparisons between epidemiology and social epidemiology provide the reader with an understanding of both and allow greater application of the concepts.

In this edition, Quaranta, Srnka-Debnar, and Lev wrote a new chapter, Chapter 5, "Educating Public Health Nurses to 'Do' the Work." In this chapter, the authors explore the education of public health nurses and the various national organizations that speak to the education required to accomplish the role of public health nurses. It highlights the need for public health nurses, the impact that public health nurses have on the health of populations, and the rigor intricate to their education. With a changing and challenging healthcare system, public health nurses can facilitate the movement from a reactive, sick-care healthcare system to a proactive, health promotion, and disease prevention agenda. Public health nursing brings to the table the skill and expertise needed to organize all components of our healthcare system to ensure improvement in health outcomes. The authors include a case study that highlights a collegiate public health nursing course, showing how the faculty and students engage in the coursework and the outcomes achieved in developing new public health nurses.

Singleton, McLeod-Sordjan, and Valery Joseph contribute their expertise to Chapter 6, "Evidenced-Based Practice from a Public Health Perspective." This chapter defines the meaning of evidence-based practice, specifically focusing on public health nurses. Through the examples and case study, the authors describe a systematic approach to finding the best available evidence. Specifically, they explore the application of evidence-based practice to the public health issues of health literacy and tobacco use. The case study allows the reader to gain insight into how a public health nurse can use an evidence-based approach to improve the health of a local community and its population.

Morris writes a whole new Chapter 7, "Informatics in Public Health Nursing," for this edition of the book, offering the reader an understanding of key concepts reflected in information technology and public health nursing practice. She describes the meaning of several key terms, such as analytic assessment, data, database, and data mining. Morris explains the use of electronic health records in public health and allows the reader to understand some of the ethical concerns that technology creates in practice. The case study reflects the use of telehealth in a rural community and how its application into practice can improve the healthcare outcomes of a particular population. This chapter also shows the evolutionary nature and incorporation of information technology and applications. For example, the World Wide Web allows rapid search of databases and evidence for healthcare practices. Linkages of personal health records, electronic health records, and regional health information exchanges provide readily accessible data for monitoring the health status of individuals, families, communities, and populations. The potential exists for the development of infrastructure that could increase worldwide access to care. Morris concludes her chapter by reminding us that public health and informatics nurses must continually develop and refine competencies, adhere to standards, and participate in development, design, use, and regulating of health information technology.

Wilson and de Chesnay contributed Chapter 8, "Considerations of Culture in the Health of the Public." In this chapter, they define the subconcepts associated with culture, compare and contrast public health issues in terms of cultural influences, and provide analysis of public health nursing interventions for selected cases in terms of cultural competence. Wilson and de Chesnay explore the meaning of culture, ethnocentrism, xenophobia, and ritual, as well as what it means to be a participant observer, and then relate these topics to the meaning of culturally competent care in public health. Throughout this discussion, they ask the reader to participate in "field observations" that allow active learning and self-reflection.

Chapter 9, "Healthcare Policy and Politics: The Risk and Rewards for Public Health Nurses," is a new contribution by Nickitas and Rome. In this chapter, these authors present issues facing the U.S. healthcare system, including rising costs; reduction in employer-based contributions; the growing ranks of the uninsured; inadequate supply of health providers; a healthcare system that is hierarchical, complex, and not well coordinated; and a system that is interdependent with the politics and policies of this country. The authors talk of the professional obligations of public health nurses as strong "influencers" of and "advocates" for the population, particularly within the context of an environment rife with debate surrounding the Affordable Care Act. They discuss many of the concepts inherent in other chapters of this book, again demonstrating the interconnectedness of healthcare reform, population health, and protection, while improving quality and controlling costs, as well as increasing access to care. Nickitas and Rome suggest that nurses look to their history and reflect on what our past leaders did during their time of practice and, at the same time, look toward our challenging future.

Chapter 10, "Social Justice and Ethics of Public Health Practice," by Selina A. Mohammed, Jamie L. Shirley, and Dan Bustillos, provides a meaningful discussion of social justice and its relationship to public health nursing practice. This new addition to this book asks the reader to explore the meaning of social justice and its effect on health care for all. The authors believe that a concern for social justice grounds the work of public health nurses. While public health nursing practice may take many forms, in a variety of settings, all interventions should ultimately be oriented toward the elimination of health inequities. The discussion offers strategies of ethical analysis that can help nurses to move beyond merely talking about social justice to developing a practice that addresses the intertwined interests of persons and communities. Using these skills, public health nurses will be able to advocate for heathier, more equitable communities.

The next five chapters of the book address the strategies found on the Intervention Wheel. These have been separated into five themes: Hitting the Pavement, Running the Show, Working It Out, Working Together, and Getting the Word Out. One of the assumptions of the Intervention Wheel is the idea that public health nurses apply the nursing process to the multiple levels of practice, including the individual/family, community, and systems (Keller & Strohschein, 2016). Each Intervention Wheel chapter explains a particular portion of the wheel and includes a vignette or case study that highlights the interventions and levels of practice. The case studies are new, reflecting the contributions of the faculty who have used the previous editions of this book. We reached out to our audience and were rewarded with a collaborative effort in developing the case studies that fit within the wheel. In this new edition, the intervention strategy chapters also include an aspect of historical research, reflecting how the particular strategy revealed itself in earlier public health nursing experiences.

Chapter 11, "Hitting the Pavement," refers to the outreach, case finding, screening, surveillance, and disease and health event investigation strategies that are found on the red wedge of the Intervention Wheel. The authors, Macali and Truglio-Londrigan, divide the discussion into several sections. The first section describes the key intervention strategies. The second section demonstrates the application of these intervention strategies within the context of several public health issues, such as tuberculosis, foodborne illnesses, rabies, and a timeline discussion about Zika. The third provides a case study to help the reader understand the process of these interventions as they are applied to the various levels of practice, including individual/family, community, and system.

In Chapter 12, "Running the Show," Dieckmann addresses three important public health interventions found in the green wedge of the Intervention Wheel: referral and follow-up, case management, and delegated functions. Dieckmann writes that these interventions have similarities, may overlap, and may be addressed in similar working objectives. All three interventions encourage the public health nurse to stretch beyond the nurse–client dyad, as the nurse seeks to add the contributions of other community services and health providers to improve the system for client support and change. At the community practice level, this means that the public health nurse participates in initiating services or expanding availability/access to meet an identified need. At the systems practice level, the public health nurse modifies organizations and policies that shape systems of care. At the individual/family practice level, the public health nurse uses interventions designed to change knowledge, attitudes, beliefs, practices, and behaviors (Rippke, Briske, Keller, Strohschein, & Simonetti, 2001).

In Drury's Chapter 13, "Working It Out," the reader returns to the settlement where Lillian D. Wald first introduced the idea of public health nursing in 1893. Drury focuses on the blue wedge of the Intervention Wheel, specifically focusing on intervention strategies that include counseling, consultation, and health teaching. The chapter defines and describes these strategies, identifies an issue in public health practice, and finally demonstrates via a case study the applying and the performing of these interventions. The case study refers to the modern-day Henry Street Settlement, now a not-for-profit social service institution located on the Lower East Side of Manhattan in New York City. The settlement supports the needs of the vulnerable populations who live in the community, and it has expanded over the years to include 19 sites such as day care centers, youth groups, workforce training, homeless shelters, mental health centers, summer camps, senior centers, and the performing arts venues. Drury uses the Henry Street Settlement and the multicultural community that it serves to illustrate the public health nursing interventions that she and her students at Pace University in New York City have brought back to Henry Street.

In Chapter 14, "Working Together," Thatcher, Park, and Kulbok present the strategies found in the orange wedge of the Intervention Wheel. The chapter explores the interventions of collaboration, coalition building, and community organizing, and devotes a separate section to each of the three interventions, and then another that discusses them as a collective action. The authors of this chapter explore how public health nurses can incorporate best practices when engaging in or supporting collective action to address health concerns. Public health professionals, while key players, also recognize that they must work with community members collectively via community organizing, collaboration, and coalition building to foster positive outcomes regarding health issues. These strategies afford the possibility of enhancing the community's capacity (Truglio-Londrigan & Barnes, 2015), as well as human, education, social, and economic capital.

In Chapter 15, "Getting the Word Out," Moscou and Murphy address the interventions found on the yellow wedge of the Intervention Wheel. These strategies include advocacy, social marketing, and policy development and enforcement of public health nursing interventions. The authors use a case study that shows how a public health nurse uses the Intervention Wheel to implement a Preexposure Prophylaxis (PrEP) program at a school-based clinic. Once the public health nurse has the relevant data, he or she can apply public health interventions of advocacy and social marketing to develop policy and enforcement strategies around the implementation of PrEP in the school-based clinic.

The final chapters move the reader from the Intervention Wheel to issues reflecting global perspectives, disaster nursing, economic issues, and environment. Here, the book draws from history, economics, and environmental health to provide a unique way of presenting the content to the reader. The use of history provides an understanding of how public health nurses responded to public health issues in the past, which can be used to inform the work that the nurses do today. In addition, the authors include a chapter that asks readers to reflect on primary health care and primary care and the relationship to public health nursing.

In Chapter 16, "Protecting, Sustaining, and Empowering: A Historical Perspective on the Control of Epidemics," Hallett traces the means by which humans have attempted to eradicate certain of those "bugs" that they consider harmful, namely, the bacteria and viruses that cause epidemic and endemic infections. She uses three case studies focusing on specific diseases appearing at specific historical moments: bubonic plague, as it appeared in the Early Modern Italian city-states during the 16th and 17th centuries; Spanish influenza, as it appeared in the cities of the United States in 1918 and 1919; and AIDS, as it appeared in the United Kingdom during the 1980s. From this historical perspective, the author explores the ways in which human societies have attempted to combat global epidemics. Readers learn the role that the nurse has played working alongside governments, doctors, and scientists in the prevention of epidemic diseases. In addition, the discussion explores the nurse's role in the treatment and care of patients with life-threatening infectious diseases at different historical moments and in different places.

In Chapter 17, "Historical Highlights in Disaster Nursing," Wall and Keeling continue to use a historical perspective as they examine the role of public health nurses in disasters. They state that "evidence for practice for disaster management logically comes from history." The chapter turns to history to impart an understanding of what has worked in the past and recognize that nurses' contributions in the past are "often overlooked" and seen as "routine." Wall and Keeling present nurses' responses to several late 19th- and 20th-century disasters, including the yellow fever epidemic of 1888, the Johnstown flood of 1889, the 1900 Galveston hurricane, the 1918 influenza pandemic, the 1947 Texas City ship explosion, and the 1964 Alaskan earthquake. The experiences learned during these disasters become a rich source of evidence for nurses addressing modern-day disasters today.

Murray authored the new Chapter 18, "Present Day Disasters and Disaster Management: Social Determinants of Health and Community Collaboration," for this book. This chapter brings the reader up to the present, exploring how public health nurses consider the social determinants of health when managing current disasters. She describes the meaning of emergency preparedness as she reflects on its role in protecting the public, and readers explore how the resilience of the individual, family, population, and community plays a part in recovery and how the burden of reliance is shifting. Murray also shows the reader how the cycle of disaster management is ongoing, and the steps overlap. Education about how to manage and mitigate the effects of disaster is required. All nurses have a role to play in how communities address disasters and must speak out on behalf of all the members of the community in which they live and work.

Another new chapter added to this book reflects on the public health and the environment. In Chapter 19, "Environment and Health," Shaner-McRae brings the environment into sharp focus as a public health issue that demands the attention of public health nurses. She examines how the physical determinants of health (including but not limited to air, water, and soil quality) effect health outcomes. The built environment as a potential facilitator effecting the health of the public is also examined. Shaner-McRae argues that there is a strong connection between environmental health and public health nursing practice and presents a midrange model/theory called the "Environmentally Responsible Clinical Practice Model (ERCPM)" as a guide for a practice.

In the final chapter, Truglio-Londrigan, Singleton, and Lewenson expand on their earlier reflection on primary health care and primary care as they relate to the health of the public and public health nursing. "Epilogue: Nursing and Primary Health Care" speaks to the challenges faced by public health nurses and other public health practitioners. In this new edition, we remind readers of the history of the terms, beginning with the Declaration of Alma-Ata, and consider what this document means in today's world. Discussion of the progress made, as well as of the progress that has yet to be made, takes shape as the reader explores successful international primary health care initiatives. This chapter includes the insights of other professionals and explores how they view primary health care initiatives that require a multisectoral collaboration. The authors show how their own view of primary health care evolved as they have included this concept in their teaching, research, and practice.

Public Health Nursing: Practicing Population-Based Care offers readers a broad view of public health nursing, encouraging all nurses to consider themselves public health nurses. It is only through the applying and performing of public health nursing that society may attain the goal expressed in the historic 1978 Declaration of Alma-Ata of "Health for All" (International Conference on Primary Health Care, 1978). This call to action reverberates throughout nursing's rich history then and now. An early public health nursing leader, Edna Foley, wrote the following in 1922:

> *Public Health means health for all. . . . Good health is the inalienable right of every citizen, man, woman, or child, and since this vague, almost unknown quality is the right of every citizen, should not good public health nursing be the concern of the laity, as well as of the handful of nurses who are struggling with this big problem? (1922/1991, p. 135)*

References

American Association of Colleges of Nursing. (2008). *The essentials of baccalaureate nursing for professional practice*. Washington, DC: Author.

American Association of Colleges of Nursing. (2011). *The essentials of master's education in nursing*. Washington, DC: Author.

Foley, E. L. (1991). Main issues in public health nursing. In N. Birnbach & S. B. Lewenson (Eds.), *First words: Selected addresses from the National League for Nursing 1894–1933* (pp. 133–137). New York, NY: National League for Nursing (Original work published 1922).

Hassmiller, S. B. (2017). Nursing's role in building a culture of health. In S. B. Lewenson & M. Truglio-Londrigan (Eds.), *Practicing primary health care in nursing: Caring for populations* (pp. 33–60). Burlington, MA: Jones & Bartlett Learning.

International Conference on Primary Health Care. (1978). *Declaration of Alma-Ata*. Retrieved from www.who.int /hpr/NPH/docs/declaration_almaata.pdf

Keller, L., & Strohschein, S. (2016). Population-based public health nursing practice: The intervention wheel. In M. Stanhope & J. Lancaster (Eds.), *Public health nursing: Population-centered health care in the community* (pp. 190–216). St. Louis, MO: Mosby-Elsevier.

Minnesota Department of Health, Division of Community Health Services, Public Health Nursing Section. (2001). *Public health interventions: Applications for public health nursing practice*. St. Paul, MN: Author.

Rippke, M., Briske, L., Keller, L. O., Strohschein, S., & Simonetti, J. (2001). Public health interventions: Applications for public health nursing practice. *Public Health Nursing Section, Division of Community Health Services, Minnesota Department of Health*. Retrieved from http://www.health.state.mn.us/divs/cfh/ophp/resources/docs /phinterventions_manual2001.pdf

Truglio-Londrigan, M., & Barnes, C. (2015). Working together: Shared decision-making. In S. B. Lewenson & M. Truglio-Londrigan (Eds.), *Decision-making in nursing: Thoughtful approaches for leadership* (pp. 141–162). Burlington, MA: Jones & Bartlett Learning.

U.S. Department of Health and Human Services. (2010). *About Healthy People*. Retrieved from www.healthypeople .gov/.2020/about/default.aspx

Wald, L. D. (1913). A Greeting: Given by Lillian Wald at the General Opening Meeting at Atlantic City, June 25, National Organization of Public Health Nursing. Lillian D. Wald Papers, 1889–1957. Writing and Speeches. Reel 25, Box 36, Folder 6, pp. 1–4. New York Public Library, Humanities and Social Sciences Library, Manuscripts and Archives Division, New York.

Notes from the Editors

Marie Truglio-Londrigan

One lesson in life that I have learned is that support and guidance from others is essential. What is equally important is to learn how to be silent and listen to what others are offering so that one can learn and integrate these lessons into one's life. As I reflect on my life, I see that there were transitional periods, and in those periods were people—nurses—who showed me what I could do and how to do it. During my undergraduate studies, it was Mathy Mezey. As I moved on and transitioned into an academic setting, it was Geraldine Valencia-Go. These individuals were icons to me and showed me what I could do as a woman and as a nurse.

There has been another individual who has left an impression on me. This individual is Sandra Lewenson. Sandy has shown me the importance of collegiality, professionalism, and most importantly friendship. It was Sandy who first suggested a partnership in which we began and completed our first book *Decision-Making in Nursing: Thoughtful Approaches for Practice*, which is now in its second edition and titled *Decision-Making in Nursing: Thoughtful Approaches for Leadership*. This partnership soon took on another challenge—the development and publication of *Practicing Primary Health Care in Nursing: Caring for Populations*. This book was and still is a labor of love. The essence of primary health care is who we are not only as individuals but also as nurses. We are firm believers in partnerships and collaboration, the idea of not just health for all Americans but quality of health for all Americans, and most importantly social, economic, legal, and educational justice. Nursing is not just the provision of compassionate care. Nursing is a social movement to ensure and assure that *all people* are aware of what is theirs and through this awareness engage in the work to assure the attainment of what is theirs. And, finally this, our third edition of *Public Health Nursing: Practicing Population-based Care* of which I am most proud. The work in the development and delivery of this book has been daunting at times. Sandy, as always, has had my back and has always been a source of encouragement through the process.

I want to take a few precious moments to thank my husband of 40 years. Yes, where did the time go, honey? My children—Paul and Leah—and my children through marriage—Jaclyn and Christopher—are continual reminders of the importance of relationships and the meaningfulness of these relationships as we grow together. To all of my children and now my grandchild Greyson—you have taught me much. I want to thank each and every one of you. You have entered into my life and I cherish all of you from deep within my soul.

Sandra B. Lewenson

This is an especially important time for us as we complete our third edition of this public health book. While I have convinced Marie to write other books, chapters, and editorials, we've had wonderful weekly meetings to discuss, write, edit, and move on. Yes, that's what it takes . . . a commitment to each other and to commit time to develop our ideas—whether it be decision making, primary health care, and (of course, both our love) public health nursing. We met weekly and have done so for many years. We both keep ourselves grounded and prepared to write! I want to acknowledge Marie as well for her support and recognition of the relevance of history to this whole process . . . and when I drift off into historical analysis, she not only remains focused, but also incorporates these ideas in a practical (and meaningful) way.

My family—all of them . . . spurs me on. My husband, not just listens to me, but offers his dental perspective. Yes, he is a dentist and I am a nurse, and somehow we have found synergy that recognizes that public health includes all health care. (And, we've been synergistically addressing this for over 46 years!) When he and his colleagues in the New York County Dental Society under the "Give Kids a Smile Program" treated elementary age children to a dental exam on the Lower East Side, right near the Henry Street Settlement, where public health nursing began, and other locations in Manhattan, his enthusiasm for health promotion and disease prevention resonated. This public health initiative provided dental screening for over 1,000 New York City public school children from vulnerable populations. The health of the public relies on all of us. So, I acknowledge all health professionals who participate in public healthcare initiatives.

My children, both grown adults, with children of their own, recognize the essential nature of health care. Whether it is special education, ballet classes, day care, home care . . . they continue to encourage me to find better solutions to the public's health. I've been clearly blessed with family, friends, and colleagues that allow me to participate in these writing projects. Thank you Marie, my family, the publishers, fellow historians, the contributors, and, of course, the readers, who make this next edition soar.

Acknowledgments

We want to thank the contributors, educators, public health nurses, readers, and students who showed enthusiasm and support for this work. We want to thank our families, too, for giving us the love and support for us to grow! We also want to acknowledge our friendship that thrived throughout the process of editing this exciting third edition. A special acknowledgment to our colleague Donna Avanecean, who served as our graduate assistant throughout the development of this book. And, finally, we want to thank our publishers who believed in this work and gave it another chance. Thank you all!

Contributors

Jane Bear-Lehman, PhD, OTR/L, FAOTA
Professor and Chair
College of Health Professions
Pace University
New York, NY
New York College of Dentistry
New York, NY

Dan Bustillos, JD, PhD
Assistant Professor
School of Nursing & Health Studies
University of Washington Bothell
Bothell, WA

Marianne Cockroft, PhD, RN
Clinical Assistant Professor
School of Nursing
The University of North Carolina at Chapel Hill
Chapel Hill, NC

Mary de Chesnay, PhD, RN, PMHCNS-BC, FAAN
Professor
Kennesaw State University
Kennesaw, GA

Janna L. Dieckmann, PhD, RN
Associate Professor
School of Nursing
University of North Carolina at Chapel Hill
Chapel Hill, NC

Shellene Dietrich, DNP, FNP-BC, RN
Maimonides Medical Center
Brooklyn, NY

Lin Drury, PhD, RN
Professor
College of Health Professions
Lienhard School of Nursing
Pace University
New York, NY

Karen S. Edwards, MD, MPH
Professor, School of Health Sciences and Practice
New York Medical College
Vice President for Education, Training
  and Research
Westchester Institute for Human Development
Valhalla, NY

Anny M. Eusebio, DNP, FNP-BC, RN
New York Presbyterian Hospital
New York, NY

Julie Fairman, PhD, RN, FAAN
Nightingale Professor of Nursing in Honor
  of Military Veterans
Chair, Department of Biobehavioral Health
  Sciences
Director Emerita, Barbara Bates Center for the
  Study of the History of Nursing
School of Nursing
University of Pennsylvania
Philadelphia, PA

Margaret Fitzgerald, JD
Associate Professor
Criminal Justice and Security
Dyson College of Arts and Sciences
Pace University
Pleasantville, NY

Coleen Francis-Jimenez, DNP, FNP-BC, RN
New York Presbyterian
New York, NY

Shirley Franco, MSN, FNP, RN
President
NP in Family Health, PC
Mahopac, NY

Tracy P. George, DNP, APRN-BC, CNE
Assistant Professor of Nursing and Coordinator
    of the Bachelor of General Studies Program
Francis Marion University
Florence, SC

Christine E. Hallett, PhD
Director of the UK Centre for the History
    of Nursing and Midwifery
Professor of Nursing History
School of Nursing
The University of Manchester
Manchester, UK

Cynthia S. Henderson, DNP, RN
Associate Professor of Nursing
College of Nursing and Health Sciences
Auburn University at Montgomery
Montgomery, AL

Marty Hucks, MN, APRN-BC, CNE
Assistant Professor of Nursing
Francis Marion University
Florence, SC

Paule Valery Joseph, PhD, FNP-BC, CTNB
Executive Director of Operations and Partnerships
Amazing Grace Children's Foundation
Washington, DC
Adjunct Professor
Pace University
New York, NY

Arlene W. Keeling, PhD, RN, FAAN
Centennial Distinguished Professor of Nursing
Associate Director, The Eleanor Crowder Bjoring
    Center for Nursing Historical Inquiry
School of Nursing
University of Virginia
Charlottesville, VA

Melida Knibbs, DNP, FNP-BC, RN
Audubon Medical Practice
New York, NY

Pamela Kulbok, DNSc, APHN-BC, RN, FAAN
Theresa A. Thomas Professor of Nursing
Coordinator of the Public Health Nursing
    Leadership program
School of Nursing
University of Virginia
Charlottesville, VA

Shai Lev
Nursing Student
Decker School of Nursing
Binghamton University
Binghamton, NY

Sandra B. Lewenson, EdD, RN, FAAN
Professor
College of Health Professions
Lienhard School of Nursing
Pace University
New York, NY

Paul Londrigan, MA
Adjunct Professor, Political Science
Dyson College of Arts and Sciences
Pace University
Pleasantville, NY

Margaret K. Macali, MSN, RN
Adjunct Faculty
School of Nursing
St. Peter's University
Jersey City, NJ

Karen Martin, MSN, FNP-BC, RN
Associate Director University Health Care Unit
Pace University
Pleasantville, NY

Renee McLeod-Sordjan, PhDc, DNP, APRN, FNP-BC, AACNP-BC, AAHIVM-S, CNL, FNAP
Clinical Assistant Professor
College of Health Professions
Lienhard School of Nursing
Pace University
New York, NY
Northwell Health Systems
Manhasset, NY

Hollie Shaner McRae, DNP, RN, MSA
Supervisor Clinical Documentation Integrity
University of Vermont Medical Center
Burlington, VT

Selina A. Mohammed, PhD, MPH, RN
Associate Professor and Associate Dean
School of Nursing and Health Studies
University of Washington Bothell
Bothell, WA

Arlene H. Morris, EdD, RN, CNE
Professor
College of Nursing and Health Science
Auburn University Montgomery
Montgomery, AL

Susan Moscou, PhD, MPH, FNP, RN
Associate Professor
Mercy College
Dobbs Ferry, NY

Nancy Murphy, PhD, NP, RN
Assistant Professor
College of Nursing and Allied Health Sciences
Howard University
Washington, DC

Sherrie Lee Murray, MS, FNP, ANP-BC
Retired Lieutenant Colonel
United States Air Force
Capital Care Family Practice
Clifton Park, NY

Donna M. Nickitas, PhD, RN, NEA-BC, CNE, FNAP, FAAN
Executive Officer and Professor
Hunter College
Graduate Center
City University of New York
New York, New York

Christopher A. Pariso, BS
Criminal Justice Technical Operations
    Coordinator
University of New Haven
Center for Analytics
New Haven, CT

Eunhee Park, PhD, APHN-BC, RN
Assistant Professor
University of North Carolina at Greensboro
Greensboro, NC

Judith Quaranta, PhD, RN, CPN, AE-C
Assistant Professor
Decker School of Nursing
Binghamton University
Binghamton, NY

Barbara Rome, MS, RN
Doctoral Candidate
Graduate Center
City University of New York
New York, NY
Queensborough Community College
Bayside, NY

Rima B. Sehl, DDS, MPA
Associate Professor & Director of Health
    Promotion
Department of Cariology and Comprehensive
    Care
New York University College of Dentistry,
    New York, NY

Jamie L. Shirley, PhD, RN
Senior Lecturer
School of Nursing and Health Studies
University of Washington Bothell
Bothell, WA

Vicki Simpson, PhD, RN, CHES
Assistant Professor
Purdue University School of Nursing
Fellow, Purdue University Teaching Academy
West Lafayette, IN

**Joanne K. Singleton, PhD, RN, FNP-BC, CNL-BC,
    FNAP, FNYAM**
Professor
College of Health Professions
Lienhard School of Nursing
Pace University
New York, NY

Frances M. Srnka-Debnar, PhD, RN
Clinical Associate Professor
Decker School of Nursing
Binghamton University
Binghamton, NY

Esther Thatcher, PhD, RN, APHN-BC
Postdoctoral Fellow
School of Nursing
University of North Carolina at Chapel Hill
Chapel Hill, NC

Marie Truglio-Londrigan, PhD, GNP, RN, FNYAM
Professor
College of Health Professions
Lienhard School of Nursing
Pace University
New York, NY

Ismael Umali, DNP, FNP-BC, RN
Montifiore Medical Center
Bronx, NY

Barbra Mann Wall, PhD, RN, FAAN
Thomas A. Saunders III Professor of Nursing
Director, The Eleanor Crowder Bjoring Center
    for Nursing Historical Inquiry
University of Virginia
Charlottesville, VA

Robin M. White, PhD, RN
Associate Professor
University of Tampa Nursing
Tampa, FL

Astrid H. Wilson, PhD, RN
Professor of Nursing Emeritus
Kennesaw University
Kennesaw, GA

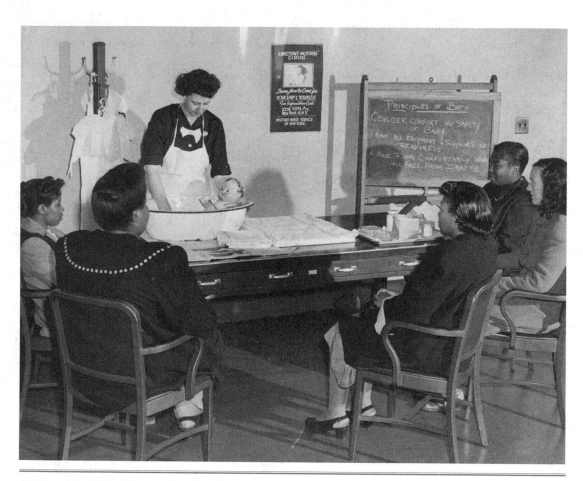

Courtesy of the Visiting Nurse Service of New York.

CHAPTER 1

What Is Public Health and Public Health Nursing?

Marie Truglio-Londrigan

Sandra B. Lewenson

. . .while the district nurse is laboring with the individual, she should also contribute her knowledge towards the study of the large general conditions of which her poor patient may be victim. Many of these conditions seem hopelessly bad, but many are capable of prevention and cure when the public shall be stimulated to a realization of the wrong to the individual as well as to the society in general if such are to persist. Therefore, her knowledge of the laws that have been enacted to prevent and cure, and her intelligence in recording and reporting the general as well as the individual conditions that make for degradation and social iniquity are but an advance from her readiness to instruct and correct personal and family hygiene to giving attention to home sanitation and then to city sanitation, an advance from the individual to the collective interest. (Wald, 1907, p. 3)

LEARNING OBJECTIVES

At the completion of this chapter, the reader will be able to:

- Define the meaning of public health and public health nursing.
- Describe what is meant by the terms *care of the public* and *population-based care*.
- Describe national health initiatives.
- Examine the 10 essential public health services in relation to the core functions of public health practice.
- Examine the role of the public health nurse within the larger context of public health.

KEY TERMS

- ❏ Assure
- ❏ Core functions of public health
- ❏ Ensure
- ❏ Essentials of public health
- ❏ Health promotion
- ❏ Maintaining health
- ❏ National health initiatives
- ❏ Preventing disease
- ❏ Public health
- ❏ Public health nursing
- ❏ Risk reduction

It never fails. Sit around a table discussing the health of the public or population-based care, and one frequently receives blank stares. What is **public health**? What does it mean when one speaks about the health of the public or population-based care? What is the role of the public health nurse within this larger framework? Who pays for public health? These questions need to be answered for those in practice, and this chapter provides answers to these questions, thus enhancing practitioners' working knowledge of the scientific discipline known as public health. Creating a professional nursing workforce that demonstrates a vigorous practice of integrating culturally congruent nursing actions based on evidence and recognizing the funding streams lay the groundwork for a strong public health infrastructure that will ultimately enhance and sustain the public's health.

Public Health Defined

To fully understand the concept of public health, it is important to review the definitions put forth over time by those in practice. This exercise will assist the reader in knowing and understanding the important characteristics and features of this discipline.

"Public health work is as old as history," wrote J. Howard Beard in 1922. Beard's article, published in *The Scientific Monthly,* charts the early progress of public health starting with the early Egyptians, who filtered mud from the Nile River to create a safer water source for citizens. Throughout history, the health of the public has been a concern for local and national governments and all members of society. The public health movement in the United States originated in Boston, Massachusetts, in the mid-1800s when Lemuel Shattuck's noted reports on the healthcare needs of the community became the "blueprint for American health organization" (Beard, 1922; Scheele, 1949, p. 293). A noted public health leader in the early 20th century, C. E. Winslow (1920), defined public health as follows:

[T]he science and the art of preventing disease, prolonging life, and promoting physical health and efficiency through organized community efforts for the sanitation of the environment, the control of community infections, the education of the individual in principles of personal hygiene, the organization of medical and nursing service for the early diagnosis and preventive treatment of disease, and the development of the social machinery which will ensure to every individual in the community a standard of living adequate for the maintenance of health. (p. 30)

The definition of public health has changed over time.

In 1988, the Institute of Medicine (IOM) defined public health as "what we, as a society, do collectively to assure the conditions in which people can be healthy" (IOM, 1988, p. 1). Society collectively works together to provide services generally to a population to prevent disease and maintain health (Buttery, 1992). The Association of Schools and Programs of Public Health

(2016) website identifies that public health "protects and improves the health of individuals, families, communities, and populations, locally and globally" (para. 1). In 2003, the IOM published *The Future of the Public's Health in the 21st Century*. This report was comprehensive in nature and spoke to partnerships; intersectoral collaboration; the strengthening of the public health infrastructure, including the building of our nation's public health workforce; and an enhanced understanding of what we mean when we speak of community and population, along with an awareness of the shifting of our demographics represented by the aging of the population. Another IOM report, titled *For the Public's Health: The Role of Measurement in Action and Accountability* (2010), looked at the critical importance of measurements in summarizing the impact that the health system has on the population, thus emphasizing the importance of outcomes. More recently, the IOM (2012) report *For the Public's Health Investigating in a Healthier Future* challenges the nation to establish a "minimum package of public health services" through the delivery of basic public health programs that are flexible, coordinated, and seamless for populations where they live, work, and play. Although brief, this information serves as a template to remind us of the progressive steps we have taken over the decades.

Populations

When one considers the preceding definitions of public health, one comes to understand that the discussion of health moves beyond the health of the individual, family, and community to the health of the population. For example, Hurricane Katrina hit the U.S. Gulf Coast, with particular destruction in Louisiana, on August 29, 2005. In the weeks that followed, healthcare professionals cared for individuals and their family members who were evacuees without shelter and who had suffered from physical and emotional distress. Brodie, Weltzien, Altman, Blendon, and Benson (2006) surveyed the experiences of the Hurricane Katrina evacuees. Their results provide valuable information for public health professionals, "highlighting challenges of effectively evacuating cities' most at-risk residents during a disaster and providing for long-term health needs of vulnerable populations in the aftermath" (p. 1407). The outcomes of this research also provided important guidelines for public health officials as they planned for future evacuations when disasters hit and discussed how to ensure the protection of the public during this evacuation. More recently, the high levels of lead discovered in the drinking water of Flint, Michigan, showed how the health of individuals, families, the entire population, and indeed the community were placed at risk (Kennedy, 2016). This occurred when Flint's water source was changed from treated Detroit water to the untreated Flint River in 2014 without due diligence as to the safety of that water. Lead from the new source seeped into the water supply, as the pipes corroded as a result of this change, placing those who drank the water, especially those most vulnerable, at risk for elevated lead levels and related health problems, so much so that President Obama called for a natural state of emergency as a result of the widespread public health issue to all concerned that emerged (Kennedy, 2016). This public health issue demonstrates the link between public health, policy, advocacy, and the media.

The concept of caring for populations can be difficult to understand and perhaps serves as a barrier to the way nurses or other healthcare workers are educated and approach care. The noted 20th-century nursing leader Virginia Henderson, when questioned on how one may care for an aggregate or population, said, "I think it impossible to nurse an aggregate effectively until you have effectively nursed individuals and acquired considerable judgment as to what helps clients or patients prevent disease, cope with it, or die with dignity when death is inevitable" (Abrams, 2007, p. 384). The question, what and who is a population, has been raised many times in hopes of understanding what a population means and what it means to care for a population. Definitions of *populations* illustrate characteristics and features specific to the particular population. Examples of these population characteristics or features are further delineated by

Warner and Lightfoot (2014) as age, gender, risk factors, disease, time, and place of employment. The American Nurses Association (2013) expands on the definition of population as those "living in a specific geographic area (e.g., town, city, state, region, nation, multinational region)" (p. 3). An example may include the nurse working with individuals diagnosed with tuberculosis living in a particular state or a nurse working with those incarcerated in a county prison system. These nurses work with the entire population and continually assess the health and wellness of the entire population within the specific environment that care is being rendered.

Henderson's concern about nursing populations versus nursing individuals may stem from her concern about the division in health care that separates the care of populations from the care of individuals. Henderson asked, "Should we have one category of health workers treating disease and another preventing it? Or should we all be trying primarily to prevent disease, and, even while treating it, to be helping the victim to prevent a recurrence?" (Abrams, 2007, p. 384). Henderson's words challenge nurses to give careful consideration to what is involved in practice in terms of the process and the strategies that must be implemented for positive health outcomes whether they are working with individuals, families, communities, or populations. These processes and strategies include health promotion and protection, risk factor identification, early detection and treatment, as well as restorative care. The important point to remember is that at whatever health point the individual, family, community, or population is, health promotion care is always essential. **Table 1-1** gives examples of how the implementation of the specific public health intervention or education may vary depending on whether the focus is on individuals, families, populations, or communities.

Prevention

Preventing disease and **maintaining health** are important strategies for public health along with emphasis on **health promotion** and **risk reduction**. To understand these concepts fully, public health nurses can turn to the historic work of Leavell and Clark (1965), who note, "The ultimate objectives of all medical, dental, and public health practice, whether carried out in the office, the clinic, the laboratory, or the community-at-large, are the promotion of health, the prevention of disease, and the prolongation of life" (p. 14).

According to Leavell and Clark's (1965) seminal work, there are three levels of prevention. The first level, *primary prevention*, includes interventions designed to promote health via health promotion strategies to specifically protect the individual and the population from disease "by providing immunizations and reducing exposure to occupational hazards, carcinogens, and other environmental health risks" (Greiner & Edelman, 2006, p. 17). These interventions take place before the presence of disease and disability, in the period known as the prepathogenesis period. *The second level of prevention*, which occurs in the period of pathogenesis, takes place once disease is present. Interventions include screening activities and early treatment to prevent the consequences of advanced disease, such as disabilities. Finally, the *third level of prevention* includes rehabilitation intervention strategies. "This is more than stopping a disease process; it is also the prevention of complete disability. . . . Its positive objective is to return the affected individual to a useful place in society and make maximum use of his remaining capacities" (Leavell & Clark, 1965, p. 26).

Today, public health nursing activities in primary, secondary, and tertiary prevention have evolved and take into consideration the idea that health is not linear. In fact, if a person requires tertiary rehabilitative services, health promotion strategies are still important. The question raised by Henderson speaks to this nonlinear approach and encourages public health nurses to think about providing care for disease while simultaneously promoting health.

Interprofessional and Intersectorial Work

The definitions of public health thus far given demonstrate the collective nature of public health and the need for multiple disciplines to work together

Table 1-1 **Examples of the Educational Interventions for Individuals, Families, Populations, and Communities**

	Individual	Family	Population	Community
	Refers to the individual, who may be part of a family, or a population, and live in a community.	Refers to a family system, which may be defined as any or all individuals who live in what they consider a family system.	Refers to a defined number of people.	Refers to individuals, families, populations, and organizations (for-profit and not-for-profit) that may or may not share the same ideas, values, beliefs, and/or physical location and may or may not intervene and network with each other.
Lyme disease prevention and early detection programs	Target the client (e.g., young adult gardeners) and provide education about Lyme disease, its cause, and methods of prevention, such as pulling socks over pants and wearing repellent. This education can be provided in a pamphlet and placed in areas where individuals may pick it up and read it, such as pharmacies and gardening supply stores.	Target families and provide education for caretakers of children about the cause of Lyme disease and methods of prevention. This information may be developed and delivered in magazines available in primary care practitioner offices or at organizations such as Boys and Girls Clubs of America.	Targeted population education about Lyme disease. This information may be developed and delivered on signs in high-risk areas (such as hiking trails) or in special service announcements on the radio or via the use of technology and social media.	A healthy community ensures that a hiking trail in their geographical area is clear of bush and that appropriate signs are posted warning of high-risk areas. A healthy community will also ensure that funding is available to sustain these endeavors.
Child car seat prevention programs	Target the child, using developmentally appropriate play strategies that illustrate use of child car seats and booster seats.	Target caretakers (e.g., parents, grandparents, day care workers), educating them about the importance of using child car seats, with pamphlets and videos in preschools.	Targeted population education through the use of billboards or other forms of or message delivery via technology, highlighting the importance of appropriate use of child car seats.	A healthy community will have strong organizations that provide programs to support use of child car seats. For example, a local hospital may stage a drive-through child car seat safety check; a fire department may install safety car seats for newborns.

Figure 1-1 The intersectoral public health system.

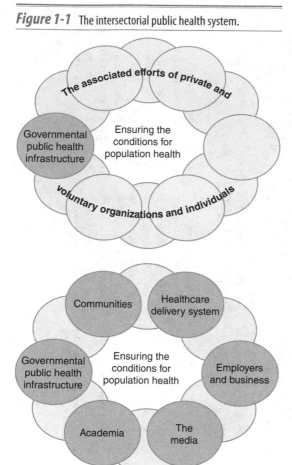

Reproduced with permission from National Academy of Sciences. (2003). *The future of the public's health in the 21st century.* Washington, DC: Author. Courtesy of the National Academies Press, Washington, DC.

in ensuring the health of the public. **Figure 1-1** is a visual depiction of this.

The IOM speaks to this collective endeavor as a process that must involve multiple individuals from various disciplines and multiple organizations. "The concept of a public health system describes a complex network of individuals and organizations that have the potential to play critical roles in creating the conditions for health. They can act for health individually, but when they

work together toward a health goal, they act as a system—a public health system" (2003, p. 28). The IOM further describes participants as actors in the public health system. Actors include the governmental public health infrastructure, such as local and state departments of health, the healthcare delivery system, academia, and communities. In turn, communities may include schools, religious organizations, and other not-for-profit organizations, just to name a few. Businesses and corporations are considered important actors because they too play a role in influencing population health with regard to the working conditions. Those involved in the media are important actors in the public healthcare system. Consider the impact that the media can have with its ability to reach populations through the various media streams. Furthermore, the layperson in the community also has a role in the intersectoral public health system as an essential active participant and collaborator. Ultimately, public health system actors, with their integrative and participatory roles, serve as a reminder of the historic Declaration of Alma-Ata International Conference (1978) that recognized primary health care as a major strategy for achieving health for all. At this historic international conference, participants expressed a need for all governments and other international organizations to engage in actions that would ensure the implementation of primary health care around the world. The Declaration of Alma-Ata International Conference (1978) described and explained primary health care as follows:

> [R]equires and promotes maximum community and individual self-reliance and participation in the planning, organization, operation, and control of primary health care, making fullest use of local, national, and other available resources; and to this end develops through appropriate education the ability of communities to participate. (para. 12)

Public health fits within a primary health care philosophical paradigm whereby elements of population-based care, community orientation, social justice, shared decision-making, collaboration, and access to and equity of healthcare services for all exist (Truglio-Londrigan & Lewenson, 2017).

Assure and Ensure the Public's Health

Public health providers **assure** the health and well-being for individuals, families, communities, and populations by **ensuring** and guaranteeing the achievement of health through the development of specific policy and laws. Working together as actors is important, but the ability to assure and ensure the health of the public is critical. How does one assure and ensure the health of the public? The involvement of the government, as an actor in the intersectorial public health system, is important in this regard. The IOM (2003) speaks to this very issue:

> *In the United States, the government's responsibility for the health of its citizens stems, in part, from the nature of democracy itself. Health officials are either directly elected or appointed by democratically elected officials. To the extent, therefore, that citizens place a high priority on health, these elected officials are held accountable to ensure that the government is able to monitor the population's health and intervene when necessary through laws, policies, regulations, and expenditure of the resources necessary for the health and safety of the public. (p. 101)*

The public cannot be healthy without strong governmental support to assure and ensure the protection of its citizens, access to health care and essential health services, and the ongoing maintenance and expansion of a strong infrastructure. The government does not do this on its own but plays a role as a broker of services by negotiating appropriate collaborations between and among those actors in intersectorial work (World Health Organization [WHO], 2008). Late-19th- and early-20th-century public health nursing leaders—such as Lillian Wald and Mary Brewster, who began the Henry Street Settlement in the Lower East Side of New York City—recognized the need to garner government support for their efforts to improve the health of the immigrant population that flooded the streets of New York during this period. As they visited the homes of the families in the community, Wald and Brewster's public health nurses wore official badges showing endorsement by the New York Board of Health (Buhler-Wilkerson, 2001). Wald, along with the other public health nurses, continued to advocate for playgrounds for children in the community, school nurses in the public schools, and votes for women as a means of ensuring the public's health (Lewenson, 2007). Suffragist and public health nurse Lavinia Dock equated the ability to vote with the ability to improve health. In an early issue of the *American Journal of Nursing*, Dock (1908) asks nurses to consider the value of the women's vote, saying, "[T]ake the present question of the underfed school children in New York. How many of them will have tuberculosis? If mothers and nurses had votes, there might be school lunches for all those children" (p. 926).

Service

Finally, the definitions of public health mention the types of services to be provided—for example, the importance of education as a service. Providing services to a population can be approached in many ways. This book, for example, features the application of the Minnesota Department of Health population-based public health nursing practice intervention wheel model. This model contains 17 intervention strategies or services that are population-based and can be applied to different levels or focused areas of practice, including individuals, families, communities, and systems. Presently this model is referred to as the intervention wheel, or simply the wheel (Keller & Strohschein, 2016).

The definitions of public health presented in this chapter highlight certain key characteristics and features. **Box 1-1** presents an overview of these key characteristics and features that are further explained in later chapters.

Public Health Nursing

Public health nurses play a central role in supporting the health of the public. Chapter 2 is dedicated to the history of public health nursing, showing the development

Box 1-1 Overview of Key Characteristics and Features of Public Health

Population based
Health Promotion and Preventing Disease
Maintaining Health
Interprofessional and Intersectoral Work
Assure and Ensure
Population-focused Services

of this role over time. *Public health nursing*, a term first coined in the late 19th century by nursing leader Lillian Wald (Buhler-Wilkerson, 1993), included the roles of health visitor, health teacher, social worker, and even health inspector (Crandall, 1922, p. 645). Crandall wrote that these roles evolved on the basis of the rich foundation of nursing (Crandall, 1922). This strong nursing background continues today as public health nursing serves the health of the public.

In a statement originally published in 1996, the American Public Health Association, Public Health Nursing Section (2013) defined public health nursing as:

> . . .*the practice of promoting and protecting the health of populations using knowledge from nursing, social, and public health sciences. Public health nursing is a specialty practice within nursing and public health. It focuses on improving population health by emphasizing prevention and attending to multiple determinants of health. . . .this nursing practice includes advocacy, policy development, and planning, which addresses issues of social justice. (para. 2)*

The Missouri Department of Health and Senior Services (2006) developed a public health nursing manual where public health nursing is defined as "the practice of promoting and protecting the health of populations using knowledge from nursing, social, and public health sciences" (p. 8). The manual further describes public health nursing practice as being a systematic process that includes an assessment of the population, families, and individuals; the development

of a plan with the defined community along with an implementation of that plan; the evaluation of that plan to determine its effectiveness and the impact on the population; and finally, based on the outcomes, the development of local and national policy to assure and ensure the health of the population. More recently, the American Nurses Association (2013) defined **public health nursing** as a practice that "focuses on population health through continuous surveillance and assessment of the multiple determinants of health with the intent to promote health and wellness; prevent disease, disability, and premature death; and improve neighborhood quality of life" (p. 2).

What the reader may glean from this is that public health nursing by definition mirrors the general definitions of public health, with an emphasis on the systematic process that nurses use to do their work. This process is the nursing process. Therefore, throughout this book, the reader will note that the nursing process is the guiding framework for assessing the population, diagnosing the needs of the population, planning interventions based in evidence using the intervention wheel, implementing those strategies, and ultimately evaluating outcomes of the population. The preceding definitions of public health nursing also stipulate how results of the process are used to influence and direct the current healthcare delivery system, thus making assurances to the public when results and outcomes are positive that these outcomes will be sustained over time. The readers of this book will find it useful to access *The Public Health Nursing: Scope and Standards of Practice* (American Nurses Association, 2013). This document serves as a detailed outline of the role and expectations of the public health nurse. This document is also helpful in that it serves as a guide and offers direction for the public health nurse's professional and noble practice.

Public Health Now

For centuries, diseases such as the Black Death, leprosy, smallpox, tuberculosis, and influenza terrorized the population with extraordinary death tolls. Similarly, for centuries it was assumed that nothing could be done about these little-understood outbreaks because they were a message from the supernatural that was, in some way, dissatisfied with humans. Since these earlier times, the scientific discipline of public health has made remarkable strides, noted by the decrease in communicable diseases along with the marked improvements in sanitation efforts (Beard, 1922).

In recent years, communicable and infectious diseases such as the Ebola virus have experienced a resurgence, along with a renewed cry to strengthen the public health infrastructure in the United States. Problems such as chronic illnesses; obesity; a healthcare system in which the cost of care is still out of control despite attempts at curbing costs, coupled with populations who continue to experience limited access to available care; health disparities; the stripping of the environment; rising mental health issues; and violence of all types clearly inform public health professionals of the need for a call to action.

Ten Essential Public Health Services

Historically, public health professionals have responded to the call to action by making changes and progress in meeting the needs of the public. One outcome was the development of the 10 essential public health services by the Public Health Functions Steering Committee (U.S. Department of Health and Human Services [DHHS] Public Health Service, 1994). This steering committee included representatives from U.S. Public Health Service agencies and other major public health organizations. Over the years, minor revisions have lead us to the more recent 10 **essentials of public health** that provide a guiding framework for the responsibilities of local public health systems and the foundation for strategy-building toward a healthy, integrated public health system capable of ensuring the health of the public. **Box 1-2** presents these 10 essential public health services, which include the key characteristics and features noted in the previous definitions of public health.

Three Core Functions

Each of these 10 essential services falls under one of the three **core functions of public health:** assessment, policy development, and assurance (Center for Disease Control and Prevention [CDC], 2015;

Box 1-2 The Ten Essential Public Health Services

1. Monitor health status to identify and solve community health problems.
2. Diagnose and investigate health problems and health hazards in the community.
3. Inform, educate, and empower people about health issues.
4. Mobilize community partnerships and action to identify and solve health problems.
5. Develop policies and plans that support individual and community health efforts.
6. Enforce laws and regulations that protect health and ensure safety.
7. Link people to needed personal health services and assure the provision of health care when otherwise unavailable.
8. Assure competent public health and personal healthcare workforce.
9. Evaluate effectiveness, accessibility, and quality of personal and population-based health services.
10. Research for new insights and innovative solutions to health problems.

Reproduced from U.S. Department of Health and Human Services, Public Health Service. (1994a). The public health workforce: An agenda for the 21st century. A report of the Public Health Functions Project. Retrieved from http://www.health.gov/phfunctions/pubhlth.pdf; Centers for Disease Control and Prevention. (2014). The public health system and the 10 essential public health services. Retrieved from http://www.cdc.gov/nphpsp/essentialservices.html

---

IOM, 1988). To assess the health of the population for early identification of health problems and/or other potential problems, a public health agency must collect and analyze data systematically. The policy development function means that public health agencies serve the public by developing public health policies, based on evidence, for the correction of issues or problems. Finally, assurance requires that public health agencies provide services directly or through other private or public agencies. In addition, assurance guarantees services for those unable to afford them. These three core functions guide the public health professional in the development, implementation, and evaluation of various public processes that assist in meeting the healthcare needs of the public (**Figure 1-2**).

Healthy People 2020

The three core functions of public health and the 10 essential public health services provide the foundation for the health agenda for the nation, known as **Healthy People**. *Healthy People 2020* is a continuation of previous initiatives that began in 1979 when the report *Healthy People: The Surgeon General's Report on Health Promotion and Disease Prevention* was released, which provided national goals for reducing premature deaths and preserving independence for older adults. *Healthy People 2020* "provides science-based, 10-year national objectives

Figure 1-2 Three core functions of public health.

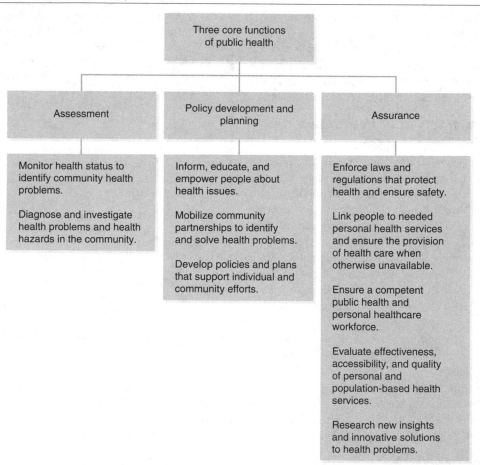

Data from Institute of Medicine. (1988); *The future of public health.* Washington, DC: National Academies Press; U.S. Department of Health and Human Services. (1994b). *The public health workforce: An agenda for the 21st century.* Washington, DC: US Government Printing Office; Centers for Disease Control and Prevention. (2015). *Core functions of public health and how they relate to the 10 essential services.* Retrieved from http://www.cdc.gov/nceh/ehs/ephli/core_ess.htm

for improving the health of all Americans" (U.S. DHHS, 2010a, para. 1). It was unveiled on December 2, 2010, and represents the ongoing work of public health through the systematic use of overarching goals, topics, and objectives that facilitate action facilitated by a vision and mission.

VISION AND MISSION

The vision and mission of the Healthy People initiative provides the direction in terms of where we wish to go as a nation regarding the health of our people and what we are going to do to get there. **Box 1-3** includes the vision and mission of *Healthy People 2020*. The vision statement is critical because it creates the point on the horizon to which all stakeholders set their sights in their combined efforts to achieve public health. The mission of *Healthy People 2020* is to identify how the vision is realized. It essentially guides the action of the stakeholders.

Box 1-3 *Healthy People 2020* Vision and Mission

Vision: A society in which all people live long, healthy lives.
Mission: *Healthy People 2020* strives to:

- Identify nationwide health-improvement priorities.
- Increase public awareness and understanding of the determinants of health, disease, and disability and the opportunities for progress.
- Provide measurable objectives and goals that are applicable at the national, state, and local levels.
- Engage multiple sectors to take actions to strengthen policies and improve practices that are driven by the best available evidence and knowledge.
- Identify critical research, evaluation, and data collection needs.

Reproduced from U.S. Department of Health and Human Services. Office of Disease Prevention and Health Promotion. (2010a). *Healthy People 2020*. Retrieved from http://www.healthypeople.gov/2020/about/default.aspx

---

OVERARCHING GOALS

The earlier *Healthy People 2010* included two goals: (1) to increase the quality of years of healthy life and (2) to eliminate health disparities. The first goal also addressed life expectancy, defined as "the average number of years people born in a given year [were] expected to live based on a set of age-specific death rates" (U.S. DHHS, 2000, p. 8). This goal speaks to the need for not only extending life but also for improving the quality of those years lived. The second goal addressed the health disparities evident among various U.S. demographic groups, including groups based on "gender, race or ethnicity; education or income; disability; geographic location; or sexual orientation" (U.S. DHHS, 2000, p. 11). An awareness of the existence of these disparities and others are still evolving; however, its importance is seen in *Healthy People 2020*, as it is highlighted as one of the four foundational heath measures (U.S. DHHS, 2010a, para. 6).

Today, *Healthy People 2020* is presented as four overarching goals, presented in **Box 1-4**. The overarching goals were developed with a twofold purpose: to develop the objectives and to assist the stakeholders in their work to achieve the stated objectives. See Box 1-4 to view these overarching goals.

Box 1-4 *Healthy People 2020*: Overarching Goals

- Attain high-quality, longer lives free of preventable disease, disability, injury, and premature death.
- Achieve health equity, eliminate disparities, and improve the health of all groups.
- Create social and physical environments that promote good health for all.
- Promote quality of life, healthy development, and healthy behaviors across all life stages.

Reproduced from U.S. Department of Health and Human Services. Office of Disease Prevention and Health Promotion. (2010a). *Healthy People 2020*. Retrieved from http://www.healthypeople.gov/2020/about/default.aspx

---

TOPICS AND OBJECTIVES

Healthy People 2020 includes 46 topic areas, each with important information such as an overview, goals, objectives, interventions, and resources as well as national snapshots (U.S. DHHS, 2010b). Public health nurses can use *Healthy People 2020* as a tool to create health initiatives to address public health concerns. Suppose a public health nurse conducts an assessment and identifies tobacco smoking as a major problem in the adolescent population they serve. An understanding of the population-based issue and the corresponding etiology is critical for public health nurses and their partners to develop initiatives to create a balanced healthcare system in which health parity rather than health disparity is the rule.

In this particular situation, the public health nurse will link into the Healthy People main web page (see **Figure 1-3**) and then click into the Topic and Objective tab. The topic and objectives list in *Healthy People 2020* is extensive, but a quick glance down the page will take the public health nurse to the topic area of Tobacco Use. Once the public health nurse clicks into the Tobacco Use topic area, they will see four tabs along the top of the screen: overview, objective, interventions and resources, and national snapshot (see **Figure 1-4**). Each of these separate tabs provides valuable information for the public health nurse and others involved in the collaborative effort to address tobacco use in the adolescent population. The overview tab provides specific information about the topic area, including why preventing tobacco use is important and a framework for ending tobacco use, as well as other important information (see Figure 1-4).

Figure 1-3 Main page of *Healthy People 2020.*

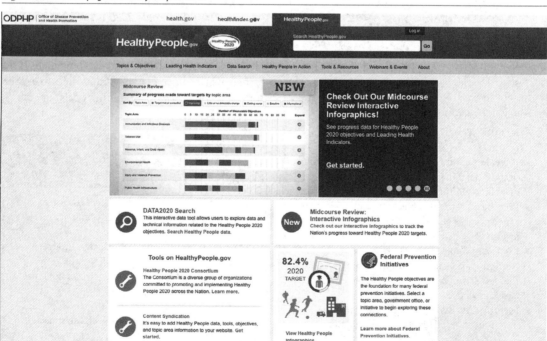

Courtesy of U.S. Department of Health and Human Services. Office of Disease Prevention and Health Promotion. (2010c). *Healthy People 2020.* Retrieved from https://www.healthypeople.gov

Figure 1-4 *Healthy People 2020* topics and objectives: Overview.

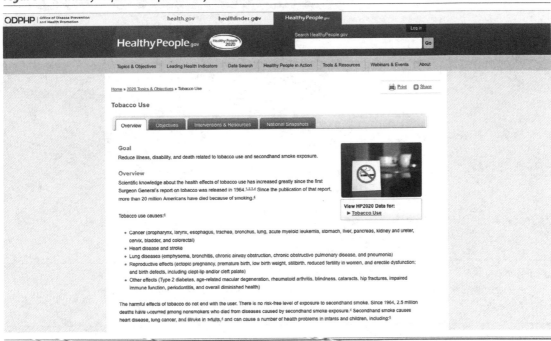

Courtesy of U.S. Department of Health and Human Services. Office of Disease Prevention and Health Promotion. (2010d). *Healthy People 2020*. Retrieved from https://www.healthypeople.gov/2020/topics-objectives/topic/tobacco-use

The objective tab presents the 21 objectives (see **Figure 1-5**). Two of the objectives specifically address the adolescent population: Tobacco Use—Objective 2: Reduce tobacco use by adolescents, and Tobacco Use—Objective 3: Reduce the initiation of tobacco use among children, adolescents, and young adults. Each of these objectives contain subobjectives. As the public health nurse enters into each of these objectives, they will see baseline, target, target-setting method, data source, and other pertinent information. It is important for the reader to note that *Healthy People 2020* is a living document and, as such, changes continually with new evidence, stakeholder interest, and participants.

Finally, the interventions and resources and the national snapshots tabs offer the public health nurse direct links to clinical recommendations for evidence-based community intervention strategies and consumer information (see **Figure 1-6** and **Figure 1-7**).

Four Foundational Health Measures

The final component of the Healthy People initiative is the Four Foundational Health Measures. These foundational measures include General Health Status, Health-Related Quality of Life and Well-Being, Determinants of Health, and Disparities. These foundational health measures are identified as way to measure what progress is being made toward the achievement of the overarching goals.

Healthy People Movement in Action

The Healthy People initiative serves as a guide for healthcare professionals and their partners as they decide collectively what types of health initiatives to engage in and how to implement and evaluate these initiatives. These partners are central to the success of the *Healthy People 2020* agenda: "Addressing the challenge of health improvement is a shared responsibility

Figure 1-5 *Healthy People 2020* topics and objectives: Objective.

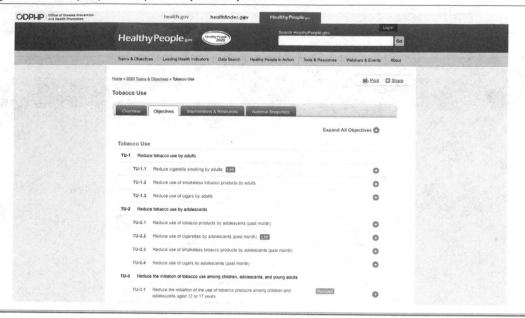

Courtesy of U.S. Department of Health and Human Services. Office of Disease Prevention and Health Promotion. (2010e). *Healthy People 2020.* Retrieved from https://www.healthypeople.gov/2020/topics-objectives/topic/tobacco-use/objectives

Figure 1-6 *Healthy People 2020* topics and objectives: Interventions and resources.

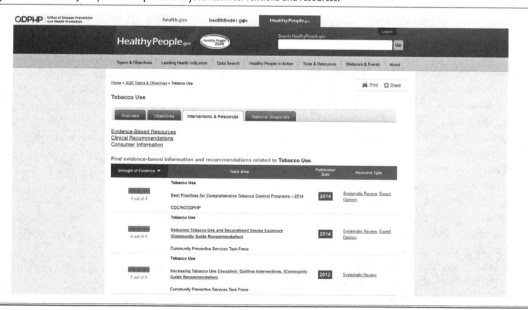

Courtesy of U.S. Department of Health and Human Services. Office of Disease Prevention and Health Promotion. (2010f). *Healthy People 2020.* Retrieved from https://www.healthypeople.gov/2020/topics-objectives/topic/tobacco-use/ebrs

Figure 1-7 *Healthy People 2020* topics and objectives: National Snapshots

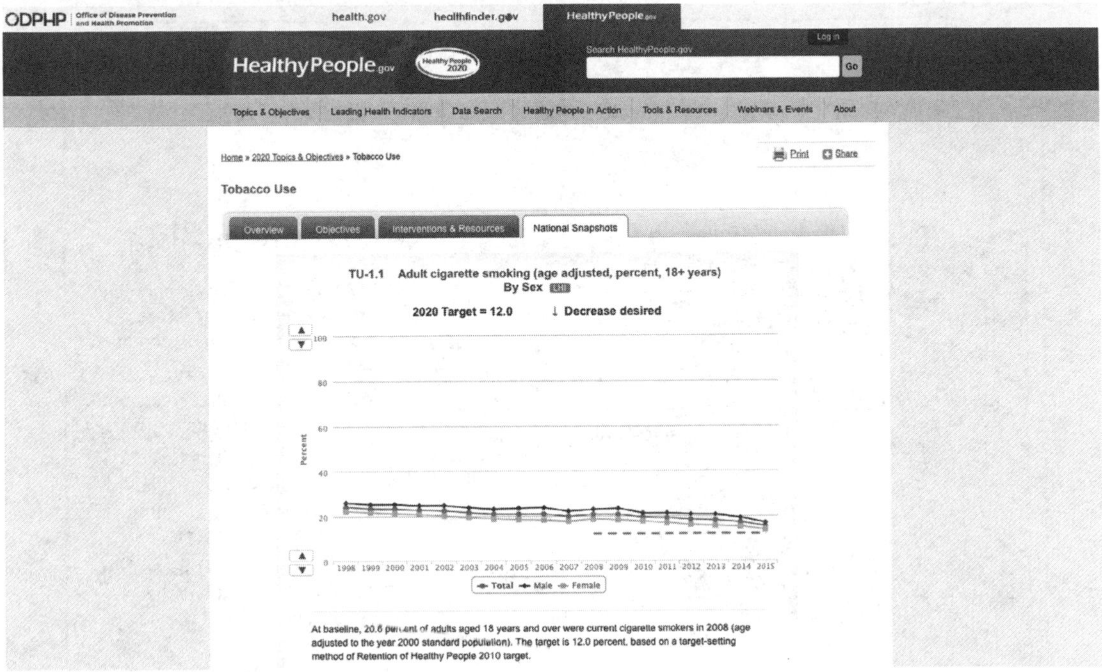

Courtesy of U.S. Department of Health and Human Services. Office of Disease Prevention and Health Promotion. (2010g). *Healthy People 2020.* Retrieved from https://www.healthypeople.gov/2020/topics-objectives/topic/tobacco-use/national-snapshot

that requires the active participation and leadership of the federal government, states, local governments, policymakers, healthcare providers, professionals, business executives, educators, community leaders, and the American public itself" (U.S. DHHS, 2000, p. 4). This resonates with the need mentioned earlier for interprofessional and intersectoral collaborative work. Public health nurses are important actors in this collaborative work and have historically been present in public health initiatives.

The *Healthy People 2020* website is interactive and a powerful tool for all stakeholders.

The graphic model, portrayed in *Healthy People 2020,* is shown in **Figure 1-8**. The graphic model portrays the determinants of health and includes physical environment, health services, social environment, individual behavior, biology, and genetics.

Although this model does not pictorially display policymaking as one of the concentric circles, policymaking is described as a determinant of health on the website (U.S. DHHS, 2010a). The authors of this text expanded the graphic model for *Healthy People 2020,* including this additional determinant of policymaking. They developed the visual depiction called the process model for *Healthy People 2020* that readers can view on the inside front cover of this book.

The multiple components of the process model depict the entire Healthy People process, not just the determinants of health as outlined in the Healthy People graphic model. The outcome of this model is the promotion and improvement of the health of the general public as well as the potential for policy change to assure and ensure the sustainability of the specific change for health.

Figure 1-8   Screenshot of the graphic model for *Healthy People 2020*.

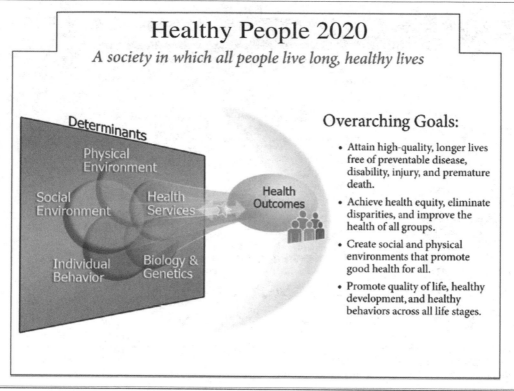

Courtesy of U.S. Department of Health and Human Services. Office of Disease Prevention and Health Promotion. (2010h). *Healthy People 2020.* Retrieved from https://www.healthypeople.gov/2020/About-Healthy-People

Application to Communities

How do public health nurses apply and use *Healthy People 2020* for a community of interest? Public health nurses and their partners can apply *Healthy People in Healthy Communities.* The U.S. DHHS (2001) presented this document in an attempt to enlist communities to apply the Healthy People initiatives to ensure a healthy population locally. A healthy community is defined as "one that embraces the belief that health is more than merely an absence of disease; a healthy community includes those elements that enable people to maintain a high quality of life and productivity" (U.S. DHHS, 2001, p. 1).

To become a healthy community and to implement *Healthy People 2020,* the public health nurse and members of the community must work together using multiple strategies. One such strategy is to use MAP-IT, a mnemonic for mobilize, assess, plan, implement, and track (U.S. DHHS, 2001). MAP-IT is a broader application of the nursing process. In addition to assessment, diagnosis, planning, implementation, and evaluation, the MAP-IT process includes the critical step of mobilization, which sets the stage for coalition, collaboration, and shared decision-making to occur. The process model depicted on the inside front cover of this book also presents the MAP-IT process and demonstrates how it is aligned with the entire process model. The first step in MAP-IT is to mobilize. One way to mobilize a group is through partnering with others and developing a coalition.

Truglio-Londrigan (2015) notes, "This coming together to work together leads to the notion of making decisions together. Working together in groups, therefore, allows individuals or organizations to come together to work toward a goal and ultimately achieve their vision via shared decision-making" (p. 142). In this case, the vision is a healthier community.

The next step in the MAP-IT technique is to assess the community of interest. Chapter 3 contains detailed information on assessment of a community and population. There are a number of ways to assess a community, both quantitatively and qualitatively. What is important is that assessment is the collection of data to identify the priority needs of the community. Those who have been mobilized, including the community participants, must look at the data collected and identify whether the issues are in line with one or more of the topic areas listed in *Healthy People 2020*. If yes, the community members can then use *Healthy People 2020* as a guide for the development of initiatives. If the issue is not identified as a topic area in Healthy People, the systematic process is still valuable for the achievement of positive health outcomes.

Once an issue is identified, the mobilized group moves on to the third step, the development of the plan. The plan takes into consideration resources such as funding, people, technology, methods of communication, and time. It is critical that those involved work with the topic areas and the objectives, with particular emphasis on the baseline, target, target-setting method, and data source for the identified topic area of need. Specific steps need to be developed, along with time frames and the clear identification of who is responsible for which portions of the plan. It is very important to include the community participants in the development of this plan, as being inclusive accounts for the various social, political, economic, and cultural factors that affect the plan. Successful plans are culturally congruent with the values, the beliefs, and the needs of the population and are based in evidence. Plan development uses the intervention strategies found on the intervention wheel.

Once the plan is identified, the next step in the MAP-IT technique is to implement the plan. Again, clear communication between and among all members is important so that every member knows who is responsible for which activities. For this communication to be effective, one must remember, "There is no 'power over' in a coalition, only 'power with.' . . . This requires equal empowerment of all members of the coalition in order for the members to communicate and work together" (Truglio-Londrigan, 2015, pp. 152–153). The application of technology to reach populations is critical to consider in the implementation phase, and the technology applied must be appropriate for the population in question. Methods for tracking progress during the implementation process are also important to consider.

The final step in the MAP-IT technique is to track progress and evaluate movement toward the outcomes. What was the original baseline? Was the target reached? Sharing success is critical. If there is a need to improve, then all members of the group, including community members, must analyze what transpired. Were the initial data collected correctly? Was the plan accessible and appropriate? What changes need to be made? How will the new plan be implemented and evaluated? These are just some questions that should be asked. As mentioned, the MAP-IT strategy is presented in the *Healthy People 2020* process model located on the inside front cover of this book. It is placed there to enhance clarity for users.

Public health nurses must become familiar with the *Healthy People 2020* website, especially the Implementing *Healthy People 2020* tab, which offers guidelines and resources for the MAP-IT process.

Conclusion

This chapter serves as a guiding framework. It discusses public health and the nation's agenda to achieve a society in which people live long and healthy lives (U.S. DHHS, 2010a). This framework demonstrates how to incorporate the public health nursing agenda into the nation's agenda. Chapter 3 uses this guiding framework to design the Public Health Nursing Assessment Tool. Later chapters are based on the intervention wheel strategies, which serve as a template for action for the profession and are models by which public health nurses can guide their own practice.

Additional Resources

U.S. Department of Health and Human Services/*Healthy People 2020* at: https://www.healthypeople.gov/

U.S. Department of Health and Human Services/Healthy People in Healthy Communities at: http://www.healthypeople.gov/2010/default.htm

Healthy Campus 2020 at: http://www.acha.org/healthycampus/

Center for Disease Control and Prevention About Healthy Places at: http://www.cdc.gov/healthyplaces/about.htm

References

Abrams, S. E. (2007). Nursing the community, a look back at the 1984 dialogue between Virginia Henderson and Sherry L. Shamansky. *Public Health Nursing, 24*(4), 382–386.

American Nurses Association. (2013). *Public health nursing: Scope and standards of practice.* Silver Springs, MD: Author.

American Public Health Association, Public Health Nursing Section. (2013). *The definition and practice of public health nursing: A statement of the public health nursing section.* Washington, DC: Author.

Association of Schools & Programs of Public Health. (2016). *What is public health?* Retrieved from http://www.aspph.org/discover

Beard, J. H. (1922). Progress of public health work. *Scientific Monthly, 14*(2), 140–152.

Brodie, M., Weltzien, E., Altman, D., Blendon, R., & Benson, J. (2006). Experiences of Hurricane Katrina evacuees in Houston shelters: Implications for future planning. *American Journal of Public Health, 96*(8), 1402–1408.

Buhler-Wilkerson, K. (1993). Bringing care to the people: Lillian Wald's legacy to public health nursing. *American Journal of Public Health, 83*(12), 1778–1786.

Buhler-Wilkerson, K. (2001). *No place like home: A history of nursing and home care in the United States.* Baltimore, MD: Johns Hopkins University Press.

Buttery, C. M. G. (1992). Provision of public health services. In J. M. Last & R. B. Wallace (Eds.), *Public health and preventive medicine* (13th ed., pp. 1113–1128). Norwalk, CT: Appleton & Lange.

Centers for Disease Control and Prevention. (2014). *The public health system and the 10 essential public health services.* Retrieved from http://www.cdc.gov/nphpsp/essentialservices.html

Centers for Disease Control and Prevention. (2015). *Core functions of public health and how they relate to the 10 essential services.* Retrieved from http://www.cdc.gov/nceh/ehs/ephli/core_ess.htm

Crandall, E. P. (1922). An historical sketch of public health nursing. *American Journal of Nursing, 22*(8), 641–645.

Declaration of Alma-Ata International Conference on Primary Care. (1978). *Primary health care.* Retrieved from http://www. who.int/hpr/NPH/docs/-declaration_almaata.pdf

Dock, L. (1908). The suffrage question. *American Journal of Nursing, 8*(11), 925–927.

Greiner, P., & Edelman, C. (2006). Health defined: Objectives for promotion and prevention. In C. Edelman & C. Mandle (Eds.), *Health promotion throughout the life span* (pp. 3–22). St. Louis, MO: Elsevier Mosby.

Institute of Medicine. (1988). *The future of public health.* Washington, DC: National Academies Press.

Institute of Medicine. (2003). *The future of the public's health in the 21st century.* Washington, DC: National Academies Press.

Institute of Medicine. (2010). *For the public's health: The role of measurement in action and accountability.* Washington, DC: National Academies Press.

Institute of Medicine. (2012). *For the public's health: Investigating in a healthier future.* Washington, DC: National Academies Press.

Keller, L. O., & Strohschein, S. (2016). Population-based public health nursing practice: The intervention wheel. In M. Stanhope & J. Lancaster (Eds.), *Public health nursing: Population-centered health care in the community* (9th ed., pp. 190–216). St. Louis, MO: Elsevier.

Kennedy, M. (2016, April 20). *Lead-laced water in Flint: A step-by-step look at the makings of a crisis.* Retrieved from http://www.npr.org/sections/thetwo-way/2016/04/20/465545378/lead-laced-water-in-flint-a-step-by-step-look-at-the-makings-of-a-crisis

Leavell, H., & Clark, A. E. (1965). *Preventive medicine for doctors in the community* (3rd ed.). New York, NY: McGraw-Hill.

Lewenson, S. B. (2007). A historical perspective on policy, politics and nursing. In D. J. Mason, J. K. Leavitt, & M. W. Chaffee (Eds.), *Policy and politics in nursing and health care* (5th ed., pp. 21–33). St. Louis, MO: Saunders Elsevier.

Missouri Department of Health and Senior Services. (2006). *Public health nursing manual.* Retrieved from http://health.mo.gov/living/lpha/phnursing/manual.pdf

Scheele, L. A. (1949). Anniversary program—150th year U.S. Public Health Service. *American Journal of Public Health and the Nation's Health, 39*(3), 293–302.

Truglio-Londrigan, M. (2015).Working together: Shared decision-making. In S. B. Lewenson & M. T. Truglio-Londrigan (Eds.), *Decision-making in nursing: Thoughtful approaches for leadership* (2nd ed., pp. 141–162). Sudbury, MA: Jones & Bartlett Learning.

Truglio-Londrigan, M., & Lewenson, S. B. (2017). In S. B. Lewenson & M. Truglio-Londrigan (Eds.), *Practicing primary health care in nursing : Caring for populations.* Sudbury, MA: Jones & Bartlett Learning.

U.S. Department of Health and Human Services Public Health Service. (1994a). *The public health workforce: An agenda for the 21st century. A report of the Public Health Functions Project.* Retrieved from http://www.health.gov/phfunctions/pubhlth.pdf

U.S. Department of Health and Human Services—Public Health Functions Steering Committee. (1994b). *The public health workforce: An agenda for the 21st Century.* Washington, DC: U.S. Government Printing Office.

U.S. Department of Health and Human Services. (2000). *Healthy People 2010, 1.* Washington, DC: U.S. Government Printing Office.

U.S. Department of Health and Human Services. (2001). *Healthy people in healthy communities.* Washington, DC: U.S. Government Printing Office.

U.S. Department of Health and Human Services. (2010a). *About healthy people—Healthy people 2020 framework.* Retrieved from http://www.healthypeople.gov/2020/about/default.aspx

U.S. Department of Health and Human Services. (2010b). *2020 topics and objectives.* Retrieved from https://www.healthypeople.gov/2020/topics-objectives.

U.S. Department of Health and Human Services. (2010c). *Healthy people.* Retrieved from https://www.healthypeople.gov/2020/default

U.S. Department of Health and Human Services. (2010d). *Tobacco use.* Retrieved from https://www.healthypeople.gov/2020/topics-objectives/topic/tobacco-use

U.S. Department of Health and Human Services. (2010e). *Objective—tobacco use.* Retrieved from https://www.healthypeople.gov/2020/topics-objectives/topic/tobacco-use/objectives

U.S. Department of Health and Human Services. (2010f). *Intervention and resources—tobacco use.* Retrieved from https://www.healthypeople.gov/2020/topics-objectives/topic/tobacco use/ebrs

U.S. Department of Health and Human Services. (2010g). *National snapshot—tobacco use.* Retrieved from https://www.healthypeople.gov/2020/topics-objectives/topic/tobacco use/national-snapshot

U.S. Department of Health and Human Services. (2010h). *About Healthy People—Healthy people 2020 framework.* Retrieved from https://www.healthypeople.gov/2020/About-HealthyPeople

Wald, L. D. (1907). Best helps to the immigrant through the nurse (A Phase of District Nursing). Lillian D. Wald Papers, 1889–1957. Writing and Speeches. Reel 24, Box 35, Folder 6, pp. 1–4. New York Public Library, Humanities and Social Sciences Library, Manuscripts and Archives Division, New York, NY.

Warner, D. D., & Lightfoot. (2014). Theoretical basis of community/public health nursing. In J. A. Allender, C. Rector, & K. D. Warner (Eds.), *Community & public health nursing: Promoting the public's health* (pp. 438–458). Philadelphia, PA: Lippincott Williams & Wilkins.

Winslow, C. E. A. (1920). The untilled fields of public health. *Science, New Series, 51*(1306), 22–33.

World Health Organization. (2008). *The world health report (2008): Primary health care now more than ever.* Geneva, Switzerland: Author.

For a full suite of assignments and additional learning activities, use the access code located in the front of your book to visit this exclusive website: **http://go.jblearning.com/londrigan.** If you do not have an access code, you can obtain one at the site.

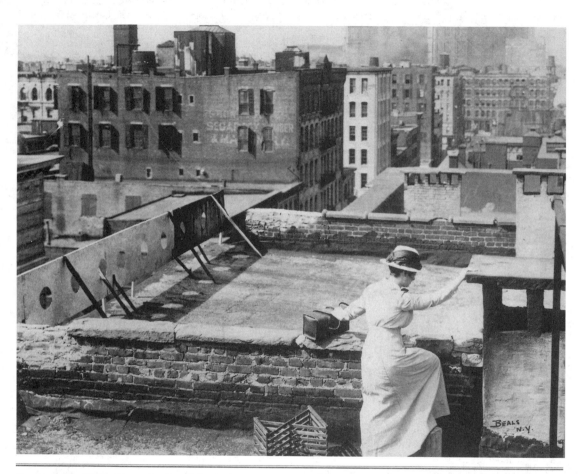

Courtesy of the Visiting Nurse Service of New York.

CHAPTER 2

Public Health Nursing in the United States: A History

Sandra B. Lewenson

The trained nurse, known under various titles, as –"the visiting nurse"- "the district nurse" – "the public health nurse", has had the obligation and the privilege of bringing, in simple form and thoroughly sympathetic approach the scientific messages of health and hygiene. The public health service, as given by the nurses, is an enlargement of the relationship of the individual nurse, patient, and physician (Wald, 1918, pp.1–2).

LEARNING OBJECTIVES

At the completion of this chapter, the reader will be able to:

- Define the various terms used to describe the work of nurses who have practiced in public health nursing over time.
- Describe the history of public health nursing.
- Explain the relevance of the history of public health nursing to current issues in public health nursing.

KEY TERMS

- ❏ Community health nurse
- ❏ District nurse
- ❏ Home care nurse
- ❏ Populations
- ❏ Public health nurse
- ❏ Visiting nurse

Hiestand (1982) called for the historian to reflect on "practice as it changed over time" because of its relevance to "understanding the nurses' experience" (p. 11). The purpose of this chapter is to reflect on the practice of public health nursing by examining the nurse's evolving experience in this role. This experience has been influenced by the type of agency where nurses worked, the community in which they served, the economic climate, the advances made in the sciences and technology, and other sociopolitical factors that shaped the kind of work being done (Bryant, 1968; Stewart & Vincent, 1968). The evolution of public health nursing reflects the response to these factors and the transformation that these nurses made in meeting the needs of individuals, families, **populations**, and communities (American Nurses Association [ANA], 2007). As the public health nursing role evolved, so did the nomenclature, leading some to question what a public health nurse is. This chapter examines public health nursing and the shift in roles as the names changed throughout the late 19th century until today. It also highlights the educational requirements for the public health nurse because as the titles and responsibilities changed to meet the needs of society, so did the educational requirements and the expectations. Although this chapter seeks to explain the history of public health nursing and address the question of what a public health nurse is, it raises more questions for the reader to consider than it provides answers.

What Is a Public Health Nurse?

Early public health nursing leader Mary Gardner raised the question of what to call the nurse who provided care in the home in the preface of her 1933 book, *Public Health Nursing*. She decided on using the term **public health nurse** throughout her book instead of the other possible terms attributed to this role. Gardner (1933) explained as follows:

Certain questions of nomenclature have arisen, chief among them the name to be given to the nurse and to her work as described in these

pages. In view of the present tendency toward more generalized methods of administration, and also because the functions of the various nurses are now so closely interwoven, the names "visiting nurse" and "visiting nursing association" have not been used in this book. "Public health nurse" and "public health nursing" have been substituted throughout to describe all types of nurses and organizations. (p. x)

Others questioned who was considered to be a public health nurse and what the activities of this nurse are. For example, Welsh (1936) wrote an article titled, "What Is Public Health Nursing?" where she exclaimed that the very need for public health nursing to define itself after 50 years of organized activity was in itself an "indication of the lack of unity within the field itself" (p. 452). Confusion about who and what a public health nurse was stemmed from the increasing specializations that public health nurses were branching into other areas, such as tuberculosis nurses, maternity nurses, infant welfare nurses, and other specialty areas aside from **visiting nurses**.

The change in names used to describe the person who provided the care in the home has perpetually confused those in health care, as well as consumers of care (Geis, 1991; Humphrey & Milone-Nuzzo, 1996; Jones, Davis, & Davis, 1987; Levin et al., 2007; Roberts & Heinrich, 1985; Welsh, 1936). In schools of nursing, for example, students take courses in public health that are often labeled community health. Faculty members debate what they consider a good community clinical experience. This debate usually includes whether a visiting nurse experience ("carry the bag"), working in a health department, incorporating public health initiatives in a shopping mall, or any number of combinations of experiences allow the student to understand the full dimension of public health nursing. This confusion stems from the faculty's orientation to this specialty and from the terminology used to describe the course: Is it public health, community health, or both? Clark (2008) poignantly asks what's in a name and tries to explicate the meaning of the various terms used to describe this specialty.

Visiting nurse with a young boy.

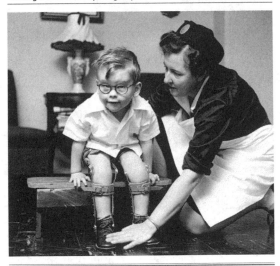

Courtesy of the Visiting Nurse Service of New York.

As the public health nursing role evolved, so did the names for this role. The changing names reflected the tensions between and among the stakeholders who shaped the work of public health nurses. The lack of cohesiveness of the various volunteer and public organizations and the separation of the preventive care from the curative aspects of the public health nurse's role led Buhler-Wilkerson (1993) to write, "it is little wonder then that the question, 'What is a public health nurse' has been debated for more than 80 years" (p. 1783). The history of public health nursing provides the reader with the origins of the various names, the educational requirements for these roles, and the insight into the debate that continues today as to what a public health nurse is.

Evolution of the Public Health Nurse

District Nurses

District nursing began in 1859 as part of an experiment where a hospital-based, trained nurse was sent to provide nursing care to the poor in a small district in Liverpool, England (Hughes, 1893/1949). From that early success, the promoter of this experiment, William Rathbone, expanded this work, dividing Liverpool into 18 districts and supplying each district with its own **district nurse** (Hughes). The adoption of this successful form of nursing spread, and various agencies began to use district nurses throughout England.

English nursing leader Florence Sara (Lees) Craven, who published under her husband's name Dacre Craven (1889/1984), wrote about the work of the district nurse in England and called Rathbone's experiment the defining incident in identifying the distinct work of the district nurse. In Craven's description of the district nurse, she includes the care of the sick poor in their homes as the main focus of a district nurse. The responsibilities of the district nurse were carefully explained in Craven's work, *A Guide to District Nursing,* first published in 1889. Craven was considered one of the first superintendents of the central home where district nurses lived together. These nurses were drawn together from "the class of gentlewomen, with a view to bringing women of higher education and refinement to grapple with the special difficulties of the work" (Hughes, 1893/1949, p. 113).

District nurses addressed the health of the poor in the community and needed to have a "real love for the poor and a desire to lessen the misery" (Craven, 1889/1984, p. 1) that was found in the homes. Concern for the family and bringing cleanliness to the patient, the family, and the environment in which the family lived was part of the district nurse's role. The district nurse needed to know about the sanitary and charitable organizations in the district where the patients lived. In this way, when sanitary problems arose, such as a defective water supply, or "untrapped" cesspools or "unemptied dustbins," the nurse would notify the appropriate "sanitary committee of the district . . . who [would] take legal steps, if necessary, to compel the landlord to put the premises into a proper sanitary condition" (Craven, 1889/1984, p. 11). The daily work consisted of care of the sick poor and enabled the nurse to observe the sanitary conditions in the home that affected the health of the patient, the family, and the community or district in which the patient lived. Craven (1889/1984) gave the following examples of the sanitary work of the district nurse:

Sometimes there is a plague of flies in the room, which can be traced to some foul or decaying animal or vegetable refuse. When the nurse carries down the dust and ashes to the dustbin she sees whether it ought to be emptied, and ascertains when this was last done. As she fetches water for the kettle she can find out whether it is from an impure and uncovered cistern, and as she empties the slops of her patient she ascertains whether the w.c. is in a good sanitary condition, and with a separate cistern from that used for drinking purposes (and she can herself occasionally flush the pan of the w.c). (pp. 11–12)

Another important role of the district nurse was to educate patients, friends, and family about the need for a sanitary environment. The nurse taught about the need for personal cleanliness and hygiene, and she herself was expected to be a role model of both. The nurse's uniform, as Craven (1889/1984) described, reflected a clean and neat appearance. The district nurse was to be a paragon of excellence in the way she cared for the sick poor, managed the sanitation of the environment, and educated others about cleanliness and sanitary principles. She also assumed the responsibility for the care of the dying patient and the dead. Craven (1893/1949) wrote that district nurses were instructed on the "best positions in which to place the dying, according to their ailment . . . so that they might breathe to the last without unnecessary effort or pain" (p. 133).

As the district nurses whom Craven (1889/1984) wrote about carried on their work, they also were responsible for keeping records of what they did. Each district nurse spent time on paperwork documenting her caseload, the time she spent, and the care she provided in each home. The nurses shared this information with the superintendent of the district nurses, who collated their reports into a monthly report. The superintendent kept a log of all the cases the nurses managed. Based on the district nurses' work, reports included the number of new cases per month, the length of visits, and the number of visits required by the patients (Craven, 1889/1984, p. 131). Superintendents rated the work done and the data collected. For example, they would use ratings such as "excellent," "good," "moderate," "imperfect," or "nil" to rank such things as the patient's status; the cleanliness of the patient, the room, utensils, and beds; and the various kinds of treatments, such as sponge baths, mouth care, precautions against bed sores, wound care, and other treatments. Records of various types of cases such as typhoid fever, diphtheria, puerperal disease, scarlet fever, obstetrical cases, and care of the newborn were also kept. In addition, the superintendent's report included an evaluation of the probationers, who acted as the district nurses, on their ability to observe the sick and manage the care of the sick (Craven, 1889/1984).

Knowledge about the work of these early district nurses in England spread to the United States. In 1893, Amy Hughes, superintendent of nurses at the Metropolitan and National Nursing Association, one of the agencies to form in London, came to the United States to speak before the International Congress of Charities, Correction, and Philanthropy in Chicago. She explained to the American audience that "district

Lillian Wald (left) and friends, 1915.

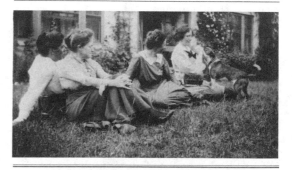

Courtesy of the Visiting Nurse Service of New York.

nursing is the technical name for the work of nursing the sick poor in their own homes" (p. 111). Interest in district nursing spread as trained nurses from the early Nightingale-influenced training schools sought ways to improve the health of those who lived in the community. Miss C. E. Somerville, from Lawrence General Hospital in Massachusetts, said, "the last quarter of the century was well advanced when America caught the reflection of England's light, and the era of trained nursing for the poor began in this country" (Somerville, 1893/1949, p. 119).

Early district nursing associations, also called visiting nurse associations, organized in the United States. Some were established along religious missionary lines that expected the care of the sick to include a religious concern for the well-being of the patient. An early example of this was the Woman's Branch of the New York City Mission and Tract Society, which in 1877 used trained nurses to provide care to the sick in the home in New York City (Lewenson, 1993; Somerville, 1893/1949). Two years later, the Ethical Culture Society offered a nondenominational visiting nurse service that rendered care to the sick poor. Both associations began almost 20 years before the secular visiting nurse service was founded by Lillian Wald and Mary Brewster in 1893 at the Henry Street Settlement. Other early district and visiting nurse associations opened in Boston, Chicago, Philadelphia, and other cities across the United States, offering care to the sick poor and those of moderate means. They shared a common goal and assumed many of the same roles as their counterpart district nurses did in England (Somerville, 1893/1949).

Nightingale's paper "Sick Nursing and Health Nursing," presented at the Chicago World Fair in 1893, described the district nurse as providing care to the sick at home, as well as someone who assumed the work as a health missioner. A health missioner required additional training in how to teach healthy behaviors to mothers in the community and in the home. Nightingale outlined some of the content that was included in their additional training in areas such as sanitary conditions in the home, management of

health of adults, women in childbearing years before and after confinement, and infants and children (Nightingale, 1893/1949, p. 41).

Nightingale (1893/1949) believed that to improve the health of infants and babies, mothers needed to learn about healthier lifestyle behaviors. Nightingale used a population focus to explain why these health missioners needed to be concerned about the health of infants and babies. She wrote that,

> *The life duration of babies is the most 'delicate test' of health conditions. What is the proportion of the whole population of cities or country which dies before it is five years old? We have tons of printed knowledge on the subject of hygiene and sanitation. The causes of enormous child mortality are perfectly well known: they are chiefly, want of cleanliness, want of fresh air, careless dieting and clothing, want of whitewashing . . . in one word, want of household care of health. (p. 29)*

Nightingale's idea about health nursing extended to the community, and she summarized this in her paper by saying, "The health of the unity is the health of community. Unless you have the health of the unity, there is no community health" (Nightingale, 1893/1949, p. 35).

The concept of health missioners or health nursing was embedded in the work of the visiting nurse in the United States, as these nurses added to their work the ideas generated by the public health movement that was calling for ways to keep communities healthy. The public health movement was ongoing in the United States since the mid-1800s, when the Shattuck commission identified the need for the creation of local health boards that would collect statistical data on the population, including records of marriages, births, and deaths. States were called on to investigate "the cause of disease, abatement of the smoke nuisance, adoption of means for public health education, and other far-reaching measures" (Beard, 1922, p. 142). Scientific discoveries about the causes of the spread of certain diseases such as yellow fever, malaria, tuberculosis, or poliomyelitis

Philadelphia visiting nurse with a family.

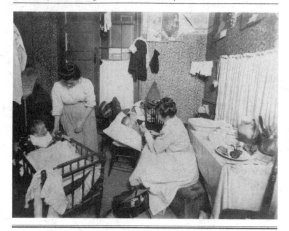

Courtesy of the Barbara Bates Center for The Study of
The History of Nursing, School of Nursing, University of
Pennsylvania.

further advanced public health initiatives. Visiting nurses cared for the sick at home and provided the families they visited with information about how to keep their families and communities healthier.

Public health nursing leader Lillian Wald attended the Chicago exposition and was greatly influenced by Nightingale's paper describing health nursing (Haupt, 1953). Haupt wrote that Wald had "accepted Florence Nightingale's concept of 'health nursing' and put the word 'public' in front of it so that all the people would know that they could use it" (p. 81). The nurses at the Henry Street Nurses Settlement, for example, cared for the sick at home and offered classes to mothers on how to keep their families healthier. Although the term health missioner is rarely seen in the literature describing public health nursing in the United States, the dimension of health promotion and disease prevention continued to be imbued in the work of public health nursing.

Visiting Nurse

Public health nursing leader Lavinia Dock and nursing educator Isabel Maitland Stewart addressed the issue of nomenclature in their text, *A Short*

History of Nursing (Dock & Stewart, 1938). Dock and Stewart wrote that the first evidence of the term **visiting nursing** was found in the early records of St. John's House, England, which began in 1848. During that period, cholera and smallpox were rampant in England and the United States, and "Anglican and Catholic sisters spent their lives in visiting the poor and caring for the sick under the most terrible conditions" (Dock & Stewart, 1938, p. 305). By the 20th century, however, the role of the visiting nurse expanded into what was to become part of the larger public health movement. Dock and Stewart (1938) wrote, "In the 20th century, visiting nursing became one part of the broadening field of 'public health nursing,' as an ideal of the visiting nurse who was teacher, sanitarian, and public-spirited citizen as well as nurse, gradually took form" (pp. 305–306). This new expanding field of public health nursing, Dock and Stewart believed, was to become the "nursing of the future" (p. 306).

As mentioned earlier, public health nurses were closely aligned with the public health movement that flourished during the early 20th century. Fitzpatrick (1975a) described the noted public health expert Charles Winslow's identification of three phases of the public health movement: "the phase of empirical environmental sanitation, the bacteriological phase, and the educational phase" (p. 6). The fact that nurses were already engaged in providing both health care and health education within communities led Winslow and others to acknowledge the value public health nurses brought to the larger public health movement (Fitzpatrick, 1975a).

Modern Nursing Movement

The history of the modern nursing movement in the United States began in 1873 as Nightingale's work influenced the opening of schools for nurses in New York, Connecticut, and Massachusetts (Lewenson, 1993). It was a time of great change for women who sought a way to financially support themselves in some kind of labor outside of the home. Women read a description about one of the new training schools that had started at Bellevue Hospital in New York City in *The Century Magazine* (North, 1882), describing nursing as a "new profession for women" (p. 38). Once a nursing student completed the apprenticeship training at one of these hospital schools, however, she was sent out as a trained nurse into the community without the security of hospital employment. Instead of hiring their graduates, hospitals typically used their next class of nursing students to staff the hospital. A trained nurse consequently had to find employment elsewhere and usually worked as a private duty nurse, caring for one patient in the home setting, or as a public health nurse, working in public or privately funded organizations with responsibilities for visiting patients in their homes and promoting health in the community.

By 1893, 20 years after the first few Nightingale-influenced training schools began, nursing superintendents of the schools that had already opened joined together with other women from around the world at the now famous Chicago World's Fair. It was at this international conference that professional nursing organizations in the United States began. The first organization to form was the American Society of Superintendents for Nurses, which was started by pioneering nursing superintendents who wanted to establish standards and control over the education and practice of nursing. These leaders banded together in 1893 and by 1912 became known as the National League of Nursing Education, which changed its name again in 1952 to the current title, the National League for Nursing (NLN). As this group formed, the leaders, Isabel Hampton Robb, Lavinia Dock, and others, saw the need to organize nurses working at the bedside. The need to control practice; lobby for state nursing registration laws, which were nonexistent at the time; and support those nurses in financial trouble led to the formation of the Nurses Associated Alumnae of the United States and Canada in 1896, which in 1911 became known as the American Nurses Association (ANA).

This need to control and standardize nursing education and practice extended to another group of nurses, marginalized because of racial bias. Many African American nurses were excluded from joining the ANA, as a result of a shift to statewide membership in the organization. Once that occurred in 1916, individual nurses no longer could join and relied on membership through their state nurses associations (Carnegie, 1991; Lewenson, 1993). Racist policies of many states, particularly in the South, prohibited African American nurses from membership and left them without the support of a professional organization. This meant issues such as control of education in their nursing schools and control of practice through state registration laws that often discriminated against them would be left unattended until 1908, when the National Association of Colored Graduate Nurses (NACGN) formed. Nursing leader Martha Franklin sought assistance from other African American nurses to establish this organization to support the needs of Black nurses in the United States. This organization lasted from 1908 until 1952, when integration into the ANA was achieved (Carnegie, 1991).

Sophia Palmer, first editor of the *American Journal of Nursing*, wrote that, "Organization is the power of the age. Without it nothing great is accomplished" (Palmer, 1897/1991, p. 297). Organizations formed throughout the country, addressing many of the Progressive Era issues touching on the social, economic, and political welfare of the population. Nurses, by virtue of their education and practice, were aware of the connection between a healthy society and the right to vote (Lewenson, 1993). Concern for women's rights extended into the discussions of the NLN and the ANA, leading to organizational support of a woman's right to vote by 1912. The NACGN also supported women's rights initiatives, as evidenced by its support of the work of the International Council of Nurses in that area. The NACGN had sent a delegation years ahead of both the NLN and the ANA to participate in discussions related to women's rights around the globe (Lewenson, 1993).

Public Health Nursing Emerges

Throughout the late 1800s and early 1900s, Lavinia Dock advocated suffrage for women and wrote extensively about this issue in the *American Journal of Nursing* and other journals of that period. Dock aligned the vote with health care and said that without it, nurses would not be able to effectively improve the health of society (Lewenson, 1993). Concern for the public's health was shared by others such as Lillian Wald and Mary Brewster, who founded the Henry Street Settlement in New York City's Lower East Side in 1893 to address the health of the people who lived there. Graduates and friends from the New York Hospital training school, Wald and Brewster opened the nurses' settlement house in 1893, two years after they had graduated from the training school, to care for the population of immigrants who flooded into the United States during the late 19th and early 20th centuries. The spread of illness became a real threat to the many Americans who lived in the overcrowded cities and experienced firsthand the diversity of those who immigrated here (Fitzpatrick, 1975a; Lewenson, 1993).

Buhler-Wilkerson (1985) said the impetus of the wealthier parts of society to improve the health of the poor stemmed, in part, from an understanding of the germ theory along with the idea that infectious diseases could be spread easily to their own families and communities by those immigrants who "sewed clothes in their filthy tenement homes or who processed food" (p. 1155). Early visiting nurses were hired by philanthropic women who sought to provide the urban poor with assistance during times of illness. According to Buhler-Wilkerson (1985), the nurses hired by these lady philanthropists were to bring their shared vision of the good society by bringing "care, cleanliness, and character to the homes of the sick poor" (p. 1155). Nurses were to teach the families they visited about the ways of American life that would lead to the prevention of disease and the promotion of health. Fear of the spread of illness prompted some of the concerns of those nurses

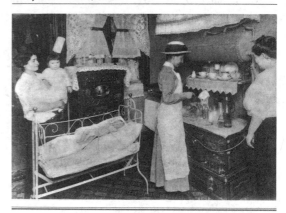

Henry Street nurses, 1903.

Courtesy of the Visiting Nurse Service of New York.

and their benefactors in bringing health care to the homes of the sick poor (Buhler-Wilkerson, 1985).

Dock worked at the Henry Street Settlement alongside Wald and other colleagues, engaging in what we now call primary healthcare activities, including visiting homes of those who needed care related to an illness, participation in well-baby clinics, case finding, health-promoting activities, surveillance, and school nurse activities. They lived within the Henry Street Settlement in the same community in which they provided nursing care. It was the comprehensive visiting nurse services like the ones delivered at Henry Street that proliferated throughout the country and offered another way for nurses to support themselves while caring for individuals, families, populations, and communities. Nursing care included the care of the sick at home, as well as well-baby classes and other health-promoting courses offered to the community.

Most nurses who graduated from the nursing schools in the late 1800s worked in private duty, providing nursing services to one patient in the home. This focus differed somewhat from that of the visiting nurse. Visiting nurses saw several patients in a day, and depending on the agency in which they worked, variable fees were attached to their visit based on the patients' ability to pay. While caring for the sick at home, they also provided much-needed health education. Often, the ability to care for the sick at home fostered a level of trust among the nurses and the families and community they served, which in turn provided them easier access to these same groups as they sought to provide health education. The work of the visiting nurse evolved into what became known as public health nursing and became a viable specialization for the graduate-trained nurse. Having coined the term public health nurses, Wald and other nursing leaders recognized a need to control the practice of this emerging specialization in nursing and founded the National Organization for Public Health Nursing (NOPHN) in 1912 (Buhler-Wilkerson, 2001).

National Organization for Public Health Nursing

The NOPHN grew out of a desire by public health nurses to control the practice and the standards of the emerging field of public health nursing. By 1912, the number of public health nurses had grown to over 3,000, and their work was supported through private and public funding (Gardner, 1933). The work was accepted by the community and extended far beyond the care provided to the sick at home. The public health nurses' role had expanded to meet the needs of a growing American urban and rural population—public health nurses visited patients in the home and provided additional primary healthcare services. In 1933, Gardner described the increasingly expanded and valued role of the public health nurse as follows:

> *We find other agencies counting not only on her help in individual cases, but upon the knowledge which she has gained from her unique position. We see that she has had her effect on state and city legislation, and has influenced public opinion to effect non-legislative reform. We find her valued as a preventive agent and health instructor by municipalities and state*

> *bodies, and the usefulness of her statistics acknowledged by research workers. We find her acting as probation officer, tenement house and sanitary inspector, county bailiff, domestic educator, and hospital social workers. She is found in the juvenile courts and the public playgrounds, in the department stores and the big hotels, in the schools and factories, in the houses of small wage-earners and in the swarming tenements of the poor. We find her in the big cities, the small towns, the rural districts and the lonely mountain regions. We find her dealing with tuberculosis, babies, mental cases, industrial workers, expectant mothers, midwifery and housing conditions. (p. 25)*

The expansion of the public health nurse's role in all facets of life grew in response to the needs of society. Visiting nurse associations proliferated throughout the early 20th century. Public health nurses worked for these newly forming visiting nurse associations throughout the country in both rural and urban settings. They provided care to the sick in their homes, educated the public on healthcare measures that would prevent illnesses such as tuberculosis and other communicable

Nurse teaching a nutrition class to a family, 1928.

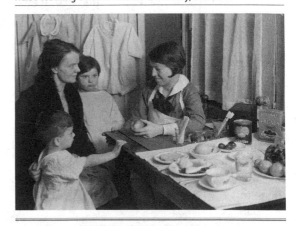

Courtesy of the Visiting Nurse Service of New York.

diseases, and promoted healthy behaviors. Each of these associations developed its own guidelines and was mostly organized by lay boards that did not have the same background as the public health nurses who founded some of the earlier visiting nurse associations, such as the Chicago Visiting Nurses Association or the Cleveland Visiting Nurse Association (Fitzpatrick, 1975a). Fitzpatrick (1975a) explained, "Until the rapid extension of public health nursing associations took place, there had been some success in upholding higher ethical and professional practices as well as a certain degree of conformity among the largest associations. This was due, in part, to the exceptional leadership ability and ideals of the early pioneers in the movement" (pp. 18–19). Yet as public health nursing associations expanded in the early 1900s, the lack of appropriate supervision and the misplaced understanding by the lay boards that ran the newly organized visiting nurse associations caused many in nursing to be worried about a real "threat to sound nursing practice itself" (Fitzpatrick, 1975a, p. 19).

Without clarity about the nursing role in public health, without understanding what the educational requirement of this nurse should be, and without standards regarding the practice, public health nursing leaders believed it imperative to organize. Public health nursing educator Ella Crandall contacted several of her peers between 1910 and 1911, asking them for their thoughts on the need for another nursing organization that specifically focused on public health nurses. Crandall found support among her colleagues; however, support for the format of such an organization varied. Although all agreed that an organization was needed, and all agreed to lay members being included, some favored becoming a committee of the already existing ANA. Crandall's idea, however, was for a separate organization that focused on setting standards and guidelines for public health nursing practice and education (Fitzpatrick, 1975a).

In 1912 Crandall's idea for a separate organization prevailed, and the NOPHN formed. Leaders in nursing, such as Lillian Wald, Mary Beard, Mary Gardner, Edna Foley, Jane Delano, and Anna Kerr, participated in the organization of this newly formed group. They addressed the issues of standardizing public health nurse requirements, such as requiring them to be graduates of nurse training schools and registered nurses in states that required registration, and they supported the idea of agency membership, which meant that non-nurses could be members of the organization, an idea that had not yet been practiced by the ANA or the National League of Nursing Education (forerunner of the NLN). The purpose of the NOPHN was to promote "sound public health nursing for the people of this country, who would be the recipients of the service" (Fitzpatrick, 1975a, p. 24).

A public health nurse weighing children, 1930.

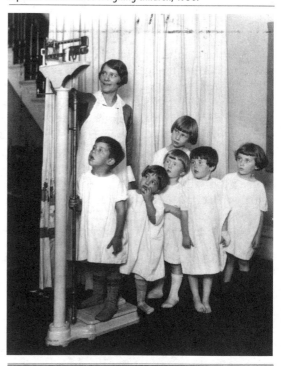

Courtesy of the Visiting Nurse Service of New York.

The architects of this new organization struggled with what to name the group. Some wanted to reflect the name of the visiting nurse, whereas others, such as Crandall, sought to use the term public health nursing in the title because public health nursing was considered to be broader than the earlier term of visiting nurse. The leaders debated the name, and when they finally came up with the title National Association of Public Health Nurses, again Crandall argued that the name needed to reflect more than nurses. Edna Foley, another public health nursing leader, suggested the name National Organization for Public Health Nursing, which was unanimously agreed upon (Fitzpatrick, 1975a). Wald was elected as the organization's first president.

One of the early NOPHN pamphlets (1914) described the public health nurse as follows:

A Public Health Nurse is a product of evolution. She has developed from the old-fashioned district or visiting nurse, who visits and nurses the sick, poor patient in his home. She is still that same visiting nurse and also, according to the demands of the community in which she serves, a public school nurse, an infant welfare nurse, a tuberculosis nurse, a hospital social service nurse, a sanitary inspector, a truant officer, a social worker, a visiting dietician, and even a midwife. Adequate preparation means special training and experience for each worker.

The idea that public health nursing evolved from the various terms to date—district nurse, visiting nurse—represented the full scope of practice that public health nurses were expected to provide. Public health nurses initially engaged in the wide range of practice, knowing that providing care in the home as visiting nurses afforded them access to where health-promoting behaviors could take place. Who paid for the care, whether the public or a privately run voluntary or business association, often determined the types of services the nurse could provide. The earlier public health nurse found

employment as school nurses, industrial nurses, visiting nurses, and in other settings where they could affect the health of a particular population; for example, they worked with mothers and babies or people with communicable diseases such as tuberculosis. Providing preventive and health promotional education in the community was all part of the work of public health nurses regardless of particular setting or agency for whom they worked.

As public health nurses became more valuable to society, their numbers and the number of settings where they worked increased, yet the tension between the privately funded visiting nurse services, which offered more of the care of the sick at home, compared with publically run health departments, which assumed more of the activities such as surveillance of communicable diseases and health education, created a separation—perhaps a false one—of the work of the public health nurse. The frequently seen overlap of the public health nurse's role created confusion in both the public and the profession's understanding of that role (Buhler-Wilkerson, 1985).

The term public health nurse was continually being defined and refined. For example, in 1919, five years after the formation of the NOPHN, Executive Director Ella Crandall wrote to George Vincent at the Rockefeller Foundation, where she sent him a corrected report of a previously shared description of the term public health nurse. Crandall (1919) wrote the following:

Term public health nurse considered for past five or six years by public health nurses and people administering visiting nurse associations as applicable to work of modern visiting nurse because (1) any nurse giving bedside care should realize opportunities for teaching health protection and hygiene; (2) individual illness not solely individual matter but lowers health standard for family, hence for community; consequently visiting nurse is a public health nurse; although usually supported by private funds, ultimate goal to have all public health nursing supported by public funds as are public school teachers, nurses employed by municipality not allowed time for bedside care; hence dependent on visiting nurse to round out her service; impossible to employ both kinds of workers in small and rural communities, therefore rural nurse must be trained in both.

There was a distinction in the work of the public health nurse based on the setting, the specialization, and the environment in which the public health nurse practiced. If the public health nurse worked in an urban setting, there were more resources in the community that addressed the various healthcare needs of the population. As a result, visiting nurses, in many instances, focused more on the care of the sick at home, whereas nurses who worked in public health departments focused more on the preventive and health-promoting kinds of education the public required. In rural settings where healthcare resources were more limited, the public health nurse would offer the full range of public health services, including the preventive and the curative.

In 1919, the NOPHN published a book presenting a description of the public health nurse that recognized that "public health nursing is a profession still in process of evolution" (Brainard, 1919, p. v). Anna Brainard (1919) wrote that although public health nurses worked in both publically and privately funded organizations, "It does not necessarily mean nursing done under the direction of a public department of health; it means nursing done for the health of the public. It does not mean merely bedside care; it means nursing care with an eye to the social as well as the medical aspects of the case" (p. 4). Her definition of a public health nurse included "any graduate nurse who is doing any form of social work in which the health of the public is concerned, and in which her training as a nurse comes into play or is recognized as a valuable part of her equipment" (p. 4).

A public health nurse with a child in Chinatown.

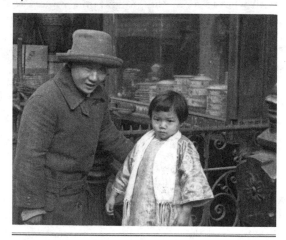

Courtesy of the Visiting Nurse Service of New York.

The idea that public health nurses were found providing bedside care in the home as well as dispensing health information to the public continued to create tension as to the role of the public health nurse. The public health nurse found herself dependent on the resources in the community. The division of the type of care the organization provided continued to be a source of concern for those in public health because it was viewed as necessary for the public health nurse to offer a full range of services to improve the health of the public.

Early Experiments in Public Health Nursing

METROPOLITAN LIFE INSURANCE COMPANY

In 1909, just before the founding of the NOPHN, the Metropolitan Life Insurance Company linked visiting nurses with home care services that were offered to millions of their policyholders. Wald was instrumental in setting the stage for the expanded role of public health nurses. Evidence of the efficacy of their care was collected by nurses through the statistics they kept of their work (Gardner, 1933).

The public, as well as the company, valued the work of the visiting nurses who participated in this program, which lasted from 1909 until 1952. Almost 20 years before this successful experiment was to end, Gardner (1933) wrote, "the tendency of the Company towards an increase in the use of the nurse's time for instructive work in the home is an interesting comment on the value of such work in the actual conservation of life" (p. 24).

The visiting nurse brought health care and healthcare education into the homes of the families she visited. The number of visits to the homes of policyholders throughout the United States rose to 1 billion home visits, making Wald's experiment one of the "first national system[s] of insurance coverage for home-based care" (Buhler-Wilkerson, 1993, p. 1782). The demise of the Metropolitan Visiting Nurse experiment, however, came about because of many factors, one of which Hamilton (1988) related to tension created by two different approaches to care: an economic concern for cost containment, as espoused by the Metropolitan Life Insurance Company, and one embodying the concern to provide nursing services to those in need regardless of the need to contain costs. In addition, by 1952, the decline in policyholders coupled with the increasing cost of nursing service led the company to close this program (Buhler-Wilkerson, 1993). Although historians such as Hamilton, Buhler-Wilkerson, and others critique the experiences of the past from a vantage point of time, Alma Haupt, who was the director of Nursing Bureau of Metropolitan Life Insurance Company from 1935 until it closed in 1952, expressed her more immediate and perhaps personal view of the program, highlighting its success. Haupt (1953) wrote the following:

> "Metropolitan Nursing Service" has provided an example of how a profession and a business organization can work together for a common goal—better health, less sickness and death, and better business. It has shown that maintaining a high standard of nursing service depends on the availability and use of the cooperation, leadership, and standards of a profession. It has shown the advantages of having the prestige, leadership, and financial and organizational backing of the Metropolitan, a company whose contributions have had marked influence on the health of a nation. (p. 84)

AMERICAN RED CROSS TOWN AND COUNTRY NURSING SERVICE

Wald's insight into the needs of populations in both the urban and rural communities led to another important experiment in public health nursing. Buhler-Wilkerson (1993) describes this experiment as the founding of the American Red Cross Town and Country, in 1912. Public health nurses were used to bring public health care to rural communities around the country. The Red Cross organized and standardized the work of these public health nurses to function in the community, providing an expanded role of public health nursing services that included home care and preventive care (Kernodle, 1949). The rural nurses who served in this role needed additional education in public health that would allow them to meet the challenges of this expanded role (Lewenson, 2015).

The American Red Cross Town and Country (whose name changed several times throughout its history) lasted until 1947, when fewer than 100 Red Cross rural public health nursing services remained. The nurses who served in these rural areas provided both the nursing care at home and the health promotion and disease prevention activities that designated the ideal role of the public health nurse (Lewenson, 2017). This dichotomy of the two roles, although combined in most rural settings because of lack of services, was mostly reflected in urban settings where the split between the visiting nurse hired by voluntary agencies and the public health nurse hired in public agencies segmented the care that nursing could have more seamlessly provided (Roberts & Heinrich, 1985). Buhler-Wilkerson (1993) speaks in depth about the repercussions of this public health nursing experiment and the reasons for its demise. Although this discussion is beyond the scope of this chapter, the reader is encouraged to explore the reasons for this change because it relates to the lack of a cohesive plan of care that would translate Wald's vision of public health nursing to the American public. The division between the curative care provided to the sick at home and the activities of health promotion and disease prevention by competing healthcare agencies contributed to the end of this experiment and perhaps contributes to the continued confusion about the role of the public health nurse.

The Evolution Continues: Public Health Nursing in the 1930s

The 1930s saw the economic depression where unemployment in all communities permeated the well-being of those who lived during this period. Between 8,000 and 10,000 nurses were unemployed during this time (Abrams, 2007a). Nurses lost private-duty positions and public health employment and found relatively few hospital jobs available (Ashmun, 1933; Fitzpatrick, 1975b). Public health nurses saw their salaries cut and their jobs lost (Abrams, 2007a). The New Deal, however, brought government-funded healthcare programs to American communities to improve economic conditions, hiring unemployed graduate nurses with or without public health experience in programs such as the Children's Bureau. Both the public health movement and the need for communities to determine their healthcare needs faced the challenging economic downturn of the 1930s. Public health nurses, however, with help from various governmental programs, endured this economic crisis, continuing to find meaning in their work in both the public and private settings.

Toward the end of the depression, in 1938, a revised copy of the *Board Members' Manual for Board and Committee Members of Public Health Nursing Services* was published by the NOPHN. The purpose of such a manual was to offer guidance to the many local community advisory boards, composed of lay and professional people, that formed in communities around the country to provide support "for public health activities of municipal and state governments" (NOPHN, 1938, p. vi). The preface of the manual reminded the reader that "at a time when some despairing folk would turn over all social activities to tax-supported agencies, it is well to remind ourselves that voluntary associations still have essential things to contribute: flexibility and willingness to experiment, standards of efficiency . . . creation of public opinion, discovery of community leaders" (NOPHN, 1938, p. vi). Community boards undertook a variety of public health services in the community, including managing finances, determining public health policies, and deciding on the type of public health nursing programs that were needed in a community, such as "public health nursing associations, American Red Cross chapters, and tuberculosis associations" (NOPHN, 1938, p. ix). The *Board Members' Manual* supported these community advisory boards as both a guide and a reference because they served both public and private organizations engaged in public health activities.

The NOPHN (1938) *Board Members' Manual* also provided a definition of the term public health nursing, stating that public health nursing includes "all nursing services organized by a community or an agency to assist in carrying out any or all phases of the public health program. Services may be rendered on an individual, family, or community basis in home, school, clinic, business establishment, or office of the agency" (NOPHN, 1938, p. 4). The role of the public health nurse by the late 1930s still included both the care of the sick at home and the broader work of community education and health promotion activities. The idea of separating the services of the public health nurse, according to the *Board Members' Manual,* would fly in the face of "efficiency and economy" (NOPHN, 1938, p. 6). The range of functions that the public health nurse was responsible for were maternity health, infant and preschool health, school health, industrial nursing, adult health, communicable diseases, tuberculosis, syphilis and gonorrhea, noncommunicable diseases, orthopedic services, vital statistics, sanitation, mental hygiene, nutrition, reports and records, and medical standing orders (NOPHN, 1938). The care moved from the concern for individuals to concern for the health of the larger community. It was recommended that each community have public health agencies to engage in some, if not all, of the above activities as part of a planned approach to provide a comprehensive public health nursing program in the community.

C. E. A. Winslow (1938a), a professor of public health at the Yale School of Medicine, recognized the need for communities to organize all nursing care in the community to meet the health needs of the public. He spoke about the need for voluntary organizations to continue to be part of communities' planned public health resources. Winslow (1938a) wrote that

good public health nursing by its very nature is a generalized family service and the ideal toward which we are working is that of a single public health nurse in a given area providing both bedside care and health education to the families under her charge. Any administrative plan which tends to separate bedside care from health instruction, or nursing for the poor from nursing for the rich is undesirable. (p. 2)

Winslow saw public health nurses as providing a wide range of nursing services, all for the purpose of fostering health.

The need for more public health nurses in the community required financial support from both the public and the private sectors. Winslow (1938a) saw a need to coordinate all nursing services in the community, including those in the hospital, private duty, and public health:

Under an organized community plan it should be possible to develop effective coordination of all the nursing forces of the community. It is obvious that duplications of work by different agencies should be avoided, unfilled needs discovered and met, and the public informed as

to the role of each agency . . . planning should make possible better service for the home and far more economical use of community resources. The respective fields of the hospital and public health nursing agency could be adequately defined and provision made for continuity of treatment upon discharge from the institution. (p. 4)

Simplistically, the coordination of community nursing services could ultimately enhance the health care of the public and could lead to such innovations as insuring the middle class with home healthcare service benefits, increasing the income of public health nurses, and ultimately supporting a "modern public health program" (Winslow, 1938a, p. 7). The need for public support of nursing education was also considered a part of the plan that Winslow saw as essential to improving and increasing the number of public health nurses.

Through the evolutionary development of community advisory boards and councils as well as the three nursing organizations (NLN, ANA, and NOPHN) and organizing the Joint Committee on Community Nursing Service (in 1934), coordination of public health nursing needs throughout the country was a goal that some believed could be established (Winslow, 1938a, 1938b). Winslow, along with others, looked toward these local and organizational councils to solve the concerns about providing for the health of the public. Winslow (1938a) wrote,

I am convinced that the development of a fully coordinated and truly effective system of community nursing, in home and in hospital, for rich and for poor, including health instruction and bedside care, is one of the most vital social problems of the present day . . . but the community councils of nursing can solve it if they have the courage and vision. (p. 8)

Nurses needed to organize and bring together the various stakeholders, hospitals, community agencies, and private-duty nurses to coordinate and advance the public health nursing services in the community.

Public Health Nursing in the Second Half of the 20th Century

By the middle of the 1900s, the kinds of nursing services that communities would need as public health and public health nursing evolved in response to advances in science, new technologies, and social legislation. The advent of new drugs, such as penicillin in the 1940s, created different challenges for public health nurses. Because people were living longer, nurses working in the community had to address the healthcare issues presented by an increasingly aging population, care for the chronically ill, and respond to cardiac diseases and cancer (Winslow, 1945, p. 989). The dramatic communicable illnesses at the beginning of the 20th century gave way to increased disabilities related to chronic illnesses later on. Even though the cost of care in the home was less than institutional-based care, the institution offered families some support from the daily responsibilities of providing care in the home (Buhler-Wilkerson, 2001).

"She's something special in a very special service." A Visiting Nurse Service of New York flier, 1950.

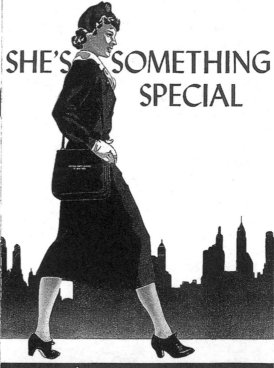

Courtesy of the Visiting Nurse Service of New York.

In the 1950s, the nursing profession underwent a transformation, as many of the earlier nursing organizations reorganized. The NOPHN, for example, was subsumed under the NLN, and public health nursing issues became one of many issues for the larger organization, which, in turn, may or may not have sufficiently addressed the needs of this important evolving nursing role. Nursing organizations sought to break down racial and gender bias in nursing, and the NACGN became extinct as it merged with the ANA in 1952. The profession also sought to move nursing education into institutions of higher learning and to encourage more men and women of diverse backgrounds into the profession (Brown, 1948). Esther Lucille Brown, author of a noted study about nursing, also acknowledged that health care was changing, and the existing barriers between healthcare institutions within the community and hospital were breaking down. Brown (1948) wrote that, "The hospital is moving out into the larger community; the community is moving into the hospital" (p. 30). The public health agencies that up to the 1940s had successfully focused on reducing morbidity and mortality rates were now poised to focus on diseases of middle age. Increasing amounts of federal funding in various statewide public health initiatives addressing the control of "venereal disease, tuberculosis, cancer, mental health, and maternal child health" (Brown, 1948, p. 31) added to a changing public health environment in which public health nurses worked. Nurses needed to meet different challenges that public health nursing afforded.

Home Health Nursing

The social upheaval of the 1960s, challenging women's rights, civil rights, as well as the U.S. military responsibility in Vietnam, also brought with it sweeping social reforms. Medicare legislation in 1965 included a home healthcare benefit to constituents that "increased the reach and visibility of home care and led to its significant growth" (ANA, 2008, p. 2). The 2008 ANA publication regarding the evolution of home health nursing refers the reader back to the founder of the modern nursing movement, Florence Nightingale, and to William Rathborn's district nursing. The evolution of the term home health nursing included similarly expressed ties to the history of public health nursing in the ANA (2007) description of public health nursing. These two terms, home health nursing and public health nursing (and this may be too simplistic), diverged as more people were discharged earlier from hospitals by the 1970s as a result of a Medicare benefit offering home care support. Acute care in the home, offered 24 hours a day, seven days a week, was an outcome of the increased home care benefits reaped by this new social legislation.

By the 1980s, home care services became essential for those people being discharged earlier and earlier from hospitals as a result of the institution of diagnosis-related groups in hospitals across the United States. Home health nursing focused on acute care of individual patients in the home, similar to the focus of early district nurses on care of the sick in the home. Two national nursing organizations formed in the 1980s to address the needs of **home care nurses**, the Visiting Nurse Associations of America and the National Association for Home Care (ANA, 2008).

A public health nurse teaching a baby class, 1942.

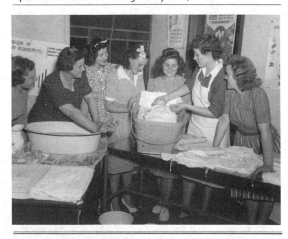

Courtesy of the Visiting Nurse Service of New York.

The ANA published the first standards in home care in 1986, which were subsequently revised in 1992, 1999, and more recently in 2008. Although the definition of home health nursing differs greatly from that of the more recent definition of public health nurse (ANA, 2007), they both share a similar history. However, this history diverged in the 1960s because of the social and political changes in healthcare benefits. The ANA (2008) definition of home health nursing describes it as providing nursing care to the "acutely ill, chronically ill, and well patients of all ages in their residences" (p. 3). The definition goes on to include that the home health nurse focuses on "health promotion and care of the sick while integrating environmental, psychosocial, economic, cultural, and personal health factors affecting an individual's and family's health status" (p. 3). This varies from the ANA (2007) definition of public health nursing, which states that "public health nursing is the practice of promoting and protecting the health of populations using knowledge from nursing, social, and public health science" (p. 5). The ANA (2007) further delineates the practice of public health nursing as "population-focused with the goals of promoting health and preventing disease and disability for all people through the creation of conditions in which people can be healthy" (p. 5). According to the ANA (2008), home health nurses assume a greater responsibility in managing the financial cost of care, and it is this aspect of their role that differentiates this specialty from other nursing specialties (p. 4). Because home health nurses work directly with both public and private payers of care, they must have knowledge of the financial systems that pay for this care to support the individuals and the families within their care. The striking difference between the two nursing specialties seems to be the breadth in which they approach the care as well as the target of their care, and yet there seems to be overlap.

COMMUNITY HEALTH NURSE

A term of more recent origin was coined by the ANA to refer to all nurses who work outside of an

A public health nurse of today.

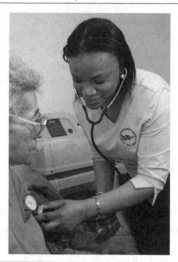

Courtesy of the Visiting Nurse Service of New York.

institutional setting such as the hospital (Clark, 2008). The term **community health nurse** refers to nursing services in the community and encompasses the work of the public health nurse (Jones et al., 1987). In the 1980s, some viewed the terms community health nurse and public health nurse as interchangeable, whereas some interpreted public health nursing to be a specialty encompassed by the term community health nurse (Levin et al., 2007). In 1985, the term community health nurse meant that any nurse who worked in a community setting, whether or not he or she was educationally prepared for public health nursing, was considered a community health nurse (Levin et al., 2007). Public health nurses, however, needed advanced education at the master's or doctoral level that was based on public health science (Levin et al.,2007). A distinction between public health nursing and other community health nurses was made in 1992, calling for public health nurses to be "community-based and population focused" (Williams, as cited by Levin et al., 2007, p. 6). The noted nursing leader of the second half of the 20th century, Virginia Henderson, questioned how one could separate "home care from public health nursing . . . and [was] puzzled at the change that has come about in the public image of the community nurse" (Abrams, 2007b, p. 385).

Public Health Nurses in the 21st Century

The title of public health nurse has been used since Lillian Wald claimed the name for the work of the visiting nurse who provided both sick care in the home and the full range of health promotion and disease-preventing activities in the community in the early part of the 1900s. Wald collected statistical data on the work of the public health nurse of Henry Street, served as an advocate for healthcare policy reforms, refined the work of the public health nurse to include school nursing, and led the many early experiments in public health nursing mentioned in this chapter. As the 20th century progressed and public and private agencies divided the kinds of nursing services provided, the role of the public health nurse was often segmented into either the care of the sick or population-based health-promoting and disease-prevention activities. By the 1970s, and perhaps beginning earlier in the 1960s, community health nursing was the term that was frequently used instead of public health nursing, and in 1973, the ANA published for the first time standards of community health nursing practice (ANA, 2007). In 1986, the ANA defined the community health nursing practice as promoting and preserving the "health of populations by integrating the skills and knowledge relevant to both nursing and public health" (ANA, 2007, p. 56). The glossary of the 1986 document, which was reprinted in the 2007 edition of the *ANA Public Health Nursing: Scope and Standards of Practice*, stated that the terms "public health nursing and community health nursing are synonymous" (ANA, 2007, p. 57).

The ANA (2007) described the distinguishing characteristic of public health nursing as population-focused with "goals of promoting health and preventing disease and disability as well as improving the quality of life" (p. 11). Public health nurses still cared for the sick at home as well as maintained an expanded role in the care of the public's health. Public health nurses were involved in eight content domains, including "informatics, genomics, communication, cultural competence, community-based participatory research, policy and law, global health, and ethics" (ANA, 2007, p. 2). The increasing complexity of the role was noted by the ANA (2007) as a result of societal and political events that signify challenges to the

A public health nurse of today.

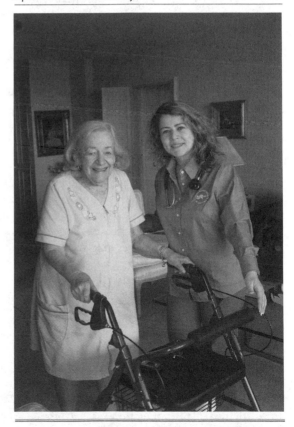

Courtesy of the Visiting Nurse Service of New York.

stability of a community, whether they are local, national, or global. The ANA (2007) identified the threats to the "health of populations as including a reemergence of communicable diseases, increasing incidence of drug-resistant organisms, overall concern about the structure of the healthcare system, environmental hazards, and the challenges imposed by the presence of modern public health epidemics such as obesity- and tobacco-related deaths" (p. 3). Public health nurses are now involved with "syndromic surveillance, mass casualty planning, and the handling of biological and chemical agents" (ANA, 2007, p. 4). Partners in the community now include law enforcement officers, communication experts, postal workers, and others involved in the safety of the community-at-large. According to the ANA (2007), the public health nurse has a greater emphasis on population-based services than ever before. The level of understanding is greater, and the demands for higher education more profound. Evidence-based practice guides public health nurses in their work with populations under duress. The current definition of the public health nurse described by the ANA (2007) has evolved into the following:

> *Public health nursing is the practice of promoting and protecting the health of populations using knowledge from nursing, social, and public health sciences (American Public Health Association, Public Health Nursing Section, 1996). The practice is population-focused with the goals of promoting health and preventing disease and disability for all people through the creation of conditions which people can be healthy. (p. 5)*

This text applies the intervention wheel as a model to guide public health nursing practice. Public health nursing, according to the Minnesota Department of Health (2007), is defined as "the synthesis of the art and science of public health and nursing" (p. 2). This science and art focuses on the development of interventions to the population as opposed to the individual. This population may be defined as a population at risk or that with a common risk

Mothers and a public health nurse with babies.

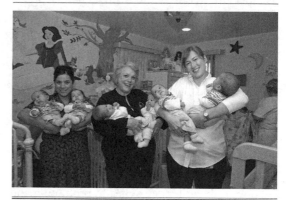

Courtesy of the Visiting Nurse Service of New York.

factor leading to the threat of a particular health issue. It also may be defined as a population of interest known as a healthy population, which may, in fact, improve its health by making certain choices that will further promote health and/or protect against disease or injury—for example, an adolescent population that engages in alternative sports and chooses to wear protective gear avoids serious injury. Although public health nurses' primary focus is working with populations, their work often extends beyond this. Minnesota Department of Health (2001) noted the following:

> *Public health nurses work in schools, homes, clinics, jails, shelters, out of mobile vans and dog sleds. They work with communities, the individuals and families that compose communities, and the systems that impact the health of those communities. Regardless of where public health nurses work or whom they work with, all public health nurses use a core set of interventions to accomplish their goals. (p. 1)*

Public health nursing still maintains the need to provide care to those in the community, and the evolution of the term continues and seems to be the term that now describes the role of those nurses who work within the community.

A public health nurse weighs a baby.

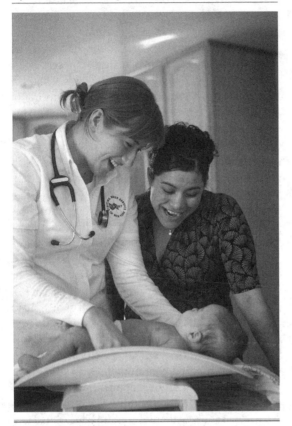

Courtesy of the Visiting Nurse Service of New York.

Education of Public Health Nurses

Although the nomenclature of public health nurses changed over time, the one constant that can be found in the literature is the need for advanced education for those who worked in this specialization. From the inception of public health nursing in the United States, early nursing leaders recognized the need for public health nurses to have more education than the three-year diploma training provided to support the work they did in this specialization. Programs such as the postgraduate course at the Instructive District Nursing

Association of Boston in 1906 and the one started at Teachers College in 1910 were designed to better prepare nurses to take up the work of nursing in the community (Gardner, 1933; Haupt, 1939). By 1915, there were approximately four postgraduate programs in public health, which grew to over 15 in 1922. By 1952, there were over 28 programs set within colleges and universities approved by the NOPHN (NLN, 1952). The various studies that examined nursing in the early 1900s, such as the Goldmark report, examined the kinds of advanced education required of public health nurses above and beyond the training they received in the three-year programs (Crandall, 1922). Later studies, such as Brown's *Nursing for the Future* (1948), recognized that "as collegiate schools of nursing have developed . . . it has come to be believed that preparation designed for beginning positions in public health nursing can and should be built into the basic curriculum" (p. 96). Nurses entering the public health nursing field would be prepared at the baccalaureate level. The American Red Cross Town and Country Nursing Service, required its public health nurses to have additional education as a public health nurse before undertaking such a responsibility (Kernodle, 1949; Lewenson, 2017).

In 1952, a joint committee consisting of the NOPHN and the U.S. Public Health Service studied the curricular needs of the public health nurse. The number of public health nurses had increased to over 24,000 in 1952 from 3,000 in 1912 (Gardner, 1933; NLN, 1952). This increase in numbers constituted a "potent force in translating public health science into service" (NLN, 1952, p. iii). As before, public health nurses were responding to the changing concepts of public health that extended into all facets of life. The joint committee developed a public health nursing curriculum guide that reflected the current thinking of that period, which was that public health was "to provide, through community effort, those services for the saving of life, the prevention of disease, and the restoration to health which the individual or family is unable to provide, or to provide as well, by individual effort" (NLN, 1952, p. iii).

The joint committee noted that the profound changes in the science of medicine, public health, psychology, education, social organization, social sciences, and public health administration called for a new and more comprehensive curriculum guide than had previously existed. Recognizing the need for public health nurses to be responsive to future changes, the curriculum guide was designed to develop the professional skills of the individual to meet the needs for the "immediate future" as well as "be able to adjust to changing situations" (NLN, 1952, p. 2). The joint committee recognized the need for advanced content to be included in its guide; however, they seemed ambivalent about specifying the level in which the public health curriculum would be instituted (NLN, 1952):

> While the Central Committee decided that an adequate basic nursing education in accordance with generally accepted standards would be assumed in the preparation of the Guide, the Committee recognized that this raised certain practical questions. The actual curriculum content that is needed to produce the knowledge and skill required of the public health nurse today or tomorrow is of course conditioned by the students' previous educational and professional background. It has not been found possible nor deemed necessary to specify at each point in the Guide where the learning should take place—in the school of nursing, in the postgraduate program of study, or through a variety of other processes of education and professional experience. (p. 6)

Associate degree programs in nursing that originated in the early 1950s, with the intent of preparing the technical nurse, began to include community and home care in the curriculum in the 1990s (NLN, 1993). In 1993, the NLN published a booklet claiming a vision for nursing education that called for a population-based focus for all nursing programs. All nursing programs accredited by the organization, including baccalaureate, associate, diploma, and practical nursing programs, would

ensure that all nurses "are prepared to function in a community-based, community-focused health care system" (NLN, 1993, p. 3). The idea that all types of entry into practice programs would include community content in their curriculum challenged the idea that this content had usually been reserved for baccalaureate and higher degree programs. Although the level of content may have varied, according to the ANA (2007) the "baccalaureate degree in nursing is the educational credential for entry into public health practice," and the master's level prepares a "nurse specialist level with specific expertise in population-focused care" (p. 10). The ANA (2007), however, acknowledges the roles that the associate degree and diploma graduate registered nurse, as well as the licensed practical nurse, have in a community setting. The graduates of these programs also practice in a community setting "where care is directed toward the health or illness of individuals or families, rather than populations" (ANA, 2007, p. 10).

The ANA (2007) describes the term advanced practice public health nurse as a master's-prepared public health nurse who functions as a clinical nurse specialist or a nurse practitioner using a population-focused care model. Doctoral education also affords additional opportunities for public health nurses to function in roles such as informatics, clinical practice, epidemiology, and education. Here too, the coursework at the doctoral level would have a population focus that translates into the work of the public health nurse.

Conclusion

The history of public health nursing tells the story of an extraordinary group of professionals who, over time, adapted to the healthcare needs of the public. Whether they cared for the sick poor or those who could pay, whether they worked in voluntary visiting nurses' organizations or in municipal health departments, or whether they were educated in postgraduate programs or in baccalaureate degree programs, these nurses provided both curative and preventive services to the population living in the community. Changing names from district nurse to public health nurse to community nurse and back again to public health nurse only typified the efforts of nurses to adjust to changes that social, political, and economic factors required. The ability to continue to work in public health, regardless of the term applied to their work, shows the resiliency of public health nursing. The tradition whereby a need to redefine itself and reflect on the kinds of care they can provide in both the public and private sector continues with us today. As we read further in the book, it is important to remember the origins of the public health nurses' role as the intervention wheel is applied and to consider the many iterations of this role and how nursing continues to evolve, serve its present day populations, and learn from its past.

Additional Resources

American Association for the History of Nursing at: http://www.aahn.org

Barbara Bates Center for the Study of Nursing History at: http://www.nursing.upenn.edu/history/Pages/default.aspx.

Eleanor Crowder Bjoring Center for Nursing Historical Inquiry at: https://www.nursing.virginia.edu/research/cnhi/

Midwest Center for the Study of Nursing History at: http://www.nursing.uic.edu/about-us/midwest-nursing-history-research-center#overview

New York Foundation of Nurses at: http://www.foundationnysnurses.org

---

References

Abrams, S. E. (2007a). For the good of a common discipline. *Public Health Nursing, 24*(3), 293–297.

Abrams, S. E. (2007b). Nursing the community, a look back at the 1984 dialogue between Virginia Henderson and Sherry L. Shamansky. *Public Health Nursing, 24*(4), 382–386.

American Nurses Association (ANA). (2007). *Public health nursing: Scope and standards of practice.* Silver Spring, MD: Author.

American Nurses Association (ANA). (2008). *Home health nursing: Scope and standards of practice.* Silver Spring, MD: Author.

Ashmun, M. (1933). The cause and cure of unemployment in the nursing profession. *The American Journal of Nursing, 33*(7), 652–658.

Beard, J. H. (1922). Progress of public health work. *Scientific Monthly, 14*(2), 140–152.

Brainard, A. M. (1919). *Organization of public health nurses.* New York, NY: Macmillan.

Brown, E. L. (1948). *Nursing for the future: A report prepared for the National Nursing Council.* New York, NY: Russell Sage Foundation.

Bryant, Z. (1968). The public health nurses' expanding responsibilities. In D. M. Stewart & P. A. Vincent (Eds.), *Public health nursing* (pp. 3–9). Dubuque, IA: Wm. C. Brown Company.

Buhler-Wilkerson, K. (1985). Public health nursing: In sickness or in health? *American Journal of Public Health, 75*(10), 1155–1161.

Buhler-Wilkerson, K. (1993). Bringing care to the people: Lillian Wald's legacy to public health nursing. *American Journal of Public Health, 83*(12), 1778–1786.

Buhler-Wilkerson, K. (2001). *No place like home: A history of nursing and home care in the United States.* Baltimore, MD: Johns Hopkins University Press.

Carnegie, M. E. (1991). *The path we tread: Blacks in nursing 1854–1990.* New York, NY: National League for Nursing Press.

Clark, M. J. (2008). *Community health nursing* (5th ed.). Upper Saddle River, NY: Pearson-Prentice Hall.

Crandall, E. P. (1919). Letter dated January 9, 1919, from Ella Crandall, Executive Secretary, National Organization for Public Health Nursing, to Dr. George E. Vincent at the Rockefeller Foundation. Collect RC, Record Group 1.1, Series 200, Box 121, Folder 1494, Rockefeller Archives, Pocantico, NY.

Crandall, E. P. (1922). An historical sketch of public health nursing. *American Journal of Nursing, 22*(8), 641–645.

Craven, D. (1889/1984). *A guide to district nursing.* London, UK: Macmillan and Company. In S. Reverby (Series Ed.), *The history of American nursing, A Garland Series.* New York, NY: Garland Publishing.

Craven, D. (1893/1949). On district nursing. In I. A. Hampton and others, *Nursing of the sick 1893: Papers and discussions from the International Congress of Charities, Correction and Philanthropy, Chicago* (published in 1949 under the sponsorship of the National League of Nursing Education, pp. 127–133). New York, NY: McGraw-Hill.

Dock, L. L., & Stewart, I. M. (1938). *A short history of nursing: From the earliest times to the present day* (4th ed. illustrated). New York, NY: G. P. Putnam's Sons.

Fitzpatrick, M. L. (1975a). *The National Organization for Public Health Nursing, 1912–1952: Development of a practice field.* New York, NY: National League for Nursing Press.

Fitzpatrick, M. L. (1975b). Nurses in American history: Nursing and the Great Depression. *American Journal of Nursing, 75*(12), 2188–2190.

Geis, M. J. (1991). Differences in technology among subspecialties in community health nursing. *Journal of Community Health Nursing, 8*(3), 161–170.

Hamilton, D. (1988). Clinical excellence, but too high a cost: The Metropolitan Life Insurance Company Visiting Nurse Service (1909–1953). *Public Health Nursing, 5*(4), 235–240.

Haupt, A. C. (1939). Thirty years of pioneering: In public health nursing. *American Journal of Nursing, 9*(36), 619–626.

Haupt, A. C. (1953). Forty years of teamwork in public health nursing. *American Journal of Nursing, 53*(1), 81–84.

Hiestand, W. C. (1982). Nursing, the family, and the "new" social history. *Advances in Nursing Science,* April:1–12.

Hughes, A. (1893/1949). The origin and present work of Queen Victoria's Jubilee Institute for Nurses. In I. A. Hampton and others, *Nursing of the sick 1893: Papers and discussions from the International Congress of Charities, Correction and Philanthropy, Chicago* (published in 1949 under the sponsorship of the National League of Nursing Education, pp. 111–119). New York, NY: McGraw-Hill.

Humphrey, C. J., & Milone-Nuzzo, P. (1996). *Orientation to home care nursing.* Gaithersburg, MD: Aspen.

Jones, D. C., Davis, J. A., & Davis, M. C. (1987). *Public health nursing: Education and practice.* Springfield, VA: U.S. Department of Health and Human Services, Public Health Service, Health Resources and Services Administration, Bureau of Health Professions, Division of Nursing.

Kernodle, P. B. (1949). *The Red Cross nurse in action 1882–1948.* New York, NY: Harper and Brothers.

Levin, P., Cary, A., Kulbok, P., Leffers, J., Molle, M., & Polivka, B. (2007). Graduate education for advanced practice public health nursing: At the crossroads. *Association of Community Health Nursing Educators,* 1–24.

Lewenson, S. B. (1993). *Taking charge: Nursing, suffrage, and feminism in America, 1873–1920.* New York, NY: Garland Publishing.

Lewenson, S. B. (2015). Town and Country nursing: Community participation and nurse recruitment. In J. C. Kirchgessner & A. W. Keeling (Eds.), *Nursing rural America: Perspectives from the early 20th century* (pp. 1–19). New York: Springer Publishing Company.

Lewenson, S. B. (2017). Historical exemplars in nursing. In S. B. Lewenson & M. Truglio-Londrigan (Eds.), *Practicing primary health care in nursing: Caring for populations* (pp. 1–17). Sudbury, MA: Jones & Bartlett Learning.

Minnesota Department of Health. (2001). *Public health interventions: Applications for public health nursing practice.* Retrieved from http://www.health.state.mn .us/divs/cfh/ophp/resources/docs/phinterventions _manual2001.pdf

Minnesota Department of Health. (2007). *Cornerstone of public health nursing.* Retrieved from http://www.health.state.mn.us/divs/cfh/ophp/resources/docs/cornerstones_definition_revised2007.pdf

National League for Nursing (NLN). (1952). *Public health nursing curriculum guide.* New York, NY: National League for Nursing Press.

National League for Nursing (NLN). (1993). *Vision for nursing education.* New York, NY: National League for Nursing Press.

National Organization for Public Health Nursing (NOPHN). (1914). Pamphlet attached to a letter sent by Ella Crandall to John D. Rockefeller on October 13, 1914, requesting funding for the organization. Collect RC, Record Group 1.1, Series 200, Box 121, Folder 1498, Rockefeller Archives, Pocantico, NY.

National Organization for Public Health Nursing (NOPHN). (1938). *Board members' manual for board and committee members of public health nursing services* (2nd ed., revised and reset). New York, NY: Macmillan.

Nightingale, F. (1893/1949). Sick nursing and health nursing: Addendum. District nursing. In I. A. Hampton and others, *Nursing of the sick 1893: Papers and discussions from the International Congress of Charities, Correction and Philanthropy, Chicago* (published in 1949 under the sponsorship of the National League of Nursing Education, pp. 24–43). New York, NY: McGraw-Hill.

North, F. N. (1882). A new profession for women. *The Century Magazine, 25*(1), 38–47.

Palmer, S. (1897/1991). Training school alumnae associations. In N. Birnbach & S. B. Lewenson (Eds.), *First words: Selected addresses from the National League for Nursing 1994–1933* (pp. 293–297). New York, NY: National League for Nursing Press.

Roberts, D. E., & Heinrich, J. (1985). Public health nursing comes of age. *American Journal of Public Health, 75*(10), 1162–1172.

Somerville, C. E. M. (1893/1949). District nursing. In I. A. Hampton et al. (Eds.), *Nursing of the sick 1893: Papers and discussions from the International Congress of Charities, Correction and Philanthropy, Chicago* (published in 1949 under the sponsorship of the National League of Nursing Education, pp. 119–127). New York, NY: McGraw-Hill.

Stewart, D. M., & Vincent, P. A. (1968). *Public health nursing.* Dubuque, IA: Wm. C. Brown Company.

Wald, L. D. (1918, June). Best Helps to the Immigrant Through the Nurse (A Phase of District Nursing). Lillian D. Wald Papers, 1889–1957. Writing and Speeches. Reel 25, Box 37, Folder 4, pp. 1–9. New York Public Library, Humanities and Social Sciences Library, Manuscripts and Archives Division, New York, NY.

Welsh, M. S. (1936). What is public health nursing? *American Journal of Nursing, 36*(5), 452–456.

Winslow, C.-E. A. (1938a). Nursing and the community. *Public Health Nursing,* April. Reprint.

Winslow, C.-E. A. (1938b). Organizing for better community services. *American Journal of Nursing, 38*(7), 761–767.

Winslow, C.-E. A. (1945). Postwar trends in public health and nursing. *American Journal of Nursing, 45*(12), 989–992.

For a full suite of assignments and additional learning activities, use the access code located in the front of your book to visit this exclusive website: **http://go.jblearning.com/londrigan**. If you do not have an access code, you can obtain one at the site.

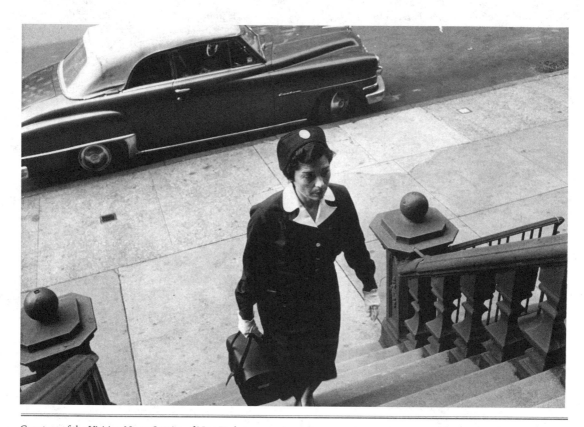

Courtesy of the Visiting Nurse Service of New York.

CHAPTER 3

Assessment: Using the Public Health Nursing Assessment Tool

Marie Truglio-Londrigan
Sandra B. Lewenson

To develop the visiting nurse service adequately, it has been necessary to consider the whole city as a hugh [sic] hospital. The districts become wards, and the staff of nurses in each district must be sufficient to meet its needs. In New York it is estimated that 90% of those who are sick remain in their homes, only 10% of them ever going to a hospital. (Wald, 1918, p. 4)

LEARNING OBJECTIVES

At the completion of this chapter, the reader will be able to:

- Identify the importance of a public health nursing assessment.
- Describe the components of the Public Health Nursing Assessment Tool.
- Apply the Public Health Nursing Assessment Tool.

KEY TERMS

- ❑ Assessment
- ❑ Determinants of health
- ❑ Disparities
- ❑ General health status
- ❑ Health-related quality of life and well-being
- ❑ The Intervention Wheel

Assessment is foundational for decision-making in health care by providing information about the health of the individual, family, community, system, and population. As a core function, assessment is identified as a key element and one of the major core competencies for public health nurses (American Association of Colleges of Nursing, 2013; American Public Health Association, Public Health Nursing Section, 2013; Quad Council Competencies for Public Health Nurses, 2011). Public health nurses recognize that communities in which the individual, family, system, or population reside influence their health and well-being. Likewise, the individual, family, system, and population affect the health of the community and each other. An assessment tool guides the public health nurse through the process of discovery. This chapter presents the Public Health Nursing Assessment Tool (PHNAT), designed by

Lewenson and Truglio-Londrigan, which uses the concepts found in *Healthy People 2020* and **the intervention wheel**. Specifically, the PHNAT uses the four foundation health measures that serve as indicators of progress toward achieving the goals of *Healthy People 2020*. These indicators include **general health status**, **health-related quality of life and well-being**, **determinants of health,** and **disparities** (U.S. Department of Health and Human Services [DHHS], 2010a, para. 4). Using the four foundation health measures helps the public health nurse determine the priority needs of the community and then develop, implement, and evaluate a plan using the intervention wheel strategies as a guide. The PHNAT also asks the public health nurse to reflect on the experience of doing a public health nursing assessment. **Box 3-1** provides an outline of the organization of the PHNAT.

Box 3-1 Public Health Nursing Assessment Tool (PHNAT)

SECTION I: FOUR FOUNDATION HEALTH MEASURES

Part 1: *General Health Status* **(Certain aspects of this portion of the PHNAT may be directed toward the individual/family.)**

A-1 Individual and Family
B-1 Population: Vital Statistics
B-2 Population: Mortality
B-3 Population: Morbidity
B-4 Population: Life Expectancy
 (with international comparisons)

B-5 Population: Healthy Life Expectancy
B-6 Population: Years of Potential Life Lost
 (YPLL) (with international comparisons)
B-7 Population: Physically and Mentally
Unhealthy Days

Part 2: *Health-Related Quality of Life and Well-Being* **(Individual/family assessment)**
A-1 Individual and Family

Part 3: *Determinants of Health*

Part 3-1 Biology and Genetics

A-1 Individual and Family Assessment
B-1 Population Assessment
B-2 Population: Age Distribution

B-3 Population: Race Distribution
B-4 Population: Gender Distribution

Part 3-2 Social Factors/Determinants

A-1 Social Determinants: Housing Conditions
A-2 Social Determinants: Transportation

A-3 Social Determinants: Workplace
A-4 Social Determinants: Recreational Facilities
 Distribution

A-5 Social Determinants: Educational Facilities
A-6 Social Determinants: Places of Worship
in Community
A-7 Social Determinants: Social Services
A-8 Social Determinants: Library Services

A-9 Social Determinants: Law Enforcement
A-10 Social Determinants: Fire Department

A-11 Social Determinants: Communication
A-12 Social Determinants: Employment

A-13 Social Determinants: Leading Industries
A-14 Social Determinants: Educational Level
of People Older Than 25 Years
A-15 Social Determinants: Family Income

Part 3-2: Physical Factors/Determinants

B-1 Physical Determinants: History of the Community
B-2 Physical Determinants: Windshield Survey
B-3 Physical Determinants: The Built Environment
B-4 Physical Determinants: Natural Environment

B-5 Physical Determinants: Physical Barriers/
Boundaries
B-6 Physical Determinants: Environmental/
Sanitation/Toxic Substances

Part 3-3: Health Services

*Types of Services

A-1 Acute Care
A-2 Home Care
A-3 Primary Care
A-4 Long-Term Care
A-5 Rehabilitative
A-6 Assistive Living

A-7 Mental Health Services
A-8 Occupational
A-9 School Health Programs
A-10 Dental
A-11 Palliative

*Access to Care

B-1 Access to Care: Using the Seven A's

Part 3-4: Policymaking

A-1 Local, State, and Federal Organizational
Structure of Community

A-2 Political Issues in the Community
A-3 Health Policies

Part 3-5: Behavior

Individual (choices for healthy living: exercise, stress reduction activities, sleep and rest, healthy diet, etc.)
Population (participation in town weight loss programs or exercise programs)

Part 4: Health Care Disparities Assessment: Frequently takes place after the collection of data, during the analysis located in Part II of this document. The public health nurse, along with partners, may note disparities from their direct observations of the environment as well as noting disparities within data collected in all of the previous sections of this document. For example, five-year cancer survival rate differences between races.

SECTION II: ANALYSIS OF HEALTH STATUS

SECTION III: PRIORITIZE PUBLIC HEALTH ISSUE

SECTION IV: PLAN AND IMPLEMENTATION USING THE INTERVENTION WHEEL

SECTION V: TRACKING AND EVALUATING

SECTION VI: REFLECTION THROUGHOUT ENTIRE PROCESS

Modified from U.S. Department of Health and Human Services. (2010a). *Healthy People 2020 framework*. Retrieved from www.healthypeople.gov/2020/about/default.aspx

Overview of the Unique Qualities of the PHNAT

The PHNAT offers a kaleidoscopic way to view the process of assessment. The authors of this chapter see this kaleidoscopic capability as essential to the public health nurses' broad practice as they work with a wide spectrum of clients. In the public health nurse's practice, clients include individuals, families, communities, systems, and populations. A tool, therefore, that permits the public health nurse to focus on each of these types of clients must be flexible. The PHNAT permits the public health nurse to assess the individual as well as simultaneously assess the family, community, population, and system. This flexibility permits the public health nurse to shift his or her view back and forth depending on the area of focus and the priority needs at that moment in time. The authors developed the PHNAT using the *Process Model for Healthy People 2020: Improving Health of Americans* (Process Model) as a guide. This process model is located on the inside front cover of this book.

The PHNAT guides the user throughout the Mobilize, Assess, Plan, Implement, and Track (MAPIT) process discussed in Chapter 1, including the mobilization of partners who work together toward ensuring the health of the public. These partners participate in the assessment, analysis, planning, implementation, tracking of data, evaluation, and reflection. A visualization of the MAP-IT process is also presented in the process model. Each part of the tool includes space for responses to questions, tables where data can be organized, and definitions for each of the foundational measures. The PHNAT prompts the user to analyze and reference the data collected. As the user becomes more familiar with the PHNAT, additional information and data may be sought, new tables formed, and original ones revised, depending on the needs of the user. For example, if the user wants to compare the findings with national or global data, he or she can do so. An online version of the PHNAT further facilitates the use of this tool and in the management of

information collected. The comprehensiveness of the PHNAT also suggests that the completion of a public health nursing assessment would lend itself to teamwork in a course or in the practice setting.

The Internet provides a wealth of data that can be incorporated into the study. Information such as geography and history of a community, as well as census track data, can also be found on the Internet and facilitates the assessment of the community. Online databases, such as those found in **Box 3-2**, are examples of important resources the public health nurse can use when completing the PHNAT. The data needed for many of the suggested tables on the PHNAT can be found through the Internet and the various databases. The public health nurse should be sure to select reliable and valid sources of information. Sharing information with the team and other community partners is essential throughout the assessment, ultimately collaborating and reaching shared decisions about the needs of the community and the people residing in that community (Truglio-Londrigan, 2017).

The various parts of the PHNAT can be completed in any sequence. This flexibility permits the team to work together in the collection of data simultaneously. Assessment is not a linear process and allows for the public health nurse to complete the process while facilitating expediency, time, and efficiency. Although this assessment tool can be completed alone, the authors encourage the use of

---

Box 3-2   Potential Databases for Data Collection

http://www.census.gov
http://www.fedstats.gov
http://cdc.gov/nchs
http://health.gov/nhic
http://www.cdc.gov/BRFSS/
http://seer.cancer.gov/
http://www.cdc.gov/nchs/ahcd.htm
http://www.cdc.gov/nchs/nhanes.htm
http://www.cdc.gov/aging/agingdata/index.html

a team approach when gathering and interpreting the data (Truglio-Londrigan, 2017).

The PHNAT can be used by public health nurses and students who work in all types of community settings such as home care, visiting nurse service, health departments, neighborhood health centers, schools, and industry. Because the PHNAT encourages mobilization and collaboration within a community, this tool can be shared and used by others in the community. The ethics of public health practice warrant that public health nurses who collect data be mindful and respectful of those they are assessing—for example, students assessing a community must schedule appointments with the various stakeholders rather than showing up unannounced. They also should carry identification and at times may find a letter of introduction from their school beneficial. Carrying out an assessment using the PHNAT lends itself to an ongoing process of discovery and rediscovery.

PHNAT Four Foundational Health Measures

General health status is one of the four foundational health measures. It refers to data that inform the public health nurse and partners in the health initiative about the health of the population and includes information located in Box 3-1 (U.S. DHHS, 2010b). Some of this information is not population-focused, such as self-assessed health status; however, this is an example of how public health nurses serve individuals in the community as well as the general population.

Another foundational health measure is *health-related quality of life*. Health-related quality of life is a complex concept and focuses on "the impact health status has on quality of life" (U.S. DHHS, 2010c). This portion of the PHNAT also focuses on the individual and again sheds light on those public health nurses who do practice on a one-to-one basis with clients in the community. The particular areas included in this portion

of the tool are (1) patient-reported outcomes measurement information system (PROMIS) tools to measure health outcomes from a patient perspective, (2) well-being measures, and (3) participation measures that also reflect an individual's perception of his or her health or ability to participate in and interact with the environment (U.S. DHHS, 2010c).

A major portion of the PHNAT includes the *determinants of health*. In this section, the public health nurse collects information pertaining to those factors that determine the health of the individual, family, and the population living in a community. The health determinants that organize this section include biology and genetics, social factors, health services, policymaking, and individual behavior (U.S. DHHS, 2010d).

Biology and Genetics

The determinant of health under *biology and genetics* may include data that are individual/family focused or population focused. The public health nurse gathers the information on the individual and family with the selected assessment tool his or her particular academic or clinical setting uses. Pertaining to the population, data such as age, race, and gender are important. Box 3-1 offers a comprehensive view of the type of information that needs to be collected. In addition, the databases listed in Box 3-2 help the public health nurse complete this section. Specific questions the public health nurse may use and reflect upon that are representative of the kaleidoscopic view of the PHNAT include:

- Who is the client/family?
- What is the health of the client/family?
- What are the client's/family's health behavior and choices?
- Do these choices support health and a healthy lifestyle?
- What are the resources in the community that facilitate the client/family/populations health?
- Where does the client/family live, work, participate in recreation, and engage in spiritual activities?

- Does the client/family have access to these resources?
- What part of the population does the client/family represent?
- What is the status of health for this population?
- Is this family's particular circumstances reflected in the population as well?

Social Factors

Social factors, the next determinant of health to be considered, include both social and physical determinants or conditions in the environment (U.S. DHHS, 2010e). Social factors that the public health nurse assesses include the client's interactions and connections representing important social supports and networks with family, friends, and organizations in the community. These interactions are important for positive health outcomes in individuals/families and a population. Social support is the type of supportive behavior offered to an individual/family or population by another person, family, or organization. The support may be emotional, instrumental as in services provided, informational such as knowledge, and appraisal such as feedback (House, 1981). Social supports may be offered informally, as in the type of support offered to an individual by a family member or a friend, or they may be more formal, as in the support offered by an agency such as Meals On Wheels. The social assessment section of the PHNAT, as shown in Box 3-1, asks for information about formal and informal support systems in the community. Some of the areas the public health nurse assesses include housing, transportation, work, recreation, education, places of worship, health care, social services, library services, law enforcement, fire protection, and communication services (U.S. DHHS, 2010e). As public health nurses assess these areas, they must pay careful attention to the Seven A's (Krout, 1986; Truglio-Londrigan & Gallagher, 2003; Williams, Ebrite, & Redford, 1991), which are discussed later in this chapter.

The second factor includes physical determinants. The public health nurse must assess the physical environment of the community at large. The physical environmental factor informs the public health nurse about the health of the community and the population that resides in that community. Generally speaking, the physical environment is represented by that which can be seen, touched, heard, smelled, and tasted. However, the physical environment also contains less visible elements such as radon, lead, and ozone. The physical environment can harm individual and community health, especially when individuals and communities are exposed to toxic substances, irritants, infectious agents, and physical hazards in homes, schools, and work sites. The physical environment can also promote good health, for example, by providing clean and safe places for people to work, exercise, and play (U.S. DHHS, 2000, p. 19). The chapter on the environment will provide the reader with a deeper account of the environment and its relationship to health.

In *Healthy People 2020,* a limited definition is offered with an extensive list of physical environment examples that can be used throughout the PHNAT. Collecting assessment data on the physical environment includes what is often referred to as a windshield survey (Gibson & Thatcher, 2016). The windshield survey reflects what one can view from a car window as one drives through a community and contains observations of various components of the community such as housing, open spaces, transportation, race, ethnicity, restaurants, and stores. In urban areas, walking through the community yields similar results. As public health nurses walk or drive through a community, they assess the physical environment using their five senses (Matteson, 1995). Are there trees, flowers, blue sky, trash, cracked asphalt, smokestacks, or garbage? Can birds, dogs, rain, car horns, screams, or traffic be heard? Can nurses smell flowers, grass, gas, or sewage? Finally, what tastes abound? In other words, is the environment clean and safe for the people, or are there hidden dangers such as radon, ozone, carbon monoxide, and lead in their homes? The PHNAT asks the public health nurse to identify the boundaries of the community, the physical characteristics in relation to topography and terrain, the history of the community, sanitation services such as garbage pickup and recycling, and environmental programs that protect air, food, water, and provide animal and vector control. Here the public health nurse can obtain the data by using the Internet and electronic databases, by walking or driving through a community, or by interviewing members of the community.

Health Services

The determinant of health known as health services is more than a listing of the physical, social, and mental health programs offered to individuals/ families or populations in a particular community (see Box 3-1). It also includes an assessment of access to these services. This access to quality care is an important part of the PHNAT. Most community- or population-based assessment tools request an assessment of health service organizations; however, the inclusion of access to care using the Seven A's is unique to the PHNAT. The Seven A's address more than the single concept of access. Whether or not there is access frequently depends on the additional factors of awareness, availability, affordability, acceptability, appropriateness, and adequacy of the service. It is essential for the public health nurse to assess and analyze each of these for whether individuals or populations can gain access to essential services that influence their health and well-being (Krout, 1986; Truglio-Londrigan & Gallagher, 2003; Williams et al., 1991).

The following Seven A's questions can assist the public health nurse in analyzing his or her findings:

- Is the population *aware* of its needs and the services in the community to meet these needs?
- Can the population gain *access* to the services that it needs?
- Is the service *available* and convenient to the population in terms of time, location, and place for use?
- How *affordable* is the service for the population in question?

- Is the service *acceptable* to the population in terms of choice, satisfaction, and cultural congruence?
- How *appropriate* is the service for the specific population, or is there a fit?
- Is the service *adequate* in terms of quantity or degree?

Policymaking

The public health nurse must also assess the laws and policies that influence the health of the individual, family, community, system, and population under study. Examples include laws and policies on seat belt use, helmet use, phone use and texting while driving, smoking, and child car seats. Each of these has had a positive influence on the health and well-being of individuals and the population at large, resulting in a decrease in deaths, disabilities, and injuries. The public health nurse must be knowledgeable about how his or her community functions with regard to the political infrastructure, and as such must assess this infrastructure to be familiar with how it works: Who are the formal and informal political leaders? How can they be reached? What initiatives have they supported in the past? What are the laws that affect the individual/family, population, and community with regard to the public's health? Are these laws upheld? Are there issues that have not been addressed. If so— what can be done to address these issues? The data collected in this section include the organizational structure of the community, a description of the political issues in the community, and an identification of some of the public health laws that affect the community and its members' health. As the public health nurse conducts this portion of the assessment, it is important to be attentive to the news media reports, meet with the local government officials, and locate the school boards or any of the governing bodies in the community. Meet the candidates if it is an election year, and listen to what the community is saying. Check websites, social networking sites, and local blogs. Using the Internet, here and throughout the PHNAT, assists the public health nurse in obtaining the necessary data and learning about the community.

Behavior (Individual and Population)

The data to be collected in this section of the PHNAT are the behaviors of individuals and families; however, population behavior may also be observed. The type of behavior an individual or population engages in reflects choices that ultimately affects health. An individual who smokes cigarettes may have a different set of health outcomes compared with an individual who does not engage in the behavior of smoking. In recent years, there have also been examples of population-based behavior; for example, towns have gathered and participated in a collective great smoke-out or weight loss program, and towns have engaged in referendums that allocate funding for building walking paths to facilitate physical activity safely. The American Nurses Association organized a 2017 Year of the Healthy Nurse resolution designed to engage nurses to improve population health through role modeling and health behavior changes (American Nurses Association, 2017). The public health nurse collects data on the individual and family that reflect their behavior and again turns the kaleidoscope to look outward to the community and population within that community. Some of the questions that provide insight into individual or population-based behavior are as follows:

- What does the assessment of the individual tell about his or her behavior?
- What types of choices does he or she make with regard to diet, physical activity, alcohol, cigarette smoking, other drug use, and so forth?
- How does the family support health choices?
- How does the community support health choices?
- Have there been community-driven health promotion initiatives, like weight loss or physical activity programs such as a walk-to-school program?

Disparity is the fourth and final foundational health measure and has been an area of focus and goal of the Healthy People initiative. According to *Healthy People 2020,* "If a health outcome is seen in a greater or lesser extent between populations, there is disparity. Race or ethnicity, sex, sexual identity, age, disability, socioeconomic status, and geographic location all contribute to an individual's ability to achieve good health" (U.S. DHHS, 2010f, para. 1). Thus, disparities are the result of the complex relationship that exists between and among all of the foundational health measures along with the presence of "discrimination, racism, literacy level, and legislative policies" (U.S. DHHS, 2010f, para. 7). Frequently, the public health nurse will note disparities as he or she makes observations within the community and analyzes the data that are being gathered. Hence, for this foundational health measure, much of the information needed is gathered throughout the PHNAT.

Analysis of Health

The public health nurse, along with other partnering members of a health initiative including the people living in the community, analyzes the information gathered during the assessment process. Many times the public health nurse will examine past data to see whether trends and patterns have emerged over time. This process of analysis takes time and reflection. The key here is that the public health nurse does not do this alone but takes part in a partnership. This process identifies issues in a community and sets priorities.

Prioritize Public Health Issues

Once the public health nurse and partners conduct the assessment, an analysis of the data elucidates which priority public health issues exist in the community. In determining the priority health issues, the public health nurse, using a population-based focus, collaborates with other public health practitioners, key informants in the community, and any organization or agency that may have a voice with regard to the population and public health issue. In population-based care, partnerships form the necessary bonds to make sustainable changes necessary for health in the particular targeted population. Those involved in the partnership work together to form a common understanding of the issue. All involved, including the population of interest residing in the community, agree on the priority issue identified; this is essential for a positive outcome. Once the priority is noted, the partners confer with the *Healthy People 2020* topic areas and corresponding objectives for guidance in creating and implementing a plan to address the issue (U.S. DHHS, 2010g).

Plan and Implementation: Applying the Intervention Wheel

In this section of the PHNAT, the public health nurse, along with any members of the partnership, develops a plan of action using the intervention wheel strategies. Again, working with members of the partnering organizations as well as other stakeholders is critical because partnering is more likely to ensure a plan that is congruent with cultural ideas, values, and beliefs. It is also important to engage in reviews to determine a plan that is based on best practice. The PHNAT involves the application of the intervention wheel, which identifies 17 nursing interventions applied to three levels of practice: individual/family, community, and system. The intervention wheel began in the mid-1990s as part of a "grounded theory process carried out by public health nurse (PHN) consultants at the Minnesota Department of Health" (Keller & Strohschein, 2016, p. 192). Questioning the contribution public health nurses made in population-based care, the consultants held a series of workshops that informed them of the work of public health nurses. Using a systematic, evidenced-based review of the literature, they analyzed the input of public health nurses who worked in a variety of community settings. This enabled the consultants to construct the wheel graph depicting the 17 intervention strategies applied to the three levels of practice (Keller & Strohschein, 2016). The intervention strategies visually depicted and color coded on the wheel are case finding, surveillance, disease and health event investigation, outreach, screening, referral and follow-up, case management, delegated functions, health

teaching, counseling, consultation, collaboration, coalition building, community organizing, advocacy, social marketing, and policy development and enforcement. The intervention wheel provides a language that can be commonly used by public health nurses across the various practice settings (Keller & Strohschein, 2016).

For the purposes of this book, these intervention strategies have been separated out into five themes addressed in specific intervention chapters:

- *Hitting the pavement* includes the strategies of case finding, surveillance, disease and health event investigation, outreach, and screening.
- *Running the show* includes the strategies of referral and follow-up, case management, and delegated functions.
- *Working it out* includes the strategies of health teaching, counseling, and consultation.
- *Working together* includes the interventions of collaboration, coalition building, and community organizing.
- *Getting the word out* includes the interventions of advocacy, social marketing, and policy development and enforcement.

These intervention chapters focus on each of the themes noted above by using case study examples from public health nurses who use the intervention wheel strategies to address public health problems experienced by individuals, families, and populations within their communities. The reader can refer to these chapters when using the PHNAT.

Overall, when selecting the intervention strategy and developing a plan of action, the public health nurse works in concert with others in the community and considers the following:

- The population to be targeted
- Short-term and long-term goal(s)
- Community resources including human, financial, time, technology, and educational resources
- Evidence that supports the intervention for the population
- Evidence that the strategy is culturally appropriate
- Evidence that the Seven A's are accounted for

- Best way to implement the strategy
- How to evaluate whether or not the outcomes are met
- How to communicate between and among all of the participants.

Tracking and Evaluation

Tracking and evaluation are critical to the entire process model outlined on the inside front cover of this book. While the partnership is determining what the plan will be and how the plan will be implemented, it is also important for the partners to determine what type of information will be collected, where it will be collected, who will collect it, where it will be stored, what kind of technology will be used, how it will be collected, and what type of resources will be needed. This is important for tracking so that the public health nurse and partners may determine if progress is being made in meeting objectives. If it is determined that there is progress, the public health nurse and partners will need to decide if the same plan and course of action will be sustained. If there are questions about the progress, changes may need to be initiated. Tracking of information and evaluation is fed back to all levels of the process model. Over time, analysis of the data may inform the public health nurse and the members of the partnership that the vision or the goals may need to change or the partners may determine that the plan is not based in evidence, the plan is not culturally congruent, or one or more of the Seven A's are not met, and that may be the reasons for the weak outcomes. The tracking and the evaluation of data are important and inform every part of the process model. In 2010, the Institute of Medicine (IOM) published a report, *For the Public's Health: The Role of Measurement in Action and Accountability,* which speaks to some of the issues related to tracking and evaluation. Some of the interesting and complex questions raised include: How do we measure our progress as a nation in our movement toward a healthier America? What measurement approaches can we implement that will help us evaluate and critique agencies'/partnership's health initiatives with regard to population-based health outcomes? What are the best ways to gather and analyze data with a focus on all of the foundational health measures? Ultimately, the entire process concludes with the development of possible laws and policies, when appropriate, to assure and ensure the ongoing implementation and funding of the strategies to sustain health outcomes. So much time, energy, and resources are spent in partnership development, assessment, prioritizing of issues, planning, and in the implementation of health initiatives. Tracking and evaluation are critical to all of these processes in that they bring us back to the three core functions of public health: assessment, policy development, and assurance.

Reflection

Reflection occurs throughout the PHNAT and reminds the public health nurse to be reflective in his or her practice. Self-reflection aids in the decision-making process (Truglio-Londrigan & Lewenson, 2015) and causes the public health nurse to be vigilant during the assessment process and in the implementation of any plans. Too often both students and public health nurses carry out this all-important work by rote for the expressed purpose of completing the task and filling in the blanks without conscious thought and questioning. To address the practice of roteness, the authors of the PHNAT sought to identify a way to teach public health nurses and students to be more conscious of providing meaningful care in the communities in which they serve. Integration of reflection throughout the PHNAT enables the public health nurse to work in partnership within the community rather than just an exercise in data collection. Using reflection provides a way for the public health nurse to channel their curiosity to mine the data for nuances, meanings, and, hopefully, shared decisions. It is important for the public health nurse to strive to come to know the community in a meaningful reflective way. Furthermore, reflective practice provides the context for collaborative partnerships where shared decision-making takes place. The following case study provides an example of why reflective practice is important.

	Reflective Practice
CASE STUDY	Marty Hucks, MN, APRN-BC, CNE; Tracy P. George, DNP, APRN-BC, CNE
	Francis Marion University

A.W. was a 23-year-old well-groomed, attractive female who presented to the rural public health clinic with painful sores on her vulva. A nurse practitioner student was working with me in a clinical rotation. The student began by obtaining the patient's history, while I answered a few phone calls. The student came to me in a few minutes, and he told me he was surprised by the patient's history. The patient admitted to past heroin use, sex with 50+ males and females in the past years, and currently was on house arrest. The student did not think that someone who looked "normal" would use IV drugs and engage in high-risk sexual behaviors.

I then completed the exam with the student. There were several painful ulcerated lesions on the vulva. The patient was tested for hepatitis C, HIV, syphilis, genital herpes, gonorrhea, and chlamydia. She had never had a Pap smear, so that test was also obtained. No rashes were noted on her body. This patient voiced interest in a contraceptive implant, which lasts for three years. She wanted to learn more about it and then make a decision.

Because of the painful lesions, the patient was treated presumptively at the clinic for herpes while awaiting all test results. We educated the patient on the implant and scheduled a follow-up visit in a week. The syphilis results came back positive with a 1:256 RPR titer and a positive confirmatory test. Usually, syphilis chancres are nonpainful, so her lesions were not typical. All the other tests were negative, so she received treatment for primary syphilis with penicillin G benzathine intramuscularly. She was counseled on safer sexual practices and the use of condoms. Partner notification and treatment was also completed. The patient also received the contraceptive implant at the office visit because of her interest in a long-acting contraceptive method.

Through this experience and working with the student to understand that one cannot rely on one's assumptions about patient's sexual practices or drug/alcohol use based on appearances. Syphilis is on the rise in the United States, and some of the rural counties in the South have very high rates of syphilis. Syphilis is an important disease to consider when caring for patients. The student also realized that they needed to continually reflect upon what they are seeing, hearing, and feeling during the assessment process and ask themselves questions about how their own worldview affected their perceptions. In other words, it is important to make decisions based upon evidence, not based upon assumptions. This also holds true when one engages in the assessment process of families as well as communities and populations.

Questions that the public health nurse may ask which facilitate reflection include: What am I observing? What am I hearing? Am I seeing and hearing all that needs to be seen and heard? What am I missing? What feelings am I experiencing during this assessment process? Are these feelings facilitating this assessment or creating a barrier to the assessment? Are these feelings hindering the development of the partnership and the development of trust? Am I engaging in activities that help in mobilizing the community of interest?

The table in the reflection section of the PHNAT asks the public health nurse to keep a record of the experience. The public health nurse can use this table to record when he or she worked on the assessment and how he or she responded to the various parts of the assessment, reflect on the group experience if the assessment was conducted in a group, or record any personal or professional reflection observed during the assessment process.

Conclusion

This chapter explains how to conduct a public health nursing assessment using the author-designed PHNAT. The unique qualities of the PHNAT include the use of the U.S. DHHS (2010a–g) foundational health measures, including general health status, health-related quality of life and well-being, determinants of health, and disparities; application of the intervention wheel strategies; and self-reflection. The application of the PHNAT provides the public health nurse with the information that needs to be analyzed and ultimately determines the priority healthcare issues for a specific population within a community. To carry out the assessment, the public health nurse uses a variety of methods to obtain the data, including observation, interviews, Internet research, census tracks, government reports, newspaper accounts, reflection, research, history, and evidence of best practice. The public health nurse collaborates with other public health practitioners, key informants in the community, and other agencies to determine the priority. Once this priority is identified, the public health nurse works with partners toward the development and implementation of a culturally congruent initiative based in evidence. The tracking and evaluation of the implemented plan is important as is the reflective piece by the public health nurse. The outcomes identified during the evaluation provide rich feedback that may potentially lead to the subsequent development of laws and policies that sustain positive health outcomes.

Additional Resources

Alliance of Nurses for Healthy Environments at: http://envirn.org/pg/pages/view/4103/assessment-tools

Centers for Disease Control and Prevention-Healthy Places at: http://www.cdc.gov/healthyplaces/hia.htm

Healthy People Database at: https://www.healthypeople.gov/2020/data-source/healthy-people-2020-database

Minnesota Department of Health Characteristics of Needs Assessment Tools at: http://www.health.state.mn.us/communityeng/needs/character.html

Center for Disease Control and Prevention-National Vital Statistics System at: http://www.cdc.gov/nchs/nvss/

University of Minnesota Data Sources at: https://hsl.lib.umn.edu/biomed/help/health-statistics-and-data-sources

---

References

American Association of Colleges of Nursing. (2013). *Public health: Recommended baccalaureate competencies and curricular guidelines.* Washington, DC: Author.

American Nurses Association (ANA). (2017). *The Year of the Healthy Nurse.* Washington, DC: Author. Retrieved from http://nursingworld.org/MainMenu Categories/ThePracticeofProfessionalNursing/2017 -Year-of-Healthy-Nurse

American Public Health Association, Public Health Nursing Section. (2013). *The definition and practice of public health nursing: A statement of the public health nursing section.* Washington, DC. Author.

Gibson, M. E., & Thatcher, E. J. (2016). Community as client: Assessment and analysis. In M. Stanhope & J. Lancaster (Eds.), *Public health nursing: Population-centered health care in the community* (9th ed., pp. 396–421). St. Louis, MO: Mosby Elsevier.

House, J. S. (1981). *Work stress and social support.* Reading, MA: Addison-Wesley.

Institute of Medicine (IOM). (2010). *For the public's health: The role of measurement in action and accountability.* Washington, DC: National Academies Press.

Keller, L. O., & Strohschein, S. (2016). Population-based public health nursing practice: The intervention wheel. In M. Stanhope & J. Lancaster (Eds.), *Public health nursing: Population-centered health care in the community* (9th ed., pp. 190–216). St. Louis, MO: Mosby Elsevier.

Krout, J. A. (1986). *The aged in rural America.* Westport, CT: Greenwood.

Matteson, P. S. (1995). *Teaching nursing in the neighborhoods: The Northeastern University Model.* New York, NY: Springer.

Quad Council Coalition. (2011). *Quad council competencies for public health nurses.* Retrieved from http://www.quadcouncilphn.org/documents-3/competencies/

Truglio-Londrigan, M., & Gallagher, L. (2003). Using the Seven A's to determine older adults' community resource needs. *Home Healthcare Nurse, 21*(12), 827–831.

Truglio-Londrigan, M., & Lewenson, S. B. (2015). Know yourself: Reflective decisionmaking. In S. B. Lewenson & M. Truglio-Londrigan (Eds.), *Decision-making in nursing: Thoughtful approaches to leadership* (2nd ed. pp. 1–12). Burlington, MA: Jones & Bartlett Learning.

Truglio-Londrigan, M. (2017). Coalitions, partnerships, and shared decision-making: A primary healthcare perspective. In S. B. Lewenson & M. Truglio-Londrigan (Eds.), *Practicing primary health care in nursing: Caring for populations* (pp. 89–108). Burlington, MA: Jones & Bartlett Learning.

U.S. Department of Health and Human Services. (2000). *Healthy people 2010* (Vol. 1). Washington, DC: U.S. Government Printing Office.

U.S. Department of Health and Human Services. (2010a). *About healthy people.* Retrieved from http://www.healthypeople.gov/2020/about/default.aspx

U.S. Department of Health and Human Services. (2010b). *General health status.* Retrieved from http://www.healthypeople.gov/2020/about/GenHealthAbout.aspx

U.S. Department of Health and Human Services. (2010c). *Health-related quality of life.* Retrieved from http://www.healthypeople.gov/2020/about/QoLWBabout.aspx

U.S. Department of Health and Human Services. (2010d). *Determinants of health.* Retrieved from http://www.healthypeople.gov/2020/about/DOHAbout.aspx

U.S. Department of Health and Human Services. (2010e). *Determinants of health social factors.* Retrieved from http://www.healthypeople.gov/2020/about/DOHAbout.aspx#socialfactors

U.S. Department of Health and Human Services. (2010f). *Disparities.* Retrieved from http://www.healthypeople.gov/2020/about/DisparitiesAbout.aspx.

U.S. Department of Health and Human Services. (2010g). *Topics and objectives.* Retrieved from http://www.healthypeople.gov/2020/topicsobjectives2020/default.aspx

Wald, L. D. (1918). Visiting Nurse, Lillian D. Wald Papers, 1889-1957. Writing and Speeches. Nurses & Nursing II, Reel 25, Box 37, Folder 4, pp. 1. New York Public Library, Humanities and Social Sciences Library, Manuscripts and Archives Division, New York, NY.

Williams, M., Ebrite, F., & Redford, L. (1991). *In-home services for elders in rural America.* Kansas City, MO: National Resource Center for Rural Elderly.

For a full suite of assignments and additional learning activities, use the access code located in the front of your book to visit this exclusive website: http://go.jblearning.com/londrigan. If you do not have an access code, you can obtain one at the site.

Public Health Nursing Assessment Tool

Designed by Sandra B. Lewenson and Marie Truglio-Londrigan

Suggestions for Table Use:

1. Use all horizontal and vertical columns to guide you in your assessment.
2. Fill in the vertical column for each table that requests information on the Seven A's. When filling in these boxes, place the most pertinent information that you think informs the assessment.
3. When completing Section I *Part 3-3(B-1)*: Access to Care. Note that this is a summary of the work that you did in Part 1. Reflect on this information, and arrive at your decisions pertaining to access to care.
4. In some instances, you need to consider collecting data on multiple years to identify trends. You can duplicate these tables and use them to collect the data on different years using census data.
5. Remember this is a working document that you, the public health nurse, can adjust and revise to meet the needs of the community you are assessing. The collection of data is more than filling in the boxes. You may need to collect additional data in a particular area, depending on what you learn as you go. For example, you may fill in the boxes about the number of schools in a community, but you may also want to know the number of students per faculty member, if a community collaborator cited that as a concern.
6. In some instances, there will be overlap of data collection. Because information for this tool will usually be collected by a group, in qualitative research the overlap may be considered a saturation of data. In the analysis section, these data will provide a variety of perspectives.

Section I: Four Foundational Health Measures

Part 1: General Health Status

Refers to information that will inform the public health nurse and partners in the health initiative about the health of the population. Some of this information is not population focused such as self-assessed health status; however, this is an example of how public health nurses serve individuals in the community as well as the general population.

A-1 Individual and Family

When appropriate, the public health nurse will include self-assessed health status as well as history, physical, genogram, ecogram, and any other tools used by his or her organization. Summarize your finding in a narrative form below.

Source of Evidence: _____

B-1 Population: Vital Statistics

	Census Tract	Community	County	State
Live births				
General deaths				

Source of Evidence: _____

B-2 Population: Mortality

Census Tract	Community	County	State

Source of Evidence: _____

B-3 Population: Morbidity

Census Tract	Community	County	State

Source of Evidence: _____

B-4 Population: Life Expectancy

Census Tract	Community	County	State	National/International

Source of Evidence: _____

B-5 Population: Healthy Life Expectancy

Census Tract	Community	County	State	National/International

Source of Evidence: _____

B-6 Population: Years of Potential Life Lost (YPLL)

Census Tract	Community	County	State	National/ International

Source of Evidence: _____

B-7 Population: Physically and Mentally Unhealthy Days

Census Tract	Community	County	State	National/ International

Source of Evidence: _____

Part 2: Health-Related Quality of Life and Well-Being (Individual/family assessment)

Health-related quality of life is a complex concept and focuses on the effect of health status on quality of life. This portion of the PHNAT also focuses on the individual and again sheds light on those public health nurses who do practice on a one-to-one basis with clients in the community.

A-1 Individual and Family*—Includes review of the following:

- Patient-Reported Outcomes Measurement Information System (PROMIS) (www.nihpromis.org /default.aspx) tools to measure health outcomes from a patient perspective.
- Well-being measures.
- Participation measures (activities of daily living, instrumental activities of daily living).

*There is no B in Section I Part 2.

Part 3: Determinants of Health
Part 3-1

Biology and Genetics

The determinants of health under biology and genetics include data that are individual/family focused or population focused. The public health nurse gathers the information on the individual and family as a client using whatever health assessment tool he or she uses in the particular academic or clinical setting. Pertaining to the population aggregate, data such as age, race, and gender would be considered important to gather.

A-1 Individual and Family Assessment

In this section, when appropriate, the public health nurse includes an assessment of the individual and family. Include the history, genogram, and ecogram. Special consideration is given to analysis of genetically defined diseases such as sickle cell anemia, cystic fibrosis, and BRCA1 or BRCA2.

B-1 Population Assessment

	Census Tract	Community	County	State
Population at last census				
Population density				
Population changes in the last 10 years				

Source of Evidence: _____

B-2 Population: Age

	Census Tract	Community	County	State
0–4				
5–9				
10–14				
15–19				
20–24				
25–29				
➤ 85				

Source of Evidence: _____

B-3 Population: Race

	Census Tract	Community	County	State
White				
Black/African American				
Hispanic				
Asian				
Native American				
Other				

Source of Evidence: _____

B-4 Population: Gender

	Census Tract	Community	County	State
Female				
Male				

Source of Evidence: _____

Part 3-2

Social Factors

Social factors, the next determinant of health to be considered, include social determinants of health and physical determinants or conditions in the environment. Social factors that the public health nurse assesses include the client's interactions and connections with family, friends, and others in their community. The second part includes physical determinants. The public health nurse must assess the physical environment of the community at large.

Social Determinants

A-1 Housing Conditions

Housing Characteristics		Total # of Units		Owner Occupied		Renter Occupied		Vacant	Housing Subsidies/ Homeless Provisions

Source of Evidence: _____

A-2 Transportation

	Description of Services: Cost, Destination of Service, Quality of Service, Condition of Services and/or Roads, Handicap Accessibility	Data Collection on Seven A's that Will Assist with Determining Adequacy or Inadequacy
Train		
Bus		
Taxi including private services		
Major roads		
Minor roads		
Volunteers providing transportation		
School buses		

Source of Evidence: _____

A-3 Workplace

List Places of Employment	Description of Workplace Professional, Industry, Factories, Schools, Town, City, County, Businesses	What Workplace Safety Measures Are in Place?	What Is the Estimated Yearly Salary Range of Employees?

Additional Questions to Ask:
- Do most people who reside in the community work in the community, or do they commute?
- If they commute, what is their mode of transportation?
- What is the cost of that commute?
- What is the time of the commute?
- Does this commute impact quality of life?

Source of Evidence: _____

A-4 Recreational Facilities

Recreational Facilities	Area Served/Services Provided, Cost, Population Served, Hours, Maintenance of Recreation Facilities (e.g., Parks, Playgrounds, Athletic Fields)	Data Collection on Seven A's that Will Assist with Determining Adequacy or Inadequacy

Source of Evidence: _____

A-5 Educational Facilities

	# of Public	# of Private (religious)	# of Private (secular)
Preschool			
Elementary			
Junior high			
Senior high			
Colleges/universities			
Early-morning programs			
Recreational programs within school system			
After-school programs			

Source of Evidence: _____

A-6 Places of Worship

Name/Address/Phone	Denomination	Services

Source of Evidence: _____

A-7 Social Services

Agency Name/Address/Phone (Food and Clothing Banks, Homeless Shelters, Adult Day Care Social Services, Child Care)	Area Served/Services Provided/Cost of Services	Data Collection on Seven A's that Will Assist with Determining Adequacy or Inadequacy

Source of Evidence: _____

A-8 Library Services

Libraries Name/Address/Phone	Area Served/Services Provided	Data Collection on Seven A's that Will Assist with Determining Adequacy or Inadequacy

Source of Evidence: _____

A-9 Law Enforcement

Law Enforcement Services	Area Served/Services Provided, Size, Equipment, Response Time, Types of Calls over Past 6 Months, Neighborhood Programs	Data Collection on Seven A's that Will Assist with Determining Adequacy or Inadequacy
Police force		
Special services (SWAT, bomb squads, emergency response teams)		
Animal enforcement		
Senior watch patrols		
Private security		
Neighborhood watches		
Vigilante groups		

Source of Evidence: _____

A-10 Fire Department

Fire Department Stations	Area Served/Services Provided, Number of Companies, Equipment, Response Time, Types of Calls over Past 6 Months, Community Programs	Data Collection on Seven A's that Will Assist with Determining Adequacy or Inadequacy
Fire fighters in company		
Special fire forces (emergency response teams)		

Source of Evidence: _____

A-11 Communication

	Description of Services (Include Whether It Is Community-based, State, or National)	Data Collection on Seven A's that Will Assist with Determining Adequacy or Inadequacy
Television (e.g., educational, relaxation, emergency response)		
Radio (e.g., educational, relaxation, emergency response)		
Newsprint (e.g., educational, relaxation, emergency response)		
Internet/social networking/text messaging (e.g., educational, relaxation, emergency response)		
Newsletters		
Bulletin boards		
Telephone chains		

Source of Evidence: _____

A-12 Employment Distribution

		# in Census Tract		# in Community		# in County		# in State
Employed persons								
Unemployed persons								

Source of Evidence: _____

A-13 Leading Industries in Community (name at least two)

Name	Address	Type	# of Employed

Source of Evidence: _____

A-14 Level of Education

	Census Tract	Community	County	State
Ninth grade and lower				
High school graduate				
Some college				
College graduate (associate's and baccalaureate)				
Median # of years of school completed				

Source of Evidence: _____

A-15 Family Income

	Census Tract	Community	County	State
$0–4,999				
$5,000–$9,999				
$10,000–$14,999				
$15,000–$24,999				
$25,000–$34,999				
$35,000–$49,999				
$50,000–$64,999				
$65,000–$79,999				
$80,000 or more				
	100%	100%	100%	100%

Source of Evidence: _____

Physical Determinants

B-1 History of the Community

Write a narrative including information about the history of the community you are assessing. Include data that describe who started the community, any interesting stories that define the community.

Source of Evidence: _____

B-2 Windshield Survey

The windshield survey reflects what the public health nurse can view from a car window while driving through a community and contains observations of various components in the community such as housing, open spaces, transportation, race, ethnicity, restaurants, and stores.

Source of Evidence: _____

B-3 The Built Environment

The built environment describes the human-made structures in the community including the kinds of stores, buildings, and sidewalks that facilitate healthy behaviors (or not). Describe your observations about this built environment and how it may be a determinant of health.

Source of Evidence: _____

B-4 Natural Environment

Write a narrative that includes data on factors such as topography, climate, terrain, topographical features, and other factors in the community.

Source of Evidence: _____

B-5 Physical Barriers/Boundaries

Write a narrative that includes data such as geographical boundaries and human-made boundaries.

Source of Evidence: _____

B-6 Environmental/Sanitation/Toxic Substances

	Description of Services (Include Whether It Is Community based, State, or National)	Data Collection on Seven A's that Will Assist with Determining Adequacy or Inadequacy
Water supply		
Sewerage supply		
Solid waste disposal		
Provisions or laws for recycling		
Air contaminants		
Vector control programs for deer, ticks, rabid animals, rodents		
Other		

Source of Evidence: _____

Part 3-3

Health Services

The determinant of health known as health services is more than a listing of the physical, social, and mental health programs offered to an individual/family or a population in a particular community. It also includes an assessment of access to these services and uses the Seven A's. The Seven A's address more than the single concept of access. Whether or not there is access frequently depends on additional concepts of awareness, availability, affordability, acceptability, appropriateness, and adequacy of the service. Each of these is essential to assess and analyze for whether individuals or populations can access essential services that can influence their health and well-being.

Source of Evidence: _____

Types of Services

A-1 Acute Care

Agency Name/Address/ Phone	Area Served/Services Provided, Cost, Hours, Population Served	Data Collection on Seven A's that Will Assist with Determining Adequacy or Inadequacy

Source of Evidence: _____

A-2 Home Care

Agency Name/Address/ Phone	Area Served/Services Provided, Cost, Hours, Population Served	Data Collection on Seven A's that Will Assist with Determining Adequacy or Inadequacy

Source of Evidence: _____

A-3 Primary Care

Agency Name/Address/ Phone	Area Served/Services Provided, Cost, Hours, Population Served	Data Collection on Seven A's that Will Assist with Determining Adequacy or Inadequacy

Source of Evidence: _____

A-4 Long-Term Care

Agency Name/Address/ Phone	Area Served/Services Provided, Cost, Hours, Population Served	Data Collection on Seven A's that Will Assist with Determining Adequacy or Inadequacy

Source of Evidence: _____

A-5 Rehabilitative

Agency Name/Address/ Phone	Area Served/Services Provided, Cost, Hours, Population Served	Data Collection on Seven A's that Will Assist with Determining Adequacy or Inadequacy

Source of Evidence: _____

A-6 Assistive Living

Agency Name/Address/ Phone	Area Served/Services Provided, Cost, Hours, Population Served	Data Collection on Seven A's that Will Assist with Determining Adequacy or Inadequacy

Source of Evidence: _____

A-7 Mental Health Services

Agency Name/Address/ Phone	Area Served/Services Provided, Cost, Hours, Population Served	Data Collection on Seven A's that Will Assist with Determining Adequacy or Inadequacy

Source of Evidence: _____

A-8 Occupational

Agency Name/Address/ Phone	Area Served/Services Provided, Cost, Hours, Population Served	Data Collection on Seven A's that Will Assist with Determining Adequacy or Inadequacy

Source of Evidence: _____

A-9 School Health Programs

Agency Name/Address/ Phone	Area Served/Services Provided, Cost, Hours, Population Served	Data Collection on Seven A's that Will Assist with Determining Adequacy or Inadequacy

Source of Evidence: _____

A-10 Dental

Agency Name/Address/ Phone	Area Served/Services Provided, Cost, Hours, Population Served	Data Collection on Seven A's that Will Assist with Determining Adequacy or Inadequacy

Source of Evidence: _____

A-11 Palliative

Agency Name/Address/ Phone	Area Served/Services Provided, Cost, Hours, Population Served	Data Collection on Seven A's that Will Assist with Determining Adequacy or Inadequacy

Source of Evidence: _____

Access to Service

B-1 Access to Services

The following Seven A's questions can assist the public health nurse in analyzing his or her findings:

- Is the population aware of its needs and the services in the community?
- Can the population gain access to the services that it needs?
- Is the service available and convenient to the population in terms of time, location, and place for use?
- How affordable is the service for the population in question?
- Is the service acceptable to the population in terms of choice, satisfaction, and cultural congruence?
- How appropriate is the service for the specific population, or is there a fit?
- Is there adequacy of service in terms of quantity or degree?

B-1 Access to Care: Using the Seven A's

	Adequate/Inadequate	Identify as a Problem Statement
Is the individual/family or population aware of its needs and services in the community?		
Can the individual/family or population gain access to the services it needs?		
Is the service available and convenient for the individual/ family or population in terms of time, location, and place for use?		
How affordable is the service for the individual/family or population?		
Is the service acceptable to the individual/family or population in terms of choice, satisfaction, and congruence with cultural values and beliefs?		
How appropriate is the service for the individual/family or population, or is there a fit?		
Is there adequacy of service in terms of quantity or degree for the individual/family or population?		

Source of Evidence: _____

Part 3-4

Policymaking

The public health nurse must also assess the policies that influence the health of the individual, family, community, system, and population under study. Examples include policies on seat belt use, helmet use, phone use and texting while driving, and child car seats. Each of these policies has had a positive influence on the health and well-being of individuals and the population at large, resulting in a decrease in disabilities and injuries. The public health nurse must be knowledgeable about how his or her community functions with regard to the political infrastructure and as such must assess this infrastructure to be familiar with how it works: Who are the formal and informal political leaders? How can they be reached? What initiatives have they supported in the past? What are the laws that affect the individual/ family, population, and community with regard to the public's health? Are these laws upheld? Are there issues that have not been addressed, and, if so, what can be done to address these issues? The data collected in this section include the organizational structure of the community, a description of the political issues in the community, and an identification of some of the public health laws that affect the community and its members' health. As the public health nurse conducts this portion of the assessment, it is important to explore what the local newspapers report, meet with the local government, and check out the school boards or any of the governing bodies in that area. Meet the candidates if it is an election year, and listen to what the community is saying. Check websites, social networking sites, and local blogs. Using the Internet, here and throughout the PHNAT, assists the public health nurse in obtaining the necessary data and learning about the community.

A-1 Local, State, and Federal: Organizational Structure of Community

In the following table, include the organizational structure of the community including political parties of leadership: governor, senators, assemblypersons, mayor, and boards.

Once you collect the data, include a narrative and an organizational chart that represents a visual model of the hierarchy.

- Titles
- Names
- Method of contact
- Initiatives supported in the past and presently
- Interview one of the officials or go to a town board meeting

Source of Evidence: _____

A-2 Political Issues

Political Issues	Action Taken/Policy

Source of Evidence: _____

A-3 Health Policies (e.g., seat belts, taxes on tobacco, smoking ordinances, cell phone and texting bans)

Health Policies	Action Taken/Policy

Source of Evidence: _____

Part 3-5

Behavior

Collect data on the individual and family that reflect their behavior, and again turn the kaleidoscope to look outward to the community and population in that community.

The public health nurse gathers the information on the individual and family as a client using whatever health assessment tool he or she uses in the particular academic or clinical setting. Some of the questions that provide insight into individual or population-based behavior are as follows:

- What does your assessment of the client tell you about his or her behavior?
- What types of choices does he or she make with regard to diet, physical activity, alcohol, cigarette smoking or other drug use, and so forth?
- How does the family support health choices?
- How does the community support health choices?
- Have there been community-driven health promotion initiatives that support health such as weight loss or physical activity programs like a walk-to-school program?

Summarize your finding in a narrative form below.

Part 4: Health Care Disparities

According to *Healthy People 2020*, "If a health outcome is seen in a greater or lesser extent between populations, there is disparity. Race or ethnicity, sex, sexual identity, age, disability, socioeconomic status, and geographic location all contribute to an individual's ability to achieve good health" (2010f, para. 1). Frequently, the public health nurse will note disparities as he or she observes within the community and analyze the data gathered. Hence, for this foundational health measure much of the information needed is gathered throughout the PHNAT. Summarize your finding in a narrative form below.

Section II: Analysis of Health Status

The public health nurse, along with other partnering members of a health initiative, analyzes the information gathered during the assessment process. Many times, the public health nurse will examine past data to see whether trends and patterns have emerged over time. This process of analysis takes time and reflection. The key here is that the public health nurse does not do this alone. It is a process that takes shape and form in the partnership. From this process the issues in a community are identified and priorities are set. Summarize your findings below identifying community needs, topics, and objectives.

Section III: Prioritize Public Health Issue

In determining the priority health issues, the public health nurse, using a population-based focus, collaborates with other public health practitioners, key informants in the community, and any organization or agency that may have a voice with regard to the population and public health issue. In population-based care, partnerships form the necessary bonds that make sustainable change for health in particular targeted populations. Those involved in the partnership work together to form a common understanding of the issue. All involved, including the population of interest residing in the community, agree on the priority issue identified. This is essential for a positive outcome. Once the priority is noted, the partnership will confer with the *Healthy People 2020* topic areas and corresponding objectives (U.S. DHHS, 2010g).

Issues	Targeted Population	Short-Term Goal(s)	Long-Term Goal(s)

Section IV and Section V: Plan and Implementation

Tracking and Evaluation

The Intervention Strategies and Levels of Practice

Interventions	Levels of Practice			Track and Outcome Evaluation				
	Individual/Family/ Population	Community	System					
Surveillance								
Disease and health threat investigation								
Outreach								
Screening								
Case-finding								
Referral/follow-up								
Case management								
Delegated functions								
Health teaching								
Counseling								

The Intervention Strategies and Levels of Practice

Interventions			Individual/Family/ Population	Community	System	Track and Outcome Evaluation			
						Levels of Practice			
Consultation									
Collaboration									
Coalition building									
Community organizing									
Advocacy									
Social marketing									
Policy development and enforcement									

Section VI: Reflection

This final section reminds the public health nurse to be reflective in his or her practice. This section can be completed throughout the PHNAT process. Some of the questions that the public health nurse may ask include the following:

- What am I observing?
- What am I hearing?
- Am I seeing and hearing all that needs to be seen and heard?
- What am I missing?
- What feelings am I experiencing during this assessment process?
- Are these feelings facilitating this assessment or creating a barrier to the assessment?
- Are these feelings hindering the development of the partnership and the development of trust?
- Am I engaging in activities that help in mobilizing the community of interest?

A. Reflection Gained During Public Health Nursing Assessment

Date	Reflection

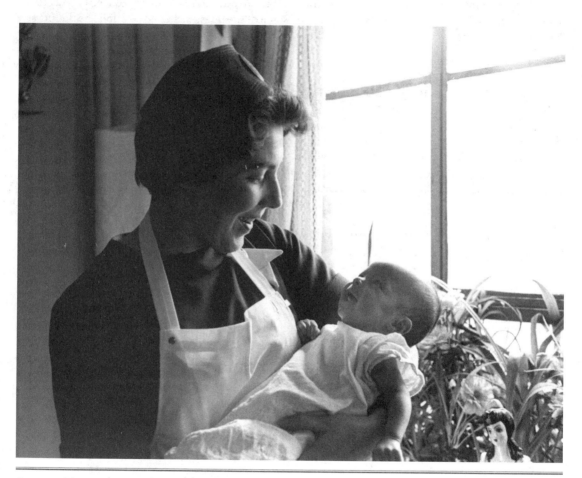

Courtesy of the Visiting Nurse Service of New York.

CHAPTER 4

Fundamentals of Epidemiology and Social Epidemiology

Susan Moscou

In community health work she has become an indispensable factor, because of her great advantage in being the natural object of people's confidence. Almost from the time when the first independent organization of visiting nurses was created to carry the greatest discoveries of science into the humblest homes of the community, its social value has been full recognized. In the numerous measures for human progress and social welfare that the last two decades have seen develop the nurse has had her share-in the protection of child life, the following up of the individual by all sorts of unified and harmonized public powers aiming at care and prevention rather than at police power and punishment, such as probation systems, children's courts, and care and segregation of feeble-minded and defectives; the early detection and treatment of mental cases as well as physical disease; the study of economic conditions and their effect on homes and the nuture [sic] of children; the supplementing of parents' imperfect efforts—in all these efforts toward health in physical, mental, and moral spheres the nurse has contributed. (Wald, 1913, June 23, n.p)

LEARNING OBJECTIVES

At the completion of this chapter, the reader will be able to:

- Describe the concepts in epidemiology and social epidemiology.
- Explain how epidemiology and social epidemiology support the public's health.
- Analyze the use of epidemiology and social epidemiology within the application of public health nursing practice.

KEY TERMS

Epidemiology Terms
- ❏ Age-specific rates
- ❏ Analytical epidemiology
- ❏ Attack rates
- ❏ Chain of infection
- ❏ Crude rates
- ❏ Descriptive epidemiology
- ❏ Epidemiological triad
  - ◯ Agent
  - ◯ Environment
  - ◯ Host
- ❏ Incidence rates
- ❏ Prevalence rates
- ❏ Rate

Social Epidemiology Terms
- ❏ Developmental and life-course perspective
- ❏ Life-course model
- ❏ Multilevel analysis
- ❏ Population perspective
- ❏ Social context
- ❏ Social determinants of health
  - ◯ Discrimination
  - ◯ Education
  - ◯ Income
  - ◯ Income inequality
  - ◯ Occupation
  - ◯ Socioeconomic position
  - ◯ Socioeconomic status

This chapter discusses the concepts of epidemiology and social epidemiology and their use in public health nursing. Nurses use epidemiological tools when they want to understand how and why disease occurs within populations instead of individuals. Examples of populations are pregnant adolescents living in a geographic area, such as the South Bronx in New York City, or in a particular demographic group, such as college-aged students with sexually transmitted diseases. Nursing students use social epidemiological tools when they want to understand how the effects of poverty, **income inequality**, and **discrimination** contribute to how and why disease occurs within specific populations. The purpose of this chapter is to present the concepts of epidemiology and social epidemiology to the public health nurse for application in his or her practice.

Epidemiology

Epidemiology is the scientific discipline that studies the distribution and determinants of diseases and injuries in human populations (Tarzian, 2005). The goal of epidemiology is to limit disease, injury, and

Florence Nightingale.

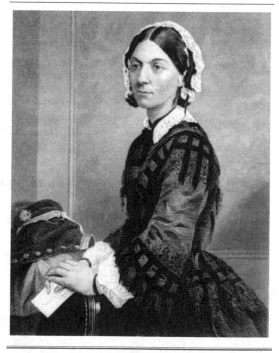

Courtesy of the National Library of Medicine.

death via specific interventions designed to prevent or limit outbreaks or epidemics (U.S. Department of Health and Human Services [DHHS] & Centers for Disease Control and Prevention [CDC], 1998, 2006). Epidemiology is concerned with the health of particular populations, whereas clinical nursing and medicine are concerned with individual health issues. The perspective of epidemiologists is to understand the source of the illness cause or exposure, ascertain who else has been exposed, if the exposure has spread beyond the initial point of contact, and prevent additional cases or recurrences (U.S. DHHS & CDC, 1998, 2006, 2011). In comparison, the clinical perspective of medicine and nursing is to obtain information about the history of the present illness, conduct a physical, make a diagnosis, prescribe treatment—issues are considered on an individual basis and are treated as a single episode. Public health nurses are more in line with the epidemiology perspective because they are educated to integrate knowledge about the environment and the community with their understanding of health and illness as experienced by the individual, family, and population. The perspective in medicine tends to be focused on individual health, whereas the perspective in epidemiology tends to be focused on the population. **Box 4-1** illustrates the various ways these clinicians, practicing within these two frameworks, would approach a situation in which a college student falls ill and is taken to the student health center.

Florence Nightingale applied this epidemiological framework when attending to soldiers in the Crimean War. Nightingale recognized that environmental

---

Box 4-1 Clinical versus Epidemiology Perspective

Picnic Scenario: Fifty college students attend a picnic. The food is served at noon, and the students eat turkey, cornbread, tuna salad, and ice cream. The students return to campus. One student becomes sick and is taken to the student health center.

Clinical Perspective (Single Episode)

- History/physical finding of present illness
- Diagnosis
- Treatment

The clinician asks about the illness, diagnoses the ailment based on symptoms, and then treats.

Epidemiologist Perspective (Possible Multiple Episodes)

- History of present illness and observation for patterns
- How many students were at the picnic?
- Who else was sick?
- Timing
- What caused the illness?
  - Food
  - Heat
- Is this an epidemic?

The epidemiologist not only asks about the illness but also wants to know how many students attended the picnic and how many became sick. The epidemiologist also explores with the students what could have caused the illness: Was it the heat or the food? The epidemiologist would also analyze the food and ask if there was mayonnaise in the tuna salad or how long had the tuna salad been sitting in the heat before it was served? Most importantly, after the epidemiologist gathers the information about the illness, he or she wants to make sure this is not an epidemic and learns how to prevent this illness in the future.

problems such as poor nutrition, sanitation, and contaminated blankets contributed to infection and increases in mortality and morbidity. Nightingale's empirical observations of her surroundings enabled her to methodically examine the factors that contributed to disease (Pfettscher, 2002). This big picture allowed Nightingale to deduce how illness occurred and what strategies reduced the spread of disease.

History

Epidemiological tenets have been used to describe and explain disease and the prevalence of these diseases since 400 BC. A brief history of epidemiological events and well-known persons who used epidemiological thinking is found in **Table 4-1**.

This epidemiological history can be viewed within the context of two revolutions (**Table 4-2**).

Table 4-1 **Epidemiological History and Events**

400 BC

Hippocrates (c. 400 BC) provided an approach to those who wanted to investigate disease.
Hippocrates's treatise, *On Airs, Waters, and Places,* noted that these elements affected health.
Hippocrates believed that knowing how these elements were similar and different in specific areas would provide the basis to understand why a disease occurred and the probability of where the disease would occur.

17th Century

John Graunt (1620–1674) from London published *Observations on the Bills of Mortality,* which quantified Britain's mortality data in 1662.
Graunt noted birth and death patterns, infant mortality, occurrences of disease, differences in disease by gender, differences in disease in urban and rural areas, and variations in disease by season.

18th Century

James Lind (1716–1794) studied scurvy (vitamin C deficiency) while sailing on a Navy ship in 1747.
In 1753, Lind published *A Treatise on Scurvy in Three Parts.*
This publication explained why scurvy occurred and the treatment for scurvy.

19th Century

William Farr (1807–1883) was responsible for the concept of surveillance data.
John Snow (1813–1858), an anesthesiologist, conducted investigations in London during the cholera outbreak.

20th Century

Joseph Goldberger (1874–1929) discovered why the disease pellagra (niacin deficiency) occurred.
The 1964 Surgeon General Report: Smoking and Health: Report of the Advisory Committee to the Surgeon General linked tobacco to lung cancer.
The Framingham Heart Study was initiated to identify factors contributing to heart disease in the United States.
The 1986 Surgeon General's Report *The AIDS Epidemic* was published.

Data from Hippocrates. (400 BCE). Translated by Francis Adams. On airs, waters, and places. Retrieved from http://classics .mit.edu//Hippocrates/airwatpl.html; The James Lind Library. (n.d.). Treatise of scurvy. Retrieved from http://www .jameslindlibrary.org/trial_records/17th_18th_Century/lind/lind_tp.html; National Library of Medicine (n.d.a.). The reports of the surgeon general: The AIDS epidemic. Retrieved from http://profiles.nlm.nih.gov/NN/Views/Exhibit/narrative/aids.html; National Library of Medicine. (n.d.b.). The reports of the surgeon general: The 1964 report on smoking and health. Retrieved from http://profiles.nlm.nih.gov/NN/Views/Exhibit/narrative/smoking.html; Office of History, National Institute of Health. (2005). Dr. Joseph Goldberger & the war on pellagra. Retrieved from http://history.nih.gov/exhibits/goldberger/index.html; Stephan, E. (n.d.). John Graunt. Retrieved from http://www.edstephan.org/Graunt/graunt.html; UCLA Department of Epidemiology School of Public Health. (n.d.). John Snow. Retrieved from http://www.ph.ucla.edu/epi/snow.html

Table 4-2 Epidemiological Revolutions

First Epidemiological Revolution (1870–1930)

The first epidemiological revolution was largely about infectious diseases. Scientists and public health practitioners discovered the causes of infectious diseases.
Immunizations discovered during this time period:

- Smallpox
- Polio
- Tetanus

    Antibiotics discovered:

- Streptomycin: effective against tuberculosis (1947)
- Penicillin

Immunizations and antibiotics accounted for only a 5% drop in mortality rates.
Greatest advances of the first epidemiological revolution:

- Water purification
- Pasteurization
    - Decrease in diarrhea
    - Decrease in gastroenteritis

Second Epidemiological Revolution (1950–Present)

The second epidemiological revolution focused on chronic diseases such as asthma, cancer, and heart disease and on understanding levels of prevention.
Epidemiologists had little understanding of noninfectious diseases until 1950. During the second revolution, epidemiologists began to understand that 38% of deaths were a result of:

- Tobacco (lung cancer and heart disease)
- Diet and inactivity (heart disease, diabetes)
- Alcohol (heart disease, liver disease)

Understanding the factors that contribute to noninfectious diseases paved the way for interventions. Clinicians use the following levels of preventions with their clients:

- Primary (prevent from the outset)
    - Immunizations
    - Health education
- Secondary (early detection of disease)
    - Screening tests
        - Pap
        - Mammogram
        - Cholesterol
        - Colonoscopy
- Tertiary (reducing mortality and morbidity of the disease)
    - Cardiac rehabilitation

Data from Bodenheimer, T. S., & Grumbach, K. (2008). *Understanding health policy: A clinical approach* (5th ed.). New York, NY: McGraw-Hill Lange Medical Books.

The first epidemiological revolution focused on infectious diseases such as influenza, plague, and tuberculosis, which were largely responsible for illnesses and death in previous centuries. It was also during these times that scientists and public health practitioners discovered that the causes of infectious diseases were poverty, overcrowding, sanitation, and contaminated food and water supplies (Breslow, 2005). From 1870 to 1930, scientists and public health practitioners began to understand the cause(s) of infectious diseases. Once epidemiologists had an understanding about why infectious diseases occurred, public health interventions and some medical advances played a role in the reduction of those diseases.

The **rates** of morbidity and mortality of infectious diseases declined in the 18th and 19th centuries because of increases in food production, which led to less malnutrition. Improvements in nutrition led to healthier adults and children. Improvements of overall living conditions were a result of improved sanitation and clean water, pasteurization of milk, and less overcrowding. Decreases in infectious disease rates occurred because of public health interventions.

The second epidemiological revolution began in 1950 when epidemiologists started to understand the causes of noninfectious diseases (e.g., heart disease, asthma, diabetes). With this understanding, public health practitioners could apply epidemiological principles to shed light on health promotion, disease prevention, and the role of risk factor identification and behavioral change in the promotion of health. Noninfectious diseases are discussed later in this chapter.

To summarize, during the first epidemiological revolution (1870–1930), scientists had little understanding about the causes of infectious diseases (e.g., tuberculosis and influenza). Reductions in infectious diseases were largely the result of public health interventions, whereas medical advances (immunizations and antibiotics) contributed to about a 5% reduction in mortality rates. During the second epidemiological revolution, beginning in 1950,

epidemiologists began to understand the causes of noninfectious diseases such as heart disease, asthma, and diabetes, which then paved the way for public health and clinical interventions (Bodenheimer & Grumbach, 2008).

Uses of Epidemiology

Why is it important to understand epidemiology, and how it is used? In this section, the reader will come to see how epidemiology is applied in public health nursing practice. This process includes the systematic collection of data and how the analysis of these data not only leads to a better understanding of a disease process but the reduction of disease. The reader will also come to understand how the epidemiological process informs the public health nurse's decision-making.

The collection and use of epidemiology data for decision-making can be viewed in the following ways. Public health nurses engage in an assessment process that informs them about the health of the individual, family, population, and community. The process of assessment provides information so the public health nurse may engage in problem identification and/or potential problem identification, as well as information that may support program development and, at times, the development of public health policy. For example, the data collected by public health nurses may be presented to policymakers to shed light about the actual and potential problems seen in the population of their targeted home communities. Examples of this information may include data that highlight health, social, or environmental problems in a particular population in a policymaker's constituency; data on risks within that constituency; the history of health problems within a particular population, showing trends such as the increase or the decrease of a particular disease; and the services available in a community. Knowing this information helps policymakers make decisions regarding the establishment of law and resource utilization and allocation.

Epidemiology plays a role in our day-to-day individual decisions pertaining to healthy behaviors such as smoking cessation, exercising, weight control, and eating healthy foods. These positive decisions are made because of epidemiological studies. Epidemiology has contributed to the fount of information about associations and causal relationships (we say causal relationships because research can never prove cause and effect) between obesity and diabetes, smoking and lung cancer, and risky sexual practices, such as engaging in unprotected sex, and sexually transmitted diseases. Without epidemiology, we would not know how a disease is transmitted or the strategies to reduce our risks of contracting the disease. Public health nurses use this evidence-based knowledge in their practice as they develop educational programs for individuals, families, and populations in an effort to offer information that assists others to make healthy lifestyle choices.

The work of public health practitioners involves public health nurses, epidemiologists, health department officials, clinicians, physicians, scientists, media experts, educators, sanitation officials, and researchers. These individuals all provide particular worldviews that, when joined collectively, complete the clinical picture needed to understand the disease, the progression and trajectory of that disease, and interventions. Completing the clinical picture is identifying what the infectious agent is, why and how the disease is transmitted to the host, where the disease is most prevalent in terms of the place or location, when the disease most makes itself known with regard to time, and who the individual is who is affected by the disease. These are known as the five W's of **descriptive epidemiology** (U.S. DHHS & CDC, 2006, 2011, p. 31). Part of this clinical picture is understanding the determinants of health. One practitioner alone is unable to be a solo artist in this endeavor because effective public health strategies require collaborative and collective efforts between and among many different professions.

Human immunodeficiency virus (HIV) is an example of how epidemiologists were able to complete the clinical picture. In the early 1980s, a strange pneumonia affected five men who identified themselves as having sex with men. *Pneumocystis*

carinii pneumonia was a relatively rare lung disease and appeared to be clustered only within this specific population (Sepkowitz, 2001). Additionally, clinicians were seeing Kaposi's sarcoma (KS), a relatively benign form of cancer, in their younger male patients who had sex with men. KS was also relatively rare in the United States; the skin lesions associated with KS were usually localized to the lower extremities and affected older people in their 70s (Hymes et al., 1981).

Because these cases appeared to be clustered within a specific population and puzzled the medical community, the cases and the laboratory results were reported to the CDC for further investigation. In 1981, the CDC provided information about the first cases of *P. carinii* pneumonia and KS among men who have sex with men (CDC referred to this group as homosexuals) to the medical community, and in 1982 the CDC named this disease acquired immune deficiency syndrome, known as AIDS. It was not until 1986 that the term human immunodeficiency virus, or HIV, was adopted by the clinical community (Sepkowitz, 2008). Once a particular disease or health event is identified, healthcare professionals make the diagnosis in individual cases, whereas epidemiologists contribute to our understanding of the natural history of the disease. Since this time, the work pertaining to HIV has been carried on by a wide and varied group of healthcare professionals. Take a few minutes and just think. Who has contributed to the knowledge of this disease and the treatment of this disease? The list is rather overwhelming, yet at the same time, it clearly presents for us the view that in order for the health of the public to be sustained there is a need for the collective wisdom of many working together. Public health nurses are a valued member of this collective group.

Finally, the search for causes is epidemiological research. This research is dedicated to the investigation of the causes and individual, societal, and environmental factors that contribute to a person's risk for contracting a disease and/or suffering injury. This research provides evidence for interventions that health professionals can use in their clinical practice, such as counseling about smoking, protective sexual practices, seat belts, child car seats, and immunizations. Public health nurses not only apply this research as evidence in their practice but raise questions for research and conduct research.

Epidemiological Approach

When we see a particular disease in our clinical practice, or if we decide to explore a particular disease, we want to know who is affected by this disease, what factors contribute to this disease (environmental, social, or personal factors), if there were other cases, when this disease became known, why some individuals are more prone to this particular disease, and what common factors do diseased individuals have in common. Epidemiologists begin with case definition as the standard criteria to guide their practice.

A case definition is that which determines if a person has a particular disease. For example, an individual is diagnosed with diabetes if his or her blood sugar levels are above the cutoff point (126 mg/dL) on two separate occasions (U.S. Preventive Services Task Force, 2008). Case definitions standardize the diagnoses of a particular disease, thus ensuring that every case is similarly diagnosed. Additionally, case definitions consist of clinical criteria, including subjective data, which are client complaints, and objective data, which are the clinician's observations inclusive of physical, environmental, and laboratory findings.

NUMBERS AND RATES

Epidemiologists are concerned about numbers and rates because it allows them to measure, describe, and compare the morbidity and mortality of a particular disease and/or injury in populations. Rates are "measures of frequency of health events that put raw numbers into a frame of reference to the size of a population. Rates are determined by statistical adjustments to the raw data, making them useful in making comparisons or examining trends" (Stotts, 2008, p. 91).

In epidemiology, the numerator is the actual number of cases or events occurring during a given time period, and the denominator is the total population at risk during the same time period. The denominator is typically converted to a standard base denominator, such as 1,000, 10,000, or 100,000, so that comparisons can be made among at-risk populations, communities, and neighborhoods (Tarzian, 2005). Rates are useful to the public health nurse because they can help the nurse identify what populations in the community are at an increased risk for a particular disease and/or injury. For example, City A has a population of 130,000 nursing home residents. City A reported 100 cases of hepatitis A among nursing home residents to the Department of Health (DOH). City B has a population of 120,000 nursing home residents. City B reported 150 cases of hepatitis A among its nursing home residents to the DOH. The DOH determined that the specific rate for hepatitis A was 7.6 cases per 10,000 persons living in a nursing home in City A and was 12.5 cases per 10,000 persons in City B. The DOH specific rate calculations for these cities are found in **Box 4-2**. This type of data helps the public health nurse think about and develop initiatives that target nursing home residents who appear to be a high-risk population for contracting hepatitis A.

In addition to the specific rates, there are many other rate definitions that measure morbidity (illness rates) or mortality (death rates) for populations at risk for contracting or dying from a particular disease, such as asthma, diabetes, or high blood pressure, or cause, such as a motor vehicle accident. Examples of these rates or statistical calculations are **incidence rates**, **prevalence rates**, **attack rates**, **crude rates**, and **age-specific rates**, as listed in **Table 4-3**.

DESCRIPTIVE EPIDEMIOLOGY

Descriptive epidemiology describes the extent of an outbreak in terms of who gets the disease, where the disease occurs, and when the disease occurred. These characteristics are described in **Table 4-4**. For example, Lyme disease was classified as a new disease

---

Box 4-2 Specific Rate Calculations for Hepatitis A Found in City A and City B

Numbers and rates permit the epidemiologist to measure, describe, and compare the morbidity and mortality of particular diseases. A rate is:

$$\frac{\text{Number of cases or events occurring during a given time period}}{\text{Population at risk during the same time period}}$$

In epidemiology, rates are changed to a common base such as 100,000 because it changes the result of the division into a quantity that permits a standardized comparison.

Example:
City A and City B saw an outbreak of hepatitis A in their nursing home residents. Each city reported these cases to the Department of Health. The Department of Health calculated the specific rates for each city using 10,000 as the standard base number. Hepatitis A specific rate for nursing home residents is calculated as follows:
City A specific rate:

$$\frac{100 \text{ cases of reported hepatitis A cases}}{130,000 \text{ City A nursing home residents}}$$

City A specific rate: 7.6, which means that in nursing homes for City A, about seven to eight residents contracted hepatitis A.
City B specific rate:

$$\frac{150 \text{ cases of reported hepatitis A cases}}{120,000 \text{ City B nursing home residents}}$$

City B specific rate = 12.5
By calculating the specific rate, the Department of Health can compare the hepatitis rates in City A and City B. Additionally, the Department of Health knows that nursing home residents are at risk for contracting hepatitis A.

Modified from U.S. Department of Health and Human Services (DHHS) & Centers for Disease Control and Prevention (CDC). (2011). *Principles of epidemiology in public health practice: An introduction to applied epidemiology and biostatistics* (3rd ed.). Atlanta, GA: Author.

---

when about 50 children were diagnosed with arthritis in Lyme, Connecticut. This cluster of arthritis in children caused an epidemiologist in Lyme, who was concerned because juvenile rheumatoid arthritis is relatively rare in children (France, 1999), to request that the CDC investigate this outbreak. The who in this outbreak were children, the where in this outbreak was a wooded hamlet at the mouth of the Connecticut River, and the when for this disease is typically during the summer and fall when people tend to spend more time outdoors and thus are more at risk for a tick bite. The collection and analysis of this descriptive information form a critical first step in the epidemiological investigatory process.

This gathering and analyzing of data in descriptive epidemiology is also called the gathering of data on person, time, and place. This information allows the public health nurse to become knowledgeable about the public health problem being studied, thus enabling the public health nurse to provide a comprehensive picture of the health of the population under study and determine who is at risk for

Table 4-3 **Rate Definitions**

Incidence Rate	Prevalence Rate	Attack Rate	Specific Rates	Crude Rate	Age-specific Rate
Applied in the study of acute diseases, a disease outbreak, or in the diagnosis of new cases. Incidence rates are the frequency with which a new condition or event occurs in a population over a period of time. Example We want to know the number of new cases of flu. In the second week of November the student Health Services diagnosed three students with the flu. The total student population is 1,600. *Calculation* three new flu cases ÷ 1,600 (student population) × 1,000 (comparison denominator) Incidence rate is 1.8.	Applied in the study of chronic disease. Prevalence rate measures the number of people in a given population who have an already existing condition at a given point in time. Example We want to know the number of existing cases of flu. There were three new cases of the flu in the second week of November and 10 old cases of the flu in the first week of November. *Calculation* 3 + 10 cases ÷ 1,600 (student population) × 1,000 Prevalence rate is 8.1.	Important for the study of a single disease outbreak or epidemic during a short time period. The number is expressed as a percentage. Example 120 people flew from New York to Los Angeles. The meal served was meatloaf. Eighty people ate the meal and 40 people chose not to eat meatloaf. Twenty of those who ate meatloaf became ill. *Calculation* 20 (ill) ÷ 80 (meatloaf pop) × 100 Attack rate is 25%.	These measure morbidity or mortality for a particular population: • Age specific • Gender specific • Income • Race/ethnicity • Infant mortality • Maternal mortality Example Age-specific diabetes mortality in 45- to 55-year-olds *Calculation* Number of diabetes deaths in 45 to 55-year-olds ÷ Population of individuals 45- to 55-year-olds × 1,000	A crude rate measures the experience of the entire population in a specific area with regard to the specific disease or condition being investigated. The crude mortality rate looks at the entire mortality rate from all causes of death for a population in a particular area during a specific time. Example NYC death rate *Calculation* The total number of NYC deaths reported during 1985 ÷ 5 million × 100,000	These rates provide age-specific information for a particular disease. Example Age-specific mortality rate is one limited to a particular age group. The numerator is the number of deaths in that age group and the denominator is the number of persons in that age group in the population. Examples include: Neonatal mortality rate Infant mortality rate

Modified from U.S. Department of Health and Human Services (DHHS) & Centers for Disease Control and Prevention (CDC). (2011). *Principles of epidemiology in public health practice: An introduction to applied epidemiology and biostatistics* (3rd ed.). Atlanta, GA: Author.

Table 4-4 Descriptive Epidemiological Variables

Person	Place	Time
Person variables are used to understand what makes a person susceptible to a disease or injury. Inherent characteristics include age, race/ethnicity, and sex. Acquired characteristics include marital status, education, occupation, living conditions, socioeconomic status, and access to health care.	Place variables describe the disease event by where the disease occurs, such as: • Place of residence • School district • Community • Country • State • Hospital unit	Time variables give information about how disease rates change over time. Time information can be reported in • Days • Weeks • Months • Years • Decades
Inherent characteristics are considered fixed or unchangeable. A person's gender makes him or her at higher risk for some diseases, such as breast cancer. However, because age varies, the person becomes more susceptible to illness as he or she ages. Acquired characteristics may be modifiable via education.	Place information also provides insight into the geographical location and what factors in that environment facilitate the disease. For example, the temperature and climate may promote a place where a particular agent may grow and multiply.	Epidemic period: when the number of cases is greater than normal. Does the disease manifest itself during certain seasons? Is the presentation of the disease predictable? If so, why? Can this information be used in the prevention of the disease?
Example A 50-year-old man develops lung cancer. He has smoked for 30 years. The smoking is considered an acquired characteristic because it is potentially modifiable with education. Behavioral changes (quitting or smoking fewer cigarettes) lead to a healthier life and prevention of lung cancer.	Example Lyme disease was first characterized in Lyme, Connecticut, because the lush wooded environment supported the agent, the host, and the environment cycle.	Example Seasonality may demonstrate disease occurrences by week or by month over the course of a year. For example, flu season typically begins in November and ends in March.

Modified from U.S. Department of Health and Human Services (DHHS) & Centers for Disease Control and Prevention (CDC). (2011). *Principles of epidemiology in public health practice: An introduction to applied epidemiology and biostatistics* (3rd ed.). Atlanta, GA: Author.

acquiring the particular disease. Another part of the epidemiological approach is known as **analytical epidemiology**, which facilitates the how and why of a particular disease.

ANALYTICAL EPIDEMIOLOGY

Analytical epidemiology illustrates the causal relationship between a risk factor and a specific disease or health condition. In other words, it seeks to answer questions about how and why disease occurs and the effects of a particular disease. Analytical studies use a comparison group to learn why one group has a disease and another does not. These groups are drawn from a healthy population living in the same community in which the disease has occurred. For example, a public health nurse was sent to a community where there was an outbreak of hepatitis A. The nurse interviewed the individuals who were diagnosed with hepatitis A and discovered they had attended a graduation party at the local high school in the neighborhood. The public health nurse learned about the food that was served at this party and asked each person what he or she had eaten at the party. The public health nurse recognized the need for a comparison group for further investigation of this hepatitis A outbreak. The comparison group in this case would be those individuals at the same party who did not eat those same foods and who were not ill. "When . . . investigators find that persons with a particular characteristic are more likely than those without the characteristic to develop a certain disease, then the characteristic is said to be associated with the disease" (U.S. DHHS & CDC, 2006, 2011, p. 46). These characteristics include demographics such as age, race/ethnicity, or sex; constitutional characteristics such as immune state; behavioral characteristics such as smoking; or other characteristics, such as living next to a waste site (U.S. DHHS & CDC, 2006, 2011).

Analytical epidemiology is used to search for causes and effects of the disease under study. Furthermore, epidemiologists discern how or why exposure to a particular agent results in the outcome of disease or no disease. Epidemiologists can study the occurrences of diseases in two ways: experimental studies and observational studies.

In an experimental study, the researcher is the one who determines the exposure status of the individual or population. The researcher does not only observe but also determines and actively initiates what the exposure is, where to deliver the exposure, how to deliver the exposure, when to deliver the exposure, and who will be the recipient of the exposure. The researcher determines recipient characteristics such as age, gender, and **socioeconomic status** (SES), which comprises education, income, and education. The researcher then carries out a research design to determine the effects of the exposure on the experimental individual or population and compares the outcomes with those not having had the exposure. Those who have not been exposed are the comparison group. This type of study is sometimes referred to as prospective because the research moves forward in time to look at the effects of the exposure. These studies rarely prove causation but often lead to more research.

Experimental studies are generally used to determine the effectiveness of a treatment such as a vaccine or a drug. These types of studies are considered the gold standard of clinical trials. Study participants in clinical trials are either given the medication or the drug under study or given a placebo such as a sugar pill. Most of the major medications used to treat chronic diseases such as high blood pressure, diabetes, and asthma were subjected to clinical trials in experimental studies.

Observational studies include cohort and case-control studies. In a cohort study, a cohort of healthy individuals who share similar experiences or characteristics are identified and classified by their exposures. For example, in a study that wishes to look at tobacco use and lung cancer, the cohort identified may be men 21 years of age who are actively engaged in smoking. This group is studied over a period of years, allowing researchers to compare the disease rates in the exposed group (those who smoked) with the unexposed group (those who did not smoke). In a case-control group, the researcher identifies a group of people who have already been diagnosed with a disease (e.g., women diagnosed with breast cancer) and a group without the disease. The researcher compares and contrasts the participants' past life experiences, characteristics, and exposures to determine patterns. Again, a comparison group is important in case-control studies. This type of research is sometimes referred to as retrospective because the researcher is looking at a situation in the present and linking it to situations or conditions in the past.

The Framingham Study is an example of a classic cohort study. Since 1949, the National Heart Institute of the U.S. Public Health Service observed men and women living in Framingham, Massachusetts, to identify factors related to developing coronary heart disease (Kannel, Schwartz, & McNamara, 1969). The Nurses' Health Study, another example of a cohort study, was started several decades ago to examine the relationship between oral contraception (birth control pills) and breast cancer (Colditz, Manson, & Hankinson, 1997).

Epidemiological Triad

The epidemiological triad (**Figure 4-1**) is the traditional model of infectious disease causation. The three components are agent, host, and environment.

Agent factors refer to an infectious organism such as a virus, bacterium, parasite, or other microbe. **Host** factors that can mediate the effect of a particular agent are age, sex, socioeconomic factors (SES) (education, income, occupation), behaviors (smoking, drinking, and exercise), and genetic factors. For example, a 95-year-old man with multiple chronic illnesses who does not get his yearly flu vaccine is more susceptible to influenza than is a healthy 20-year-old college student who does not get a flu shot. These host factors are also known as intrinsic factors. **Environmental** factors are known as extrinsic factors and include physical factors such as geography, climate, and physical surroundings (e.g., homeless shelters); biological factors such as insects that transmit the agent (e.g., mosquito transmits malaria); and socioeconomic factors such as sanitation and available health services that can determine the spread of a particular disease (e.g., tuberculosis increases with overcrowding) (U.S. DHHS & CDC, 2006, 2011).

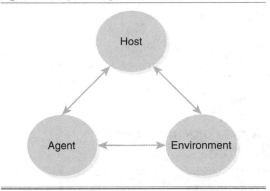

Figure 4-1 Epidemiological triad.

Modified from U.S. Department of Health and Human Services & Centers for Disease Control and Prevention. (2011). *Principles of epidemiology in public health practice: An introduction to applied epidemiology and biostatistics* (3rd ed.). Atlanta, GA: Author.

Again, Lyme disease is an excellent example of the epidemiological triad. A particular deer tick infected with the bacterium *Borrelia burgdorferi* (the agent) infects a person (the host). The bacteria enter the skin at the bite site only after the infected tick has been in the host for 36 to 48 hours. The initial symptoms felt by the host are primarily the result of the body's response to this invasion. Specific factors such as exposure to heavily wooded areas (environment), the season (infection is most likely contracted during the summer and fall), age (most common in children and young adults), and location (90% of cases occur in the coastal Northeast as well as in Wisconsin, Minnesota, California, and Oregon) predispose the host to contracting Lyme disease (Depietropaolo, Powers, & Gill, 2005).

Chain of Infection

Diseases are classified as communicable or noncommunicable. *Communicable diseases* are considered infectious because they can be transmitted by an infected person to a noninfected person. The common cold, HIV, and tuberculosis are examples of communicable diseases. Diseases come about when the body (host) is exposed to an infectious agent (virus or microorganism), and the organism or virus grows within the body. If the organism or virus is able to grow within the host, the host at some point in time might become infectious and then can transmit the particular disease to another susceptible host. *Noncommunicable diseases* such as diabetes, asthma, and heart disease cannot be transmitted by the person who has that particular diagnosis. The contributing factors of noncommunicable diseases are genetics (e.g., Tay-Sachs disease), environmental factors (e.g., Love Canal), and behaviors such as overeating.

The **chain of infection** (**Figure 4-2**) shows that infectious diseases result from their interaction with the agent, host, and environment. Transmission, direct or indirect, of an infectious agent takes place after the agent leaves its reservoir (host) by a portal of exit such as the mouth when coughing. The agent then enters the susceptible host via a

Figure 4-2   The chain of infection.

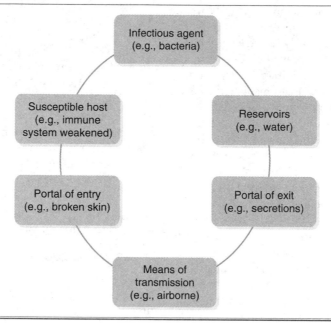

Data from U.S. Department of Health and Human Services & Centers for Disease Control and Prevention. (2011). *Principles of epidemiology in public health practice: An introduction to applied epidemiology and biostatistics* (3rd ed.). Atlanta, GA: Author.

portal of entry, such as a skin wound, to infect the susceptible host (U.S. DHHS & CDC, 2006, 2011).

Direct transmission modes are the immediate transfer of the disease agent between an infected person and a susceptible person. Examples of direct transmission modes are direct contact via touching, kissing, and direct projection, which includes a large short-range spray of droplets via sneezing or coughing. Indirect transmission takes place as an agent is carried from a reservoir to a host via air particles and gains access to the portal of entry via respiratory tract systems (e.g., mouth and nose). Vehicle-borne transmissions are contaminated materials or objects (fomites) in which communicable diseases are transferred (e.g., children's toys in a day care center) and vector-borne transmission methods transfer the disease by a living organism (e.g., mosquito) (U.S. DHHS & CDC, 2006, 2011).

Public Health Surveillance Data

Public health surveillance data are used by public health nurses and other health officials to understand disease prevalence and disease patterns. Surveillance data are critically analyzed and used by these individuals to make decisions about policy, funding, research, and program initiatives. Surveillance as an intervention strategy is discussed later in this book.

Social Epidemiology

Social epidemiology is the study of social conditions such as poverty, socioeconomic status (SES), and discrimination and their role and influence in the health of populations (Honjo, 2004). Social epidemiology goes beyond the analysis of individual risk factors such as age and gender to include the study of the social context or societal implications in which the health–disease phenomenon occurs (Krieger, 2002). Social epidemiology measures the impact of the social environment on health outcomes, whereas epidemiology is more concerned with the impact of the physical environment on health outcomes (Berkman & Kawachi, 2014). Galea, Tracey, Hoggatt, DiMaggio, and Karpati (2011) examined the literature about social factors and health outcomes from 1980 to 2007 and then calculated the deaths attributable to each social factor in the United States in 2000. Galea et al. (2011) found that the deaths attributed to low education numbered 245,000, racial segregation was 176,000, low social support was 162,000, impoverished individuals was 133,000, income inequality was 119,000, and area-level poverty accounted for 39,000. Although these numbers may vary in later years, the take-home message is that social factors play a large role in preventable deaths in the United States.

Social epidemiology attempts to address social inequality's role in disease causation. Social epidemiologists investigate social conditions responsible for patterns of health, patterns of disease, and the well-being of populations, as well as examine how social inequality in the past and present has a role in the health or disease of populations (Krieger, 2001a; Pavalko & Caputo, 2013). Social epidemiologists investigate the gradient of income on the health status of lower-income, middle-income, and upper-income classes in society. By looking at the health status at each income level, social epidemiologists can examine how income exerts an influence, either positive or negative, on health outcomes (Krieger, 2001b). For example, people growing up in poorer communities have worse health outcomes than those growing up in wealthier communities. Once a social epidemiologist teases out variations in health status by different income groups, the relationship between individual income, which is considered an individual factor, and income inequality, which is considered a contextual factor, can be explored (Subramanian, Kawachi, & Kennedy, 2001).

The concepts guiding social epidemiology are as follows:

- **Population perspective**, which means that because individuals are rooted in society, their risks for disease or staying healthy are situated with the population in which they belong.
- **Social context** of behavior, which means that certain behaviors such as smoking, drinking, and voter participation are shaped by social influences. For example, children who see their parents smoke are more likely to smoke when they get older, or communities with ample resources such as parks, grocery stores, and health clinics are more likely to inculcate healthier behavior.
- **Multilevel analysis**, which means that health outcomes are understood within the perspective of individual factors such as income and education, along with contextual factors that assess environmental exposures at the community, state, national, and global level.
- **Developmental and life-course perspective**, which means the early life experiences of an individual contribute to his or her susceptibility to disease later in life (**Table 4-5**).

Population Perspective

The population perspective is a guiding concept in social epidemiology. As discussed, the population perspective illustrates that an individual's risk for health problems cannot be isolated from the community in which he or she resides or from the population or society in which he or she belongs. Murray (2011) noted that "a population focus that addresses the social determinants of health is an essential component of primary health care" (p. 3); as such, an individual's risk for disease must be seen in the context of where he or she lives. For example, breast cancer survival rates in the population of Japanese women are higher than in the population of Japanese immigrants living in America and Japanese Americans. One explanation for the improved survival rate is the low dietary fat intake of Japanese

Table 4-5 **Guiding Perspectives in Social Epidemiology**

Population	Social Context of Behavior	Multilevel Analysis	Developmental and Life Course
This perspective examines an individual's health in the context of the population where the person resides. Example Breast cancer survival rates for women in Japan are higher than for Japanese women who become U.S. immigrants.	This perspective makes the case that risky behaviors such as smoking and drinking tend to be clustered in particular communities. The residents in these communities typically have less education, are more socially isolated, and have less access to health-promoting environments. This perspective recognizes that social environments have a large role in positive or negative health behaviors. Example Communities with higher rates of smoking exist in areas where smoking is heavily advertised.	This perspective encourages a larger analysis of the problem by assessing all factors that contribute to disease. This analysis assesses the levels of exposures found at the community, state, national, and global level. If we understand the relationship between the individual and the community level, we gain a larger understanding of health outcomes for the individual. Example A person lives in a community that does not have grocery stores with fresh food, but there are several fast food restaurants on every block. Eating fast food almost every day might contribute to becoming overweight and might lead to diabetes in the future.	This perspective examines the cumulative risk of health status based on early life exposures. This perspective recognizes that disadvantages in one's early life may facilitate disease later in life. Example A child grew up in a poor neighborhood next to a medical incinerator. Additionally, several family members smoked cigarettes. The family did not have health insurance until the child was 10 years old. The child, however, was healthy and did not need medical attention. The child went to college and became quite wealthy. The early life experience of deprivation for this child, however, may contribute to developing asthma when older even though the new environment is less conducive to developing asthma.

Data from Berkman, L. F., & Kawachi, I. (2014). A historical framework for social epidemiology. In L. F. Berkman, I. Kawachi, & M. M. Glymour (Eds.), *Social epidemiology* (2nd ed., pp. 1–16). New York, NY: Oxford University Press.

women (Pineda, White, Kristal, & Taylor, 2001). This means that when a Japanese woman moves from Japan to the United States, her breast cancer survival rate would be less than if she lived in Japan.

Social Context of Behavior

The social context of behavior is a guiding concept of social epidemiology. As discussed, the social context of behavior addresses individual behavioral risk factors, such as smoking and drinking, and examines these behaviors in a larger social context or by the

social influences or conditions that contribute to specific behaviors. For example, the number of green spaces such as parks and supermarkets in a neighborhood often determines the choices the person has to make to maintain health and reduce his or her susceptibility to disease. If the neighborhood offers few healthy choices, it becomes more difficult for individuals to create and maintain healthy lifestyles.

Public health nurses working in the South Bronx, a part of one of the five boroughs of New York City, where many of the adults are overweight and at risk for diabetes or high blood pressure, recommend diet and exercise regimens for these individuals, but because there are few green space areas, no access to walking paths, no gym facilities, and the neighborhood feels less safe in the evening, many of these individuals are unable to adhere to the diet and exercise recommendations.

Social conditions often determine an individual's actions and play a role in how susceptible a person is to disease. Growing up in poverty or wealth determines the type of neighborhoods where people can live (unsafe versus safe), the environmental exposures in certain neighborhoods (lead), how people in these neighborhoods access health care (emergency room versus private healthcare office), and the levels of educational attainment (high-school degree versus college degree). For example, people living in poorer communities face increased risks of environmental exposures such as living near a medical incinerator, which might cause more asthma; lack of adequate housing might lead to overcrowding, which can increase the prevalence of tuberculosis; reduced availability of medical resources might lead to the increased use of the emergency room versus seeing a primary care clinician; and lower educational attainment might create the context for detrimental behaviors such as smoking and drinking, which contribute to disease later in life such as lung cancer, cirrhosis of the liver, or emphysema.

Social conditions do not create disease but generate a susceptibility to disease. Social epidemiology takes into account that the continued exposure to adverse social conditions has a role in how well the host can resist disease, and these exposures often lay the groundwork for poorer health in the future (Berkman & Kawachi, 2014; Kasper et al., 2008).

In summary, the whole notion of social context of behavior may also be viewed from a positive perspective in which the population's strengths are identified and engaged. In other words, how healthcare practitioners work with the population in shaping the social context of where they live can enhance health. Carthon (2011) engaged in a historical inquiry focusing on two civic associations that functioned in Philadelphia during the early 1900s. The population of individuals consisted of primarily black Americans who lived in economically and medically underresourced communities, which accounted for poorer health rates. The utilization of community and social networks provided the population with resources needed to effect change.

The above is also an exemplar of social capital at work. Social capital structures are systems of networks, norms, and trust relationships that allow communities to address common problems (Pronyk et al., 2008). Putnam (1995) has defined social capital as social relationships (interpersonal trust norms of reciprocity and civic responsibilities) within communities that act as resources for individuals and facilitate collective action for a mutual benefit. Residents of a community with high social capital may provide one another with greater instrumental and psychosocial support than residents of a community with low social capital. Furthermore, the community's level of interconnectedness and trust may reduce or increase barriers to care (Perry, Williams, Wallestein, & Waitzkin, 2008).

Multilevel Analysis

Multilevel analysis is a guiding concept of social epidemiology. As discussed, multilevel analysis is necessary to understand all factors that contribute to disease at the group and individual levels. It is an approach that permits simultaneous examination of group- and individual-level variables on individual-level outcomes (Diez-Roux, 2000). It has already been noted that individuals are influenced by their social context. Therefore, using a multilevel analysis will assist those in public health to look at independent and interacting effects of individual-level factors as well as group-level factors on health outcomes. An example of this is noted by Diez-Roux (2000):

Within this field, one of the main research areas in which multilevel models have been applied is the investigation of the effects of neighborhood

*social environments on health outcomes. . . .
A key issue in investigating neighborhood effects on health is separating out the effects of neighborhood characteristics (context) from the effects of individual-level attributes that persons living in certain types of areas may share (composition). Because neighborhoods can be thought of as groups or contexts with individuals nested within them, multilevel models have been used to investigate how neighborhood factors, individual-level factors, and their interactions influence health. (p. 181)*

Life-Course Model or Perspective

The life-course perspective is a guiding concept in social epidemiology. The **life-course model** puts forward that the **socioeconomic position** of the family during childhood affects the child's health status, educational opportunities, and occupation choices in the future. Children growing up in families with less economic means or a lower socioeconomic position might have more health problems than do children growing up in families with more economic means or a higher socioeconomic position. For example, children growing up in poverty might have more health problems such as asthma, which then might contribute to a lower level of education because frequent asthma episodes result in more school absences, which in turn leads to less occupational choices because they did not do well enough in school to attend college, and less education results in lower income levels that can precipitate downward mobility (Dike van de Mheen, Stronks, & Mackenbach, 1998). Children, however, growing up in more prosperous neighborhoods tend to have better health outcomes than do children in economically disadvantaged communities because they attend better schools, have access to health care, and their parents are better educated and therefore have better jobs (Acevedo-Garcia, Lochner, Osypuk, & Subramanian, 2003). Economic disadvantages in early life can set in motion negative consequences that build up over time to produce disease after 20, 30, 40, or 50 years of being disadvantaged (Berkman & Kawachi, 2014).

Multilevel Approaches to Understanding Social Determinants of Health

Social determinants of health refer to the interaction of environmental and social systems that can affect individuals making them more susceptible to a disease and lead to health disparities. These interactions are frequently in evidence where the individuals live, work, learn, and play (Dean, Williams, & Fenton, 2013; Hassmiller, 2017; Huang, Cheng, & Theise, 2013; Robert Wood Johnson Foundation, 2014). For example, a child is exposed to secondhand smoke and develops asthma when he or she is 6 years old. Additionally, this child might even develop lung cancer later in life because of the continued exposure to secondhand smoke and the early development of lung disease. We know that early life experiences can contribute to subsequent health outcomes, good or bad. Solving the direct effects of material and environmental conditions such as pollution, malnutrition, and housing are important, but the person might still be at risk for health problems depending on how long he or she was exposed to the offending agent or experienced economic or social deprivation.

Socioeconomic factors such as income, education, occupation, medical care, healthcare barriers, language, environmental exposures, discrimination, and so forth are all correlated with health outcomes in one context or another (Dean, Williams, & Fenton, 2013; Sadana & Blas, 2013). The public health nurse considers the above variables to bring about a better understanding of health disparities noted in individuals, families, populations, and communities. Additionally, analyzing the interaction between socioeconomic factors, health, and discrimination gives the public health nurse a framework to develop interventions for specific individuals, families, or populations in specific areas. What follows is a discrete and detailed discussion of these social determinants of health.

Socioeconomic Status and Socioeconomic Position

The relationship of SES and health status has been well documented (Adler & Newman, 2002; Lipowicz, Koziel, Hulanicka, & Kowalisko, 2007; Lynch & Kaplan, 2000; Mirowsky, Ross, & Reynolds, 2000; Sadana & Blas, 2013; Berkowitz, Traore, Singer, & Atlas, 2015). Socioeconomic status consists of family income, educational level, and occupation. Additionally, SES determines an individual's socioeconomic position within society. How much money, level of educational attainment, and the occupation a person has have a bearing on and reflect his or her socioeconomic position or standing in society. Additionally, populations have a socioeconomic position, and this is based on the economic resources available to the community. Like SES, the relationship between the socioeconomic position of a person or population and health status has been well established. The effects of SES and socioeconomic position on health have been consistent with regard to health outcome disparities across different time periods, different geographical areas, and in nearly all measurements used to assess health and disease (Condliffe & Link, 2008; Lantz et al., 2001).

An individual's SES and socioeconomic position in society are based on his or her educational level, annual income, occupation, and level of assets such as stocks, bonds, and home ownership. A person's SES and socioeconomic position matter to health status because living in a relatively poor community can be bad for one's health, whereas living in a relatively affluent community can be good for one's health. The SES or socioeconomic position of an individual or population contributes to positive or negative health behaviors (Stringhini et al., 2010). For example, individuals growing up in lower socioeconomic circumstances are more likely to live in areas where there may be health-damaging exposures, such as living near a sewage treatment plant, as opposed to individuals in upper socioeconomic circumstances who are more likely to grow up in communities with health-enhancing resources, such as supermarkets containing fresh fruits and vegetables (Kaiser et al., 2016; Piccolo, Duncan, Pearce, & McKinlay, 2015). The SES and socioeconomic position of an individual or population reflect the social and economic risks, for example, living in unsafe neighborhoods, or rewards, for example, living in safe neighborhoods, of that particular class in society (Herd, Goesling, & House, 2007; Mirowsky et al., 2000).

Income

One of the most significant determinants of good health is **income**; therefore, many have suggested that economic policy is a powerful form of health policy (Dean, Williams, & Fenton, 2013). By increasing a person's income, you increase the health status for everyone in society (Kaplan, 2001). Income matters in society because income gives a person access to resources that are necessary to maintain health (Braveman, Cubbin, Egerter, Williams, & Pamuk, 2010; Kawachi, 2000; Wilkinson, 1999). For example, stress has been shown to have a negative impact on one's health, so being able to relieve stress is an important resource (Kasper et al., 2008). A 55-year-old executive is able to relieve stress during the day because she has access to a gym in her office, whereas a 55-year-old bus driver does not have that resource available. The bus driver's inability to relieve stress makes him more susceptible to health problems.

Public health nurses work with individuals, families, and populations who experience stressors daily. How one responds to a particular stressor sets in motion physiological, behavioral, and psychological responses in the person. Additionally, how one handles a particular stressor depends on his or her coping mechanisms, support systems, and personality (Marmot, 2000; Schneiderman, Ironson, & Siegel, 2005). Sister Callista Roy, although not a social epidemiologist but a nursing theorist, recognized that adaptation to a particular stimuli is shaped by perceptions of the event and interpretation of the event. How the person interprets an event brings about a particular adaptive response. This response could have been formed by earlier life experiences.

The Roy Adaptation Model puts forth that adaptation mechanisms used by a person have health consequences in the present and possibly in the future (Badr Naga & Al-Atiyyat, 2013; Phillips, 2002). This example is presented for the reader in an attempt to demonstrate that public health nurses must also bring into their practice nursing's own unique body of knowledge.

Income Inequality

Income inequality describes where wealth is concentrated and who controls the wealth in society. Income inequality measures the degree of income variation in a population, and income inequality on a community level contributes to the loss of social capital. Social capital refers to social resources such as parks, medical facilities, schools, and economic investments that are needed to ensure that communities have the resources to maintain health (Pollack et al., 2013; Kawachi, 1999). Hence, communities with higher income are more likely to have higher social capital or resources—such as parks for their population to enjoy and enhance health—as opposed to communities with lower income and lower social capital. Income inequality also influences the average life expectancy for citizens in society.

Income inequality is either relative or absolute. Relative income inequality (growing up poor in a rich society versus growing up poor where everybody is poor) has health consequences because individuals' perceptions of the social and material world can trigger biological processes, for example stress, which can lead to a current illness such as a headache or a future illness such as heart disease. For example, a child who is from a lower-income family attends an expensive preparatory school on scholarship. This child is surrounded by students who have money and privilege. Furthermore, the child's classmates vacation in Europe, wear the latest fashions, and see a movie every weekend. The child often feels sad because he or she does not have the money to buy new clothes, go to the movies, or travel. Had this child, however, gone to the local school with children of similar economic means, he or she might have better health outcomes in the present and the future. This model posits that socioeconomic inequalities as experienced by this child may activate psychosocial factors that contribute to health and illness (Case, Darren, & Paxson, 2002; Wilkinson, 1999).

Education

Education is positively associated with employment and is an important variable in understanding the social determinants of health. For example, an individual with a college degree is more likely to have employment that is more secure, higher paying, with health benefits and has limited environmental exposures to hazards than an individual with a high-school diploma. *The New York Times* reported that staying in school for a long period of time and not smoking resulted in the best outcomes; thus, extreme education has a role in longevity (Kolata, 2007). Adults with more years of education are less likely to engage in risky health behaviors such as smoking and drinking. Additionally, more education leads to a greater sense of personal efficacy. Simply put, the number of years of schooling an individual attains has a significant effect on that persons health status (Robert Wood Johnson Foundation, 2011). Of note, educational attainment and income returns vary over time and often differ by gender, race, and ethnicity. For example, what this means is even though women may have the same educational degree and same occupation, they earn less than men because they are paid less for the same work.

Occupation

Occupation is studied less by researchers in the United States but is still an important indicator in health outcomes; Great Britain uses occupation in its analysis of health outcomes. A person's occupation tells us about his or her educational opportunities, economic independence, environmental exposures, and likely health stressors. For example, a coal miner in West Virginia has limited educational opportunities and less economic independence because he or she has skills that are unique to coal mining.

These same individuals are exposed to coal dust, which affects their lungs and can lead to illnesses such as asthma, emphysema, and chronic respiratory infections. Furthermore, coal miners experience a multitude of on-the-job stressors. Existing health problems may be worsened by stress because coal miners have less autonomy in their job and are unable to control or relieve their stress levels. A white-collar worker or executive has more education; thus his or her job is considered more prestigious. The more prestigious jobs are more likely to be held by individuals who are healthier, wealthier, and have more autonomy, which contributes to feelings of control. Furthermore, autonomy or how well one controls his or her life can improve social status and social supports and lead to better health status (Marmot & Wilkinson, 2006).

DISCRIMINATION, DISPARITY, AND HEALTH

Studies of racial and ethnic disparities find that being a member of a minority group is a risk factor for less intensive and lower quality of healthcare services (Mead, Cartwright-Smith, Jones, Ramos, Woods, & Siegel, 2008; Institute of Medicine, 2002). Racial and ethnic disparities have been consistently noted in cardiovascular procedures (LaVeist, Arthur, Plantholt, & Rubinstein, 2003), cancer diagnosis and treatment, and colorectal cancer (Cooper, Yuan, & Rimm, 1997; Shavers & Brown, 2002; Ward et al., 2004). Thinking about how discrimination harms health requires the public health nurse to consider the different experiences of those considered a dominant group, such as white men, and those considered a subordinate group, such as women. Social epidemiology considers that discrimination has an adverse effect on health, and some social epidemiologists hypothesize that discrimination actually creates a biological pathway for disease to occur in the body.

Social epidemiologists posit "inequality hurts and discrimination harms health" (Krieger, 2000, p. 36). How discrimination affects one's health status necessitates a conceptual framework that provides measurements and methods that permit an analysis of how discrimination can affect health in the present and in the future. Discrimination is the process by which people are treated differently because they are members in a particular group. Particular *isms* such as racism (bias against racial and ethnic groups), sexism (bias against women), ageism (bias against elders), heterosexism (bias against gays and lesbians), ableism (bias against disabled), and classism (bias against lower incomes) are forms of discrimination. How these *isms* become pathways for poor health is called the ecosocial theory of disease distribution. Ecosocial theory seeks to integrate the biological and social mechanisms of discrimination within a historical and multilayered analytical perspective. Ecosocial theory leads social epidemiologists to develop knowledge about (1) how a person embodies disease or how disease grows within the body, (2) the social and biological pathways that contribute to this embodiment, and (3) the cumulative interaction between exposure, susceptibility, and resistance to disease (Krieger, 2001c). Additionally, ecosocial theory examines the biological and social mechanisms of discrimination and how they become expressions for disease or poor health.

The public health nurse assesses discrimination on an individual level and a population level. The individual level examines indirect or unobserved forms of discrimination (how clinicians treat their clients differently based on race or gender) and direct forms of discrimination as reported by the client, then links these to an observable outcome measure such as uncontrolled high blood pressure, as noted in **Figure 4-3**.

On the population level, institutional discrimination is examined. Institutional discrimination refers to policies that are part of the standard working relationships of institutions. An example is corporate policies that often make it difficult for women or people of color to advance into upper management even though they are qualified. The public health nurse should always consider how the individual level and population level of discrimination contribute to poorer health outcomes as evidenced by increases in morbidity and mortality rates.

Figure 4-3 Conceptual model to understanding discrimination.

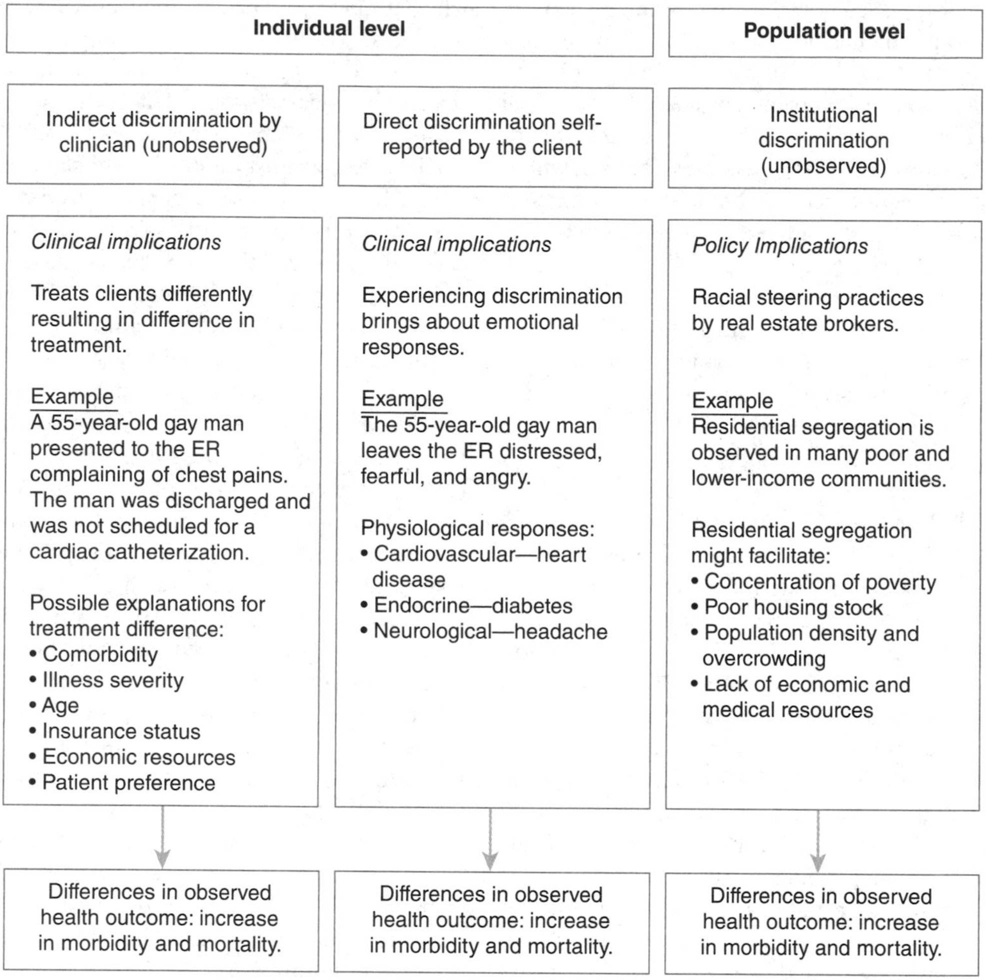

Individual level		Population level
Indirect discrimination by clinician (unobserved)	Direct discrimination self-reported by the client	Institutional discrimination (unobserved)
Clinical implications Treats clients differently resulting in difference in treatment. Example A 55-year-old gay man presented to the ER complaining of chest pains. The man was discharged and was not scheduled for a cardiac catheterization. Possible explanations for treatment difference: • Comorbidity • Illness severity • Age • Insurance status • Economic resources • Patient preference	*Clinical implications* Experiencing discrimination brings about emotional responses. Example The 55-year-old gay man leaves the ER distressed, fearful, and angry. Physiological responses: • Cardiovascular—heart disease • Endocrine—diabetes • Neurological—headache	*Policy Implications* Racial steering practices by real estate brokers. Example Residential segregation is observed in many poor and lower-income communities. Residential segregation might facilitate: • Concentration of poverty • Poor housing stock • Population density and overcrowding • Lack of economic and medical resources
Differences in observed health outcome: increase in morbidity and mortality.	Differences in observed health outcome: increase in morbidity and mortality.	Differences in observed health outcome: increase in morbidity and mortality.

Data from Krieger, N. (2000). Discrimination and health. In L. F. Berkman, I. Kawachi, & M. M. Glymour (Eds.), *Social epidemiology* (2nd ed., pp. 36–75). New York, NY: Oxford University Press.

Discrimination can tell the public health nurse how groups are treated differently. Racism is a subset of discrimination. Jones (2001) developed a framework for understanding racism on three levels: institutionalized, personally mediated, and internalized.

- Institutionalized racism describes resources that are available to certain groups in society and

their ability to access them. For example, the wait times in the emergency room in a private hospital are less than the wait times in a public hospital. Additionally, a wealthy community will have more grocery stores with fresh food than a poorer community.

- Personally mediated racism describes prejudice and discrimination as experienced by particular

Figure 4-4 Impact of racism on health outcomes.

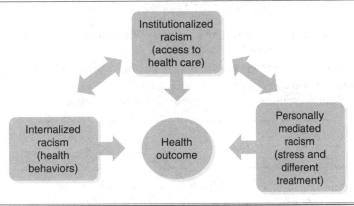

Data from Jones, C. P. (2001). Race, racism, and the practice of epidemiology. *American Journal of Epidemiology, 154*(4), 299–304.

groups of people because of their race. This type of racism can be intentional or unintentional. For example, a black student attending Yale might experience feelings of racism when a classmate asks if he or she was accepted into Yale because of the affirmative action program.

- Internalized racism describes how members of a stigmatized race accept or internalize the negative messages about their abilities. Manifestations of internalized racism might be hopelessness, self-devaluation, and other actions that reflect loss of self-esteem. For example, a child of color may play only with a white doll.

Understanding how racism exemplifies itself on all three levels gives the public health nurse an understanding of the resulting health outcomes for individuals, families, populations, and communities. **Figure 4-4** illustrates the relationship between and among the three.

Conclusion

A historical review of epidemiology looked at special events in history that facilitated the need for epidemiological practices. Furthermore, epidemiological practices evolved after each significant revolution, for example, infectious disease control versus noninfectious disease control. Today, public health nurses and other public health practitioners apply epidemiological principles and tools to systematically collect health-related data, analyze these data, interpret these data, and recommend public health actions in terms of policy initiatives that address preventing and controlling disease(s) in particular populations and communities. Descriptive and analytical epidemiology was described and explored as well as the epidemiological triad and the chain of infection. Examples were offered throughout the reading to bring this material to life for the readers.

Social epidemiology makes the case that social determinants of health, which consists of SES (income, occupation, and education), socioeconomic position, and discrimination can influence health outcomes in the future. Additionally, it is the economic and educational advantages of an individual that facilitate better health outcomes. Social epidemiologists study how social equality and inequalities contribute to the biological expression of disease and positive or negative health outcomes.

Additional Resources

Centers for Disease Control and Prevention/Principles of Epidemiology in Public Health Practice at: http://www.cdc.gov/ophss/csels/dsepd/ss1978/

World Health Organization/Epidemiology at: http://www.who.int/topics/epidemiology/en/

Robert Wood Johnson Foundation Building a Culture of Health at: http://www.rwjf.org/en/library/features /culture-of-health-prize.html?cid=xps_other_pd_ini%3Aprize2017_dte%3A20160902-2b

References

Acevedo-Garcia, D., Lochner, K. A., Osypuk, T. L., & Subramanian, S. V. (2003). Future directions in residential segregation and health research: A multilevel approach. *American Journal of Public Health, 93*(2), 215–221.

Adler, N. E., & Newman, K. (2002). Socioeconomic disparities in health: Pathways and policies. *Health Affairs, 21*(2), 60–76.

Badr Naga, B. S. H., & Al-Atiyyat, N. M. (2013). Roy adaptation model: A review. Middle East Journal of Nursing, 7(1), 58–61.

Berkman, L. F., & Kawachi, I. (2014). A historical framework for social epidemiology. In L. F. Berkman, I. Kawachi, & M. M. Glymour (Eds.), *Social epidemiology* (2nd ed. pp. 1–16). New York, NY: Oxford University Press.

Berkowitz, S. A., Traore, Y., Singer, D. E., & Atlas, S. J. (2015). Evaluating area based socioeconomic status indicators for monitoring disparities within health care systems: Results from a primary care network. *Health Services Research, 50*(2), 398–417.

Bodenheimer, T. S., & Grumbach, K. (2008). *Understanding health policy: A clinical approach* (5th ed.). New York, NY: McGraw-Hill Lange Medical Books.

Braveman, P. A., Cubbin, C., Egerter, S., Williams, D. R., & Pamuk, E. (2010). Socioeconomic disparities in health in the United States: What the patterns tell us. *American Journal of Public Health, 100*(S1), S186–S196.

Breslow, L. (2005). Origins and development of the International Epidemiological Association. *International Journal of Epidemiology, 34*, 725–729.

Carthon, M. B. (2011). Making ends meet: Community networks and health promotion among blacks in the city of brotherly love. *The American Journal of Public Health, 101*(8), 1392–1401.

Colditz, G. A., Manson, J. E., & Hankinson, S. E. (1997). The Nurses' Health Study: 20-year contribution to the understanding of health among women. *Journal of Women's Health, 6*(1), 49–62.

Condliffe, S., & Link, C. R. (2008). The relationship between economic status and child health: Evidence from the United States. *American Economic Review, 98*(4), 1605–1618.

Cooper, G. S., Yuan, Z., & Rimm, A. A. (1997). Racial disparity in the incidence and case-fatality of colorectal cancer: Analysis of 329 United States counties. *Cancer, Epidemiology, Biomarkers, & Prevention, 6*, 283–285.

Dean, H. D., Williams, K. M., & Fenton, K. A. (2013). From theory to action: Applying social determinants of health to public health practice. *Public Health Reports, 128*(Suppl. 3) 1–4.

Depietropaolo, D. L., Powers, J. H., & Gill, J. M. (2005). Diagnosis of Lyme disease. *American Family Physician, 72*(2), 297–303.

Diez-Roux, A. V. (2000). Multilevel analysis in public health research. *Annual Review of Public Health, 21*, 171–192.

Dike van de Mheen, H., Stronks, K., & Mackenbach, J. P. (1998). A lifecourse perspective on socioeconomic inequalities: The influences of childhood socioeconomic conditions and selection processes. In M. Bartley, D. Blane, & G. D. Smith (Eds.), *The sociology of health inequalities* (pp. 193–216). Oxford, UK: Blackwell.

France, D. (1999, May 4). Scientists at work: Allen C. Steere; Lyme disease expert developed the big picture of tiny tick. *The New York Times.* Retrieved from http://www.nytimes.com/1999/05/04/health/scientist-at-work-allen-c-steere-lyme-expert-developed-big-picture-of-tiny-tick.html

Galea, S., Tracy, M., Hoggatt, K. J., DiMaggio, C., & Karpati, A. (2011). Estimated deaths attributable to social factors in the United States. *American Journal of Public Health, 101*(8), 1456–1465.

Hassmiller, S. B. (2017). Nursing's role in building a culture of health. In S. B. Lewenson & M. Truglio-Londrigan (Eds.), *Practicing primary health care in nursing: Caring for populations.* (pp. 33–60). Burlington, MA: Jones & Bartlett Learning.

Herd, P., Goesling, B., & House, J. S. (2007). Socioeconomic position and health: The differential effects of education versus income on the onset versus progression of health problems. *Journal of Health and Social Behavior, 48*(3), 223–238.

Hippocrates. (400 BC). *On airs, waters, and places,* (F. Adams, Trans.). Retrieved from http://classics.mit.edu//Hippocrates/airwatpl.html

Honjo, K. (2004). Social epidemiology: Definition, history, and research examples. *Environmental Health and Preventive Medicine, 9,* 193–199.

Huang, K. Y., Cheng, S., & Theise, R. (2013). School contexts as social determinants of child health: Current practices and implications for future public health practice. *Public Health Reports, 128*(Suppl. 3) 21–28.

Hymes, K. B., Cheung, T., Greene, J. B., Prose, N. S., Marcus, A., Ballard, H., . . . Laubenstein, L. J. (1981). Kaposi's sarcoma in homosexual men—A report of eight cases. *Lancet, 318*(8247), 598–600.

Institute of Medicine. (2002). *Unequal treatment: Confronting racial and ethnic disparities in health care.* Washington, DC: Author.

The James Lind Library. (n.d.). *Treatise of scurvy.* Retrieved from http://www.jameslindlibrary.org/trial_records/17th_18th_Century/lind/lind_tp.html

Jones, C. P. (2001). Race, racism, and the practice of epidemiology. *American Journal of Epidemiology, 154*(4), 299–304.

Kaiser, P., Auchincloss, A. H., Moore, K., Sanchez, B. N., Berrocal, V., Allen, N., & Roux, A. V. (2016). Associations of neighborhood socioeconomic and racial/ethnic characteristics with changes in survey-based neighborhood quality, 2000-2011. *Health Place, 42,* 30–36.

Kannel, W. B., Schwartz, M. J., & McNamara, P. M. (1969). Blood pressure and risk of coronary heart disease: A Framingham study. *Chest, 56*(1), 43–52.

Kaplan, G. A. (2001). Economic policy is health policy: Findings from the study of income, socioeconomic status, and health. In J. A. Auerbach & B. K. Krimgold (Eds.), *Income, socioeconomic status, and health: Exploring the relationships* (pp. 137–149). Washington, DC: National Policy Association.

Kasper, J. D., Ensminger, M. E., Green, K. M., Fothergill, K. E., Juon, H. S., Robertson, J., & Thorpe, R. J. (2008). Effects of poverty and family stress over three decades on the functional status of older African American women. *Journal of Gerontology, 63B*(4), S201–S210.

Kawachi, I. (1999). Social capital and community effects on population and individual health. *Annals of New York Academy of Sciences, 896,* 120–130.

Kawachi, I. (2000). Income inequality and health. In L. F. Berkman & I. Kawachi (Eds.), *Social epidemiology* (pp. 76–94). New York, NY: Oxford University Press.

Kolata, G. (2007, January 3). A surprising secret to long life: Stay in school. *The New York Times.* Retrieved from http://www.nytimes.com/2007/01/03/health/03aging.html

Krieger, N. (2000). Discrimination and health. In L. F. Berkman & I. Kawachi (Eds.), *Social epidemiology* (pp. 36–75). New York, NY: Oxford University Press.

Krieger, N. (2001a). Theories for social epidemiology in the 21st century: An ecosocial perspective. *International Journal of Epidemiology, 30,* 668–677.

Krieger, N. (2001b). Historical roots of social epidemiology: Socioeconomic gradients in health and contextual analysis. *International Journal of Epidemiology, 30,* 899–900.

Krieger, N. (2001c). A glossary for social epidemiology. *Journal of Epidemiology and Community Health, 55,* 693–700.

Krieger, N. (2002). A glossary for social epidemiology. *Epidemiological Bulletin, 23*(1). Retrieved from http://www.paho.org/English/SHA/be_v23nl-glossary.htm

Lantz, P. M., Lynch, J. W., House, J. S., Lepkowski, J. M., Mero, R. P., Musick, M. A., & Williams, D. R. (2001). Socioeconomic disparities in health change in a longitudinal study of U.S. adults: The role of health-risk behaviors. *Social Science and Medicine, 53,* 29–40.

LaVeist, T. A., Arthur, M., Plantholt, S., & Rubinstein, M. (2003). Explaining racial differences in receipt of coronary angiography: The role of physician referral and physician specialty. *Medical Care Research and Review, 60*(4), 453–467.

Lipowicz, Koziel, S., Hulanicka, B., & Kowalisko, A. (2007). Socioeconomic status during childhood and health status in adulthood: The Wroclaw growth study. *Journal of Biosocial Science, 39*(4), 481–491.

Lynch, J., & Kaplan, G. (2000). Socioeconomic position. In L. F. Berkman & I. Kawachi (Eds.), *Social epidemiology* (pp. 13–35). New York, NY: Oxford University Press.

Marmot, M. (2000). Multilevel approaches to understanding social determinants. In L. F. Berkman & I. Kawachi (Eds.), *Social epidemiology* (pp. 349–367). New York, NY: Oxford University Press.

Marmot, M., & Wilkinson, R. (2006). *Social determinants of health* (2nd ed.). Oxford, UK: Oxford University Press.

Mead, M., Cartwright-Smith, L., Jones, K., Ramos, C., Woods, K., & Siegel, B. (2008). *Racial and ethnic disparities in U.S. health care: A chartbook* (Publication No. 1111). New York, NY: Commonwealth Fund.

Mirowsky, J., Ross, C. E., & Reynolds, J. (2000). Links between social status and health. In C. E. Bird, P. Conrad, & A. M. Fremont (Eds.), *Handbook of medical sociology* (pp. 47–78). Upper Saddle River, NJ: Prentice Hall.

Murray, L. R. (2011). Public health and primary care: Transforming the U.S. health system. *The Nation's Health, 41*(5), 3.

National Library of Medicine (n.d.). *The reports of the surgeon general: The AIDS epidemic.* Retrieved from http://profiles.nlm.nih.gov/NN/Views/Exhibit /narrative/aids.html

National Library of Medicine. (n.d.). *The reports of the surgeon general: The 1964 report on smoking and health.* Retrieved from http://profiles.nlm.nih.gov/ NN/Views/Exhibit/narrative/smoking.html

Office of History National Institute of Health. (2005). *Dr. Joseph Goldberger & the war on pellagra.* Retrieved from http://history.nih.gov/exhibits /goldberger/index.html

Pavalko, E. K., & Caputo, J. (2013). Social inequality and health across the life course. *American Behavioral Scientist, 57*(8), 1040–1056.

Perry, M., Williams, R. L., Wallerstein, N., & Waitzkin, H. (2008). Social capital and health care experiences among low-income individuals. *American Journal of Public Health, 98*(2), 330–336.

Pfettscher, S. A. (2002). Florence Nightingale: Modern nursing. In A. M. Tomey & M. R. Alligood (Eds.), *Nursing theorists and their work* (5th ed., pp. 65–83). Philadelphia, PA: Mosby.

Phillips, K. D. (2002). Sister Callista Roy: Adaptation model. In A. M. Tomey & M. R. Alligood (Eds.), *Nursing theorists and their work* (5th ed., pp. 269–298). Philadelphia, PA: Mosby.

Piccolo, R. S., Duncan, D. T., Pearce, N., & McKinlay, J. B. (2015). The role of neighborhood characteristics in racial/ethnic disparities in type 2 diabetes: Results from the Boston Area Community Health (BACH) survey. *Social Science Medicine, 130,* 79–90.

Pineda, M. D., White, E., Kristal, A. R., & Taylor, V. (2001). Asian breast cancer survival in the U.S.: A comparison between Asian immigrants, U.S.-born Asian Americans, and Caucasians. *International Journal of Epidemiology, 30,* 976–982.

Pollack, C. E., Cubbin, C., Sania, A., Hayward, M., Vallone, D., Flaherty, B., & Braveman, P. A. (2013). Do wealth disparities contribute to health disparities within racial/ethnic groups? *Journal of Epidemiology and Community Health, 67*(5), 439–45.

Pronyk, P. M., Harpham, T., Morison, L. A., Hargreaves, J. R., Kim, J. C., Phetla, G.,. . . Porter, J. D. (2008). Is social capital associated with HIV risk in rural South Africa? *Social Science and Medicine, 66*(9), 1999–2010.

Putnam, R. D. (1995). Bowling alone: America's declining social capital. *Journal of Democracy, 6,* 65–78.

Robert Wood Johnson Foundation. (2011). *Issue brief series: Exploring the social determinants of health— education and health.* Retrieved from http://www .rwjf.org/en/library/research/2011/05/education -matters-for-health.html

Robert Wood Johnson Foundation. (2014). *Time to act: Investing in the health of our children and communities.* Retrieved from http://www.rwjf.org/en/library /research/2014/01/recommendations-from-the -rwjf-commission-to-build-a-healthier-am.html

Sadana, R., & Blas, E. (2013). What can public health programs do to improve health equity? *Public Health Reports, 128*(Suppl. 3) 12–20.

Schneiderman, N., Ironson, G., & Siegel, S. D. (2005). STRESS AND HEALTH: Psychological, Behavioral, and Biological Determinants. *Annual Reviews Clinical Psychology, 1*, 607–628.

Sepkowitz, K. A. (2001). AIDS—The first 20 years. *New England Journal of Medicine, 344*(23), 1764–1772.

Sepkowitz, K. A. (2008). One disease, two epidemics—AIDS at 25. *New England Journal of Medicine, 354*(23), 2411–2414.

Shavers, V. L., & Brown, M. L. (2002). Racial and ethnic disparities in the receipt of cancer treatment. *Journal of the National Cancer Institute, 94*(5), 334–357.

Stephan, E. (n.d.). *John Graunt*. Retrieved from http://www.edstephan.org/Graunt/graunt.html

Stotts, R. C. (2008). *Epidemiology and public health nursing*. Clifton Park, NJ: Delmar Cengage Learning.

Stringhini, S., Sabia, S., Shipley, M., Bruner, E., Nabi, H., Kivimaki, M., & Singh-Manoux, A. (2010). Association of socioeconomic position with health behaviors and mortality. The Whitehall II study. *Journal of American Medical Association, 303*(12), 1159–1166.

Subramanian, S. V., Kawachi, I., & Kennedy, B. P. (2001). Does the state you live in make a difference? Multilevel analysis of self-rated health in the U.S. *Social Science & Medicine, 53*, 9–19.

Tarzian, A. J. (2005). Epidemiology: Unraveling the mysteries of disease and health. In F. A. Maurer & C. M. Smith (Eds.), *Community/public health nursing practice: Health for families and populations* (3rd ed., pp. 150–174). St. Louis, MO: Elsevier Saunders.

UCLA Department of Epidemiology School of Public Health. (n.d.). *John Snow*. Retrieved from http://www.ph.ucla.edu/epi/snow.html

U.S. Department of Health and Human Services (DHHS) & Centers for Disease Control and Prevention (CDC). (1998). *Principles of epidemiology: An introduction to applied epidemiology and biostatistics* (2nd ed.). Atlanta, GA: Author.

U.S. Department of Health and Human Services (DHHS) & Centers for Disease Control and Prevention (CDC). (2011). *Principles of epidemiology: An introduction to applied epidemiology and biostatistics* (3rd ed.). Atlanta, GA: Author.

U.S. Preventive Services Task Force. (2008). *Guide to clinical preventive services: Recommendations of the U.S. Preventive Services Task Force*. Rockville, MD: Agency for Healthcare and Research Quality.

Wald, L. (1902). The nurses' settlement in New York. *American Journal of Nursing, 2*(8), 567–575.

Wald, L. D. (1913, June 23). Visiting nurses? NOPHN ? First annual meeting, Atlantic City, June 23, 1913. [The title of this paper is handwritten and accompanied by a question mark]. Found in Lillian D. Wald Papers, 1889-1957. Writing and Speeches. Reel 25, Box 36, Folder 6, p. 1. New York Public Library, Humanities and Social Sciences Library, Manuscripts and Archives Division, New York.

Ward, E., Jemal, A., Cokkinides, V., Singh, G. K., Cardinez, C., Ghafoor, G., & Thun, M. (2004). Cancer disparities by race/ethnicity and socioeconomic status. *CA Cancer Journal for Clinicians, 54*, 78–93.

Wilkinson, R. (1999). Income distribution and life expectancy. In I. Kawachi, B. Kennedy, & R. Wilkinson (Eds.), *The society and population health reader: Income inequality and health* (pp. 28–35). New York, NY: The New Press.

For a full suite of assignments and additional learning activities, use the access code located in the front of your book to visit this exclusive website: http://go.jblearning.com/londrigan. If you do not have an access code, you can obtain one at the site.

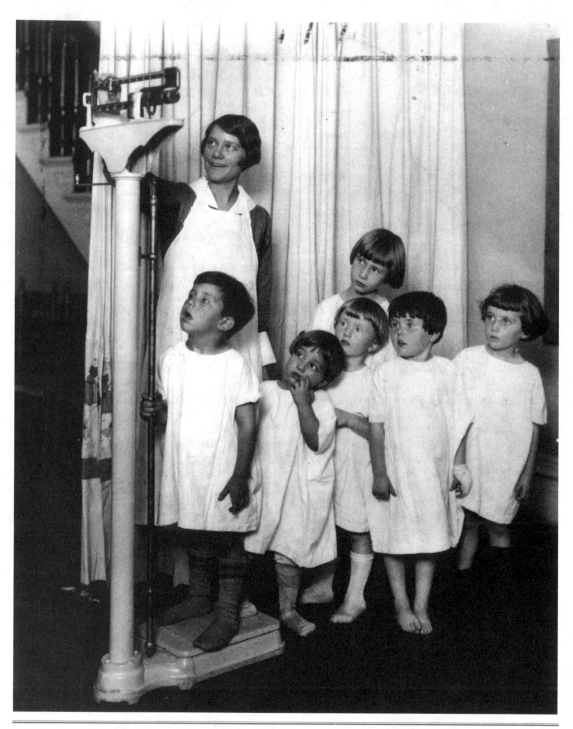

A public health nurse weighing children, 1930. Courtesy of the Visiting Nurse Service of New York.

CHAPTER 5

Educating Public Health Nurses to Do the Work

Judith Quaranta
Fran Srnka-Debnar
Shai Lev

. . . the nurse no longer feels herself qualified to care for people unless she has been trained to recognize and report symptoms other than those of her patient. Instruction in measures for protection and relief in housing, on labor legislation, on school laws, is a necessary part of her equipment, and above and beyond all is the personal and spiritual attitude, and the realization that she is not only serving the individual, but promotion the interests of collective society. (Wald, 1913, June 25, p. 2)

LEARNING OBJECTIVES

At the completion of this chapter, the reader will be able to:

- Describe public health nursing education.
- Identify challenges to public health nursing and public health nursing education.
- Analyze the relationship between interprofessional education and public health nursing education.
- Examine the benefits of participating in community-engaged learning.

KEY TERMS

- ❑ Community engaged learning
- ❑ Community partnerships
- ❑ Interprofessional education
- ❑ Nursing's social policy statement
- ❑ Population-focused care
- ❑ Public health nursing education
- ❑ The Association of Community Health Nursing Educators (ACHNE)
- ❑ Quad Council

State of Public Health

The U.S. healthcare system is facing many unique challenges that threaten the well-being of the population. Although antibiotics and vaccine development have minimized the impact of infectious disease in the past, we are now faced with antibiotic-resistant diseases and newly emerging infectious diseases. Zika, pandemic flu, *Escherichia coli* O104:H4, Ebola, resistant tuberculosis, and gonorrhea are some of the conditions greatly influencing the health of populations. Environmental factors, both natural and man-made, create hazards throughout the lifespan. Lead toxicity, as reported in Flint, Michigan, highlights the severe health risks posed, potentially impacting more than 26,000 children (Save the Children, 2016). In addition, lifestyles of modern society have created unprecedented levels of obesity for both adults and children, impacting nearly one-third of adults and 17% of children. This leads to chronic disease development and the need for health-promoting behavior, prevention, and better management (Ogden, Carroll, Kit, & Flegal, 2014). War and terrorism have challenged our healthcare system, with increasing incidence of posttraumatic stress disorders, as well as severe physical impairments, including traumatic amputations, sensory deficits, and disfiguring injuries. Nearly 4 million veterans reported a service-related disability in 2014 (U.S. Census Bureau, n.d.). It is striking that in today's society, gun violence is a leading cause of premature death, resulting in almost 30,000 deaths and 60,000 injuries each year (American Public Health Association, 2016).

Health promotion and disease prevention have taken the forefront as healthcare costs have soared, highlighting the need to gain control of these issues. In addition, lack of affordable health insurance with the consequent large number of uninsured individuals poses challenges to achieving good health outcomes. Public health nurses are well situated to address these crises and promote health and wellness for our communities. It is imperative that nurses and nursing students are well versed in these areas and understand the overreaching impact they have on these all-encompassing problems facing us today.

Table 5-1 **Centers for Disease Control 2016 Health Threats**

Ebola	Antibiotic resistance
Global health security	Smoking and tobacco use
Prescription drug overdose	Lab safety

Data from Centers for Disease Control and Prevention. (2015). *2015: What kept us up at night and what will keep us busy in 2016.* Retrieved from http://www.cdc.gov/media/dpk/2015/dpk-eoy.html

See **Table 5-1** for Centers for Disease Control and Prevention 2016 Health Threats.

What Is Public Health Nursing?

The practice of public health nursing promotes and protects the health of populations by using knowledge from nursing, social, and public health sciences. It is a specialty practice that embodies knowledge about advocacy, policy development, and planning (American Public Health Association, Public Health Nursing Section [APHA], 2013).

Population-focused care, the defining characteristic of public health nursing, provides interventions, using an ecological framework and systems approach, to individuals, families, communities, populations, and the systems that impact their health (APHA, 2013). A thorough understanding of the environmental, social, and physical determinants guides the public health nurse address inequities and provide focus on improving population health.

Implementation of the Patient Protection and Affordable Care Act (PPACA) impacts public health nursing. Public health nurses are called upon to provide the skills and the leadership necessary to implement the health promotion and prevention requirements of the PPACA (Quad Council, 2012). As the focus of the healthcare arena will be primary health care, positions requiring the expertise of public health nurses will be needed in acute care and community agencies. The public health nurse will be instrumental in providing population-focused care, addressing the needs for self-managing chronic diseases, and advocating health promotion interventions. The educational preparation of public health nurses position these professionals to facilitate the collaborative efforts needed to bring all key players to the table—including the population—to form a proactive team. Public health nurses are well versed in partnering with not only members of the health-care team but with their clients as well, including individuals, families, communities, and populations.

Status of Public Health Nurses in the United States

The need for a strong public health nursing workforce has become increasingly evident in recent years. This need has occurred because of ongoing national events that have demonstrated the importance of emergency preparedness along with renewed attention on health promotion, risk factor reduction, and early detection of diseases and emerging infections in all areas. These events call for a stronger public health infrastructure requiring more and better educated public health nurses (American Public Health Association, 2014a). An alarming statistic, according to both the 2000 U.S. Census and the 2008 American Community Survey, less than 1% of nurses work in a public health setting. However, this does represent a 23% increase from 2000 to 2008 (Health Resources and Services Administration [HRSA], 2013).

Public health nursing comprises the largest discipline within the public health work force. At this time, the current public health nursing workforce shortage is the worst ever experienced in the United States. The ratio of public health nurses to population has decreased by more than 25% between 1980 and 2000 (Quad Council, 2013). The estimated total employment of registered nurses by local health departments decreased by approximately 5,000 full-time equivalent employees between 2008 and 2013 (National Association of County and City Health Officials, 2013).

Many factors contribute to the public health nursing workforce shortage. Already challenged by a general nursing shortage nationally, lower public health nurses' salaries are not competitive with salaries for nurses in acute care, resulting in fewer graduates seeking public health nursing as a career option. The low percentage of baccalaureate-prepared nurses in the overall nursing workforce, compounded by a shortage of faculty prepared to teach this specialty, add to the difficulty of meeting the needs for public health. Additionally, a lack of promotional and training opportunities challenges recruitment and retention of qualified public health nurses (National Association of County and City Health Officials, 2015; Quad Council, 2013). To compound the issue, nursing is confronted with an aging workforce. About one third of the nursing workforce is older than 50, with the average age of nurses increasing by almost two years, raising the issue of impending retirements and a decreased workforce (HRSA, 2013).

Public Health Nursing Education

The American Public Health Association (2014b) recommends integration of **public health education** into undergraduate curricula, which is supported by the 2003 Institute of Medicine (IOM) report. These core curricula include introductory coursework in public health, epidemiology, and global health, using integrative interdisciplinary approaches. In addition, local public health practitioners should participate in the teaching of these undergraduate courses. This will result in graduates having skills to critically examine public health issues, understand the importance of public health interventions, and be able to develop public health messages in the media geared to targeted populations. Many schools have reflected upon their traditional community health nursing courses and, based on recommendations from leaders in the field and various organizations, altered not only the content of their course but delivery as well. This evolution of course work represents the changing definitions of public health nursing as well as the maturing educational pedagogy of our time. The following case study provides such an example.

Example of Reflections and Evaluation Leading to Course Evolution

CASE STUDY	**Population Health Teaching Strategies: Enhancing the Relevance** Vicki Simpson, PhD, RN, CHES Assistant Professor Purdue University School of Nursing Fellow, Purdue University Teaching Academy

As healthcare transitions from acute care settings to the community, helping nursing students understand and apply population health concepts and approaches is vital. A BSN program in the Midwest had noted that students taking the school's public health science course alongside junior-level medical-surgical courses did not see the content as relevant to nursing. This course provided support for a senior-level public health nursing course and was generally rated poorly by students. Additionally, faculty for the senior-level public health nursing course indicated that students did not appear to retain the content taught the previous year. To address these issues further, faculty decided to revise the course and teaching strategies while an overall curriculum revision was underway. To increase student understanding and application of population health principles in their approach to nursing practice, faculty made three major changes.

The first change was to move the course from the junior year to the sophomore year based on the hope that provision of the content earlier in the curriculum would allow the students time to apply the concepts as they began their foundational nursing courses. Second, using current literature and national guidelines, the course was renamed "population health." Last, based upon the learning styles and preferences of the student population and with the support of a university-wide initiative, faculty decided to use active learning strategies to improve student engagement.

Faculty designed the course as a flipped design; material traditionally provided in class is completed online as preparation for in-class activities. Online content is delivered via multiple methods, including voice-over PowerPoints, videos, web quests, and text readings. Students attend class every other week, taking a quick five-point quiz using iClicker at the start of class to ensure the prep work has been completed. Classrooms used for the class are designed to support active learning strategies and include small group tables with computer access, whiteboards, and enhanced technology. During class, students are randomly assigned to groups of four to five to complete in-class activities while faculty circulate around the room answering questions and challenging the students to think critically and use a population frame of reference. In-class activities include web quests, case studies, and guided use of public health data using sites such as *Healthy People 2020* and County Health Rankings. At the end of each class, students share content learned with the entire class, using tools such as prezi.com and bubbl.us. Additionally, throughout the course, reflective journaling is used to encourage the students to critically think about complex issues such as social determinants, health disparities, environmental health, and global health challenges.

Since the revision, course ratings have dramatically increased. Students report they enjoy working together in class to learn the content. Students additionally indicate that the class supports a stronger understanding of population health issues and their relevance to nursing practice. Although this approach initially requires time to develop, faculty involved also report increased satisfaction with the course.

Recommended educational preparation for entry-level public health nurses is the baccalaureate degree (ACHNE, 2009; APHA; 2013; Quad Council of Public Health Nursing Organizations, 2011). However, only 55% of the RN workforce holds a bachelor's or higher degree (HRSA, 2013). *The Essentials of Baccalaureate Education for Professional Nursing Practice* (American Association of Colleges of Nursing [AACN], 2008) specify the educational framework for the preparation of professional nurses and emphasize the fundamental concepts needed for public health nursing practice. These include clinical prevention; population health; healthcare policy, finance, and regulatory environments; and interprofessional collaboration. Nursing students will graduate from their programs with the ability to conduct population and community assessments and apply principles of epidemiology.

Advanced degrees in nursing are encouraged. Nurses with master's degrees or higher have the knowledge and the expertise required for leadership positions. Competencies include interprofessional collaboration, health policy and advocacy, population assessment, prevention strategies, and program planning and evaluation. The doctor of nursing practice (DNP) provides executive leadership, systems development, and translation of research into practice. The doctor of philosophy (PhD) develops the science relevant to public health nursing and generates evidence needed to guide practice (APHA, 2013). Certification in public health nursing is available through the American Nurses Credentialing Center (ANCC) through portfolio submission. Eligible candidates must have practiced two years (or equivalent) as a registered nurse, hold a graduate degree, practiced a minimum of 2,000 hours in advanced public health nursing, and completed a minimum of 30 continuing education hours in advanced public health applicable to nursing in the past three years. Successful candidates earn the credentials of APHN-BC (ANCC, 2016).

Unfortunately, gaps exist in the education and training of public health nurses.

In state and local health departments, 29% of individual nurses do not hold a bachelor's degree in nursing, the entry-level qualification for public health nursing practice. Approximately 12% of nurses in state and local health departments have an advanced degree at the master's level and less than 1% hold a doctoral degree (APHA, 2014c; University of Michigan, 2013).

The Association of Community Health Nursing Educators

The Association of Community Health Nursing Educators (ACHNE) developed *Essentials of Baccalaureate Nursing Education for Entry Level Community/Public Health Nursing Practice* (ACHNE, 2009). Objectives of this document are: (1) to provide a framework for nursing educators in planning and implementing baccalaureate nursing curricula relevant to 21st-century healthcare systems and (2) to communicate to the nursing, public health, and other communities, the theoretical and clinical practice underpinnings necessary for community/public health nursing education and practice (p. 3). The core competencies, which are community and population focused, are based on a synthesis of the science, values, and practice of nursing and public health, with emphasis on global health, disaster preparedness, emerging and reemerging infections, and environmental health (p. 4). Furthermore, in 2007, ACHNE developed *Graduate Education for Advanced Practice Public Health Nursing: At the Crossroads.* This position paper offers a vision for graduate education for the advanced practice public health nursing (APPHN). The complexity of our contemporary society along with the burgeoning public health issues presents a very real need for nurses with advanced knowledge and skills to address these issues. Examples of content for the APPHN include population-centered nursing theory and practice, leadership, biostatistics, epidemiology, environmental health sciences, health policy, social and behavioral sciences, public health informatics, genomics, communication, community-based participatory research, and ethics and law (ACHNE, 2001).

The Quad Council of Public Health Nursing Organizations—Quad Council

The Quad Council of Public Health Nursing Organizations is composed of ACHNE, the Association of State and Territorial Directors of Nursing (ASTDN), APHA public health nursing section, and the American Nurses Association's Congress on Nursing Practice and Economics (ANA). The Council was founded in the 1980s to address priorities for public health nursing education, practice, leadership, and research, and to be the voice for public health nursing. In 2010, revision of the core competencies for public health nursing was undertaken. These competencies are applicable to agencies employing public health nurses, as well as educational institutions and other agencies involved in educating public health nurses (Quad Council, 2011).

The Quad Council Core Competencies covers both generalist and advanced public health nursing practice by incorporating three tiers of practice: basic or generalist (tier 1), specialist or midlevel (tier 2), and executive or multisystem (tier 3). The tiers are defined on a continuum, so public health nursing practice in each tier assumes mastery of the competencies of the previous tier. In addition, there are eight domains, which include analytic assessment, policy development/program planning, communication, competency, community dimensions of practice, basic public health science, financial planning and management, and leadership and systems thinking. The domains include specific tasks and duties for each of the three tiers. These competencies reflect the standards for public health nursing practice. They are written to be demonstrable and measurable and reflect the minimum competency at each of the three tiers of practice (Cravetz, Krothe, Reyes, & Swider, 2011; see **Table 5-2**).

Table 5-2 **Examples of Competencies for Selected Domains**

Tier 1	Tier 2	Tier 3
Analytic and Assessment Skills		
Identifies determinants of health and illness of individuals and families.	Assesses health status of populations; partners with stakeholders to interpret data.	Conducts comprehensive system/organizational assessment related to population health.
Policy Development		
Identifies policy issues relevant to the health of individuals, families, and groups.	Identifies data relevant to health policies and uses policy analysis to address specific public health issues.	Establishes methods to collect and analyze public health and public policy information.
Public Health Sciences Skills		
Incorporates public health and nursing science in delivery of care to individuals, families, and groups.	Utilizes public health and nursing science in practice at population and community level.	Serves as an expert in utilizing public health and nursing science in the design of public health practice environments.
Financial Management		
Describes interrelationships among local, state, tribal, and federal public health and healthcare systems.	Collaborates with relevant public and/or private systems for managing programs in public health.	Identified funding sources and support to meet community and population health needs.

Data from Quad Council of Public Health Nursing Organizations. (2011). Quad Council competencies for public health nurses. *Quad Council of Public Health Nursing Organizations.*

Tier 1 core competencies apply to generalist public health nurses, not in management positions, who carry out daily functions in state and local public health organizations. These functions include clinical, home visits, and population-based services. Responsibilities of the public health nurse may include working directly with at risk populations, carrying out health-promotion programs at all levels of prevention, basic data collection and analysis, field work, program planning, outreach activities, programmatic support, and other tasks in their organization. Public health nurses apply these skills and competencies in the care of individuals, families, or groups (Cravetz et al., 2011).

Tier 2 core competencies apply to public health nurses with responsibilities for program implementation, management, and/or supervisory responsibilities of generalist public health nurses. These responsibilities may include implementation and oversight of personnel; clinical, family-focused and population-based health services; program and budget development; establishing and managing community relations; establishing timelines and work plans; and presenting recommendations on policy issues. These skills and competencies reflect practice primarily with communities or populations (Cravetz et al., 2011).

Tier 3 core competencies apply to public health nurses who are at an executive/senior management level or in leadership roles in public health organizations. They are responsible for oversight and administration of programs or operation of an organization. This would include setting the vision and the strategy for an organization and its structural units. They are at a high level of positional authority within the organization and possess a higher level knowledge, an advanced education, and more experience than tier 2 public health nurses. They reflect organizational- and systems-level public health nursing leadership (Cravetz et al., 2011).

Public Health Nursing Education, Nursing's Social Policy Statement, Code of Ethics

The essence of public health nursing is embedded within **Nursing's Social Policy Statement** (American Nurses Association, 2010). One of the six key areas of health care addressed in the document is provision for the public's health. This area focuses attention on the health promotion, disease prevention, and environmental measures interventions needed to assist self-help measures by the individual, family, group, community, or population.

Nursing has a long history of concern for the welfare of the ill, injured, and vulnerable as well as for social justice. This is embodied in the provision of nursing care to individuals, families, groups, the population, and communities for the prevention of illness protection and promotion of health. *The Code of Ethics for Nurses*, developed by the American Nurses Association, forms the foundation to guide public health nurses in their decisions and conduct (Fowler, 2008). Nursing has historically engaged in socially relevant, social justice-type activities since Lillian Wald's Henry Street Settlement (Lewenson & Nickitas, 2016).

The principles that guide public health nursing include autonomy, dignity, and the rights of individuals. Assuring confidentiality and applying ethical standards are critical in advocating for health and social policy. Serious disparities in health exist in the United States and at the global level. To address these disparities, public health is shifting to focus on disparities and the underlying social determinants of health such as poverty. Public health nurses have an obligation to care for the well-being of others and protecting the public. Critical to meeting that role requires an understanding of healthy populations, which in turn entails a concern for healthy individuals. In a restructured healthcare system that engages new advances in technology and genetics, it further underscores the imperative to provide ethical care and respect human rights. Public health nurses must be in the forefront of providing care that reflects an ethical base and a rights-based approach to practice with populations (Savage et al., 2016).

Interprofessional Education

In the late 1960s and early 1970s, the term *interdisciplinary education* began to be discussed in the medical and nursing journals (Fairman, 2016). Fairman explains that, "Its meaning has changed over time from one profession teaching another, to learning together or from each other in informal settings, to our current, more structured, and formal understanding" (p. 110). The World Health Organization (WHO) defines the term **interprofessional education** as two or more students from different professions learning about, from, and with each other to enable effective collaboration and improve health outcomes. The goal of interprofessional education is to produce a health workforce prepared to collaborate in new and different ways to yield positive impacts on the health of individuals, the communities in which they live, and the health systems that care for them (WHO, 2010). The American Association of Colleges of Nursing, American Association of Colleges of Osteopathic Medicine, American Association of Colleges of Pharmacy, American Dental Education Association of American Medical Colleges, and Association of Schools of Public Health, comprising the Interprofessional Educational Collaborative, developed interprofessional competencies for health professions students to ready them for team-based care, envisioning this collaborative

preparation as key to safe, high-quality, accessible, patient-centered care. **Box 5-1** provides a listing of these competencies.

Interprofessional learning prepares health professions students to deliberatively and with intention work together with the common goal of building a safer and better patient-centered and community/population-oriented U.S. healthcare system. Collaborative practice occurs when health workers from different professional backgrounds provide comprehensive services by working with patients, their families, caregivers, and communities to deliver the highest quality of care across settings (Interprofessional Educational Collaborative [IPEC], 2011). These competencies highlight the realization that in order to achieve improvement in health, collaboration with professionals well versed in public health needs to occur to facilitate addressing environmental and social determinants of health, prevention, and early detection with both a patient-centered and community/population health orientation. See the following case study for an example of a global interprofessional educational initiative.

Box 5-1 Principles of Interprofessional Competencies

- Patient/family centered
- Community/population oriented
- Relationship focused
- Process oriented
- Linked to learning activities, educational strategies, and behavioral assessments that are developmentally appropriate for the learner
- Able to integrate across the learning continuum
- Sensitive to the systems context/applicable across practice settings
- Stated in language common and meaningful across the professions
- Outcome driven

Reproduced from Interprofessional Education Collaborative Expert Panel. (2011). *Core competencies for interprofessional collaborative practice: Report of an expert panel.* Washington, DC: Association of American Medical Colleges.

<table>
<tr><td>**CASE STUDY**</td><td>Sustainable Interdisciplinary and Interprofessional Approaches to Clean Water in Developing Countries
Vicki Simpson, PhD, RN, CHES
Assistant Professor
Purdue University School of Nursing</td></tr>
</table>

Global health problems are very complex and challenging. Developing sustainable solutions to global health problems such as access to clean water must be addressed from multiple perspectives. A group of faculty and students from a Midwestern university (graduate and undergraduate) took on the challenge of providing access to clean water for a poor rural community in the Dominican Republic. In an effort to address all aspects of this issue, the group included students and faculty from engineering (civil, industrial, environmental, and ecological), nursing, agricultural economics, food science, and biological sciences. This student-driven service learning class worked with a nongovernmental organization (NGO) to find a community in need. In collaboration with the population residing within that community, an assessment was completed to determine the needs of the community and the population within that community, how they interacted with and accessed water, the cleanliness of water being used for drinking and cooking, and the current health issues being faced by the population and community. The assessment identified multiple health issues, particularly for women and children, related to unclean water and a large economic impact due to the cost of purchasing water for drinking and cooking, most of which tested positive for bacteria and parasites. In addition, the faculty/student group identified many local leaders, families, and healthcare providers at the local community clinic who were interested in being involved in the development of a system to provide clean water for the community.

Over a span of three years, many trips were made by the faculty/students to establish a relationship and develop trust with the community, which are so crucial to projects such as this. During these visits, the students and faculty spent long days interacting with the people residing within the community; community members provided lunches and dinners as well as many events to involve us in activities that were important to them and reflected their culture. Over this time, with our support, they developed a governance structure (El Patronato) for the water system and identified a location at the community's primary school. With the help of the university group and the funding they obtained, a water system was built using locally available materials and labor. The system was designed to require minimal maintenance and generate enough water to support the school and the nearby community. Excess water could be sold to the surrounding community at a cost far lower than most were currently paying for water, with the funds generated by the sales supporting the maintenance of the system. A ribbon-cutting ceremony and celebration were held with the community to taste the first water generated by the system. Several other ideas were carried out in tandem with this project: 1) a health curriculum concerning safe water use and hygiene for the children was developed and provided to the teachers at the school; 2) the governance group was trained on use of the system including maintenance; 3) the population residing within the community was taught about bacteria, viruses, and parasites that are common in the water in that region along with the signs and symptoms of water-related illnesses as well as safe water use and storage; and 4) a collaboration was created with the local community health clinic to monitor for any changes in health outcomes. This system has been running now for two years. There have been some issues, predominantly related to communication and the taste of the ground water used by the system as compared with the rainwater which they often drink. The children adapted rather quickly to the taste difference, whereas the adults have been much slower to adjust, with many refusing to drink the water from the system. This was an issue that the university group had not considered and one that we continue

(continues)

to address with the community; we are currently collaborating with the community to bring rainwater into the system in addition to ground water.

A great deal was learned by the community, faculty, and students from the completion of the first water system. We continue to learn as we enter our fourth year of the project. This knowledge is being used as we continue with plans to build three more systems at other schools in the region and as we continue to work with the existing system so that it is used to its full capacity. Community members from the original site are collaborating with us as we develop relationships with the nearby communities. It is our hope to build a network of water systems so that these communities can work together to provide access to clean water for all.

We have gained far more than we have given throughout this project. Students and faculty have worked together to obtain awards and grant funding to support travel and purchase of the materials and labor needed to build the water systems. The students have gained grant writing, presentation, teamwork, and leadership skills. They have learned to value the contributions of multiple professions and disciplines to projects such as these, truly working as a team to build and implement these water systems. Above all, we have gained humility and respect for the people of the Dominican Republic who have allowed us to work with them and experience true collaboration with a global community.

Public health nurses are vital to the interprofessional teams to ensure and assure that all people have equitable access to high-quality care and health environments. Their assessment skills, primary prevention focus, and system-level perspectives can assure that programs are coordinated and communities are engaged (APHA, 2013). Nursing education focusing on public health intersects with the emphasis on chronic disease management and behavioral change put forth by the ACA and Institutes of Medicine reports (IPEC, 2011). With public health nurses now embedded within communities, they are well positioned to enact the goals of the ACA, including improving the health of populations and reducing the cost of health care.

Inadequate interprofessional preparation of health professionals has been implicated in many adverse outcomes, including lower provider and patient satisfaction, greater numbers of medical errors and patient safety issues, low workforce retention, system inefficiencies resulting in higher costs, and suboptimal community engagement. Unfortunately, the health, welfare, and social care sectors often have been slow to implement team-based care and interprofessional education that is necessary to support and improve collaboration (IOM, 2015).

The American Association of Colleges of Nursing (AACN) has integrated interprofessional collaboration behavioral expectations into its *Essentials* for baccalaureate (2008), master's (2011), and doctoral education for advanced practice (2006). *Baccalaureate Essential VI* focuses on interprofessional communication and collaboration for improving patient health outcomes (AACN, 2008), emphasizing that communication and collaboration among healthcare professionals are critical to delivering high-quality and safe patient care. The *Faculty Tool Kit for the Essentials of Baccalaureate Education for Professional Nursing Practice* suggests strategies and activities for achieving this outcome. **Box 5-2** contains some of these strategies. *Master's Essential VII* focuses on interprofessional collaboration for improving patient and population health outcomes. This *Essential* recognizes that the master's-prepared nurse, as a member and leader of interprofessional teams, communicates, collaborates, and consults with other health professionals to manage and coordinate care. The master's-degree graduate is educated to be a member and a leader of interprofessional healthcare teams, understanding others profession's scope of practice, employing collaborative strategies for patient-centered care (AACN, 2011).

Box 5-2 Strategies to Address Essential VI Baccalaureate Education: Interprofessional Communication and Collaboration for Improving Patient Health Outcomes

- Case studies with various healthcare and other professionals.
- Grand rounds, community coalition meetings.
- Interprofessional and intraprofessional teams for course assignments and simulation labs.
- Interprofessional community projects.

Modified from American Association of Colleges of Nursing. (2009). *Nurse faculty tool kit for the implementation of the Baccalaureate Essentials.* Retrieved from http://www.aacn.nche.edu/education-resources /BacEssToolkit.pdf

DNP *Essential VI* expands on the master's essential, again focusing on interprofessional collaboration for improving patient and population health outcomes. DNP graduates have preparation in methods of effective team leadership to play a central role in establishing interprofessional teams, participating in the work of the team, and assuming leadership of the team when appropriate (AACN, 2006).

Several challenges confront implementation of interprofessional education. Top administrative support is needed to create the experiences essential for interprofessional education. Access to other professional schools interested in integrating interprofessional education into their curriculums is crucial. Scheduling and finding time to bring students together across the professions can be problematic. Health professions faculty need training to become effective interprofessional educators. The content and process of interprofessional learning differ from other academic content they teach. There is also a need for assessment instruments to evaluate interprofessional experience. In addition, there is a lack of regulatory expectations by accrediting bodies for health professions that would reinforce the need to establish interprofessional education within their institutions (IPEC, 2011).

Community-Engaged Learning

Community-engaged learning provides students hands-on, real-life experiences while benefitting the community and its health. Community engagement, or service learning, is experiential learning consisting of mutually beneficial collaboration between institutions of higher education and the communities. It is a teaching and learning strategy that integrates community service with instruction and reflection to enrich the learning experience, teach civic responsibility, and strengthen communities. Community engagement enriches scholarship, research, and creative activities, as well as enhancing teaching and learning, offering community partners opportunities to address significant needs. Students participating in community-engaged learning develop a strengthened sense of civic responsibility with a greater ability to address critical societal issues (New England Resource Center for Higher Education, n.d.; Vanderbilt University, 2016). These community-campus partnership relationships are relationship focused and committed to mutual learning and are based in specific principles outlined in **Box 5-3**.

Outcomes for this relationship must be tangible and relevant, including eliminating health disparities with a greater sense of social justice (CCPH Board of Directors, 2013).

Community-engagement learning occurs within courses through projects that have both learning and community action goals. Projects meet the needs of not only the learner but also the community partner as well, with the design of the project the result of collaboration between faculty, students, and community partners. The project allows students to apply course content to community-based activities. This gives students experiential opportunities to learn in real-world contexts and develop skills of community engagement while offering community partners opportunities to address significant needs (Vanderbilt University, 2016). At the end of this chapter, there is an extensive example of a community-engagement service learning course along with student outcomes.

Box 5-3 Principles of Community-Campus Partnerships

1. The partnership forms to serve a specific purpose.
2. The partnership agrees upon goals, measurable outcomes, and processes for accountability.
3. The relationship between partners is characterized by mutual trust, respect, genuineness, and commitment.
4. The partnership builds upon identified strengths and assets.
5. Partners make clear and open communication an ongoing priority in the partnership by striving to understand each other's needs and self-interests, and developing a common language.
6. Principles and processes for the partnership are established with the input and agreement of all partners, especially for decision-making and conflict resolution.
7. There is feedback among all stakeholders in the partnership, with the goal of continuously improving the partnership and its outcomes.
8. Partners share the benefits of the partnership's accomplishments.
9. The partnership values multiple kinds of knowledge and life experiences.

Modified from Community-Campus Partnerships for Health, CCPH Board of Directors. (2013). Position statement on authentic partnerships. Retrieved from https://ccph.memberclicks.net/principles-of-partnership

---

Box 5-4 Faculty Benefits in Teaching Community-Engaged Service Learning Courses

Encourage interactive teaching methods and reciprocal learning between students and faculty.

Add new insights and dimensions to class discussions.

Lead to new avenues for research and publication.

Promote students' active learning; engage students with different learning styles.

Promote students' opportunities to directly apply course content to theory, thus creating a deeper level of understanding.

Boost course enrollment by attracting highly motivated and engaged students.

Foster relationships between faculty and community organizations, which can open other opportunities for collaborative work.

Provide firsthand knowledge of community issues; provide opportunities to be more involved in community issues.

Modified from Center for Civic Engagement at Binghamton University (2015). Benefits of using engaged learning. Retrieved from https://www.binghamton.edu/cce/faculty/engaged-teaching/course-development/benefits.html

---

Positive student outcomes have been associated with community-engaged learning (Curtin, Martins & Schwartz-Barcott, 2015; Foli, Braswell, Kirkpatrick, & Lim, 2014; Groh, Stallwood, & Daniels, 2011; O'Neill, 2016). These positive findings include an increase in the quality of the students' communication capabilities pertaining to listening, awareness, building community, leadership, stewardship, moral development, and empathy, as well as professionalism, teamwork, collaboration, and problem-solving to name a few. This type of learning positively affects students' ability to work with others. In addition, community-engaged learning improves cultural and racial understanding, resulting in an increased sense of social responsibility and citizenship skills. Students engaged in this type of learning are more likely to be involved with their communities after graduation and demonstrate an understanding of the complexities of problem analysis, critical thinking, and cognitive development. In addition, community-engaged learning contributes to career development. Students engaged in this type of learning report stronger faculty relationships and improved satisfaction with college; these students are more likely to graduate.

College students participating in community-engaged learning demonstrated increases in their plans for future civic action, assessments of their own interpersonal problem-solving and leadership skills, and social justice. These students also reported greater satisfaction with their courses, reporting higher levels of learning about the academic field and the community than did students not participating in service learning (Moely, McFarland, Miron, Mercer, & Ilustre, 2002). Faculty too benefit from teaching community-engaged learning courses. **Box 5-4** offers a list of these faculty benefits.

Nursing 499: Community-Engaged Service Learning Course and Student Outcomes

Introduction to a Selected Public Health Issue and a Vulnerable Population

Childhood asthma continues to be a major public health problem for the pediatric population. In 2014, 8.6% of children less than 18 years of age had asthma, with a dramatic increase when looking at the age group of 5–14 years with a 10.3% prevalence. Race and poverty worsen outcomes for this age group, with 13.4% of black non-Hispanic children and 10.4% of people below the poverty level having higher asthma rates compared with 7.6% for white non-Hispanic children and 6.3%

not in poverty. For children less than 18 years old with an asthma diagnosis, 48% had one or more asthma attack. More children are hospitalized for asthma, as seen with rates of 18.3 per 10,000 compared with 13 per 10,000 for adults. In 2013, asthma accounted for 13.8 million school days lost (Centers for Disease Control, 2016). These startling statistics highlighted not only the need for expanded asthma education for parents and the children diagnosed with asthma, but also the need for qualified health professionals competent in the knowledge and skill to teach asthma education per the evidence-based guidelines of the Expert Panel Report 3 (National Heart, Lung, & Blood Institute, 2007), which spurred the creation of our course.

Overview of Nursing 499

The title of Nursing 499 is *Asthma Interventions in the Community*. It was developed to: (a) address the major issues associated with asthma; (b) increase undergraduate nursing students' knowledge of asthma and how best to intervene to improve asthma outcomes; (c) foster undergraduate nursing students' interest and confidence in conducting research; (d) increase the number of nursing students who will choose public health nursing as their area of practice upon graduation and successful completion of NCLEX-RN; (e) create interest in pursuing advanced research degrees in nursing with evidenced-based applications, which has the potential to address the nursing faculty shortage.

This course was first offered in the spring 2015 semester after receiving approval to run as a nursing elective. The course targets undergraduate nursing students but welcomes non-nursing students to attend. It was, and remains, the hope that students will enroll in the course each semester until graduation and continue to develop a research trajectory that will propel them to graduate school. While the majority of students enrolled were already admitted into the nursing major, there were several who had other majors and many who were hoping to transfer into the nursing program. Response from these students was overwhelming. Initially with an enrollment cap of 10, this had to be increased incrementally until the course was closed with 41 students registered. The course has subsequently been offered each semester since, with approximately 50% of the students returning each semester. Presently enrollment is limited to 20.

Students in this course are immersed in the research process. All the students complete the mandated federal training for research investigators. Data are collected with each asthma program implemented. A rigorous training process is conducted for all studies done within the course to make sure all the students deliver the same message to the participants. Additionally, class time is devoted to asthma content. It was vital that the students were well versed in asthma management and understood the medications as well as the underlying pathophysiology. This was challenging as not all of our students were nursing students, and some of those who were had not yet started the nursing program.

An imperative for this course was for students to understand that without dissemination of findings, research becomes a meaningless dead end. To this end, groups of students self-selected a topic pertinent to asthma. Each semester, the students were involved with manuscript preparation. To date, integrated reviews have been completed for five topics; abstracts have been developed and submitted with poster presentations at two local conferences, and students have been introduced to data entry and analysis using SPSS. Several students were accepted for oral presentation at the 2016 APHA Annual Meeting and Expo. Future plans include submitting the integrated reviews for publication. It is the goal of the course and faculty that each student participate in a research study from beginning to end, contribute to a manuscript, and submit for publication.

Interprofessional Education

Nursing 499 provides interprofessional education and experiences. Students from different undergraduate foci of study work together in the implementation of the requirements for this course. Students must learn to communicate with each other, understand different perspectives to solve problems, learn empathy for each other's knowledge and experience base, and find common ground to work as a cohesive group. Students also worked with the Graduate School of Education in the implementation of the *Wee Breathers* program. Nursing students implemented the asthma teaching; education students provided educational activities for the children while the parents attend the asthma teaching.

Community–Campus Partnership

This course would not have been possible without **community partnerships**, which includes local elementary schools and Head Start programs. Working closely with these organizations that advocate for children, families, and health optimizes the possibility to implement our asthma intervention and research opportunities. Our activities support the missions of our community partners, allowing for that mutually beneficial relationship that benefits both the community and our students. Children with asthma have the potential for better outcomes, and our students gain valuable hands-on experience with usually vulnerable populations. Self-efficacy, self-confidence, self-awareness, and cultural competence increase for our nursing students throughout the semester. Our local elementary schools and Head Start agencies have been wonderful collaborators, facilitating implementation of our asthma initiatives.

Specific Course Content

Several research initiatives were carried out since the inception of the course. Each semester, additional projects were instituted to maintain the interest of the students and to encourage reenrollment. All of the interventions were validated, evidenced-based programs for asthma management for children with asthma and their parents. The following describes the specific programs delivered by students in Nursing 499.

OPEN AIRWAYS FOR SCHOOLS

The American Lung Association's *Open Airways for Schools* is a program that educates and empowers children through a fun and interactive approach to asthma self-management. The program teaches children with asthma ages 8 to 11 how to detect the warning signs of asthma, avoid their triggers, and make decisions about their health. It is the most widely recognized asthma management program for children in the nation. It is a proven, effective way to improve asthma self-management skills, decrease asthma emergencies, and raise asthma awareness among families and school personnel (American Lung Association, 2016)

All students were trained as American Lung Association Open Airways for Schools facilitators. This was accomplished through online activities as well as classroom instruction. Students worked in groups to present one of the *Open Airways* modules in class. This allowed further familiarization with all the modules before implantation in the schools. Each student was assigned a specific school and a group of children with asthma to present the entire curriculum over a five-week period.

The students enrolled in the course participated in data collection. Asthma knowledge pretests and posttests were administered to determine if participation in this program changed asthma management. In addition, the Asthma Control Test for Children Ages 4–11 years was also completed before attending *Open Airways* and at completion of the program. Significant increases in the child's asthma management knowledge were found as well as increases in the level of asthma control. Unfortunately, no differences were found for the parents.

Wee Breathers

Wee Breathers is an interactive program developed by the Asthma and Allergy Foundation of America (AAFA) and the Centers for Disease Control and Prevention (CDC)—Cooperative Agreement EH10-007 764-05 (**Figure 5-1**). This program provides a curriculum for health professionals to teach parents of young children about managing asthma. It is designed to be used during home visits, one-on-one, or in-group classes for parents in child care centers. The program as written consists of seven lessons on asthma management,

Figure 5-1 Wee Breathers.

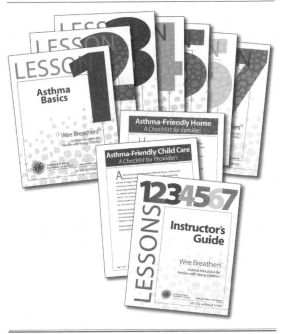

Developed by the Asthma and Allergy Foundation of America (AAFA) and the Centers for Disease Control and Prevention (CDC)—Cooperative Agreement EH10-007 764-05.

a home asthma trigger checklist, an asthma trigger checklist for child care centers, and an instructor's guide (AAFA, 2016).

As with the *Open Airways* program, to ensure rigor for data collection, all students presented segments of the program to their fellow classmates. To increase participation of the families in Wee Breathers, the seven original modules were condensed into four sessions. Students were assigned to a family with the intent of implementing the programs. The students from the 499 class were to give the parents pretests and posttests after each module to determine if their level of knowledge about asthma changed with the implementation of the program. Students from the graduate school of education provided educational activities for the children while the family participated in the asthma sessions.

A IS FOR ASTHMA

Sesame Workshop developed the project Sesame Street *A is for Asthma* to help children with asthma lead fun and active lives. *A is for Asthma* is geared toward both children and adults, showing children with asthma what to do when they have trouble breathing and explaining to the adults in their lives what they can do to help (Sesame Workshop, n.d.). A video highlighting Sesame Street characters delivers the content in a developmentally appropriate manner for young children. The students in Nursing 499 presented the video to Head Start programs in the local area. Content included how to deal with an asthma attack: "Sit down, stay calm, and get a grown up to help." The students reinforced the content of the video with the students, then had them listen to their lungs with stethoscopes.

Challenges with Nursing 499

There were many challenges in the implementation of these initiatives. Coordinating the students' schedule was problematic. Finding a common time when the students in the groups could implement the program took hours of coordination. It was also extremely difficult to match our students' schedules with the schedule that the schools determined would work for their children. In addition, it was very difficult to contact the parents as well as get them to complete the pretests and posttests.

Transportation was also a major obstacle for our course. Many students did not have access to a vehicle. Public transportation was limited to the main city. As we utilized outlying schools, we were constantly negotiating rides, carpools, and taxis. This also added to the expense of running the courses.

Students' Reflections

Students submitted a reflection paper of their experience in the course. This reflection addressed how Nursing 499 has (or has not) impacted future professional goals, including consideration of obtaining advanced degrees after graduation; feelings about participating in research; and how, if at all, attitudes toward research changed because of participation in Nursing 499. Common themes included a desire for continuing education after graduation, an increased interest in conducting research, and a sense of expertise in working with individuals and groups with asthma. Students also discussed their increased confidence and self-efficacy in providing these interventions in the community. See **Box 5-5** for a reflection from a student enrolled in Nursing 499.

Course Outcomes

This course embodies the core professional values and competencies of the *Essentials of Baccalaureate Nursing Education for Entry Level Community/Public Health* (ACHNE, 2009). These include community/population as client, prevention, partnership, and health promotion and risk reduction. Also embraced are the assumptions of *The Essentials of Baccalaureate Education for Professional Nursing Practice* (American Association of Colleges of Nursing, 2008): The professional nurse must be able to practice in an evidence-based environment. Nursing 499 fulfills the required essentials for public health nursing practice, specifically Essential III,

Working with children in a community-based asthma program.

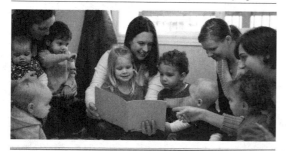

© FatCamera/E+/Getty

Box 5-5 Student Reflections on Nursing 499

When I first heard about the asthma research class in my nursing school, I thought it would be a good way to learn something new about the disease that is the cause of the most missed school days for children. Coming from a family with an asthmatic, I have seen inhalers throughout the house, as well as the occasional use of the nebulizer. Before attending this course, I thought all research happened in a lab with test tubes, but I now understand that research, especially in the realm of public health nursing, largely involves interactions with the community.

Along with a few other classmates, I went to an elementary school and worked with nine children who have asthma between the ages of 8 and 10 years old. We worked with *Open Airways for Schools*, a curriculum that teaches youngsters to manage their symptoms. Each week, we touched on a different aspect of this chronic illness, including a brief understanding of the disease, triggers, medications, and ways to prevent attacks and to continue with normal daily activities. Part of teaching each week included taking the concepts I learned in the classroom and translating them into terms that were easily understandable. Throughout all this, my team needed to find a way to communicate effectively so that the children's attention was on the topic at hand and our time together ran smoothly.

Another part of this course involved working with the parents of children with asthma. This experience showed me that there is always more to learn. With a fellow student, I visited the home of a first grader with asthma. We felt we made a difference by suggesting new ways to manage triggers, such as vacuuming the bedroom each night before going to sleep and washing stuffed animals weekly.

For the research portion of this class, I investigated adverse childhood events and their impact on asthma through a literature review. We submitted an abstract and presented a poster at our university and at a local hospital. Working on both aspects of this project introduced me to a realm which was totally unfamiliar—that of researching in the field through interactions, surveys, focus groups, and incorporating this information into already known material. This is how new information becomes something that can be a contribution to the public. This is also how nurses can introduce new topics to the community and to the region.

Community and public health nursing are facets of the profession that were unfamiliar to me before taking this course. I learned how to take the content I learned in the classroom and incorporate it into a practical and comprehensible way. This is a way to transmit information to bigger groups of people and to make an impact on both the local area and on the community as part of the population. I look forward to continuing research as part of my education as a student and my practice as a nurse and future nurse practitioner.

Shai Lev, Decker School of Nursing, Class of 2017

which states, "Professional nursing practice is grounded in the translation of current evidence into one's practice" (American Association of Colleges of Nursing, 2008, p. 3). In addition, the course also fulfills Essential VIII, which states, "Professionalism and the inherent values of altruism, autonomy, human dignity, integrity, and social justice are fundamental to the discipline of nursing" (American Association of Colleges of Nursing, 2008, p. 4).

Conclusion

This chapter highlights the ongoing need for public health nurses, the impact that public health nurses have on the health of populations, and the rigor intricate to their education. With a changing and challenging healthcare system and a recognition of the multiple and complex determinants of health, public health nurses are well positioned to facilitate the movement from a reactive, sick care health system to a proactive, health promotion and disease prevention agenda. It is essential that all registered nurses are educated with this professional preparation. Public health nursing brings to the table the skills and the expertise to organize all components of our healthcare system (providers, health systems, individuals, families, populations, and the community) to ensure improvement in health outcomes.

Additional Resources

American Public Health Association at: http://www.apha.org/

American Public Health Association—Public Health Nursing at: https://www.apha.org/apha-communities/member-sections/public-health-nursing

Association of Community Health Nursing Educators at: http://achne.org/i4a/pages/index.cfm?pageid=1

American Nurses Credentialing Center at: http://www.nursecredentialing.org/certification.aspx

National Student Nurses' Association at: http://www.nsna.org/

Quad Council Coalition—Public Health Nursing Organizations at: http://www.quadcouncilphn.org/

References

American Association of Colleges of Nursing. (2009). *Nurse faculty tool kit for the implementation of the Baccalaureate Essentials.* Retrieved from http://www.aacn.nche.edu/education-resources/BacEssToolkit.pdf

American Association of Colleges of Nursing. (2008). *The essentials of baccalaureate education for professional nursing practice.* Retrieved from www.aacn.nche.edu/education-resources/BaccEssentials08.pdf

American Association of Colleges of Nursing. (2006). *The essentials of doctoral education for advanced nursing practice.* Retrieved from www.aacn.nche.edu/dnp/Essentials.pdf

American Association of Colleges of Nursing. (2011). *The essentials of master's education in nursing.* Retrieved from www.aacn.nche.edu/education-resources/MastersEssentials11.pdf

American Association of Colleges of Nursing. (2015). *Nursing faculty shortage fact sheet.* Retrieved from http://www.aacn.nche.edu/media-relations/fact-sheets/nursing-faculty-shortage

American Association of Colleges of Nursing. (2016). *Special survey on vacant faculty positions for academic year 2015-2016.* Retrieved from http://www.aacn.nche.edu/leading-initiatives/research-data/vacancy15.pdf

American Lung Association. (2016). *Open Airways for Schools.* Retrieved from http://www.lung.org/lung-health-and-diseases/lung-disease-lookup/asthma/asthma-education-advocacy/open-airways-for-schools/

American Nurses Credentialing Center. (2016). *Advanced public health nursing portfolio.* Retrieved from http://www.nursecredentialing.org/AdvancedPublicHealthNurse-Portfolio

American Public Health Association. (2014a). The *impact of a public health nursing shortage on the nation's public health infrastructure.* Retrieved from http://www.apha.org/policies-and-advocacy/public-health-policy-statements/policy-database/2014/07/03/09/18/the-impact-of-a-public-health-nursing-shortage-on-the---nations-public-health-infrastructure

American Public Health Association. (2014b). *Integration of core public health education into undergraduate curricula.* Retrieved from https://www.apha.org/policies-and-advocacy/public-health-policy-statements/policy-database/2014/07/22/09/58/the-integration-of-core-public-health-education-into-undergraduate-curricula

American Public Health Association. (2014c). *Strengthening public health nursing in the United States.* Retrieved from https://www.apha.org/policies-and-advocacy/public-health-policy-statements/policy-database/2014/07/23/11/02/strengthening-public-health-nursing-in-the-united-states

American Public Health Association. (2016). *Gun violence.* Retrieved from https://www.apha.org/topics-and-issues/gun-violence

American Public Health Association, Public Health Nursing Section. (2013). *The definition and practice of public health nursing.* Washington, DC: Author.

Association of Community Health Nursing Educators (ACHNE). (2009). *Essentials of Baccalaureate nursing education for entry level community/public health nursing.* Retrieved from http://www.achne.org/i4a/pages/index.cfm?pageid=1

Association of Community Health Nursing Educators (ACHNE). (2007). *Graduate education for advanced practice public health nursing: At the crossroads.* Retrieved from http://achne.org/i4a/pages/index.cfm?pageid=3325

Asthma and Allergy Foundation of America. (2016). *Educational programs for teaching patients.* Retrieved from http://www.aafa.org/page/asthma-allergy-education-programs-teach-patients.aspx#WeeBreathers

Bureau of Labor Statistics. (2014). *BLS fast facts: Nursing instructors and teachers, postsecondary.* Retrieved from http://www.bls.gov/careeroutlook/2014/interview/nursing-instructor.htm

CCPH Board of Directors. (2013). *Position Statement on Authentic Partnerships. Community-Campus Partnerships for Health.* Retrieved from https://ccph.memberclicks.net/principles-of-partnership

Center for Civic Engagement. Binghamton University. (2015). *Benefits of using engaged learning.* Retrieved from https://www.binghamton.edu/cce/faculty/engaged-teaching/course-development/benefits.html

Centers for Disease Control and Prevention. (2015). *2015: What kept us up at night and what will keep us busy in 2016.* Retrieved from http://www.cdc.gov/media/dpk/2015/dpk-eoy.html

Centers for Disease Control and Prevention. (2016). *Most recent asthma data.* Retrieved from http://www.cdc.gov/asthma/most_recent_data.htm

Cravetz, M., Krothe, J., Reyes, D., & Swider, S. M. (2011). *Quad council competencies for public health nurses.* Retrieved from www.quadcouncilphn.org/documents-3/competencies/

Curtin, A., Martins, D. C., & Schwartz-Barcott, D. (2015). A mixed methods evaluation of an international service learning program in the Dominican Republic. *Public Health Nursing, 32*(1): 58–67.

Eyler, J., Giles, D. E., Jr., Stenson, C. M., & Gray, C. J. (2001). *At a glance: What we know about the effects of service learning on college students, faculty, institutions, and communities, 1993–2000* (3rd ed.). Nashville, TN: Vanderbilt University.

Fairman, J. (2016). Interprofessional learning: An old idea in a new package. *Nursing History Review, 24,* 110–116.

Foli, K., Braswell, M., Kirkpatrick, J., & Lim, E., (2014). Development of Leadership Behaviors in Undergraduate Nursing Students: A Service-Learning Approach. *Nursing Education Perspectives, 35*(2), 76–82.

Fowler, M. D. (Ed.). (2008). Provision four. *Guide to the code of ethics for nurses: interpretation and application* (Provision 4). Silver Spring, MD: Nursebooks.org.

Groh, C. J., Stallwood, L. G., & Daniels, J. J. (2011). Service learning in nursing education: its impact on leadership and social justice. *Nursing Education Perspectives, 32*(6), 400–405.

Health Resources and Services Administration. (2013). *The U.S. nursing workforce: Trends in supply and education.* Retrieved from http://bhpr.hrsa.gov/healthworkforce/reports/nursingworkforce/nursingworkforcefullreport.pdf

Institute of Medicine. (2015). *Measuring the impact of interprofessional education on collaborative practice and patient outcomes.* Washington, DC: National Academies Press.

Interprofessional Education Collaborative Expert Panel. (2011). *Core competencies for interprofessional collaborative practice: Report of an expert panel.* Washington, DC: Interprofessional Education Collaborative.

Lewenson, S. B. & Nickitas, D. M. (2016). Nursing's history of advocacy and action. In D. Nickitas (Ed.), *Policy and politics and policy for nurses and other health professionals* (2nd ed. pp. 3-13). New York, NY: Springer.

Moely, B. E., McFarland, M., Miron, D., Mercer, S., & Ilustre, V. (2002). Changes in college students' attitudes and intentions for civic involvement as a function of service-learning experiences. *Michigan Journal of Community Service Learning, 9*, 18–26.

Monteiro, L. (1985) Florence Nightingale on public health nursing. *American Journal of Public Health, 75* (2), 181–186. doi:10.2105/AJPH.75.2.181

National Association of County and City Health Officials. (2013). *2013 National Profile of Local Health Departments Study*. Retrieved from http://www.nac cho.org/topics/infrastructure/profile/upload/2013 -National-Profile-of-Local-Health-Departments -report.pdf

National Association of County and City Health Officials. (2015). *Statement of policy: Education and recruitment of public health nurses*. Retrieved from https://www.naccho.org/uploads/downloadable -resources/Education-and-Recruitment-of-Public -Health-Nurses.pdf

National Heart, Lung, and Blood Institute. National Asthma Education Program. Expert Panel on the Management of Asthma. (2007*). Expert Panel report 3 guidelines for the diagnosis and management of asthma*. Bethesda, MD: U.S. Department of Health and Human Services, National Institutes of Health, National Heart, Lung, and Blood Institute.

New England Resource Center for Higher Education (n.d.*). Carnegie Community Engagement Classification : How is community engagement defined?* Retrieved from http://nerche.org/index. php?option=com_content&view=article&id=341 &Itemid=92#CEdef

Ogden C. L., Carroll, M. D., Kit, B. K., & Flegal, K. M. (2014). Prevalence of childhood and adult obesity in the United States, 2011-2012. *JAMA, 311*(8):806-814. doi:10.1001/jama.2014.732

O'Neill, M. (2016). Policy-focused service-learning as a capstone: Teaching essentials of Baccalaureate

nursing education. *Journal of Nursing Education, 55*(10), 583–586.

Quad Council of Public Health Nursing Organizations. (2011). Quad Council competencies for public health nurses. *Quad Council of Public Health Nursing Organizations*.

Quad Council of Public Health Nursing Organizations. (2012). *Strategic priority: Advancing public health nursing education*. Retrieved from http://www .achne.org/files/quad%20council/quadcouncil policybrief_advancingphneducation.pdf

Quad Council of Public Health Nursing Organizations. (2013*). Strategic priority—Improving the public health nursing infrastructure*. Retrieved from http://www.achne.org/files/Quad%20Council /QuadCouncilPolicyBrief_PHNInfrastructure Jan2013.pdf

Savage, C. L., Kub, J. E., & Groves, S. L. (2016). *Public health science and nursing practice caring for populations*. Philadelphia, PA: F. A. Davis Company.

Save the Children.org. (April 7, 2016). *Flint, Michigan, water poisoning crisis: Response and recovery plan*. Fairfield, CT: Save the Children.

Sesame Workshop. (n.d.). *United States: A is for asthma*. Retrieved from http://www.sesameworkshop.org /what-we-do/our-initiatives/a-is-for-asthma/

Swider, S. M., Krothe, J., Reyes, D., & Cravetz, M. (2013). Competencies for public health nursing. *Public Health Nursing, 30*(6), 519–536. doi:10.1111/ phn.12090

University of Michigan Center for Excellence in Public Health Workforce Studies. (2013). *Enumeration and Characterization of the Public Health Nurse Workforce: Findings of the 2012 Public Health Nurse Workforce Surveys*. Ann Arbor, University of Michigan.

U.S. Census Bureau. (n.d.) *Service-connected disability-rating status and ratings for civilian veterans 18 years and over universe: civilian veterans 18 years and over. 2014 American Community Survey 1-year estimates*. Retrieved from http:// factfinder.census.gov/faces/tableservices/jsf/pages /productview.xhtml?src=bkmk

Vanderbilt University. (2016). *What is service learning or community engagement?* Retrieved from https://cft.vanderbilt.edu/guides-sub-pages /teaching-through-community-engagement/

Wald, L. D. (1913, June 25). *A Greeting: Given by Lillian Wald at the General Opening Meeting at Atlantic City, National Organization of Public Health Nursing.* Lillian D. Wald Papers, 1889–1957. Writing and Speeches. Reel 25, Box 36, Folder 6, pp. 1–4. New York Public Library, Humanities and Social Sciences Library, Manuscripts and Archives Division, New York NY.

Wallerstein, N. B., Yen, I. H., & Syme, S. L. (2011). Integration of social epidemiology and community-engaged interventions to improve health equity. *American Journal of Public Health, 101*(5), 822-830 9p. doi:10.2105/AJPH.2008.140988

World Health Organization (WHO). (2010). *Framework for action on interprofessional education & collaborative practice.* Geneva, Switzerland: Author. Retrieved from http://apps.who.int/iris/bitstream/10665/70185/1/WHO_HRH_HPN_10.3_eng.pdf?ua=1

For a full suite of assignments and additional learning activities, use the access code located in the front of your book to visit this exclusive website: **http://go.jblearning.com/londrigan**. If you do not have an access code, you can obtain one at the site.

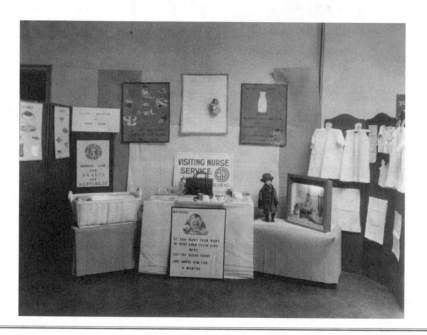

Courtesy of the Visiting Nurse Service of New York.

CHAPTER 6

Evidence-Based Practice From a Public Health Perspective

Joanne K. Singleton
Renee McLeod-Sordjan
Paule Valery Joseph

It would be an interesting and possibly valuable piece of work if a morbidity study could be made through the hospital records and a similar study of sickness in the homes. Henry Street makes an analysis of the cases that have been under its care and we feel it a pity that these figures are not made more use of. The pneumonia experience alone showed many interesting and telling facts, especially regarding home care for the children. (Wald, 1917, np)

LEARNING OBJECTIVES

At the completion of this chapter, the reader will be able to:

- Define evidence-based practice.
- Describe the systematic approach to finding best available evidence.
- Explore the application of evidence-based practice to public health issues of health literacy and tobacco use.

KEY TERMS

❑ Evidence-based medicine
❑ Evidence-based practice

❑ Health literacy
❑ Tobacco use

Introduction to Evidence-Based Practice and Public Health

"In a world where public health threats range from AIDS and bioterrorism to an epidemic of obesity, the need for an effective public health system is as urgent as it has ever been" (Gebbie, Rosenstock, & Hernandez, 2003, p. 1). This quotation comes from an Institute of Medicine (IOM, 2002) report, *Who Will Keep the Public Healthy? Educating Public Health Professionals for the 21st Century*. Although this report is aimed primarily at schools of public health, it includes recommendations for schools of nursing and medicine as well. For schools of nursing, the recommendations address the inclusion of an ecological perspective of health in nursing curricula, collaboration among all public health professionals from a variety of disciplines, and the provision of clinical experiences in the public health arena. The 2011 IOM report, *The Future of Nursing: Leading Change, Advancing Health* considers key messages and recommendations that pertain to nursing. One of the key messages specifically addresses the improvement of nursing education to ensure the delivery of "safe, quality, patient-centered care across all settings, especially in such areas as primary care and community and public health" (p. 6). Lipstein, Kellermann, Berkowitz, Sklar, and Thibault (2016) noted in the latest document from the National Academy of Medicine that the very workforce being educated today must be competent in evidence-based practice that is cost-effective.

An important aspect of these recommendations is the acknowledgment of **evidence-based practice (EBP)**. The IOM published *Health Professions Education: A Bridge to Quality* (Griener & Knebel, 2003), which included the following vision for all health professions education: "All health professionals should be educated to deliver patient-centered care as members of an interdisciplinary team, emphasizing evidence-based practice, quality improvement approaches, and informatics" (p. 3). This challenge was answered in 2006 with the Quality and Safety Education for Nurses (QSEN) initiative funded by the Robert Wood Johnson Foundation (Quality and Safety Education

for Nurses [QSEN], 2007). This initiative sought to identify the knowledge, competencies, and attitudes that nurses need to know to practice with quality and safety in mind. The six major areas of practice include patient-centered care, teamwork and collaboration, evidence-based practice, quality improvement, safety, and informatics (Cronenwett et al., 2007).

What Is an Evidence-Based Practice Lens for Viewing Population-Based Health Issues?

The term evidence based was first used by medicine in 1992 by Gordon Guyatt, a Canadian physician from McMaster University, and the Evidence-Based Medicine Working Group. Although the term **evidence-based medicine** originated within the medical profession as a new paradigm for medical practice (Oxman, Sackett, & Guyatt, 1992), the essence of this paradigm—using research evidence as the best evidence to guide professional decision-making—has recently spread to other professions both within and outside the healthcare arena. Singleton, Levin, and Keefer (2007) discussed several examples from the disciplines of law, education, and management. In addition, Cullum, Ciliska, Haynes, and Marks (2008) cite the use of the term evidence based in professions such as physiotherapy and police science.

Regardless of the field or discipline in which this paradigm or model is applied, EBP has several conceptual and process components that cross disciplinary boundaries. Evidence-based practice is a framework for decision-making that uses the best available evidence in conjunction with the professional's expertise and the client's, customer's, or consumer's values and preferences to guide problem-solving and judgments about how to best approach a situation to achieve desired outcomes (Melnyk & Fineout-Overholt, 2011; Straus, Richardson, Glasziou, & Haynes, 2005). The key to the EBP model is the systematic approach to finding the best available evidence to answer a focused question and to implement the answer in practice as follows:

1. Ask and frame a clinical question.
2. Find the evidence to answer the question.

3. Appraise the evidence for validity, source reliability, and applicability to practice.
4. Select and synthesize the best evidence for use.
5. Implement the evidence-based intervention in practice.
6. Evaluate the intervention and results.

The search for and retrieval of this evidence is not always approached in the systematic way advocated in the EBP paradigm, which is to try to find the highest level of evidence first and then proceed methodically through the hierarchy of evidence that exists to answer the focused question. Some types of evidence carry more weight than other types of evidence. For example, a single study carries less weight than a systematic review because a systematic review combines the results of several studies on the same clinical question or questions. The highest level of evidence available should be used to guide our clinical practice. Health professionals, therefore, have developed schemata that rank evidence according to levels. The higher the level of evidence, the more confidence we are able to have in a study's validity. There are many different schemata for ranking the level of a piece of evidence. Based on the work of others, Melnyk and Fineout-Overholt (2011) present seven levels in the hierarchy of evidence (see **Box 6-1**).

Although it is important to determine the levels of evidence upon which a recommendation for practice is based, it is also important to assess the quality of that evidence, whether it is a study or expert opinion. The quality of evidence depends on the critical appraisal of the study or the background of and resources used by an expert panel. The schema shown in **Box 6-2** provides one

---

Box 6-1 Levels of Evidence

Level I: Systematic reviews and/or meta-analysis of randomized controlled trials (RCTs) assessed to be relevant
Level II: Well-designed RCTs
Level III: Nonrandomized, well-designed, controlled trials
Level IV: Well-designed, case-controlled, and/or cohort studies
Level V: Systematic reviews of descriptive and qualitative studies
Level VI: Single descriptive or qualitative studies
Level VII: Expert opinion of individuals or committees

Data from Melnyk, B. M., & Fineout-Overholt, E. (2011). *Evidence-based practice in nursing and healthcare: A guide to best practice* (2nd ed). Philadelphia, PA: Lippincott.

Box 6-2 Quality Ratings

A: A very well-designed study/project (Stetler et al., 1998)
B: A well-designed meta-analysis with at least 5 studies but fewer than 12; well-designed meta-analysis with large sample but some flawed studies*; individual studies in level IV, which may have a large sample size but are secondary analyses of previously conducted randomized clinical trials (Singleton, Levin, Feldman, & Truglio-Londrigan, 2005)
C: Well-designed individual studies with small sample sizes (Singleton et al., 2005)
D: Study/project has a major flaw that raises serious questions about the validity of the findings (Stetler et al., 1998)

*For example, use of nonrandomized trials in a meta-analysis seeking to answer questions of treatment effectiveness. Reproduced from Singleton, J., Levin, R. F., Feldman, H. R., & Truglio-Londrigan, M. (2005).Evidence for smoking cessation: Implications for gender-specific strategies. *Worldviews on Evidence-Based Nursing, 2*(2), 1–12. © 2005. Reprinted by permission of the publisher, John Wiley and Sons; Stetler, C. B., Morsi, D., Rucki, S., Broughton, S., Corrigan, B., Fitzgerald, J.,... Sheridan, E. A. (1998). Utilization-focused integrative reviews in a nursing service. *Applied Nursing Research, 11*(4), 195–205.

approach for assigning a quality rating to a piece of evidence. Using this approach, a rating for any level of evidence may range from A to D and reflects the basic scientific credibility of the overall study/project or other type of evidence.

Leveling schemes and quality ratings may differ according to the agency, organization, or author. Under any circumstances, however, the leveling and determination of the quality of evidence are essential components of this model. Some evidence-based guidelines, such as the tobacco-dependence guidelines introduced later in this chapter, identify and define the strength of evidence for the specific guideline. When reading EBP guidelines, therefore, it is important to identify the criteria used to assess the level, quality, or strength of evidence. This is the approach we have taken in providing readers with the best available evidence on two very important public health challenges: helping people to stop smoking and increasing the health literacy of our population.

Healthy People 2020—Public Health Conditions: An Evidence-Based Perspective

Healthy People 2020 is a federal government initiative that contains health objectives for the citizens of our nation (U.S. Department of Health and Human Services [U.S. DHHS], 2010a). This document is built on past government initiatives intended to guide action that would improve the nation's health. *Healthy People 2020* addresses many objectives. This chapter focuses on two health conditions from a public health perspective: health literacy and tobacco addiction. We discuss the national incidence, prevalence, morbidity, and mortality of these health conditions; the evidence to guide or develop population-focused interventions for these conditions; and specific public health interventions in action for health literacy and tobacco addiction.

The first topic that will be highlighted in this chapter is health communication and health communication technology. This topic, along with its specific objectives, may be viewed in its entirety under the Healthy People tab 2020 Topics and Objectives (U.S. DHHS, 2010b). Under this topic area there are 13 objectives. One of the specific objectives for this topic area focuses on literacy:

HC/HIT-1: (Developmental) Improve the health literacy of the population.

The second issue to be highlighted is under the topic area of tobacco use. This topic, along with specific objectives, may be viewed in its entirety under the Healthy People tab 2020 Topics and Objectives (U.S. DHHS, 2010b). There are a total of 21 objectives under the topic area of **Tobacco Use**. Two of the specific objectives for tobacco use are:

TU-1: Reduce tobacco use by adults.
TU-2: Reduce tobacco use by adolescents.

The focus of this chapter is on an evidence-based approach to these two very important public health topics: health literacy and tobacco use. Before discussing these two public health topics and introducing the EBP approach to understanding them, an overview of population-based concepts will help to put the subsequent discussions about specific public health issues in context.

Health Literacy as a Public Health Condition: Overview and Definition

Before the 1990s, the impact of literacy on population health in the United States was either unappreciated by health professionals or was generally thought of as a problem of an individual; literacy was not considered to be a public health condition. Today, it is known that literacy and its healthcare counterpart, health literacy, have far-reaching effects on both the individual with low health literacy and the U.S. population as a whole (Shohet & Renaud, 2006). *Healthy People 2020* has formally included health literacy as one of the defined objectives for study and intervention for 2010 through 2020 (U.S. DHHS, 2010b).

The definition of **health literacy** is continually being refined. The most widely accepted definition states that health literacy is "the degree to which individuals have the capacity to obtain, process, and understand basic health information and services needed to make appropriate health decisions" (Nielsen-Bohlman, Panzer, & Kindig, 2004, p. 32; CDC, 2015a). This definition was expanded to reflect the even broader impact that health literacy has on individual lives. "Literacy facilitates access; to information and enables individuals to make informed health decisions, to influence events, and to exert greater control over their lives" (Shohet & Renaud, 2006, p. 10). In more concrete terms, health literacy impacts an individual's ability to access health care, to make choices in obtaining appropriate health insurance coverage, to seek out high-quality facilities to obtain evidence-based health screening and illness care, as well as comprehend health information about disease prevention or self-care of chronic disease. Nine out of 10 English-speaking patients lack proficiency to comprehend everyday health communication (Nielsen-Bohlman et al., 2004; U.S. Department of Health and Human Services, Office of Disease Prevention and Health Promotion, 2010c). In addition, if an individual is the caregiver of children or elderly family members, the individual needs to advocate and make decisions for those in his or her care. Clearly, health literacy has far-reaching effects on individuals, families, communities, and the U.S. population as a whole.

INCIDENCE, PREVALENCE, MORBIDITY, AND MORTALITY

Incidence and Prevalence

Although low health literacy is now widely recognized to have a significant negative impact on both the individual and public health, tools to measure health literacy and strategies to improve care of the low literacy population have been developed only recently. For the third time in as many decades, the National Center for Education Statistics (2006)

measured the English literacy of the U.S. population in the 2003 National Assessment of Adult Literacy. This survey was the first to include measurement of health literacy in addition to overall U.S. English literacy, and it remains the most current assessment. The National Assessment of Adult Literacy surveyed a representative sample of 19,000 U.S. households as well as 1,200 persons in prisons. For the purpose of this study, health literacy was defined using the previously quoted IOM definition (National Center for Education Statistics, 2006).

Health literacy was measured using the three literacy measures used in the overall English literacy assessments by the 2003 National Assessment of Adult Literacy survey: prose, document, and quantitative measures. *Prose literacy* is defined as the ability to search, comprehend, and use information from continuous text. *Document literacy* is defined as the ability to search, comprehend, and use information from noncontinuous text (e.g., application forms or maps). *Quantitative literacy* is defined as the ability to identify and perform computation using numbers embedded in print materials (e.g., balancing a checkbook). In addition, three domains specific to health literacy were identified and measured: clinical, prevention, and navigation of the health system. The *clinical domain* was defined as the activities involved in the provider–patient interaction, such as completing forms and understanding medication dosages. The *prevention domain* was defined as activities related to disease prevention and self-management of illness. Navigation of the health system included activities such as understanding health insurance plans and consent forms.

Results of the 2003 adult health literacy survey showed that 36% of the U.S. population, or approximately 87 million adults, had either below basic (14%) or basic (22%) health literacy levels, defined as

- Below basic: No more than the most basic and concrete literacy skills.
- Basic: Skills necessary to perform simple and basic everyday activities.

Disparities among particular subpopulations were also noted. Hispanic populations had the lowest percentage of health literacy among ethnic groups. More men (16%) than women (12%) had below basic health literacy levels. Persons who did not speak English before attending primary school had lower health literacy than those who spoke English at early ages, and adults over age 65 had lower health literacy than other age groups. Educational attainment was significantly associated with below basic health literacy: 49% of individuals who did not complete either high school or a general educational development (GED) program had below basic health literacy scores. Adults living in poverty had lower health literacy levels than other socioeconomic groups, as did persons who had self-perceived overall health at lower ratings. Persons who had no health insurance or had Medicaid/Medicare had lower health literacy levels. Those who obtained their basic health information from television or radio had lower health literacy than those who obtained information from print media (National Center for Education Statistics, 2006).

Data from the 2003 NAAL continued to be released through 2010. In 2011–12, another large-scale assessment of adult skills called the Program for the International Assessment of Adult Competencies (PIAAC) was administered. The PIACC is the most current indicator of national progress in adult skills in literacy, numeracy, and problem-solving in technology-rich environments. Although a global initiative, involving 24 countries, the data set sample size from the United States included 5,000 subjects, of which 1,300 were prisoners (USDOE, 2016). Data continues to be analyzed, but less than 15% of young adults aged 16 to 24 demonstrate the highest level of literacy proficiency.

Low health literacy may contribute significantly to the notable health disparities across specific populations in the United States. One of the overarching goals of *Healthy People 2020* (U.S. DHHS, 2010d) is to reduce these health disparities, which lead to increased morbidity and mortality as well as inefficient and ineffective use of public resources. Estimates of the cost of low health literacy to U.S. society range from $106 to $238 billion annually (Vernon, Trujillo, Rosenbaum, & DeBuono, 2007). When future and indirect costs are accounted for, this estimate increases to a range from $1.6 to $3.6 trillion annually (Vernon et al., 2007). Clearly, low health literacy is a public health condition of great consequence.

Morbidity, Mortality, and Level of Evidence

Many studies have documented how low health literacy impacts a person's ability to obtain preventive screening services and manage one's chronic diseases. Based on the level of evidence ratings in Box 6-1, the following evidence is reported. In a systematic review of the literature, Berkman, Sheridan, Donahue, Halpern, and Crotty (2011) found that patients with low health literacy used health resources less frequently than their higher literacy counterparts (level I). Maniaci, Heckman, and Dawson (2008) found that patients with lower levels of health literacy were found to have less medication knowledge after hospital discharge (level IV). In addition, patients with type 2 diabetes mellitus and low health literacy were found to have higher HgA1c levels and higher rates of retinopathy than those with higher health literacy levels (Schillinger et al., 2002) (level IV). Patients with low health literacy were less likely to use preventive services (IOM, 2004) (level V). Higher mortality rates were also associated with lower health literacy scores (Baker et al., 2007) (level IV). Patients with low health literacy have higher rates of hospitalizations, complications, and higher emergency room use (Baker et al., 2002; Baker, Parker, Williams, & Clark, 1998) (level IV). Among elderly patients 65 and older, low health literacy was associated with increased hospitalizations, higher emergency room utilization, poor medication adherence, and impaired ability to interpret health messages (Berkman et al., 2011a) (level I). Moreover, patients with low health literacy were two to three times more likely to experience poor outcomes (DeWalt, Berkman, Sheridan, Lohr, & Pignone, 2004) (level I).

EVIDENCE TO GUIDE POPULATION-FOCUSED INTERVENTIONS

Evidence on the morbidity and mortality related to health literacy provides guidance on population-focused interventions. The burden of low health literacy on the health of society mandates action to improve the problem. Population-focused interventions occur within the national, state, and local arenas.

In 2010, President Obama signed the Plain Writing Act of 2010, which was designed to promote communication that the public can understand. In response, the U.S. DHHS released a National Action Plan to Improve Health Literacy (U.S. Department of Health and Human Services, Office of Disease Prevention and Health Promotion, 2010e). The National Action Plan aims to eliminate complex medical jargon in health communication. The National Action Plan suggests a universal precautions approach to health literacy and communication. By adopting universal precautions, health professionals use clear communication that is culturally appropriate regardless of the perceived health literacy skills of the client. Health information comes from various sources across multiple disciplines (e.g., websites and social media; health professionals, caregivers, and public health officials; schools; television and radio). As a result of multiple health messages, national evidence-based strategies must be adopted to improve clear communication.

An exemplar health literacy intervention that addresses communication is the three-pronged strategy adopted by The Joint Commission (Murphy-Knoll, 2007). The first strategy makes clear communication an organizational priority. The second strategy mandates that clear communication needs to be addressed across the continuum of care, from the acute care to the primary care setting. The third strategy states that policy changes must be pursued to improve provider–patient communication. Health Literacy Innovations is a computer-based software system used by the National Institutes of Health to improve the readability of health information by translating technical information into simpler terms.

Another national intervention involves increasing access to healthcare coverage for the entire population. During 2010, 50.7 million persons in the United States under the age of 65 were uninsured (DeNavas-Walt, Proctor, & Smith, 2011). An estimated 32 million Americans have been insured by the Affordable Health Care for America Act (ACA), H.R. 3962 (Patient Protection and Affordable Care Act, 2010). The law includes provisions to communicate healthcare information clearly, promote prevention, promote patient-centered interventions and create healthy homes, ensure equity and cultural competence, and deliver high-quality care. The ACA provides that language within state programs must be readable for those with low health literacy as well as culturally and linguistically appropriate.

The ACA also establishes workforce training opportunities to improve the patient–provider interaction. This interaction could be improved by increasing basic health literacy education of primary care providers. The ACA pushes for curriculum changes to teach health professionals skills for communicating with persons of low health literacy. Methods such as *teach back* (Pfizer Clear Health Communication Initiative, 2008) and *ask me three* (National Patient Safety Foundation, 2008) have been shown to improve patient comprehension and ability for self-care. Healthcare providers need to be educated that health education materials should be written in easy-to-use formats, with large font, short sentences, and action-oriented content to improve readability and patient comprehension (CDC, 2014; Doak, Doak, & Root, 1998). Curriculums in health-related professions need to reflect training in culturally diverse education techniques. In a study by Volandes and colleagues (2008), specific teaching techniques were shown to enhance decision-making ability regarding end-of-life care preferences. At the time of writing this chapter the future of ACA remains in question.

Statewide initiatives in health literacy are overseen by the U.S. DHHS Office of Disease and Health Promotion. State and local collaborations between academic, government, and nonprofit organizations with a health literacy focus are funded across five priorities:

1. Incorporate health literacy improvement in mission, planning, and evaluation.
2. Support health literacy research, evaluation, training, and practice.
3. Conduct formative, process, and outcome evaluations to design and assess materials, messages, and resources.
4. Enhance dissemination of timely, accurate, and appropriate health information to health professionals and the public.
5. Design health literacy improvements to healthcare and public health systems that enhance access to health services.

For example, the Institute for Healthcare Advancement (2017) is a not-for-profit, privately operating California initiative that provides translation of patient education materials, delivers primary care in a community health setting, and also provides outreach services within the community.

Within communities, impaired health literacy negatively impacts the self-esteem of individual clients. The literature suggests that individuals do not access health care because of the shame related to their literacy problems. Organizations and healthcare providers can make changes to reduce this negative impact by creating shame-free environments. Providing written materials at low literacy levels and offering assistance for those completing intake forms are suggested methods to remove barriers to care for those with low health literacy. It is important at a local level to assess the learning needs of disparate communities in a culturally competent manner. Multiple instruments (e.g., Newest Vital Sign, Test of Functional Health Literacy in Adults) exist to assess the health literacy of disparate communities and should be incorporated into daily practice to tailor individualized learning plans (Hanchate, Ash, Gasmararian, Wolf, & Paasche-Orlow, 2008; McLeod-Sordjan, 2011; Weiss et al., 2005).

HEALTH LITERACY AND TOBACCO USE: SPECIFIC PUBLIC HEALTH INTERVENTIONS (CASE STUDY)

An organization reviews the current tobacco use health education materials it provides to nonsmoking adolescent clients (e.g., Did you know that tobacco addiction is one of the hardest habits to break?). These education materials could be evaluated for both reading level, using the Simplified Measure of Gobbledygook (McLaughlin, 2008), or Fry formula (Doak et al., 1998), and readability, using the suitability of assessment materials, or SAM, tool (Doak et al., 1998). When designing materials for adolescents in particular, it is important that patients see themselves in the illustrations on the material. The SAM tool gives very valuable guidelines that improve design for health education materials that are targeted to a specific audience. Revision of an organization's existing tobacco use materials to reduce reading level, improve readability, and clearly target a specific population is one example of a low-cost and effective means to begin a system-wide movement toward clear communication.

FUTURE PROJECTIONS

Unfortunately, the problem of low health literacy may worsen in the United States across racial and generational groups. Kutner et al. (2007) reports 66% of adults aged 65 and older were classified with low health literacy. It is projected that Hispanics aged 65 and older are estimated to increase to 19.8% of the U.S. population by the year 2050 (Heron & Smith, 2007). If healthcare systems and individual providers do not make health literacy and clear communication a priority, public health outcomes can be expected to decline over future decades.

Tobacco Dependence as a Public Health Condition: Overview and Definition

Tobacco, a green leafy plant that grows in warm climates, has a long history in the United States.

Figure 6-1 Cigarette health warnings.

> SURGEON GENERAL'S WARNING: Smoking
> Causes Lung Cancer, Heart Disease,
> Emphysema, and May Complicate Pregnancy.

> SURGEON GENERAL'S WARNING: Quitting Smoking
> Now Greatly Reduces Serious Risks to Your Health.

> SURGEON GENERAL'S WARNING: Smoking
> by Pregnant Women May Result in Fetal Injury,
> Premature Birth, and Low Birth Weight.

> SURGEON GENERAL'S WARNING: Cigarette
> Smoke Contains Carbon Monoxide.

Public Law 98–474, Comprehensive Smoking Education Act, 1984. Smoking Tobacco & Health, Centers for Disease Control and Prevention.

Dating back to the first American settlers in 1621 in Jamestown, Virginia, tobacco was the first crop grown for money in North America. Tobacco is dried and can be smoked or chewed. There are over 4,800 chemicals in tobacco and its smoke; nicotine is the chemical that makes tobacco addictive. Although the first settlers used tobacco in small amounts, the invention of the cigarette-making machine in 1881 resulted in widespread cigarette smoking. Nevertheless, it was not until 1964 that the Surgeon General of the United States reported on the dangers of cigarette smoking, identifying that the nicotine and tar in cigarettes may cause lung cancer. The U.S. Congress in 1965 passed the Cigarette Labeling and Advertising Act that required every cigarette pack to carry on its side the warning "Cigarettes may be hazardous to your health." This was followed by later legislation in 1971 banning radio and television advertising of cigarettes. Cigarette companies responded to the government warnings about the hazards of smoking related to tar: By the 1980s, cigarette companies made, sold, and promoted low- and ultra-low-tar cigarettes. Congress passed another law in 1984, the Comprehensive Smoking Education Act, which created four different warning labels (**Figure 6-1**) and required cigarette companies to rotate among these warnings every three months.

Federal, state, and local governments, as well as private companies, have been taking action since the 1980s to restrict and ban smoking in public places. The American Lung Association tracks and reports tobacco control trends in the United States (see http://stateoftobaccocontrol.org). As of 2010, the American Lung Association's smoke-free map reveals that only 27 states plus the District of Columbia have enacted comprehensive smoke-free laws to protect their citizens. One hundred million Americans remain unprotected by a lack of comprehensive smoke-free laws. On June 12, 2009, President Obama signed the Family Smoking Prevention and Tobacco Control Act (H.R. 1256) into law. The U.S. Food and Drug Administration (FDA) was granted the authority to regulate the sales, advertising, and ingredient content of all tobacco products marketed in the

United States. The law also limits advertising to youth and requires graphic cigarette warning labels to cover 50% of the front and rear of the cigarette pack. In addition, the law created a new prevention and public health fund expanding smoking cessation coverage for pregnant Medicaid beneficiaries and offering financial incentives to states that encourage prevention initiatives for Medicaid beneficiaries (DHHS, 2010). As of the writing of this chapter, there are issues surrounding graphic warning labels that are being challenged in the courts.

INCIDENCE, PREVALENCE, MORBIDITY, AND MORTALITY

In the United States, cigarette smoking continues to be identified as the most avoidable cause of death and disability (Centers for Disease Control and Prevention [CDC], 2016). Tobacco use begins in adolescence, with first use almost always occurring before 18 years of age. Cigarette smoking carries a significant disease burden for the primary smoker that may result in respiratory diseases, lung cancer, and/or cardiovascular disease; may have harmful reproductive effects; and results in more than 480,000 deaths per year in the United States (CDC, 2016). Exposure to secondhand smoke for the nonsmoker creates a significant health risk, especially for individuals with respiratory or cardiac conditions, and can result in premature death and disease. In addition, 16 million Americans live with a significant tobacco-related illness (CDC, 2016). According to a CDC (2016) report, direct medical costs in the United States from tobacco dependence are more than $170 billion per year, with an additional $156 billion resulting from lost productivity.

Although most smokers report a desire to quit, most quit attempts fail. New smokers from adults to children are continually recruited. Not only are interventions critical to help those who already smoke to quit, interventions to prevent people, especially children, from starting to smoke are essential to eliminating smoking-related illnesses.

About 45 million adults (21%) in the United States smoke, and each day about 3,200 children ages 12 to 17 smoke their first cigarette, with about 2,100 becoming addicted to tobacco (CDC, 2016) In 25 Gallop poll surveys taken since 1977, 74% of smokers continually say they want to quit smoking. Eighty-five percent of smokers say they have tried at least once to quit, and 45% say they have tried at least three times to quit (Newport, 2013).

Adolescent tobacco use had declined over the past 40 years, yet in 2015, 4.7 million students in middle school and high school were reported to use tobacco (DHHS, 2016). Among high school students, white high school students have a higher incidence of smoking than their black or Hispanic peers (DHHS, 2016). There is a greater prevalence of smoking among high school students who live in nonmetropolitan areas, in the South, and in the Midwest (DHHS, 2016; Keeling, Lusk, & Kulbok, 2017). Teens who smoke report interesting findings. Two-thirds say they would like to quit, while 40% have tried to quit and failed, and 70% say that if they had to do it over they would not choose to smoke. Teens who smoke two to three cigarettes a day can become addicted in as short as two weeks. Quit attempts in adolescents are usually unassisted and unplanned, yet those who enroll in quit programs are twice as likely to succeed as those who are not enrolled (McCuller, Sussman, Wapner, Dent, & Weiss, 2006). It is encouraging that based on the 2012 Tips From Former Smokers campaign, the CDC reports that 100,000 smokers are expected to have achieved permanent smoking cessation (2015b).

An estimated 6 million youths will die prematurely from cigarette-related deaths (U.S. DHHS, 2010e). Over the past 50 years, the prevalence of smoking in the United States has decreased by about 50%, to about one fifth of the population. Men smoke more than women (19% vs. 15%). Native American/ Native Alaskans smoke more (29%) than blacks and whites (both at 18%), Hispanics (15%), and Asians/ Pacific Islanders (9.5%). In 2005, 19 million adults attempted to quit, but only 4% to 7% are estimated to have been successful (CDC, 2016). In 2009, the rates of teen smoking declined to 20%, yet monitoring teen smoking is important because 80% of adult smokers began before the age of 18 (CDC,

2010b). Although there is a strong evidence-base for first-line smoking cessation interventions, the United States has yet to achieve its goal of tobacco use being a rare behavior (DHHS, 2014).

EVIDENCE TO GUIDE POPULATION-FOCUSED INTERVENTIONS

Enormous health-related disparities exist in second-hand smoke exposure. Among the highest exposed are children aged 4 to 11 and low-income individuals at 61% and 63%, respectively (CDC, 2008b). Not only does decreasing smoking in public places protect nonsmokers from the effects of secondhand smoke, but it may also promote smoking cessation by restricting smoking behavior. Comprehensive multicomponent strategies to enforce no-smoking policies within organizations were found to be the most effective strategies to decrease smoking in public places. The ACA of 2009 granted the FDA authority to regulate tobacco products to prevent illness within the population. The law creates a prevention and public health fund that provides states with financial incentives to encourage healthy behaviors among Medicaid recipients (U.S. DHHS, 2010e).

The evidence for tobacco cessation is reviewed in *Ending the Tobacco Problem: A Blueprint for the Nation* (IOM, 2007). This publication endorses innovative social policies that translate the scientific evidence into action. Sample interventions include:

- counter-marketing youth-targeted smoking cessation mass advertising,
- adopting comprehensive smoke-free laws,
- increasing healthcare access to smoking cessation programs,
- restricting smoking-related advertisements, and
- increasing the federal excise tax on cigarettes.

A moderate effect was found with the use of educational material and posted warnings to enforce no-smoking policies (Serra, Bonfill, Pladevall, & Cabezas Pena, 2008). Increasing the federal excise tax on cigarettes has shown national benefit. As of June 2016, the following nine states had set excise tax rates of $3 or more per pack: New York ($4.35),

Rhode Island ($3.75), Minnesota ($3.00), Connecticut ($3.65), Massachusetts ($3.51), Guam ($3.00), Vermont ($3.08), Washington ($3.03), and Hawaii ($3.20). For every 10% increase in the price of tobacco products, consumption falls by approximately 4% overall, with a greater reduction among youth. In 2009, the ACA enactment of the 62-cent federal cigarette excise tax increase is projected to prevent initiation of smoking by nearly 2 million children, cause more than 1 million adult smokers to quit, and prevent nearly 900,000 smoking-attributed deaths (U.S. DHHS, 2010e). The long-term healthcare savings by reducing tobacco-related healthcare costs is estimated to be $44 billion.

Mass media interventions are used as part of a comprehensive tobacco cessation program, and they can be effective strategies for adults (Bala, Strzeszynski, & Cahill, 2008). Mass media interventions, such as those delivered by leaflets, booklets, posters, billboards, newspapers, radio, and television, are used to promote smoking cessation. One example of this type of intervention is the media campaign initiated by the New York City Department of Mental Health and Hygiene. In 2006, the department launched a television advertising blitz with disturbing images and graphic descriptions of the health consequences of smoking. One vignette showed a man speaking with a robotic voice after a laryngectomy made necessary by throat cancer. This campaign reduced smoking rates overall among men and Hispanic New Yorkers (CDC, 2007). A prominent national campaign resulted in approximately 450,000 fewer adolescents initiating smoking (Farrelly, Nonnemaker, Davis, & Hussin, 2009). A cost-utility analysis found that the campaign recouped the $234 million in media-related costs and just under $1.9 billion in medical expenses averted for society over the lifetimes of the youth who did not become smokers (Holtgrave, Wunderink, Vallone, & Healton, 2009).

In May 2008, the U.S. Public Health Service released the updated guidelines on tobacco use, treatment, and dependence (Fiore et al., 2008). These evidence-based guidelines recommend treatment for individuals who are tobacco dependent. Recommendations from the guidelines represent strength of evidence with A through C ratings. The strongest recommendations, Level A, are based on multiple, well-designed, randomized trials that are directly relevant to the recommendation. Level B ratings indicate that some evidence from randomized clinical trials supported the recommendation, but the scientific support was not optimal. Level C ratings are "reserved for important clinical situations in which the panel achieved consensus on the recommendation in the absence of relevant randomized controlled trials" (Fiore et al., 2008, p. 15). According to the guidelines, "It is difficult to identify any other condition [than tobacco dependence] that presents such a mix of lethality, prevalence, and neglect despite effective and readily available interventions" (Fiore et al., 2008, p. 2).

The guidelines strongly recommend that clinicians screen and document patients' tobacco use status and deliver evidence-based tobacco dependence treatment (strength of evidence A) (Fiore et al., 2008). Simple reminders, such as chart stickers or electronic prompts, can be instituted within an organization to remind clinicians to ask about smoking status. For smokers who are not currently interested in quitting, motivational techniques can be used to encourage a future quit attempt (strength of evidence B). Clinicians and clinicians-in-training should be taught effective smoking cessation strategies to assist individuals who want to make a quit attempt and those who are not yet motivated to do so (strength of evidence B). Furthermore, because the tobacco-dependence treatments identified in the guidelines are cost effective, they should be offered to all smokers (strength of evidence A). Counseling for tobacco-dependent adolescents has been found to be effective and, therefore, is recommended (strength of evidence B). Web-based interventions may be useful in assisting tobacco cessation (strength of evidence B). Cessation counseling has been found to be effective with parents to help protect children from secondhand smoke (strength of evidence B).

More recently, the U.S. DHHS (2010e) strategic plan *Ending the Tobacco Epidemic, A Tobacco Control Strategic Action Plan* focuses on improving American health by strengthening existing EBPs as well as stimulating new tobacco cessation research. This comprehensive, evidenced-based practice plan represented the first-ever national strategic plan for tobacco control. It included 21 action step featured pillars to improve public health and advance research knowledge. In September 2011, the Centers for Disease Control and Prevention (CDC) awarded more than $100 million in community transformation grants for tobacco control initiatives. Moreover, the Food and Drug Administration (FDA) awarded $33 million in contracts to 37 states to diminish tobacco marketing, sale, and distribution to adolescents at retail locations (Koh & Sebelius, 2012).

WHAT DOES ADDITIONAL EVIDENCE TELL US ABOUT ADOLESCENTS?

The evidence indicates that tobacco advertising and promotion increase the likelihood that non-smoking adolescents will become smokers at a later time. The three most heavily branded cigarette companies accounted for 80% of adolescent cigarette brands. Joe the Camel was an example of an advertising strategy that was specifically directed to promote adolescent smoking (CDC, 2012b).

The National Cancer Institute (2008) concluded that there is a causal relationship between smoking initiation in teens and exposure to media depictions of smoking. In a 2010 meta-analysis of four studies, Millett and Glantz found that viewing tobacco use in movies contributed to a 44% rate of smoking initiation among pediatric populations. This prospective relationship between exposure to smoking in movies and smoking initiation was supported by a national cohort of 2,341 adolescents (Dal Cin, Stoolmiller, & Sargent, 2014). Overall, there is weak evidence that mass media can be effective in preventing young adults from starting to smoke, yet media depictions of smoking aimed at predominantly ethnic minorities were associated with higher rates of tobacco risk behaviors (Upson, 2015). Mass media campaigns that developed and focused their message based on their target audience were more effective than those that did not use this strategy. Campaigns of greater intensity and duration were more successful than those that were not (Sowden, 1998).

Media communications has played a key role in branding cigarettes and creating an image for adolescents. Adolescents experience tremendous social marketing and peer pressures that can promote risky behaviors such as smoking. In 2005, tobacco industries spent $13.5 billion in advertisements (National Cancer Institute, 2008). Tobacco advertisers targeted adolescents by aiming their message at the emotional developmental needs of this age group, such as popularity, peer acceptance, and positive self-image. Tobacco print and media ads create the perception that smoking will satisfy these needs.

Many population studies have documented decreases in teen smoking when social media interventions are combined with public health initiatives. In 2000, the American Legacy Foundation began the largest social media effort to prevent teen smoking, entitled "truth" (National Institute for Health Care Management [NIHCM], 2009). Farrelly et al. (2009) concluded that the truth campaign accounted for approximately a 22% decline in adolescent smoking. An example of a media campaign targeting young adults was the billboard advertising in New York City featuring star athletes from various local sports teams. The slogan, "I don't smoke, do you?" was prominently displayed along major highways throughout the city.

Other interventions are directed toward the selling of tobacco. It is believed that if young people are unable to purchase cigarettes, this may reduce the number who start to smoke. Although warnings and fines levied against retailers to discourage the illegal sale of cigarettes were shown to be effective in decreasing sales, the outcome of this intervention has not shown a clear effect (Stead & Lancaster, 2005). Furthermore, it is believed that the behavior of a child's/adolescent's family may influence the likelihood of the child/adolescent starting to smoke. Although there is evidence that

family interventions may prevent adolescents from smoking, other evidence showed neutral or negative outcomes (Thomas, Baker, & Lorenzetti, 2007).

Do school-based programs prevent children who are nonsmokers from becoming smokers? Thomas and Perera (2006) reviewed 23 high-quality, randomized controlled trials. The interventions in these studies included information giving, social influence approaches, social skills training, and community interventions. Information giving alone was not supported by the evidence as an effective intervention, and there was limited evidence for the effects of the other interventions. Peterson et al. (2009) demonstrated the effect of motivational interviewing on teen smoking cessation. In a randomized control trial of 50 high schools in Washington, abstinence from smoking increased 4% in teenagers who received personalized telephone calls and motivational interviews.

Through increased implementation of evidence-based interventions, tobacco dependence in adolescents declined 40% from 1997 to 2003. Before 2009, progress stalled, possibly because of decreased state funding for tobacco-dependence prevention programs, increased tobacco industry marketing, and decreased effectiveness of mass media campaigns (CDC, 2007). In 2009, the National Youth Tobacco Survey still revealed a decline in smoking among middle school and high school students. The prevalence of current tobacco use among middle school students declined (15.1% to 8.2%), as did current cigarette use (11.0% to 5.2%) and cigarette smoking experimentation (29.8% to 15.0%). Similar trends were observed for high school students (current tobacco use: 34.5% to 23.9%; current cigarette use: 28.0% to 17.2%; cigarette smoking experimentation: 39.4% to 30.1%). The CDC (2010a) reports that despite the decline in teenage smoking by interventions, state programs remain underfunded. The tobacco epidemic in the United States is an example of how utilizing EBP public health measures at a national level can stop this epidemic and accelerate declines in the related morbidity and mortality associated with tobacco dependence.

PUTTING EVIDENCE INTO PRACTICE

Traditional smoking cessation counter-marketing strategies employed a wide range of efforts, including paid television, radio, billboard, print, and web-based advertising at the state and local levels; media advocacy through public relations efforts, such as press releases; and local events, media literacy, and health promotion activities (Fiore et al., 2008). In today's technologically dependent society, social media has emerged as a popular source of health information. Innovations in tobacco cessation health communication should include targeting smoking audiences through personal communication devices (e.g., text messaging) and online networking environments, as well as fostering dissemination of health messages through innovative channels (such as weblogs or blogs).

Approximately 62% of the U.S. population report that they use the Internet, with greater than 50% of adults reporting health-related information searches (CDC, 2010b). Internet-based interventions provide an excellent public health opportunity to impact tobacco use at a population level. There is a positive association between web-assisted tobacco interventions and successfully quitting (An et al., 2008). A systematic review of web-based interventions demonstrated a 17% increase in six-month tobacco abstinence (Shabab & McEwen, 2009).

An exemplar of a web-assisted, EBP smoking social networking site is QuitNet. QuitNet is an Internet-based intervention that provides telephone intervention, 24-hour social networking, smoking cessation medication, and email support. QuitNet first launched on the World Wide Web in 1995. Dr. Nathan Cobb created the concept, which was later adopted by Join Together, a project of Boston University School of Public Health. With the university's help, QuitNet.com, Inc. was formed in 2000 to take on the role of expanding QuitNet into a self-supporting service operating worldwide. QuitNet is utilized in several statewide smoking initiatives, including Utah and North Dakota. Utah has the lowest smoking rate in the country at 8.8%

(Utah Department of Health, 2010). In 2011, 860 Utahans per month were served with free tailored interventions by QuitNet and telephone-based quit interventions. Structured interventions that reach the entire community have shown to improve smoking cessation in Utah: 93% of Utahans have implemented rules against smoking in their homes, and 98% of Utah children are without secondhand exposure in their homes (Utah Department of Health, 2010). Clearly, more research needs to be done to explore outcomes with Internet-based smoking programs, yet web-based interventions are important in population-based strategies for tobacco cessation. The Internet programs can be self-tailored and are an inexpensive way to deliver to large population because they require low personnel costs.

TOBACCO DEPENDENCE: FUTURE DIRECTIONS THROUGH BEST PRACTICES

According to the U.S. DHHS (2010e), the most effective evidence-based, population-based approaches result from the synergistic effect produced by putting into place the following program components: state and community interventions, health communication interventions, cessation interventions, surveillance and evaluation, and administration and management. The IOM (2007) put forth the goal of reducing smoking so that it is no longer a significant health problem for our nation. The IOM believes, based on substantial evidence, that this can be achieved through state tobacco control programs that are comprehensive, integrated, and maintained over time. The most cost-effective, worldwide strategy to reduce tobacco use has been raising taxes (WHO, 2015). In the past 25 years, cigarette prices rose 350% because of a sixfold increase in federal cigarette tax and a fivefold increase in state tax (WHO, 2015). In this same era, the adult smoking population decreased by nearly 33%, and the number of cigarettes smoked per capita decreased by more than 50% (WHO, 2015). Putting into practice national evidence-based interventions is an example of how to curtail a public health condition such as the tobacco epidemic in the United States.

Additional Resources

Center for Disease Control and Prevention—Smoking & Tobacco Use—State and Community Resources at: http://www.cdc.gov/tobacco/stateandcommunity/

Center for Disease Control and Prevention—Smoking & Tobacco Use—Data and Statistics at: https://www.cdc.gov/tobacco/data_statistics/

Center for Disease Control and Prevention—Health Literacy at: http://www.cdc.gov/healthliteracy/

National Assessment of Adult Literacy at: https://nces.ed.gov/naal/

Agency for Healthcare Research and Quality—Clinical Guidelines and Recommendations at: http://www.ahrq.gov/professionals/clinicians-providers/guidelines-recommendations/index.html

U.S. Preventative Services Task Force at: https://www.uspreventiveservicestaskforce.org/

References

An, L. C., Schillo, B. A., Saul, J. E., Wendling, A. H., Klatt, C. M., Berg, C. J., & Luxenberg, M. G. (2008). Utilization of smoking cessation informational, interactive, and online community resources as predictors of abstinence: Cohort study. *Journal of Medical Internet Research, 10*(5), e55.

Baker, D. W., Gamarazian, J. A., Williams, M. V., Scott, T., Parker, R. M., Green, D., . . . Peel, J. (2002). Functional health literacy and the risk of hospital admission among Medicare managed care enrollees. *American Journal of Public Health, 92*(8), 1278–1283.

Baker, D. W., Parker, R. M., Williams, M. V., & Clark, W. S. (1998). Health literacy and the risk of hospital admission. *Journal of General Internal Medicine, 13*(12), 791–798.

Baker, D. W., Wolf, M., Feinglass, J., Thompson, J. A., Gasmaranian, J. A., & Huang, J. (2007). Health literacy and mortality among elderly persons. *Archives of Internal Medicine, 167*(14), 1503–1509.

Bala, M., Strzeszynski, L., & Cahill, K. (2008). Mass media interventions for smoking cessation in adults. *Cochrane Database of Systematic Reviews* (Issue 1), Art. No.: CD004704. doi:10.1002/14651858.CD004704.pub2

Berkman, N., Sheridan, S., Donahue, K., Halpern, D., & Crotty, K. (2011a). Low health literacy and health outcomes: An updated systematic review. *Annals of Internal Medicine, 155*(2), 97–107.

Centers for Disease Control and Prevention. (2007). *Best practices for comprehensive tobacco control programs—2007*. Atlanta, GA: U.S. Department of Health and Human Services, Centers for Disease Control and Prevention, National Center for Chronic Disease Prevention and Health Promotion, Office on Smoking and Health.

Centers for Disease Control and Prevention. (2008a). Smoking-attributable mortality, years of potential life lost, and productivity losses—United States, 2000–2004. *Morbidity and Mortality Weekly Report, 57*(45), 1226–1228.

Centers for Disease Control and Prevention.(2008b). Disparities in secondhand smoke exposure—United States, 1988–1994 and 1994–2004. *Morbidity and Mortality Weekly Report, 57*(27), 744–747.

Centers for Disease Control and Prevention. (2010a). Tobacco use among middle and high school students—United States, 2000–2009. *Morbidity and Mortality Weekly Report, 59*(33), 1063–1068.

Centers for Disease Control and Prevention. (2010b). Vital Signs. Retrieved from http://www.cdc.gov/vitalsigns/tobaccouse/smoking/latestfindings.html

Centers for Disease Control and Prevention. (2012a). *Preventing Tobacco Use Among Youth and Young Adults: A Report of the Surgeon General*. Atlanta, GA: U.S. Department of Health and Human Services.

Centers for Disease Control and Prevention. (2012b). *National Center for Chronic Disease Prevention and Health Promotion (U.S.) Office on Smoking and Health*. Atlanta, GA: Author.

Centers for Disease Control and Prevention. (2015a). *Learn about health literacy*. Retrieved from http://www.cdc.gov/healthliteracy/learn/

Centers for Disease Control and Prevention. (2015b). Current Cigarette Smoking Among Adults—United States, 2005–2014. *Morbidity and Mortality Weekly Report, 64*(44), 1233–1240.

Center for Disease Control and Prevention. (2016). *Smoking and tobacco*. Retrieved from http://www.cdc.gov/tobacco/data_statistics/fact_sheets/youth_data/tobacco_use/index.htm

Cronewett, L., Sherwood, G., Barnsteiner, J., Disch, J., Johnson, J., Mitchell, P., & Warren, J. (2007). Quality and safety education for nurses. *Nursing Outlook, 55*(3), 122–131.

Cullum, N., Ciliska, D., Haynes, R. B., & Marks, S. (2008). *Evidence-based nursing: An introduction*. Hong Kong and Singapore: Blackwell.

Dal Cin, S., Stoolmiller, M., & Sargent, J. D. (2013). Exposure to smoking in movies and smoking initiation among black youth. *American journal of preventive medicine, 44*(4), 345–350.

DeNavas-Walt, C., Proctor, B., & Smith, J. (2011).*U.S. Census Bureau, Current Population Reports, P60-239, Income, Poverty, and Health Insurance Coverage in the United States: 2010*. Washington, DC: U.S. Government Printing Office.

DeWalt, D. A., Berkman, N. D., Sheridan, S., Lohr, K. N., & Pignone, M. P. (2004). Literacy and health outcomes: A systematic review of the literature. *Journal of General Internal Medicine, 19*(12), 1228–1239.

Doak, L., Doak, C., & Root, J. (1998). *Teaching patients with low literacy skills*. Philadelphia, PA: Lippincott.

Farrelly, M., Nonnemaker, J., Davis, K., & Hussin, A. (2009). The influence of the national truth® campaign on smoking initiation. *American Journal of Preventive Medicine, 36*(5), 379–384.

Fiore, M. C., Jaén, C. R., Baker, T. B., Bailey, W. C., Benowitz, N. L., Curry, S. J., & Wewers, M. E. (2008). *Treating tobacco use and dependence: 2008 update*. Rockville, MD: U.S. Department of Health and Human Services.

Gebbie, K., Rosenstock, L., Hernandez, L. M., & Committee on Educating Health Professionals for the 21st Century, Board on Health Promotion and Disease Prevention, Institute of Medicine of the National Academies. (Eds.). (2003). *Who will keep the public healthy? Educating public health professionals for the 21st century*. Washington, DC: National Academies Press.

Griener, A. C., Knebel, E, & Committee on the Health Professions Summit, Institute of Medicine of the National Academies. (Eds.). (2003). *Health professions education: A bridge to quality*. Washington, DC: National Academies Press.

Hanchate, A. D., Ash, A. S., Gasmararian, J. A., Wolf, M. A., & Paasche-Orlow, M. K. (2008). The Demographic Assessment for Health Literacy (DAHL): A new tool for estimating associations between health literacy and outcomes in national surveys. *Journal of General Internal Medicine, 23*(10), 1561–1566.

Heron, M., & Smith, B. (2007). *Deaths leading causes for 2003. National Vital Statistics Reports*. Washington, DC: Centers for Disease Control and Prevention.

Holtgrave, D., Wunderink, K., Vallone, D., & Healton, C. (2009). Cost-utility analysis of the national truth® campaign to prevent youth smoking. *American Journal of Preventive Medicine, 36*(5), 385–388.

Institute for Healthcare Advancement. (2017). Retrieved from https://www.iha4health.org/

Institute of Medicine. (2002). *Who will keep the public healthy? Educating public health professionals for the 21st century*. Washington, DC: The National Academies Press

Institute of Medicine. (2004). *Health literacy: A prescription to end confusion*. Washington, DC: National Academies Press.

Institute of Medicine. (2007). *Ending the tobacco problem: A blueprint for the nation*. Washington, DC: The National Academies Press.

Institute of Medicine. (2011). *The future of nursing: Leading change, advancing health*. Washington, DC: National Academies Press.

Keeling, A. W., Lusk, B., & Kulbok, P. K. (2017). Culturally sensitive primary healthcare interventions: Three exemplars. In S. B. Lewenson & M. Truglio-Londrigan (Eds.), *Practicing primary health care in nursing: Caring for populations* (pp. 161–176). Burlington, MA: Jones & Bartlett.

Koh, H. K., & Sebelius, K. G. (2012). Ending the tobacco epidemic. *Journal of American Medical Association*, *308*(8), 767–768.

Kutner, M., Greenberg, E., Jin, Y., Boyle, B., Hsu, Y., & Dunleavy, E. (2007). *Literacy in everyday life: Results from the 2003 National Assessment of Adult Literacy* (NCES 2007-490). Washington, DC: National Center for Education Statistics, Institute for Education Sciences, U.S. Department of Education.

Lipstein, S. H., Kellermann, A. L., Berkowitz, B., Sklar, D., & Thibault, G. (2016). *Workforce for 21st Century Health and Health Care: A Vital Direction for Health and Health Care* (Discussion Paper). Washington, DC: National Academy of Medicine's Vital Directions for Health and Health Care Initiative.

Maniaci, M., Heckman, M., & Dawson, N. (2008). Functional health literacy and understanding of medicines at discharge. *Mayo Clinic Proceedings, 83*(5), 554–558.

McLaughlin, G. H. (2008). *Simplified measure of gobbledygook*. Retrieved from http://www .harrymclaughlin.com/SMOG.htm

McLeod-Sordjan, R. (2011). Assessing functional health literacy: Strategy to reduce health disparities among elderly Hispanic patients with chronic disease. *Journal of Nurse Practitioners, 7*(10), 839–846.

Melnyk, B. M., & Fineout-Overholt, E. (2011). *Evidence-based practice in nursing and healthcare: A guide to best practice* (2nd ed.). Philadelphia, PA: Lippincott.

Millett, C., & Glantz, S. (2010). Assigning an "18" rating to movies with tobacco imagery is essential to reduce youth smoking. *Thorax, 65*, 77–78.

Murphy-Knoll, L. (2007). Low health literacy puts patients at risk. *Journal of Nursing Care Quality, 22*(3), 205–209.

National Cancer Institute. (2008). *Tobacco control monograph 19: The role of the media in promoting and reducing tobacco use*. Bethesda, MD: U.S. Department of Health and Human Services, National Institutes of Health, National Cancer Institute. Retrieved from http://www.cancercontrol. cancer.gov/tcrb/monographs/19/index.html

National Center for Education Statistics. (2006). *The health literacy of America's adults: Results from the 2003 National Assessment of Adult Literacy*. Retrieved from http://nces.ed.gov/pubs2006/2006483.pdf

National Institute for Health Care Management. (2009, March). *Recommended adolescent health care utilization: How social marketing can help*. (NIHCM Foundation Issue Brief). Retrieved from http://www.nihcm.org/component/content /archive/2009/3

National Patient Safety Foundation. (2008). *Ask me three*. Retrieved from http://www.npsf.org/askme3/PCHC/

National Youth Tobacco Survey. (2009). Retrieved from http://www.cdc.gov/mmwr/preview /mmwrhtml/mm5412a1.htm

Newport, F. (2013). *Most U.S. Smokers Want to Quit, Have Tried Multiple Times*. Retrieved from http:// www.gallup.com/poll/163763/smokers-quit-tried -multiple-times.aspx

Nielsen-Bohlman, L., Panzer, A., & Kindig, D. (Eds.). (2004). *Health literacy: A prescription to end confusion*. Washington, DC: National Academies Press.

Oxman, A., Sackett, D., & Guyatt, G. (1992). Evidence-based medicine workgroup. *Journal of the American Medical Association, 268*(9), 1135–1136.

Patient Protection and Affordable Care Act, Pub. L. No. 111-148, §2702, 124 Stat. 119, 318–319 (2010).

Peterson, A., Kealey, P., Mann, S., Marek, P., Ludman, E., Liu, J., & Bricker, J. (2009). Group-randomized trial of a proactive, personalized telephone counseling intervention for adolescent smoking cessation. *Journal of the National Cancer Institute, 101*(20), 1378–1392.

Pfizer Clear Health Communication Initiative. (2008). *Help your patients succeed: Tips for improving communication with your patients*. Retrieved from http:// clearhealthcommunication.com/public -health-professionals/tips-for-providers.html

Plain Writing Act of 2010 (H.R. 946), Public Law 111–274—October 13, 2010 124 STAT. 2861 Retrieved from https://www.gpo.gov/fdsys/pkg/PLAW -111publ274/pdf/PLAW-111publ274.pdf

Quality and Safety Education for Nurses. (2007). *Overview* [Online]. Retrieved from http://qsen.org /about/overview/

QuitNet. (n.d.). Retrieved from http://www.quitnet.com

Schillinger, D., Grumbach, K., Piette, J., Wang, F., Osmond, D., Daher, C., . . . Bindman, A. B. (2002). Association of health literacy with diabetes outcomes. *Journal of the American Medical Association, 288*(4), 475–482.

Serra, C., Bonfill, X., Pladevall-Vila, M., & Cabezas Pena, C. (2008). Interventions for preventing tobacco smoking in public places. *Cochrane Database of Systematic Reviews, (3),* CD001294.

Shahab, L., & McEwen, A. (2009). Online support for smoking cessation: A systematic review of the literature. *Addiction, 104*(11), 1792–1804. doi: 10.1111/j.1360-0443.2009.02710.x.ADD2710

Shohet, L., & Renaud, L. (2006). Critical analysis on best practices in health literacy. *Canadian Journal of Public Health, 97,* S10.

Singleton, J., Levin, R. F., Feldman, H. R., & Truglio-Londrigan, M. (2005). Evidence for smoking cessation: Implications for gender-specific strategies. *Worldviews on Evidence-Based Nursing, 2*(2), 1–12.

Singleton, J. K., Levin, R. F., & Keefer, J. (2007). Evidence-based practice. Disciplinary perspectives on evidence-based practice: The more the merrier. *Research and Theory in Nursing Practice, 21*(4), 213–216.

Sowden, A. J. (1998). Mass media interventions for preventing smoking in young people. *Cochrane Database of Systematic Reviews, (4),* CD001006.

Stead, L. F., & Lancaster, T. (2005). Interventions for preventing tobacco sales to minors. *Cochrane Database of Systematic Reviews, (1),* CD001497.

Stetler, C. B., Morsi, D., Rucki, S., Broughton, S., Corrigan, B., Fitzgerald, J., . . . Sheridan, E. A. (1998). Utilization-focused integrative reviews in a nursing service. *Applied Nursing Research, 11*(4), 195–205.

Straus, S. E., Richardson, W. S., Glasziou, P., & Haynes, R. B. (2005). *Evidence-based medicine: How to practice and teach EBM* (3rd ed.). Edinburgh, UK: Elsevier.

Thomas, R. E., Baker, P. R. A., & Lorenzetti, D. (2007). Family-based programmes for preventing smoking by children and adolescents. *Cochrane Database of Systematic Reviews, (1),* CD004493.

Thomas, R., & Perera, R. (2006). School-based programmes for preventing smoking. *Cochrane Database of Systematic Reviews, 19,* 3.

Upson, D. (2015). Social determinants of cigarette smoking. In *The tobacco epidemic 42* (pp. 181–198). Basel, Switzerland: Karger Publishers.

U.S. Department of Education (U.S. DOE). (2016). *U.S. Program for the International Assessment of Adult Competencies (PIAAC) 2012/2014: Main Study and National Supplement Technical Report.* Retrieved from: http://nces.ed.gov/pubs 2016/2016036.pdf

U.S. Department of Health and Human Services (U.S. DHHS). (2010a). *About healthy people.* Retrieved from http://www.healthypeople.gov /2020/about/default.aspx

U.S. Department of Health and Human Services (U.S. DHHS). (2010b). Healthy People 2020 *topics and objectives.* Retrieved from http://www.healthypeople .gov/2020/topicsobjectives2020/default.aspx

U.S. Department of Health and Human Services (U.S. DHHS), Office of Disease Prevention and Health Promotion. (2010c). *National Action Plan to Improve Health Literacy.* Washington, DC: Author. Retrieved from http://www.health.gov /communication/HLActionPlan/

U.S. Department of Health and Human Services (U.S. DHHS). (2010d). Healthy People 2010 *framework.* Retrieved from http://www.healthypeople.gov/2020 /Consortium/HP2020Framework.pdf

U.S. Department of Health and Human Services (U.S. DHHS). (2010e). *Ending the tobacco epidemic: A tobacco control strategic action plan for the U.S. Department of Health and Human Services.* Washington, DC: Office of the Assistant Secretary for Health.

U. S. Department of Health and Human Services. (2014). *The Health Consequences of Smoking—. 50 Years of Progress.* Retrieved from http://www .surgeongeneral.gov/library/reports/50-years-of -progress/exec-summary.pdf

U. S. Department of Health and Human Services. Office of Adolescent Health. (2016). *Substance Abuse.* Retrieved from http://www.hhs.gov/ash/oah /adolescent-health-topics/substance-abuse/tobacco /trends.html#

Utah Department of Health. (2010). *Behavioral Risk Factor Surveillance System (BRFSS).* Salt Lake City: Utah Department of Health, Center for Health Data.

Vernon, J. A., Trujillo, A., Rosenbaum, S., & DeBuono, B. (2007). *Low health literacy: Implications for national health policy.* Partnership for Clear Health Communication. Retrieved from http://npsf.org/askme3 /pdfs/Case_Report_10_07.pdf

Volandes, A., Paasche-Orlow, M., Gillick, M. R., Cook, E. F., Shaykevich, S., Abbo, E. D., . . . Lehmann, L. (2008). Health literacy not race predicts end-of-life care preferences. *Palliative Medicine, 11*(5), 754–762.

Wald, L. D. (1917, May 10). The care of sick children in the home. Paper delivered by Lillian D. Wald at the Academy of Medicine, Section on Pediatrics. Lillian D. Wald Papers, 1889–1957. Writing and Speeches. Nurses & Nursing, Reel 25, Box 37, Folder 3, np – 3 pages of the speech. New York Public Library, Humanities and Social Sciences Library, Manuscripts and Archives Division, New York, NY.

Weiss, B. D., Mays, M. Z., Martz, W., Castro, K. M., DeWalt, D. A., Pignone, M. P., & Hale, F. A. (2005). Quick assessment of literacy in primary care: The newest vital sign. *Annals of Family Medicine, 3,* 514–522.

World Health Organization. (2015). *WHO report on the global tobacco epidemic, 2015: raising taxes on tobacco.* Retrieved from https://escholarship.org/uc/item/1fh1f32m

For a full suite of assignments and additional learning activities, use the access code located in the front of your book to visit this exclusive website: **http://go.jblearning.com/londrigan**. If you do not have an access code, you can obtain one at the site.

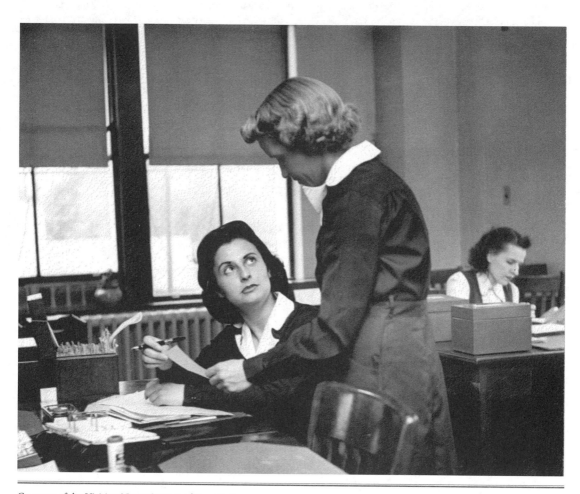

Courtesy of the Visiting Nurse Service of New York.

CHAPTER 7

Informatics in Public Health Nursing

Arlene H. Morris

The application of science has lagged behind its development, chiefly because of the vast difficulty of the problem of bringing its many sidedness to bear on the infinite varieties of our present-day social network. The necessity for practical application of medical and sanitary knowledge, however, is now recognized and admitted because of the inter-relation of all parts of society. (Wald, 1918, p. 1)

LEARNING OBJECTIVES

At the completion of this chapter, the reader will be able to:

- Define terminology related to informatics as used in public health.
- Describe current and potential applications of information technology (IT) in public health nursing.
- Differentiate various uses of informatics in public health nursing.
- Relate examples of situations and select most appropriate data for public health nursing.
- Identify potential ethical issues related to use of healthcare information technology and the future of informatics in public health nursing.

KEY TERMS

- ❏ Analytic assessment
- ❏ Data
- ❏ Database
- ❏ Data mining
- ❏ Electronic health records (EHR)
- ❏ Ethical issues
- ❏ Informatics

- ❏ Investigation
- ❏ Monitoring
- ❏ Nursing Informatics
- ❏ Personal health records (PHR)
- ❏ Public health informatics
- ❏ Regional health information exchanges
- ❏ Telehealth

In these rapidly changing times, all nurses are confronted with a myriad of sources for communication and data management. The challenge becomes determining the most effective and ethical use of communication, data collection, and resources to most accurately assess, plan, and coordinate care, and evaluate care for individuals, families, populations, communities, and systems. Required skills include ensuring accurate input of information using the most relevant of recently developed information systems tools, accurate analysis and application of aggregated data to guide planning, and selection of most appropriate technology to best implement and evaluate outcomes.

Historically, nursing as a profession can most certainly link its beginning to careful observation, data collection, and use. During Florence Nightingale's experience caring for soldiers during the Crimean War (1854–1856), Nightingale used the pie graphs and charts to show how cleaning the hospital walls and providing good nutrition to the wounded supported an improvement in morbidity and mortality rates. In a similar manner, Lillian Wald, noted public health nurse and founder of Henry Street Nurses Settlement on the Lower East Side of New York City in 1893, compared data collected by the Henry Street nurses and New York City hospitals to reveal that care in the home setting as compared with hospital setting resulted in improved outcomes (Wald, 1915). Wald explained that the data the visiting nurses at Henry Street collected facilitated the comparison between the quality and safety of care in the home versus the care in hospitals.

> *Our records show that in 1914 the Henry Street staff cared for 3, 535 cases of pneumonia of all ages, with a mortality rate of 8.05 percent. For purposes of comparison four large New York hospitals gave us their records of pneumonia during the same period. Their combined figures totaled 1,612, with a mortality rate of 31.2 percent. (Wald, 1915, p. 38)*

As public health developed, nurses continued to assess the health of individuals, families/groups, populations, and communities. In 1912, the National Organization for Public Health Nursing was formed, and subsequently a template for documentation on handwritten record cards was designed to facilitate national comparison of information and statistics. Further developments

for comprehensive public health included recording, interpreting, and publishing essential facts of births, deaths, and reportable diseases (Freeman, 1950).

Information Technology in Public Health Nursing

In the current century, health care has evolved to use of **electronic health records (EHR)**, **personal health records (PHR)**, web-based health education, and **telehealth**. Passage of legislation such as the U.S. Federal Health Information Technology for Economic and Clinical Health (HITECH, 2009) Act prompted the development and use of certified EHRs to allow sharing of health information across systems. EHRs can include health information such as demographics, assessment findings, flow sheets, diagnoses, treatments, medication profile of previous and current medications, diagnostic test results, an order-entry system, and decision support. EHRs can be used simultaneously by multiple providers, and it allows for more rapid and efficient data entry than use of paper charts. Additionally, individuals can enter their own information (e.g., blood sugar level, heart rate, exercise type and time) into a PHR that can be linked to an EHR. Multiple EHRs can be linked within **regional health information exchanges** that provide access to health data across a regional system. These exchanges can improve public health surveillance (Dixon, Jones, & Grannis, 2013).

The American Nurses Association (ANA) specifies use of data and associated knowledge and skills in technology as a competency for all nurses (ANA, 2010), for public health nurses in particular (2013), and for the specialty of nursing informatics (2015). Information technology assists nurses to access information, to provide and document care and outcomes, to communicate interprofessionally, and for research. Advances in public health include more sophisticated methods to integrate information technologies that provide real-time data entry and immediate information access to multiple stakeholders. The future of nursing and public health nursing in particular will include further changes, implications, and ethical issues not previously imagined.

Public health nurses must document assessment, intervention, and evaluative information related to care of individuals, families/groups, communities, populations, and systems. **Data** are objective measurements and facts that provide essential information. However, the data have not yet been interpreted. An example of a datum would be an individual case of a disease such as presence of the Zika virus in a blood sample, which is required to be reported to the Centers for Disease Control and Prevention (CDC) and the World Health Organization (WHO). Data such as vital statistics, morbidity and mortality reports, interventions and responses across all settings of care, geographic regions, and ages can be compared in databases. **Databases** are computerized systems into which data can be entered and then analyzed for patterns and trends through comparisons of such data through programs that permit queries and allow identification and extraction of information (McGonigle & Mastrian, 2012). Thus, data become information through organizing or structuring the facts for interpretation. However, various users may have access to data within databases, yet interpret information differently. Accurate use of databases is critical for accurate interpretation. Examples of types of databases are provided in **Box 7-1.**

Box 7-1 Examples of Databases

International Databases:

United Nations Statistics Division at: http://unstats.un.org/unsd/

World Health Organization Statistical Information Systems (WHOSIS) at: http://www3.who.int/whois/en

Collaboration of U.S. Federal Agencies, Organizations and Health Science Laboratories:

Partners in Information Access for the Public Health Workforce

Healthy People 2020 **Structured Evidence Queries at:** https://phpartners.org/hp2020/

Databases from U.S. Federal Agencies:

Agency for Healthcare Research and Quality (AHRQ) at: http://www.ahrq.gov

AHRQ is the federal agency charged with supporting research to improve quality of healthcare, reduce cost, improve patient safety, decrease medical errors, and broaden access to services.

Home site for U.S. Government's Open Data at: https://www.data.gov/

The following websites provide access to data prepared by the Centers for Disease Control and Prevention (CDC):

Behavioral Risk Factor Surveillance System (BRFSS) at: http://www.cdc.gov/brfss/

BRFSS tracks health risks of adults in the U.S. Emerging Infectious Diseases (EID) at: www.cdc.gov/eid/

The Morbidity and Mortality Weekly Report (MMWR) at: http://www.cdc.gov/mmwr/

Data in the weekly MMWR are based on reports from state health departments:

National Notifiable Disease Surveillance System (NNDSS) at: http://www.cdc.gov/epo/dphsi/nndsshis.htm

NNDSS aggregates infectious disease reports from state health departments

National Vital Statistics System at: http://www.cdc.gov/nchs/nvss.htm

The National Center for Health Statistics collects and provides data about official U.S. official records of births, deaths, fetal deaths, marriages, divorces.

State and Local Data:

Alabama Department of Public Health at: http://www.adph.org/

Modified from National Network of Libraries of Medicine and National Library of Medicine (2013). *Public health information and data tutorial.* Retrieved from https://phpartners.org/tutorial/01-si/index.html

Databases may be created by an individual nurse or at a system level for data entry and retrieval. Products such as Microsoft Excel or Access can help organize data. Data can then be monitored to analyze developments, track trends, and analyze anticipated implication of the trends. For example, public health nurses enter information regarding influenza immunizations, then track and compare data for subsequent evaluation of number and locations of influenza outbreaks to help determine effectiveness of the current-year influenza vaccine. Another example is public health nurses' use of reportable laboratory results, services provided, and related client/population demographic information. As time passes and additional data are entered, comparisons can provide information about potential communicability or containment of documented health concerns.

Monitoring is observation of a population, specific group(s), or individuals while continuously making adjustments to what is occurring. Thus, monitoring involves tracking data and is a vital aspect of public health nursing. Data from various systems may be used in the monitoring or tracking efforts such as birth certificate registries, immunization records; laboratory results, assessment of needs of individuals, families/groups, communities, and populations, along with documentation of interventions and treatments and evaluation of outcomes. Tracking of data assists public health nurses to analyze trends, improve decisions, and more effectively plan for needs as they arise. The information is also used as evidence to present to policymakers. **Analytic assessment** is the process of identifying appropriate data and information sources (National Network of Libraries of Medicine website, 2013). **Data mining** involves searching through computerized data to determine useful patterns in the data that can be helpful for identifying trends. Data must be clean, which means accurate and free of errors that could skew relationships or patterns, such as multiple names for similar terms, misspelled words, or abbreviations. Software packages can be purchased to scrub the data by removing inconsistencies. Automatic processes are then used to mine large

data sets in order to identify patterns and hidden relationships to gain information and knowledge that can impact nursing care and nursing as a science. Difficulties are encountered if different terms are used for assessment findings, interventions, or outcomes. Standardized language and coding promotes more accurate identification of relationships and ultimately impacts the quality of care.

Monitoring and data mining for analysis is provided in the following example. The public health department in one state was aware of a high infant mortality rate. Initial responses included increasing prenatal care in all regional offices and carefully monitoring outcomes of mothers and infants. Although a drastically higher rate of mothers of all ages received high-quality prenatal care, the infant mortality rate decreased only slightly. Continued monitoring allowed tracking of the mothers across multiple pregnancies. Data analysis revealed that although prenatal care was received, health status of mothers between pregnancies had a greater impact. Regional health department interventions to encourage exercise, improved nutrition, folic acid intake, avoidance of nicotine, and reduced abuse of other substances gradually influenced the delivery of healthier infants. The challenge continues for public health nurses to work collaboratively with the interprofessional healthcare team across settings to foster development of infrastructure that allows opportunity to make healthier choices. Interventions such as access to fresh fruits and vegetables in convenience stores, incorporating safe areas for walking, biking or other exercise in community development efforts, increasing public safety, and education about risks of tobacco, alcohol, and substance abuse are required. Continued monitoring across settings of care and across time can provide data to measure outcomes of mother and infant health.

Accurate documentation is the foundation for trustworthy data. Information is developed when data are interpreted and organized. Knowledge is formed when relationships are identified among information. When knowledge is used appropriately to solve human problems, wisdom is developed. Information technology assists with this development of knowledge for making decisions, evaluating the outcomes of those decisions, and developing wisdom (ANA, 2015).

Informatics is the use of information and technology to communicate, manage knowledge, mitigate error, and support decision-making (Quality and Safety Education for Nurses, 2010). **Nursing informatics (NI)** is defined as "a specialty that integrates nursing and computer science to assist in decision for the patient" (The Healthcare Information and Management Systems Society [HIMSS] website, 2016a, para. 2). Nursing informatics is further defined by the American Nurses Association (2015) as

> *the specialty that integrates nursing science with multiple information management and analytical sciences to identify, define, manage, and communicate data, information, knowledge, and wisdom in nursing practice. NI supports nurses, consumers, patients, the interprofessional healthcare team, and other stakeholders in their decision-making in all roles and settings to achieve desired outcomes. This support is accomplished through the use of information structures, information processes, and information technology. (pp. 1–2)*

According to the American Association of Colleges of Nursing (AACN, 2011, pp. 17-18), informatics and healthcare technologies encompass the following five broad areas:

1. Use of patient care and other technologies to deliver and enhance care.
2. Communication technologies to integrate and coordinate care.
3. Data management to analyze and improve outcomes of care.
4. Health information management for evidence-based care and health education.
5. Facilitation and use of electronic health records to improve patient care.

Moreover, the ANA (2015) addresses the functional roles of nurses related to information technology at various levels of preparation and scope of practice. Entry-level clinical nurses must have basic computer

competencies, information literacy competencies, and information management competencies as defined by Technology Informatics Guiding Education Reform (TIGER). The Healthcare Information and Management Systems Society (HIMSS, 2016c) website provides the TIGER competencies, which may be explored at http://www.himss.org/professionaldevelopment/tiger-initiative.

Additionally, academic accrediting agencies specify competencies for graduates at various levels of education. Essential IV of the AACN's Baccalaureate Essentials (2008) specifies:

> *Graduates must have basic competence in technical skills, which includes the use of computers, as well as the application of patient care technologies such as monitors, data gathering devices, and other technological supports for patient care interventions. In addition, baccalaureate graduates must have competence in the use of information technology systems, including decision support systems, to gather evidence to guide practice. Specific introductory level nursing informatics competencies include the ability to use selected applications in a comfortable and knowledgeable way. (p. 17)*

Master's-prepared nurses "must have the knowledge and skills to use current technologies to deliver and coordinate care across multiple settings, analyze point-of-care outcomes, and communicate with individuals and groups, including the media, policymakers, other healthcare professionals, and the public" (AACN, 2011, p. 18). Furthermore, the AACN (2006) specifies that

> *Knowledge and skills related to systems/technology and patient care technology prepare the DNP graduate to apply new knowledge, manage individual and aggregate level information, and assess the efficacy of patient care technology appropriate to a specialized area of practice. DNP graduates also design, select, and use information systems/technology to evaluate programs of care, outcomes of care, and care systems . . . DNP graduates must also be proficient in the use of information*

systems/technology resources to implement quality improvement initiatives and support practice and administrative decision-making. (pp. 12–13)

Thus, nurses develop abilities to use information technologies across practice levels for increasingly more complex and analytical purposes.

Collaboration of nurses at various scopes of practice is relayed in the following example. In one state that experiences frequent tornado and hurricanes, public health department nurses collaborated with nurses in all counties of this state and adjacent states to document available health resources into a database. The database includes the number of beds in hospitals and long-term care settings, emergency departments, and other large facilities that could temporarily provide shelter in time of emergency evacuation. At any point in time, data regarding availability and number of individuals who could be received are immediately accessible. Thus, weather alerts can prompt relocation of those in the anticipated path of severe weather to areas that are available and prepared to receive the ones being transported to provide the appropriate level of care. Doctoral-prepared nurses created the information systems while collaborating with nurses of other levels to identify the number and type of facilities throughout the state.

Informatics in Public Health

American Public Health Association Public Health Nursing Section (2013) defines **public health nursing** as "the practice of promoting and protecting the health of populations using knowledge from nursing, social, and public health sciences" (para. 2). In the early 1980s, the Quad Council was established to represent interests of public health nursing and subsequently developed competencies for public health nurses along three tiers of practice: basic or generalist, midlevel or specialist, and executive or multisystem. In addition, eight domains were developed. Pertinent within *Domain 1 Analytic and Assessment Skills*, a public health nurse must have competencies to collect and develop systems to support collection and use of valid information and to identify gaps in

data. Within *Domain 3 Communication*, public health nurses must effectively communicate electronically. Included in *Domain 6 Public Health Science Skills* is competency to identify a variety of sources to access public health information (Quad Council, 2011). Increasingly, **public health informatics** courses involve graduate-level library science, public health, and healthcare professionals (Yu et al., 2015).

Public health nurses rely on infrastructure that easily allows accurate input of data, safe storage, rapid access, and facilitates management of data for various purposes. Information systems must convey data among various points to prevent the need for repeated input of the data. Reeder, Hills, Demiris, Revere, and Pina (2011) recommend the formalization of standard design methods for public health informatics that will allow for interoperable public health information systems. The National Environmental Public Health Tracking Program developed by the Centers for Disease Control and Prevention (CDC, 2016b, c) provides an example of a system that links environmental hazards such as air and water pollution with chronic diseases, and implements technology such as satellites and geographic information systems (GIS). Rababah, Curtis, and Drew (2014) suggest establishing multidisciplinary collaborative teams to further use GIS for research.

Public Health Interventions

It is obvious that informatics is critical to the following functions of public health nurses. **Investigation** is the search for health data, using skills for assessing individuals, families/groups, and populations, and skills in informatics to access information regarding a particular need. For example, screening involves methods to find previously unknown cases or existence of potential or current health concerns. Surveillance relates to comparing population health status before and after health events. Surveillance can be a process to track cases and to collect and analyze health data. Population-based interventions are focused on those who have common risks or exposures and the potential for health improvement, based on assessment of the community's determinants of health and prevention. Public health nurses care for individuals, and thus population-based, individual-focused practice refers to the care of individuals and those in a family, class, or group that is identified as being part of a population at risk. Population-based, community-focused practice relates to assessment and interventions such as community attitudes and behaviors and are measured by changes. Population-based, systems-focused practice involves organizations and systems that influence health through power, policies, or laws (Keller & Strohschein, 2016; Rippke, Briske, Keller, Strohschein, & Simonetti, 2001).

Early on, the Minnesota Department of Health (2001) provided a circular intervention wheel model to specify 17 types of actions carried out by public health personnel, and it is useful to also differentiate the level of practice as related to individuals/families, community, or systems rather than by location of the visit. Within the wheel, five wedges include interventions at each level of a population-based focused practice (Keller & Strohschein, 2016; Rippke et al., 2001). Today, this model is referred to as the intervention wheel (Keller & Strohschein, 2016).

Red: Surveillance, disease and health event investigation, outreach, screening.
Green: Delegated functions, case management, referral and follow-up.
Blue: Consultation, counseling, health teaching.
Orange: Community organizing, coalition building, collaboration.
Yellow: Advocacy, social marketing, policy development and enforcement.

This book uses the intervention wheel strategies to explicate the work of public health nurses.

An example of use of informatics in public health nursing is noted in **Box 7-2** by Cyndy Henderson, a public health nurse, and will be followed by an application of the intervention wheel.

Although this situation is still in process, and the actual implementation of telehealth connections at regional health departments has not been fully achieved, it provides an example of the services that can potentially be provided (Wicklund, 2016). Of the many who anticipate easier access to care without undue burden on family for transportation and care coordination, one case will illustrate the tremendous impact. One wounded warrior was unable to leave Walter Reed Medical Center and return home to be with and receive support from family because of unavailability of consultation resources in the rural area of Alabama. Family or friends would have needed to take an absence from work to transport the patient several hours away at frequent intervals in order to receive the level of surveillance and consultation needed. Through telehealth, public health nurses will be able to better accomplish the interventions of surveillance, disease and health event investigation, outreach, and screening (red wedge). They will be able to perform functions delegated from providers located in any number of areas across the country or internationally, improve case management, referral, and follow-up (green wedge). Internet connections such as Skype and FaceTime will allow for consultation, counseling, and health teaching at a distance and not require several of hours of travel for frequent follow-up (blue wedge). Establishment of the bandwidth and other computer systems required collaboration among healthcare providers, information technology specialists, and many others. Thus, this situation is an example of collaboration, coalition building, and community organizing (orange wedge). Advocacy, social marketing, and policy development and enforcement (yellow wedge) were needed to get support of legislators; city, county, and state officials; and business owners and foundations for financial support and development.

The future will most likely include development of smart homes, in which computerized applications or robots are used to monitor and direct activities that support care for individuals such as older adults, children, or those with need for functional assistance (De Silva, Morikawa, & Petra, 2012; Reeder et al., 2013). Automated retrieval of information such as medication times and doses, nutrition, mobility, or falls can be linked to PHRs or EHRs. Telehealth may be used to help caregivers provide more effective care

---

Box 7-2 Telehealth/Telemedicine

Cynthia S. Henderson, DNP, RN
Associate Professor of Nursing, College of Nursing and Health Sciences, Auburn University at Montgomery

Health disparities for people living in rural areas are a current force influencing nursing and by extension transforming healthcare. These disparities include reduced access to healthcare/specialist care, prevalence of underserved population, and decreased transportation. **Telehealth** is the "use of technology to deliver health care, health information, or health education at a distance" (U.S. Department of Health and Human Services [HRSA], 2016, p. 1), whereas telemedicine "refers only to clinical applications of technology" (HRSA, 2016b, p. 1). The availability of telehealth and telemedicine is a positive external factor impacting health in the rural South.

In Alabama, 10 rural hospitals have closed since 2009, prompting the creation of a health care improvement task force with a subcommittee to address access to care and telemedicine. The Alabama Department of Public Health (ADPH) created an infrastructure to support the telemedicine program, lead the charge to change the law suspending the rule requiring first-time visits between patients and physicians be face to face (F2F), and began strengthening partnerships with providers and specialists (ADPH, 2016). The infrastructure changes included extending the bandwidth capacity to all 67 county health departments, providing technical expertise (IT), improving clinic exams to include digital technologies (real-time two-way video and audio), a full-spectrum of medical services (patient assessment, diagnosis, and consultation), and peripheral exam tools such as Bluetooth stethoscope, handheld exam camera, and ultrasound (2016).

The implications for the population of individuals and families living in rural Alabama are life altering for high-risk pregnancies, wounded veterans, and those with chronic illnesses requiring close frequent medical monitoring. Traveling to healthcare sites can be expensive, long, and, depending on the condition of the roads and/or weather, difficult. Alabama's delivering hospitals can be anywhere from 50 to over 100 miles away. Using digital technologies to connect high-risk pregnant women to specialized services has the potential to reduce low-birth-weight babies, cesarean sections, and infant mortality. Providing a full spectrum of healthcare services locally to wounded veterans would allow their return home from out-of-state veteran hospitals faster, thus improving both their physical and mental recovery and providing a method for chronically ill patients to be quickly and conveniently monitored. Telemedicine provides quality care; decreases hospitalizations, emergency room visits, and the cost of services; and ultimately produces better health outcomes.

Challenges include the need for public health nurses to be instructed in using the peripheral exam tools and digital technologies; telemedicine practice experience performing actual clinical exams to provide medical services; and proactive and provide opportunities to learn about and experience telemedicine.

---

for vulnerable and hard-to-reach populations and deal with stress (Wicklund, 2015). Storfjell, Marion, and Brigell (2017) reflect on its usefulness for "hard-to-reach" populations, including those with serious mental illness. They found that developing telehealth programs to reach these populations where they live serve the purpose of improving access to care, continuity of care, and the potential for improved health outcomes. Their program, one of the American Academy of Nursing's Edgerunners, provides another example of a public-nurse-run telehealth initiative.

Additionally, geographic information systems may impact resource distribution around the world (Lin, Yen, Chiu, Chi, & Liou, 2015).

Ethical Concerns

Ethical issues include confidentiality, accurate data entry and analysis, and cybersecurity for electronic health records. For example, text messaging health information over unsecured networks can lead to breaches in confidentiality and increase the risk that the text may be sent to the wrong number. Diligence and collaborative effort by all contributors to the current and future healthcare system and all users of healthcare informatics will be needed to promote accuracy in data entry, mining, and analysis.

Continued diligence must be focused on reducing the inappropriate use of search engines for monitoring status of individuals on social media or blogs, analysis of queries for information retrieval, or health marketing (Eysenbach, 2009). Although the Internet provides access to information at a rapid speed, efforts to monitor quality and accuracy must continue. All nurses and specifically public health nurses have the opportunity to teach how to evaluate the quality of information on the Internet.

Access to information technology is not equally available to all individuals because of economic, geographic, social, or political issues, and thus this creates a health disparity because of the lack of technology availability. Ethical issues related to global health requires skills in cultural competence, communication, advocacy, health policy, research, collaboration, and public health ethics.

Conclusion

The progress of public health in the past century can be described as phenomenal. From Nightingale's and early U.S. nurses' hand-documentation of data, changes include developments in information technology and applications. The World Wide Web allows for the rapid search of databases and evidence for healthcare practices. Linkages of personal health records, electronic health records, and regional health information exchanges provide readily accessible data for monitoring the health status of individuals, families, groups, communities, and populations. Potential exists for development of infrastructure that could increase worldwide access to care. Public health and informatics nurses must continually develop and refine competencies, adhere to standards, and participate in the development, design, use, and regulation of health information technology.

Additional Resources

Alliance for Nursing Informatics at: http://allianceni.org

American Academy of Ambulatory Care Nursing (AAACN) at: http://aaacn.org

American Nurses Association at: http://nursingworld.org

American Nurse Credentialing Center at: http://nursecredentialing.org

Association of Community Health Nurse Educators at: http://www.achne.org/i4a/pages/index.cfm?pageid=3277

Future of Nursing: Campaign for Action Coalition at: http://thefutureofnursing.org

Healthcare Information and Management Systems Society (HIMSS) at: http://www.himss.org/about-himss

Quality and Safety Education for Nurses (QSEN) at: http://qsen.org

Technology Informatics Guiding Education Reform (TIGER) Initiative Foundation at: http://thetigerinitiative.org

---

References

Alabama Department of Public Health. (2016). *Telemedicine at Alabama department of public health county health departments.* Retrieved from http://adph.org/ALPHTN/assets/TelemedicinePPT2.pdf

Alanee, S., Dynda, D., Levault, K., Mueller, G., Sadowski, D., Wilber, A., . . . Dynda, M. (2014). Delivering kidney cancer care in rural central and southern Illinois: A telemedicine approach. *European*

Journal of Cancer Care, 23, 739–744. doi:10.1111 /ecc.12248

American Association of Colleges of Nursing. (2006). *Essentials of doctoral education for advanced nursing practice.* Washington, DC: Author.

American Association of Colleges of Nursing. (2008). *Essentials of baccalaureate education for professional nursing practice.* Washington, DC: Author.

American Association of Colleges of Nursing. (2011). *Essentials of master's education in nursing.* Washington, DC: Author.

American Nurses Association. (2010). *Scope and standards of practice* (2nd ed). Washington, DC: Author.

American Nurses Association. (2013). *Public health nursing: Scope and standards of practice.* Silver Spring, MD: Author.

American Nurses Association. (2015*). Nursing informatics; Scope and standards of practice* (2nd ed). Washington, DC: Author.

American Public Health Association, Public Health Nursing Section. (2013). *The definition and practice of public health nursing: A statement of the public health nursing section.* Washington, DC: American Public Health Association. Retrieved from http://achne.org /files/public/Draft2013PHNDefinitionByAPHA _PHNSection.pdf

Centers for Disease Control and Prevention. (2016a). *Diseases and conditions.* Retrieved from http://www .cdc.gov/datastatistics/

Centers for Disease Control and Prevention. (2016b). *National Environmental Public Health Tracking Network.* Retrieved at http://ephtracking.cdc.gov /showHome.action

Centers for Disease Control and Prevention. (2016c). *National Environmental Public Health Tracking Network Health Impact Assessments.* Retrieved from http://ephtracking.cdc.gov/showHealthImpact Assessment.action

De Silva, L. C., Morikawa, C., & Petra, I. M. (2012). State of the art of smart homes. *Journal of Engineering Applications of Artificial Intelligence, 25,* 1313–1321. doi:10-1016/j.engappai.2012.05.002

Dixon, B. E., Jones, J. F., & Grannis, S. J. (2013). Infection preventionists' awareness of and engagement in health information exchange to improve public health surveillance. *American Journal of Infection Control, 41,* 787–792. doi:10.1016/ajic.2012.10.022

Eysenbach, G. (2009). Infodemiology and infoveillance: Framework for an emerging set of public health informatics methods to analyze search, communication and publication behavior on the Internet. *Journal of Medical Internet Research, 11*(1), e11. doi:10.2196'jmir.1157

Freeman, R. B. (1950). *Public health nursing practice.* Philadelphia, PA: Saunders.

Healthcare Information and Management Systems Society (HIMSS). (2016a). *Nursing informatics.* Retrieved from http://www.himss.org/site-search? search_api_views_fulltext=what+is+nursing +informatics

Healthcare Information and Management Systems Society (HIMSS). (2016b). *Nursing informatics video 101.* Retrieved from http://www.himss.org /nursing-informatics-video-101?ItemNumber=26511

Healthcare Information and Management Systems Society (HIMSS). (2016c). *TIGER initiative.* Retrieved from http://www.himss.org /professionaldevelopment/tiger-initiative

Iwasiw, C., & Goldenberg, D. (2015). Gathering data for an evidence-informed, context-relevant, unified curriculum. In *Curriculum development in nursing education* (3rd ed., pp. 143–176). Burlington, MA: Jones & Bartlett Learning.

Keller, L. O., & Strohschein, S. (2016). Population-based public health nursing practice: The intervention wheel. In M. Stanhope & J. Lancaster (Eds.), *Public health nursing: 190-Population-centered health care in the community* (9th ed., pp. 190–216). St. Louis, MO: Elsevier.

Lin, S. W., Yen, C. F., Chiu, T. Y., Chi, W. C., & Liou, T. H. (2015). New indices for home nursing care resource disparities in rural and urban areas, based on geocoding and geographic distance barriers: a cross-sectional study. *International Journal of Health Geographics, 14,* 28. doi:01.1186/s12942-015-0021-9

McGonigle, D., & Mastrian, K. (2012). *Nursing informatics and the foundation of knowledge.* Sudbury, MA: Jones & Bartlett Learning.

Minnesota Department of Health, Division of Community Health Services, Public Health Nursing Section. (2001). *Public health interventions: Application for public health nursing practice.* Minneapolis, MN: Author. Retrieved from http://www.health.state .mn.us/divs/opi/cd/phn/docs/0301wheel_manual.pdf

National League for Nursing (NLN) Commission for Nursing Education Accreditation (CNEA). (2016). *Accreditation standards for nursing education programs.* Washington, DC: Author.

National Network of Libraries of Medicine and National Library of Medicine. (2013). *Public health information and data tutorial.* Retrieved from https://phpartners.org/tutorial/01-si/index.html

Quad Council of Public Health Organizations. (2011*). Quad council competencies for public health nurses.* Retrieved from http://www.achne.org/files/quad%20coun cil/quadcouncilcompetenciesforpublichealthnurses.pdf

Quality and Safety Education for Nurses (QSEN). (2010). Retrieved from http://qsen.org

Rababah, J., Curtis, A., & Drew, B. (2014). Informatics: Integrating a Geographic Information System into Nursing Research: Potentials and Challenges. *Online Journal of Issues in Nursing, 19*(2), 8.

Reeder, B., Hills, R. A., Demiris, G., Revere, D., & Pina, J. (2011). Reusable design: A proposed approach to Public Health Informatics system design. *BMC Public Health, 11*, 116. Retrieved from http://www .biomedcentral.com/1471-2458/11/116

Reeder, B., Meyer, E., Lazar, A., Chaudhuri, S., Thompson, H. J., & Demiris, G. (2013). Framing the evidence for health smart homes and home-based consumer health technologies as a public health intervention for independent aging: A systematic review. *International Journal of Medical Informatics, 82*, 565–579. doi:10.1016/ijmedinf.2013.03.007

Rippke, M., Briske, L., Keller, L. O., Strohschein, S., & Simonetti, J. (2001). *Public health interventions: Applications for public health nursing practice.* St. Paul: Minnesota Department of Health Division of Community Health Services, Public Health Nursing Section.

Rutledge, C. M., Haney, T., Bordelon, M., Renaud, M., & Fowler, C. (2014). Telehealth: Preparing advanced practice nurses to address healthcare needs in rural and underserved populations. *International Journal of Nursing Education Scholarship, 11*, 1–9. doi:10.1515 /ijnes-2013-0061

Sabesan, S., & Kelly, J. (2014). Are teleoncology models merely about avoiding long distance travel for patients? *European Journal of Cancer Care, 23*, (pp. 745–749). doi:10.1111/ecc.12251

Siminerio, L., Ruppert, K., Huber, K., & Toledo, F. G. S. (2014). Telemedicine for reach, education, access, and treatment (TREAT): Linking telemedicine with diabetes self-management education to improve care in rural communities. *The Diabetes Educator, 40*, 797–808. doi:10.1177/0145721714551993

Storfjell, J. L, Marion, L. N., & Brigell, E. (2017). Integrated health care without walls: Technology-assisted primary health care. In S. B. Lewenson & M. Truglio-Londrigan (Eds.), *Practicing primary health in nursing: Caring for populations.* (pp. 125-138). Burlington, MA: Jones & Bartlett Learning.

Technology Informatics Guiding Education Reform (TIGER) Initiative Foundation. (2016). Retrieved from http://thetigerinitiative.org

U.S. Department of Health and Human Services Administration. (2016a). *Telehealth.* Retrieved from: http://www.hrsa.gov/healthit/toolbox/Rural HealthITtoolbox/Telehealth/whatistelehealth.html

U.S. Department of Health and Human Services Administration. (2016b). *How does telehealth differ from telemedicine?* Retrieved from http://www .hrsa.gov/healthit/toolbox/ruralhealthittoolbox /telehealth/howdoestelehealthdiffer.html

Wald, L. D. (1918, June 20). Public health nursing. To be read at the Pan-American Congress on Child Welfare. Lillian Wald Papers. Writings & Speeches, Nurses & Nursing II, Reel 25, Box 37, Folder 4, pp. 1–12. New York Public Library, Humanities and Social Sciences Library, Manuscripts and Archives Division, New York, NY.

Wicklund, E. (2015). Using telehealth to care for the caregiver. *mHealth Intelligence.* Retrieved from http://mhealthintelligence.com/about-us

Wicklund, E. (2016). Tying telehealth to better rural health outcomes. *mHealth Intelligence.* Retrieved from http://mhealthintelligence.com /about-us

Williams, C. A., & Highriter, M. E., (1978). Community health nursing–population and practice. *Public Health Reviews, 7*(4), 201.

Yu, X., Xie, Y., Pan, X., Mayfield-Johnson, S., Whipple, J., & Azadbakht, E. (2015). Developing an evidence-based public health informatics course. *Journal of the Medical Library Association, 103*(4), 194–197. doi:10.3163/1563-5050.103.4.024

For a full suite of assignments and additional learning activities, use the access code located in the front of your book to visit this exclusive website: http://go.jblearning.com/londrigan. If you do not have an access code, you can obtain one at the site.

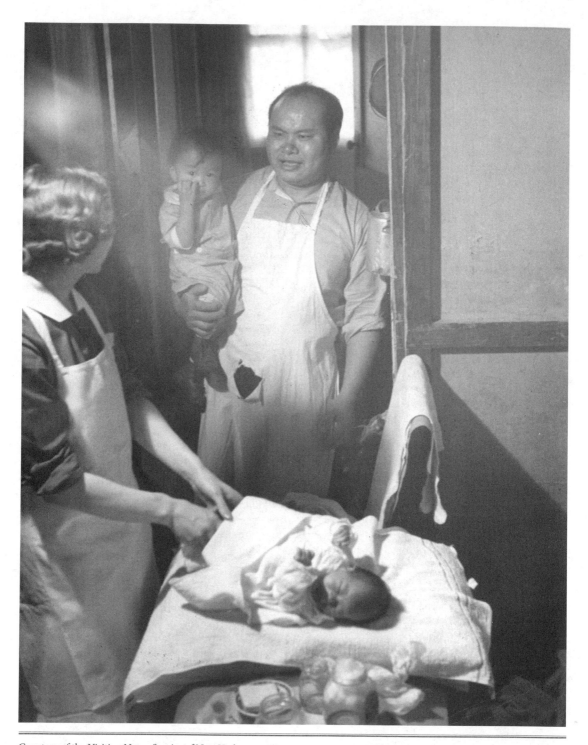

Courtesy of the Visiting Nurse Service of New York.

CHAPTER 8

Considerations of Culture in the Health of the Public

Astrid Hellier Wilson
Mary de Chesnay

Throughout the twenty years of my residence in the foreign quarter of the city, I have been challenged by various critics, anti-democratic, anti-social and political reactionaries, to defend the presence of the immigrant. (Wald, 1913, p. 1)

LEARNING OBJECTIVES

At the completion of this chapter, the reader will be able to:

- Define culture.
- Describe the subconcepts associated with culture.
- Explore the strategy of participant observation to the practice of public health nursing.
- Compare and contrast three public health issues in terms of cultural influences.
- Analyze public health nursing interventions for selected cases in terms of cultural competence.

KEY TERMS

- ❏ Culture
- ❏ Culturally competent care
- ❏ Ethnocentrism
- ❏ Participant observation
- ❏ Racism
- ❏ Ritual
- ❏ Stereotyping
- ❏ Xenophobia

This chapter presents a culturally based framework for public health nursing interventions. Although community health nurses certainly provide care to individuals and families, public health nursing generally addresses aggregate service, with heavy reliance on health-promoting and prevention strategies directed toward populations along with collaboration. The chapter provides a cultural context for health care that maximizes respect for cultural diversity while accomplishing the objectives of best practices. In the first part of this chapter, basic concepts of culture are defined and related to important aspects of public health nursing. In the second part of the chapter, model programs are presented that are examples of providing culturally competent care to populations.

Culture

Anthropologists specialize in the study of **culture**: the lifeways, folkways, rituals, taboos, and practices of a group of people who share symbols, values, and patterns of behavior. These shared aspects of living are socially determined and taken for granted by members of the culture. Cultural practices are learned and become ingrained in the subconscious to the extent that they become automatic. A common example is how members of the culture greet each other. In Russia, men might kiss each other on both cheeks. In corporate America, executives shake hands with a firm grip. In Mediterranean countries, women hug each other.

There are, however, many variations within cultural groups, particularly racial subcultural groups, and it is inappropriate to assume that all members of a group react the same in all situations. To generalize to all members of a group is considered **stereotyping**. For example, low-income, inner-city African Americans probably have more in common with low-income, inner-city whites and Hispanics than they do with upper-class African Americans regardless of where they live. In this

case, the culture of those living in poverty may dominate that of race.

Cultural beliefs are learned and shared without conscious thought or analysis of the logic behind them. Studies that demonstrate the power of cultural beliefs are easily found in the literature (Bornstein, Putnick, & Lansford, 2011; Keeling, Lusk, & Kulbok, 2017; Maupin & Ross, 2012). Some of these studies highlight differences (Koffman, Morgan, Edmonds, Speck, & Higginson, 2008; Lin, Furze, Spilsbury, & Lewin, 2008), and at the same time, there are studies that highlight the similarities among cultural groups that upon first glance might seem to be at odds with each other. For example, Cassar (2006) studied cultural expectations about pregnancy with groups of orthodox Jews and Muslims living in the United States and found similarities in need for modesty, special diet, limited spousal role in delivery, and beliefs specific to the newborn. The two groups differed on same-sex provider, period of postpartum confinement, consulting with religious leaders, and observing the Sabbath. In Keeling, Lusk, and Kulbok's (2017) work, they examine three exemplars, two from a historical perspective on Navajo Indians and public health nurses, women diagnosed with breast cancer in the 1950s, and a more contemporary example of rural youth substance abuse. In each of these exemplars, the ability to provide culturally sensitive care also rests with societal attitudes. In the second historical exemplars referring to women with breast cancer, the authors noted that "these women—in hospital and at home, young and old, of every race and ethnicity—were linked through their culture of fear, cancer phobia, and radical mastectomy" (Keeling, Lusk, & Kulbok, 2017, p. 166). The way society viewed women and this dreaded disease influenced the care received and the information shared with this particular cultural group.

Interpretation of the world according to the norms of one's own culture is called **ethnocentrism**, and it involves the belief that the way things are done within one's own culture is the right way. Bizmic, Duckitt, Popadic, Dru, and Krauss (2009) saw ethnocentrism as being common, expressed by individuals who see their particular groups or culture as superior to others, thereby creating a sense of self-centeredness. Ethnocentrism is neither good nor bad but rather a shared perception by members of a group who have in common a set of values and mores. Ethnocentrism, however, can interfere with the ability of a person to respect different ways of doing things. For example, dogmatic assertions that prescribed rituals must be followed to maintain social control can interfere with a person's empathy for individuals who do not share one's cultural beliefs.

Ethnocentrism carried to the extreme of **racism** has resulted in oppression throughout history. The violence associated with racism appears to be justified on the basis of false conclusions about the actions and intentions of others. For example, stereotypes of African Americans as a high-crime population might lead one to fear and avoid all African Americans on the basis that some might be dangerous. A few years ago, one of the authors had a young research assistant who was African American. This young man was careful to dress up for interviews (coat and tie) and to carry a briefcase to convey an image of respectability, yet he was repeatedly stopped by the police while traveling to interviews in predominantly white neighborhoods. Because he gave no signals that he might be dangerous, and because he took pains to blend in with the white middle-class neighbors, the police actions can most reasonably be interpreted as racism—by some.

Carried to an extreme, ethnocentrism can result in violence against those who simply do not share the cultural beliefs of the dominant power. For example, imagine a black man and white woman trying to raise a family in a particular community that is unable to embrace the idea of families of mixed race or the violence that frequently is experienced by members of the lesbian, gay, bisexual, and transgender (LGBT) community.

Strict rules about gender-appropriate behavior apply in many countries. Women who break these rules or who are perceived by the abuser to break the rules are subjected to sanctions that often include beatings and torture. Furthermore, throughout the world, violence against women is an ongoing public health issue. Social norms such as patriarchal social structures that perpetrate rules and social norms of oppression and subordination place woman at risk for physical, sexual, or psychological abuse, torture, and death (Hossain & Rashid Sumon, 2013; Pandey & Shrestha, 2014).

Closely related to the concept of ethnocentrism is **xenophobia**, a term that describes a conscious fear of foreigners. Foreigners can be interpreted as anyone of a different ethnic or racial group than one's own and can reside in close proximity to the group. Xenophobia is distinguished from racism in that the phenomenon does not necessarily apply to people of minority groups. Indeed, it can be the minority group that is xenophobic about others in the community. For example, Tsai (2006) reported an ethnographic study of Taiwanese immigrant youth who settled in a Mandarin-speaking neighborhood of Seattle and who experienced xenophobia in relation to their American neighbors, excluding them from their play groups. Although people of any age might experience xenophobia toward any group, particular attention should be paid to young people who are impressionable and who have not yet formed critical thinking skills. In a large friendship network of adolescents, researchers found significant correlations between both positive and negative attitudes of friends toward immigrants and xenophobia. The results of this study demonstrated that friends' tolerance predicted a corresponding increase in adolescents' tolerance, and friends' xenophobia predicted a corresponding increase in adolescents' xenophobia. Hence, these outcomes demonstrate the power of friends among adolescents and also leads the public health nurse to question what interventions can be developed to enhance tolerance (Van Zalk, Kerr, van Zalk, & Stattin, 2013).

Critical to the study of culture is to understand the rituals associated with the culture. A **ritual** is a type of action that might be as simple as shaking hands when greeting a newcomer or as complex as those found in religious ceremonies. Rituals and traditions associated with key life events can enhance joy in the case of celebratory traditions such as weddings and holidays, provide a sense of comfort in the case of death and dying, and promote a gracious lifestyle, as noted in table manners and the offering of food to guests. For example, Grigoriadis et al. (2009) conducted a systematic review of the literature on postpartum practices and rituals and their relationship to postpartum depression. The outcome of this systematic review did not conclude that all rituals prevented postpartum depression. The systematic review did find, however, that social support rituals within certain contexts could be beneficial. Yet another example concerns the religious and social dimensions of death rituals present in various cultural traditions (Venhorst, 2013). In these situations, it is important for the public health nurse, as well as other providers, to be aware of these rituals and practice in a culturally sensitive way that is congruent with the individual, family, and population's beliefs.

Rituals also protect health and are especially important in public health nursing. Consider what would happen if aseptic techniques are not practiced when providing care in homes. What would happen if the sterile techniques used to package medications were not followed? Contamination of foods and drugs has been responsible for many deaths that might have been prevented if the rituals and rules about mass production were followed.

There is evidence that rituals can reduce anxiety. Often associated with religious practices, rituals provide a measure of comfort to the person who practices them. In a study of 30 Catholic college students, Anastasi and Newberg (2008) found that reciting the rosary significantly lowered anxiety as measured by the State-Trait Anxiety Inventory. In an Alcoholics Anonymous meeting, the ritual of pronouncing, "My name is _____, and I am an alcoholic," serves to let people know they are not alone.

Previously in this chapter, culture was described as the set of lifeways, rituals, and values associated with a group of people who share ethnicity and geographic territory, for example, Navajo residents of a reservation, Bantu of Africa, and Bedouin tribes of the Middle East. We also conceptualize culture, however, as transcending geographic boundaries when people share the aspects that define culture. For example, the profession of nursing might be viewed as a culture. Nurses around the world often seem more alike than different in terms of their shared commitment to their patients and their common goals to heal and prevent illness and injury. Although some countries have higher standards of education, governance, and practice, it seems reasonable to state that nursing practice in widely diverse settings has the common origin of meeting the health needs of the community. The culture of the country of origin of the nurse, however, also has great influence over their culturally defined practice.

This idea of subcultures within a dominant culture can be further delineated. For example, other groups that might be viewed as subcultures within a dominant culture include patients with similar illnesses, such as HIV/AIDS, the chronically mentally ill, disabled children, pregnant adolescents, and those with heart disease. Groups of people living in close proximity can also be considered subcultures when they are a tightly knit group with shared values and rules, such as street gangs, retirees living in a gated golf community, expatriate Americans living in Oaxaca, and migrant workers on California ranches. More recently, there has been discussion about redefining subculture in a way that would provide for a more flexible understanding of subcultures that considers the interaction of multiple factors such as geographical factor, political factor, social factor, region, time, and language just to name a few. This new way of considering subculture allows for greater understanding of cultural identities that are more hybrid in nature (Pyrah & Fellerer, 2015).

Participant Observation: A Skillful Technique in the Process of Becoming Culturally Competent

A key skill of public health nurses is the ability to observe and make sense of their surroundings. In a clinical sense, **participant observation** is a technique in which the nurse makes careful observations of specific processes, actions, or communications while providing care as a participant in the activity. Usually, participant observation techniques are used in ethnographies conducted over time—often a year or more or in the participatory action research. The technique, however, can be useful to public health nurses who need to pay close attention to subtle changes in their client, family, and the population and group interactions (Zhao & Yingchun, 2014).

The ethnographic research method facilitates the discovery of the meaning of health and illness as experienced, for example, by an individual or family. What meaning is derived is often as a result of cultural ideas, values, and beliefs (Streubert Speziale & Rinaldi Carpenter, 2007). Participatory action research is also an effective research method as it can lead to the design of a new population-based health program. Action research involves community members in all phases of the design, planning, implementation, and the evaluation of programs targeting a particular community and population (Lucas Breda, 2015; Roye & Truglio-Londrigan, 2017).

The literature has many examples of participant observation in research, but reviewing the technique can be helpful to students who are learning observation skills to understand culture in any setting. The following are some examples, from the research literature that demonstrate how culture can be learned by an outsider. In an ethnographic study involving both participant observation and interviews, Stevens (2006) studied 15 adolescent female parents about what being healthy meant to them. A key finding was that although the girls were aware of public health messages about health, their fundamental needs of safe living conditions, finding food, and paying bills took precedence over practicing health promotion. For example, the girls' attention was focused on their own needs, and the key concepts that emerged from the data related to how the young mothers were going to meet their own basic needs and the basic needs of their infants.

An example of how participant observation is a powerful supplement to interviewing in Stevens' study was food shopping. Although it seemed clear from interviews that adolescent mothers understood that good nutrition involved eating fruits and vegetables, the pressures of long hours at work and exhaustion at taking care of an infant made fast food a much easier choice. Participant observation demonstrates exactly how and under what conditions the mothers shopped for food rather than what they stated they should buy.

In an ethnographic study of 30 rural African American women who used cocaine, Brown and Smith (2006) found that the women tended to be either child-focused or self-focused, with a wide range of responses to explain their drug use. For example, through interviews and participant observation conducted over 4 years, the researchers found that living in a rural area or small town created a sense of boredom among some of the women, who used drugs for something to do. It is one thing for someone living in a small town to say they have nothing to do but quite another for the researcher to live there and experience first-hand what it feels like to be socially isolated.

Again, participant observation makes clear to the researcher what it is like to live under the conditions required of the population being studied, and at times, the issues are more complex than what may be initially observed. Imagine a working single mother who arises at 5:00 a.m., goes to work at 6:00 a.m. as a waitress in a café until 3:00 p.m., picks up her children from school, helps them do homework, and then has to fix dinner and get them to bed by

8:00 p.m. while doing laundry and getting clothes ready for the next day. At what point in this busy day does she have time to shop for healthy food, take care of her own needs, and indulge in relaxing activities such as exercise or reading? Is boredom the single defining factor that places these young mothers at risk for cocaine use?

Similarly, in public health nursing, having a client say she is bored or overwhelmed by the demands of a growing family is much more meaningful if the nurse spends long hours in the community and sees as well as experiences firsthand there are no social outlets for young mothers or social supports and social networks. An example of how the public health nurse might use this information is to establish close, trusting, and working relationships with the people in the community—the mothers themselves. Working with the mothers, asking them their opinions, and listening to their responses is an important first step. What is it that they see as the priority issue? What do they see as a way to resolve the issue? What types of supports do they need? Do they want to have a role? What type of role do they see for themselves? What do these young mothers see as potential barriers and facilitators? One way a public health nurse can start is by developing a series of group meetings for the young mothers where child care is provided. The point is that any successful intervention program can be made culturally specific by focusing on the needs and the interests of the population served. Complete the exercises in **Box 8-1** as part of your learning.

A final example of participant observation is seen in the following community participatory action research that took place in the Dominican Republic (Foster, Chiang, Hillard, Hall, & Heth, 2010, p. 312). In this research initiative, a cross-cultural team was developed. This team consisted of midwife researchers, Dominican nurses, and members of the Dominican community. The research was designed to allow for an understanding of the community perceptions

> ### Box 8-1 Participant Observation Exercise 1
>
> Choose one of the following, and keep field notes about your observations and interpretations. Field notes are a journal in which you document the date and the setting of the observation period and then describe your observations.
>
> 1. Identify a cultural group within your community, and visit the neighborhood in which they live, work, or carry out some activity. Some examples might be an Amish farm, a Native American reservation, a juvenile court detention center, or a homeless shelter. Document your observations and discuss.
> 2. Visit a health clinic, and observe the rituals of signing in, waiting room behavior, and payment processes. Document your observations and discuss.

of the maternity services given the observation that many pregnant women failed to go to the hospital until they were very ill. The processes that the researchers and community members developed facilitated a true collaborative effort where the approach was open, and all members of the team participated in all of the steps of the research process from training, recruitment, data collection and analysis, evaluation, and the dissemination of information upon completion of the initiative. An important strategy used throughout the entire initiative was participant observation by the community health workers who came from the neighborhoods of interest. Furthermore, the community health workers volunteered and were leaders who were known as honest and cared about the community. Throughout the initiative, community health worker participant observation yielded information about the process of prenatal care. Without the community health workers' deep emersion into the community and the prenatal care, valuable information would have been lost. For example, the community health workers made notes about wait times, clinic inefficiencies, and the physical space where care was rendered, noting that there was insufficient seating and a lack of adequate fans for ventilation given the climate (Foster, Chiang, Hillard, Hall, & Heth, 2010, p. 312). Taken together, the strategy of participant observation is an approach that public health nurses may find useful given their work out in the neighborhoods as they provide care to individuals, families, and populations.

Culturally Competent Care

Keeling, Lusk, and Kulbok (2017) identified public health nurses' interest in cultural competence early on in the development of public health nursing starting with Lillian Wald in 1893. These authors provide two historical exemplars of where cultural awareness and public health nursing intersect—the first exemplar, "Nurses on the Navajo Reservation, 1920s–1950" (p. 162) and the second, "Nurses Caring for Women Following Radical Mastectomy, 1950–1960" (p. 166). The body of literature on cultural competence has continued to grow throughout the 20th and 21st centuries. At its most basic level, cultural competence and **culturally competent care** are a set of attitudes and behaviors by the public health nurse to take into account that the client or population has cultural beliefs, values, health practices, and ways of behaving in social interactions that may differ widely from expectations of the health providers. The public health nurse uses knowledge of the culture, along with information obtained from key informants—those individuals or organizations in the community of interest—to accomplish the goals of care without violating the rights of the client or population so as to maintain their cultural traditions.

The American Association of Colleges of Nursing (AACN, 2008) emphasized the importance of including cultural material in baccalaureate nursing education in the document *Cultural Competency in Baccalaureate Nursing*. Similarly, the AACN (2009) document *Establishing a Culturally Competent Master's and Doctorally Prepared Nursing Workforce* was developed, also emphasizing the importance of cultural competence to provide culturally congruent care. In addition, cultural competency tool kits have been developed for both baccalaureate and graduate nursing students. These tool kits present detailed information that will enhance the student's knowledge about culture and cultural competency. The end of this chapter posts several of the website links presented in these tool kits. Finally, Douglas et al. (2011) developed the *Standards of Practice for Culturally Competent Nursing Care*.

Several theorists (Campinha-Bacote, 2002; Giger, 2012; Jeffreys, 2015; Kim-Godwin, Clarke, & Barton, 2001; Leininger & McFarland, 2006; Purnell, 2000, 2002, 2014; Purnell & Paulanka, 2008) have published extensively on the topic. The point being made here is that the literature is extensive in the area of culture, cultural awareness, cultural competence, cultural sensitivity, and cultural congruent care. Racism, discrimination, health disparity, and healthcare disparity—issues we face as a nation—requires further work in research along with the translation of the best evidence into practice.

Regardless of how theories and concept are viewed, best practice in providing culturally competent care should involve the most fundamental characteristic of respect (de Chesnay, Peil, & Pamp, 2008). Respect for differences on the part of both provider and population leads to open communication about customs and values, and openness in the relationship leads to problem-solving about how best to meet the health needs of the population. A good rule of thumb is to be as respectful, polite, and considerate as one can under the rules of one's own culture. In this way, most clients of diverse populations understand the nurse's intentions as honorable and respond accordingly. Keeling, Lusk, and Kulbok (2017) reinforce these ideas as they conclude that "listening to these unique cultures and actively obtaining the population's involvement, not only guides our practice but also gives necessary dignity and importance to individuals and their community. . ." (p. 175).

CULTURAL COMPETENCE AND CONFLICTS

It is all well and good to say we should practice cultural competence, but what if the rights of the population conflict seriously with the values or morals of the provider? The practice of female circumcision is an example. Abhorrent to Western practitioners, female circumcision affects millions of girls and is widely practiced in some cultures. Members of these cultures often immigrate to the United States. The United Nations has called for an end to the practice of female circumcision, also called female genital mutilation. The World Health Organization (2016) has studied the public health consequences of the procedure, and research as well as the scholarly literature about female mutilation has been carried by numerous individuals (Mulong, McAndrew, & Hollins Martin, 2014; Muteshi, Miller, & Belizan, 2016; Ogunsiji, 2015). These articles discussed the effects of hemorrhage, abscesses, sepsis, long-term problems with voiding, painful intercourse, and childbirth difficulties as well as mental health needs of these women. Despite these efforts, there is limited evidence that suggests best practice on interventions (Muteshi, Miller, & Belizan, 2016). Furthermore, a systematic review on healthcare providers' ability to prevent and treat female genital mutilation yielded only two articles that met their inclusion criteria, collectively yielding limited evidence. This demonstrates the need to further develop educational interventions for providers to improve both knowledge and attitudes (Balfour, Abdulcadir, Say, & Hindin, 2016).

From a public health standpoint, it is a legitimate argument that eliminating the practice of genital mutilation is essential policy in order to assure and ensure the health of women. Support for the procedure, however, is ingrained in the culture and the attitudes of millions of poor families who do not have access to educational programs on the public health issues and who perpetuate the practice by using a variety of nonpractitioners such as elder women and even some medical personnel (World Health Organization, 2008).

Even for male circumcision, which does not have the stigma associated with female circumcision, the unsterile use of implements exacerbates the spread of one of the world's most virulent pandemics, HIV/AIDS, in areas where traditional healers and religious leaders practice cutting rituals. These rituals are not only for circumcision but also for symbolism (family bonding) and marking (curing illness), and often many boys are cut by the same tools in a short time period (Merli, 2010; Ndiwane, 2008). The cutting leads to sepsis and scarring if left untreated.

The world is becoming less a set of individual countries that are autonomous and more a global village in which there is extensive immigration and sharing of resources. Consequently, it is increasingly likely that healthcare providers and their patients find their cultural values in conflict. Respect for differences needs to be negotiated on a personal basis when providers come into conflict with clients over health issues, and education about each other's culture can certainly help prevent misunderstandings. Open discussion of these issues while maintaining the rights of the other to hold differing views is both respectful and culturally appropriate.

One way to look at whose cultural values take precedence is to view the relationship between provider and client/population as a contract in which the client/population comes to the provider as an expert to provide a specific service. The two then agree to disagree on anything not relevant to the contract. For example, a public health nurse in an inner-city immigrant neighborhood of Somali refugees wants to design a program to address diabetes management. Everyone agrees that diabetes is a major health issue for the population, but this is also a population in which female circumcision is practiced. For the nurse to try to get the women to stop this practice may not be initially the way to proceed because female circumcision is a health issue that is not part of the contract. However, being open to discussing with key leaders of the population the health risks without judging or trying to eliminate the cultural practice might be well received and a way to introduce the topic. This approach facilitates gradual trust building, thus opening doors for future programs and initiatives that otherwise may be impossible to initiate.

Complicating the issue of whose culture takes precedence is the dissonance between the rights of localities and the rights of the federal government. In a situation in which the cultural practices of a population are in conflict with U.S. law, the law takes precedence. For example, polygamy is illegal in the United States. Similarly, undocumented immigrants have no legal rights in certain states that have enacted legislation designed to criminalize actions taken to help them, for example, in the provision of health care. In the case of undocumented workers who need health care, these laws have been designed to eliminate the delivery of services, thereby creating a paradoxical effect and some say an ethical issue and moral distress for providers. For example, if free clinics are banned from serving the undocumented worker, where will they go? Many may go to emergency rooms at a cost of more than 10 times the costs of the clinics (de Chesnay & Chambers, 2011), and what of those who do not find an emergency room? With changes in the federal government beginning in January 2017, the legal status of illegal immigrants is yet to be known. But based on campaign promises regarding laws applying to the illegal immigrant and the Affordable Care Act have the potential to adversely affect health outcomes.

LEARNING PROCESS ON BECOMING CULTURALLY COMPETENT

Learning to provide culturally competent care is a complex process and starts with the respect for cultural differences that is fundamental to interaction with people of a different culture than one's own. One of the best ways to learn about different cultures is immersion in which a professor takes a group of students to a foreign country or medically underserved area of the United States to practice. There are many examples of programs in which this is an integral part of nursing education (Bennett & Holtz, 2008; de Chesnay, 2005; Larson, Ott, & Miles, 2010; Nauright, 2005; Nauright & Wilson, 2012).

Although it is certainly desirable to be proficient in the language of the group with whom one is working, lack of language skill should not be used as an excuse not to interact with people, even in immersion programs in foreign countries. Adequate translators are often available in communities with large ethnic populations, and sometimes younger members of a family can translate for older members, although this practice is not often the best choice. Taking the time to learn a few words or phrases helps greatly in establishing trust and rapport.

Other approaches to consider in the process of learning and designing culturally competent programs include:

- Project directors read as much as possible about the population and have informal conversations with key informants. Key informants are members of the group or population of interest who are trusted members of the representative culture and who are willing to educate the staff in how best to approach community leaders and stakeholders in a respectful way.
- Key project staff members meet with community leaders and the stakeholders. Stakeholders include all those who have a vested interest in the project. These stakeholders include consumers who generally are the recipients

of the interventions. Stakeholders also include gatekeepers, individuals who give permissions for access to a community such as ministers for their congregations.

- Other staff members meet with community leaders and stakeholders to identify issues they see as priorities. An excellent way to talk about issues is in focus groups. Focus groups are conducted with small homogeneous groups of people within the target population. The focus group leader asks specific questions to elicit the group's perceptions to design appropriate aspects of the program.
- Staff members meet with community leaders and stakeholders on an ongoing basis to share developments and to plan, implement, and evaluate the unfolding process of the program together.
- Staff members put in place evaluation measures that capture the perceptions of the stakeholders. It is important to note that many times this work is a partnership between the project director, staff members, and people from the community of interest.

Complete the exercises in **Box 8-2** as part of your learning.

Culture and Public Health Nursing

Cultural considerations for public health nurses extend beyond the individual and family to include communities and populations (American Nurse Association, 2013; American Public Health Association Public Health Nursing, 2013). The skill set necessary to integrate culture in providing culturally competent and congruent health care is extended to identifying diverse cultures found in different communities. Examples include working with the Navajo on the reservation (Keeling, Lusk, & Kulbok, 2017), domestic violence (Alhabib, Nur, & Jones, 2010), those experiencing substance abuse (Blum, 2016; Hopson & Steiker, 2008; Kulis et al., 2005; Lange, 2007; Walle, 2004), poverty (Anakwenze & Zuberi, 2013; Gaskinet et al., 2014;

> **Box 8-2** On Becoming Culturally Competent Exercise 2
>
> 1. Interview a client who represents a particular population on what it means to him or her to have a provider who is culturally sensitive to the client's needs. Reflect on the client's words and how this information will alter your practice.
> 2. You are developing a diabetes education program with two different populations. Describe these two different populations in terms of their similarities and differences—consider the social determinants of health. Given this information, how would you design and implement the programs considering cultural similarities and differences?

Pearson, 2003; Wood, 2003), the prison population (Cervantes, Ruan, & Duenas, 2004; Devieux et al., 2005), and those living in rural communities (Hartley, 2004; Jensen & Royeen, 2002; Keeling, Lusk, & Kulbok, 2017; Savage et al., 2006; U.S. Department of Health and Human Services, 2008). There are many themes noted throughout all of these publications; however, one of the most common is an emphasis on cultural considerations and the culturally congruent strategies the public health provider carries out with the specific population.

Migrant farm workers make a valuable contribution to the everyday lives of the American people, yet they experience poor working and living conditions, poor health, illnesses due to contact with chemicals and pesticides as well as food insecurity and overall disparities in health (Holmes, 2006; Keeling, 2015). The children of migrant workers also experience poor health such as elevated blood pressure, obesity, food insecurity, stunting, anemia, and decrease access to health care (Nichols, Stein, & Wold, 2014). Research conducted among migrant workers and children of migrant farm workers provides insight into their perceptions about health and priority issues that the public health nurse may incorporate into their practice. Knowledge of the culture of migrant farm workers enables public health nurses to work with this vulnerable population to develop and implement community projects based on the chosen priorities of this population.

Domestic violence is no stranger to public health nurses and is present in most societies and age groups. Unfortunately, the signs of violence often go unrecognized while multiple acts of physical and psychological abuse are continually perpetrated. A systematic review conducted by Alhabib, Nur, and Jones (2010) noted that domestic violence against women is present in all societies and that no racial, ethnic, or socioeconomic population is immune. Studies have demonstrated there are certain factors that may place women at risk for violence. Examples of these factors include limited education, alcohol consumption by husband, and past witness of father beating mother, which, along with deep-seated cultural norms and beliefs, lead to acceptance of abuse (Tenkorang, Owusu, Yeboah, & Bannerman, 2013). Given that educational level is associated with increased acts of violence findings suggest the possibility of educating girls as a potential for preventing domestic abuse (Babu & Shantanu, 2009; Ergin, Bayram, Alper, Selimoglu, & Bilgel, 2005). Considering this information, what can a public health nurse do, and in what ways can they use this information as they work with populations and communities when the issue of domestic violence takes center stage? The need to consider individual differences in women of any culture when planning programs for domestic violence must always be remembered.

Substance is a major problem nationally and globally and afflicts many different populations, and corresponding interventions have been developed to reflect the cultural norms and values of these populations (Blume, 2016). Substance abuse as an issue and the corresponding interventions to combat this major problem have focused on Native Americans (Walle, 2004), Native American Indian adolescents (Patchell, Robbins, Lowe, & Hoke, 2016), Hispanic men (González-Guarda, McCabe, Leblanc, De Santis, & Provencio-Vasquez, 2016), older adults (Blow & Barry, 2014), and women learning to care for themselves (Lange, 2007), just to name a few. The literature abounds with studies that describe the issue, specific populations affected, and varying culturally congruent strategies sensitive to the needs of the specific populations. The key to remember is that each of these interventions are sensitive to the cultural norms and values of the specific population being targeted. For instance, two evidence-based substance abuse prevention programs targeted students in alternative schools (Hopson & Steiker, 2008) and middle school students with a Mexican heritage (Kulis et al., 2005). Both programs emphasized the importance of culturally grounded curriculums. It is unlikely that curriculums will be implemented or sustained if interventions are not culturally congruent with those receiving the intervention. For example, Hopson and Steiker (2008) allowed students in alternative schools to read workbook exercises and reword them to capture their lifestyles and culture to facilitate student participation. More recently, a culturally tailored program was developed and implemented for the specific population of Plains Indian adolescents. In this program, a native tribal circle was the intervention that was based on tribal values and beliefs (Patchell et al., 2016). Another intervention program for adolescent juvenile offenders provides insight into the ability to decrease recidivism and increase substance abuse resistance (Cervantes et al., 2004). Much of the success of the Program Shortstop was attributed to cultural sensitivity aimed at Hispanic youth who came from low-income immigrant families. There were four prevention/intervention sessions using videos, homework, legal education, a simulation incarceration, activities to improve family communication and conflict resolution, drug information, self-esteem-building drills, parent workshops on family communication, legal rights and responsibilities, and youth mentoring. Eighty-nine percent of the youth who completed the program were not rearrested within one year. Also, the participants gained legal knowledge and effective ways to deal with substance abuse and delinquency at school. In a follow-up study, most parents reported that their child's high-risk behavior had decreased. A final example was a study that examined the differences among African American and Cuban American adolescent juvenile offenders, predominately male, related to preventing drug and sexually risky behaviors while focusing on culture. These researchers examined levels of drug and sexually risky behaviors to determine if there were any differences among the two groups. Language in the focus groups and in-depth interviews was culturally sensitive, using the local terminology of the participants. The results in part indicated that both groups of youth engaged in risky behaviors that could lead to HIV infection and had about the same level of sexual activity and number of partners. The Cuban participants in this sample had higher levels of unprotected sex and higher levels of sex while using drugs than the African American youth. Some of the differences in this sample may be related to acculturation, communication with parents, and media-targeted efforts. Adolescents who are more acculturated tend to engage earlier in risky sexual behaviors, and Hispanic youth may not talk about risky behaviors at home. Specific-media, protective health messages may have been targeted more toward the African American youths than Cuban American youths (Devieux et al., 2005).

Another vulnerable population are children living in foster care, who number over 400,000 in the United States. These children have emotional, developmental, mental, social, and behavioral needs, and there is a notable increase of mental health diagnoses compared with children not in foster care. In addition, these children frequently receive behavioral health care and psychotropic medication (Deutsch et al., 2015; Scozzaro & Janikowski, 2015; U.S. Department of Health and Human Services, 2010). Of prime importance when working with this population is to establish and maintain a strong safety culture. Safety culture in child welfare can be focused on more effective interventions and ongoing support rather than just safety and risk assessment (Pecora, Chahine, & Graham, 2013). Ways to prevent harm to children and families within the child welfare system are paramount and need to be pursued (Vogus, Cull, Hengelbrok, Modell, & Epstein, 2016).

One final example is presented here. It is well established that rural communities have limited resources and inadequate numbers of healthcare providers, making care unavailable, and even if care is available, there is limited access to that care. This limited access alone places the rural population at risk for disparities, but there are other factors placing this population at risk. According to the National Rural Health Association (2016), "Economic factors, cultural and social differences, educational shortcomings, lack of recognition by legislators, and the sheer isolation of living in remote rural areas place rural Americans at risk for health disparities" (para. 1). Furthermore, Americans residing in geographically rural areas have higher death rates from chronic obstructive pulmonary disease, unintentional injuries, and suicide compared with urban Americans and have negative health outcomes (Downey, 2013; Eberhardt & Pamuk, 2004). In addition, modifiable risk factors, such as obesity and smoking, are common (Eberhardt & Pamuk, 2004). Rural youth especially show high rates of smoking and alcohol use (Keeling, Lusk, & Kulbok, 2017). A challenge, therefore, for healthcare providers is identifying how to locate and provide health services for vulnerable populations in rural areas.

Researchers have described interprofessional collaborative partnerships as best practice in rural health projects (Jensen & Royeen, 2002). Public health nurses can be leaders in implementing population-based partnership models for improving the quality of health care in rural communities, with particular emphasis on the unique cultural aspects of each community and population. Furthermore, public health nurses are uniquely positioned to participate in community-based participatory research in that they subscribe to the four principles of building trust, collaboration, excellence in science, and ethics associated with community-based participatory research (Keeling, Lusk, & Kulbok, 2017; Roye & Truglio-Londrigan, 2017; Savage et al., 2006).

Case Studies

Three case studies are presented below as examples of programs in which culturally competent interventions are predominant. Each of the case studies have populations who are targeted in *Healthy People 2020* because of health disparities. Lack of availability and access to health services, lack of insurance, limited language access, and physical environments contribute to their health disparities. Culturally competent interventions in each case study are aimed at better health outcomes consistent with *Healthy People 2020*.

1. Migrant family project.
2. Summer Camp for children in foster care.
3. Project IDEAL— diabetes.

A description of the specific project and discussion about cultural considerations precedes a corresponding Case Study Exercise Box with field activities for students.

Migrant Farm Workers and Their Families—Case Study 1

The Farm Worker Family Health Program (FWFHP) has been in existence for over 20 years in a rural area of southern Georgia. The program is a health-focused academic community partnership where faculty and students provide health screening and referrals. Additionally, community organizations provide access for migrant farm workers at their work sites and trailer parks where they live and to their children attending a county summer school program. The local Farmworker Health Clinic provides client health records, assessment forms for documentation, and some medications and serves as the referral source for clients requiring follow-up treatment from the FWFHP.

The two-week cultural immersion program provides a unique interprofessional opportunity for students (undergraduate nursing, nurse practitioner, dental hygienists, physical therapy, and pharmacy) to gain needed cultural awareness and sensitivity while providing health-related screenings to this uninsured at-risk population. Since the inception of the program, about 15,000 episodes of care have been provided to migrant farm workers and their families. Adult screening includes vital signs, hemoglobin and glucose tests, dental screening, BMI, episodic care for health problems, and physical therapy if indicated and desired. The most frequent diagnoses among adults are low back pain, skin problems/rashes, dental caries, and diabetes, which is on the rise in this vulnerable population.

The child health screenings include a physical examination, height and weight/BMI measurements (body mass index), hearing and vision screening, glucose screening if indicated by increased body mass index, and hemoglobin screening. In addition, nursing students present health classes to migrant children in prekindergarten to ninth grade related to basic hygiene, dental care, nutrition, and smoking risks, among other topics. The teaching strategies include discussion, lecture, videos, handout materials, games, and poster presentations. The most frequent diagnoses among the children were dental caries, anemia, obesity, and vision problems.

Other students also participate. Dental hygiene students perform dental checks and fluoride treatments on all children and tooth sealants to retard decay. If needed, children are referred to a local dentist. Physical therapy students assess gross and fine motor development.

Since the FWFHP moved to Emory, several research projects have been conducted aimed at improving knowledge about health and health outcomes for the migrant workers and their families. Projects include pesticide levels in children; knowledge, attitudes, and perceptions about Chagas disease; and heat stress.

CULTURAL CONSIDERATIONS

The FWFHP developed specific cultural considerations for this particular population:

- Making available training materials to all faculty and students to enhance their understanding of the history and culture of migrant farm workers and their families.
- Addressing communication barriers by having an interpreter available at all screenings to assist with clients who did not speak English.
- Offering programs and services in the evening and at work sites considering the migrant farm workers who are unable to leave work to seek health care during the day.
- Providing educational materials in Spanish.

IMPACT ON PUBLIC HEALTH

The impact of this culturally congruent public health initiative included the following:

- Provided health care to this uninsured, vulnerable population. Even though the program runs only two weeks in the summer, other health programs are provided throughout the year by the local Farmworker Health Clinic. The health services are positively received by the migrant farm workers and their children.
- Assured and ensured community participation and resources for this uninsured population

and for the faculty and students. Different churches in the area provide chairs and tables for the screenings and lunch for the students, faculty, and other volunteers.

- Facilitated student understanding of the Hispanic and rural cultures. Specifically, this experience can be used in students' future practice when encountering patients with a Hispanic or migrant farm worker background.
- Established a medical health record that is available year after year for those children who return and attend the summer program. Parents are provided with health records related to screenings and immunization schedules and are encouraged to immunize their children at appropriate times.
- Developed a referral system that enables the healthcare providers to arrange future health care in the community. One example was a man who presented with a deep laceration that had become infected and led to septicemia. The man was taken to the emergency department at a local hospital at once and treatment began immediately, thus preventing a potential amputation or death. Ultimately, the wound began healing.

Complete the exercises below **Box 8-3** as part of your learning.

Summer Camp for Children in Foster Care—Case Study 2

A unique summer camp opportunity for children ages 6 to 12 living in foster homes has been held for a number of years in south Georgia. The camp is a partnership between a faith-based organization (FBO) and a regional social services organization (SSO). There is a great emphasis on the culture of safety for the children attending camp. The SSO selects children they believe will benefit from a week at camp and stipulates rules to maintain the safety of these children, whereas the FBO raises needed funds for the children to attend camp and

Box 8-3 Case Study Exercise 3

1. Interview a person whose first language is not English about experiences with healthcare professionals who do not speak his or her language. What feelings do these experiences evoke?
2. Develop a brief training module for migrant workers or their children on a topic similar to one of the following: dental hygiene, foot care for the elderly, HIV/AIDS prevention, prenatal nutrition, infant bathing, child immunizations, anxiety prevention, substance abuse, or domestic violence. In what way(s) would you ensure that the individual or population's particular cultural values and beliefs are addressed?
3. Conduct a participant observation session at a clinic that serves the migrant population. Observe rituals, values, and folk practices. For example, who speaks for the family to the healthcare professional? How are children disciplined? Are they told to sit still or allowed to run around? Are any foods brought in, and if so, what are they? What language is spoken?

implements the camp activities, including SSO rules, to maintain a culture of safety.

The volunteer personnel for camp include two directors, two clinical nurse specialists in child and adolescent psychiatric mental health nursing, up to three registered nurses, big campers (the word *counselor* is not used because these children have counselors from SSO), activity director and staff, chapel director and staff, a professional photographer, and numerous volunteers for specific tasks. There is significant preparation for all volunteers, including background checks; classroom training; an online module titled *Protect My Ministry Child Sexual Abuse Prevention Training Course,* which includes an examination that leads to a certificate of completion; and a review of all camp rules pertaining to interactions with campers such as having two adults at all times when in the company of one camper, never allowing a camper to sit or lay on anyone else's bed or the big camper's bed, no cameras or videos, giving safe hugs (side-to-side and not face-to-face), no piggyback rides or sitting on laps, and no sharing of personal addresses, phone numbers, or electronic addresses. The precamp training supports a culture of safety for both campers and adults and focuses on providing love and caring to these children.

Camps have had up to 70 campers with 90 volunteers. The big campers are responsible for their campers the entire time at camp; therefore, each big camper is only assigned two campers. The campers arrive at camp on buses and are greeted by volunteers, matched with their big camper, and then shown to their cabin. The activities at camp include swimming, fishing, canoeing, archery, nature walks, rock-climbing walls, arts and crafts, a special dress-up tea for the girls, karate for the boys, and chapel. Chapel is designed to present age-appropriate lessons to foster a future and a culture of hope. Campers can pursue spiritual questions with their big campers if desired. Another activity is a group birthday party designed especially for those campers who have not had birthday celebrations. Bags with presents are provided, and thanks to a local business, each camper receives a two-wheel bicycle when they return from camp.

A professional photographer is busy throughout the week taking pictures of each child during camp activities. Near the end of the week, photo albums are prepared for each child and presented on the last day of camp to take home. The albums can be useful in capturing lasting memories, fostering self-worth, and give a hope for the future.

CULTURAL CONSIDERATIONS

The summer camp for children living in foster homes facilitates specific cultural considerations for this particular vulnerable population:

- Ensuring safety for all campers attending camp via background checks, as well as classroom training on working with children who may have been abused, and an online module consisting of an examination.
- Understanding that each child has unique experiences in their past that may include abuse and neglect that could affect their behavior at camp.
- Understanding the developmental process occurring in school-age children ages 6 to 12.
- Implementing a culture of safety throughout the camp experience.

IMPACT ON PUBLIC HEALTH

The impact of this culturally congruent public health initiative included the following:

- Provided a meaningful summer camp experience that encourages healthy growth and development delivered by a successful community partnership approach.
- Provided much needed services to a vulnerable population of children.
- Enhanced the socialization between and among children in foster homes who have been separated from their parents.
- Provided a loving and caring atmosphere from all volunteers.
- Ensured the spiritual needs of this vulnerable population in a sensitive way.

Complete the exercises below in **Box 8-4** as part of your learning.

Project IDEAL Diabetes—Case Study 3

Project IDEAL is a program of the WellStar School of Nursing at Kennesaw State University that began

---

Box 8-4 Case Study Exercise 4

1. Interview a case manager from social services, and ask about the challenges children face when placed in a foster home and the challenges foster parents face. Compare the responses, and determine how the challenges can be met to benefit both children and parents.
2. Identify programs in your community that serve foster children and describe them. Consider volunteering your services where appropriate.
3. Conduct a literature search to determine long-term effects on children living in multiple foster homes such as health issues, developmental delay, school performance, mental health issues, and any other long-term effects.

---

in 2003 and is focused on providing diabetes prevention and self-management education for Latinos. Latinos have a high risk for developing diabetes, and as many as 1 in 10 Latinos may have diabetes. There are ways to prevent or postpone diabetes by maintaining a healthy lifestyle, such as eating healthy foods and exercising.

Classes are conducted in small groups and focus on maintaining a healthy lifestyle, needed medications, meal planning, blood sugar monitoring, and exercise. This is done informally now through the *promotores de salud* who are trained by the nurse and dietitian faculty and in partnership with WellStar Health System. *Promotores de salud* provide education and health coaching. *Promotores de salud* are also active members of the health ministry at each of the faith settings they serve and assist nurses in the periodic health fairs conducted in the faith settings.

Project IDEAL also provides a forum for educators and healthcare providers to study the concepts of diabetes self-management education and the American Diabetes Association criteria for recognition. Included in the program are materials for diverse Latino groups, prediabetes education materials, consultation with a Latino healthcare educator, and program development consultation and oversight.

Cultural Considerations

Project IDEAL facilitates specific cultural considerations for this particular population:

- Understanding and respecting the cultural of this specific vulnerable population.
- Understanding and respecting the demonstrative use of hugs in welcoming.
- Identifying the participants' perceptions and value of health to best foster behavioral change to prevent diabetes or in the self-management of diabetes.
- Understanding and appreciating that there are differences within Latino groups.
- Considering eating habits and the cultural names of different foods in different Latino populations. The words *naranja* and *chino* can both mean orange. The use of the metric system and traditional systems can be found among Puerto Ricans, such as measuring height in inches and weight in kilograms, and the Mayans measure height in centimeters and weight in kilograms. This cultural information is essential when teaching nutrition classes such as weighing food for diets.
- Appreciating the differences in how people best like to obtain information. For example, the oral tradition or word-of-mouth method in Latino populations is embraced.
- Knowing that some members in the Latino groups may trust individuals within their own cultural group over a physician's word or teachings. In other words, family and friends who have diabetes are trusted more than a

healthcare provider, and information is sought from them.
- Providing healthcare providers who speak Spanish.

Impact on Public Health

The impact of this culturally congruent public health initiative included the following:

- Reduced the HbA1c levels among participants with diabetes.
- Provided a service to an underserved population.
- Provided an opportunity for nursing students to work with a vulnerable population and develop culture competence skills.
- Helped participants maintain their weight throughout the program delivery.
- Offered diabetes prevention and education to children and teens participating in the program.
- Improved the quality of life for those participating in the program who live with diabetes.

Complete the exercises below in **Box 8-5** as part of your learning.

Discussion of Cultural Issues in the Community Projects

The three projects presented are diverse and meet different health needs of selected populations, yet there are common cultural issues evident in the projects. Cultural competence is needed among those providing care to these populations. Cultural themes in common with all three projects are respect, immersion, and communication.

Respect for the recipients of care encompasses allowing them to express themselves and finding ways to incorporate their desires into the plan of care and in many situations actually being a partner in the development of the plan, implementation, and the evaluation of the plan of care. One example of respect is being sensitive to special dietary needs,

---

Box 8-5 Case Study Exercise 5

1. Identify a program in your own community that addresses chronic illness and self-management. Ask to observe several intake interviews. How do the individual clients respond to the healthcare provider? How does the program reach out to the specific population being served?

2. Eat several meals at a local restaurant frequented by members of the population, and examine the types of foods on the menu. Describe the country and the locale the menu reflects. Prepare a nutritional analysis of these foods.

3. Identify a cultural group of interest and a particular health issue experienced by this group. Attend a support group meeting that addresses this particular issue, and prepare a summary of the themes of the discussion.

---

clothes, and other cultural norms. Considering the farm workers' schedules by providing services in the evening and acknowledging their need for materials in Spanish illustrates respect.

Immersion in a culture helps healthcare providers understand the cultural traditions that can assist in the planning and delivering of culturally congruent and appropriate health care. Gaining an understanding of diverse cultures enhances one's own ability to practice in an appropriate culturally sensitive manner. Much of the success of Project IDEAL can be attributed to the in-depth understanding of the variations in Latino culture and paying attention to participants' perceptions and values about health to best foster management of their diabetes.

Communication is essential and is critical for the establishment of trust. The actual planning of health care and services for diverse populations can be a challenge because of the many barriers that impede the process of communication. Communication barriers are addressed in the case studies by the use of interpreters, hiring bilingual staff, and acknowledging the differences within Latino groups. In addition, understanding how people like to get information, such as the word-of-mouth or the oral tradition method as seen in the Latino populations, and in using key informants the population trusts are helpful in facilitating desired communication. In other populations, the use of technology may be the preferred method of communication. Whichever the case may be, cultural considerations found in the case studies are essential for the health of the public.

Conclusion

The purpose of this chapter is to provide a cultural framework for public health nursing to best promote culturally competent and congruent health care to diverse populations. Several case studies were presented that demonstrate aspects of cultural considerations in implementing population-based projects. Public health nurses are encouraged to make use of participant observation and participatory action research methods to design programs that are culturally relevant to the stakeholders. Taking the time to learn the cultural lifeways, values, and traditions of the populations served is critical to providing health care, not only to patients and their families but also to populations.

Acknowledgments

We gratefully acknowledge the contributions of the project staff who shared information about their programs.

Additional Resources

Transcultural Nursing Society at: http://www.tcns.org/

Madeleine Leininger at: http://www.madeleine-leininger.com/index.shtml

Transcultural C. A. R. E. Associates at: http://transculturalcare.net/

Transcultural Nursing Standards of Practice at: http://www.tcns.org/TCNStandardsofPractice.html

European Transcultural Nursing Association at: http://europeantransculturalnurses.eu/

National Rural Health Association at: http://www.ruralhealthweb.org/

Royal College of Nursing Transcultural Health Care Practice: An Educational Resource for Nurses and Health Care Practitioners at: https://www2.rcn.org.uk/development/learning/transcultural_health/transcultural

References

American Association of Colleges of Nursing. (2008). *Cultural competency in baccalaureate education.* Washington, DC: Author.

American Association of Colleges of Nursing. (2009). *Establishing a culturally competent master's and doctorally prepared nursing workforce.* Washington, DC: Author.

American Nurses Association. (2013). *Public health nursing: Scope and standards of practice.* Silver Springs, MD: Author.

American Public Health Association, Public Health Nursing Section. (2013). *The definition and practice of public health nursing: A statement of the public health nursing section.* Washington, DC: Author.

Anastasi, M., & Newberg, A. (2008). A preliminary study of the acute effects of religious ritual on anxiety. *Journal of Alternative and Complementary Medicine, 14*(2), 163–165.

Anakwenze, U., & Zuberi, D. (2013). Mental health and poverty in the Inner City. *Health & Social Work, 38*(3), 147–157.

Alhabib, S., Nur, U., & Jones, R. (2010). Domestic violence against women: Systematic review of prevalence studies. *Journal of Family Violence, 25,* 369–382.

Babu, B. V., & Shantanu, K. J. (2009). Domestic violence against women in eastern India: A population-based study on prevalence and related issues. *BMC Public Health, 9,* 129–144.

Balfour, J., Abdulcadir, J., Say, L., & Hindin, M. J. (2016). Interventions for healthcare providers to improve treatment and prevention of female genital mutilation: A systematic review. *BMC Health Services Research, 16*(1), 409–415.

Bennett, D., & Holtz, C. (2008). Building cultural competence: A nursing practicum in Oaxaca, Mexico. In C. Holtz (Ed.), *Global health care* (pp. 601–614). Sudbury, MA: Jones and Bartlett Publishers.

Bizumic, B., Duckitt, J., Popadic, D., Dru, V., & Krauss, S. (2009). A cross-cultural investigation into a reconceptualization of ethnocentrism. *European Journal of Social Psychology, 39,* 871–899.

Blow, F. C., & Barry, K. L. (2014). Substance misuse and abuse in older adults: What do we need to know to help? *Generations—Journal of the American Society on Aging, 38*(3), 53–67.

Blume, W. (2016). Advances in substance abuse prevention and treatment interventions among racial, ethnic, and sexual minority populations. *Alcohol Research: Current Reviews, 38*(1), 47–54.

Bornstein, M. H., Putnick, D. L., & Lansford, J. E. (2011). Parenting attributions and attitudes in cross-cultural perspectives. *Parenting: Science and Practice, 11,* 214–237.

Brown, E. J., & Smith, F. B. (2006). Rural African American women who use cocaine: Needs and future aspirations related to their mothering role. *Community Mental Health Journal, 42*(1), 65–76.

Campinha-Bacote, J. (2002). The process of cultural competence in the delivery of health care services: A model of care. *Journal of Transcultural Nursing, 13*(3), 180–184.

Cassar, L. (2006). Cultural expectations of Muslims and Orthodox Jews in regard to pregnancy and the post-partum period: A study in comparison and contrast. *International Journal of Childbirth Education, 21*(2), 7–30.

Cervantes, R. C., Raun, K., & Duenas, N. (2004). Program Shortstop: A culturally focused juvenile intervention for Hispanic youth. *Journal of Drug Education, 34*(4), 385–405.

de Chesnay, M. (2005). Teaching nurses about vulnerable populations. In M. de Chesnay (Ed.), *Caring for the vulnerable*, (pp. 349–356). Sudbury, MA: Jones and Bartlett Publishers.

de Chesnay, M., Peil., R., & Pamp, C. (2008). Cultural competence, resilience and advocacy. In M. de Chesnay & B. Anderson (Eds.), *Caring for the vulnerable*, (pp. 25–35). Sudbury, MA: Jones and Bartlett Publishers.

de Chesnay, M., & Chambers, D. (2011, March 27–April 1). *Free clinics as a solution to healthcare for undocumented Immigrants.* Paper presented to the Society for Applied Anthropology, Seattle, WA.

Deutsch, S. A., Lynch, A., Zlotnik, S., Matone, M., Kreider, A., & Noonan, K. (2015). Mental health, behavioral and developmental issues for youth in foster care. *Current Problems Pediatric Adolescent Health Care, 45*, 292–297.

Devieux, J. G., Malow, R. M., Ergon-Perez, E., Samuels, D., Rojas, P., Khushal, S. R., & Jean-Gilles, M. (2005). A comparison of African American and Cuban American adolescent juvenile offenders: Risky sexual and drug use behaviors. *Journal of Social Work Practice in the Addictions, 5*(1/2), 69–83.

Douglas, M. D., Uhl Pierce, J., Rosenkoetter, M., Pacquiao, D., Clark Callister, L., Hattar-Pollara, M., . . . Purnell, L. (2011). Standards of practice for culturally competent nursing care: 2011 update. *Journal of Transcultural Nursing, 22*(4), 317–333.

Downey, L. H. (2013). Rural populations and health: Determinants, disparities, and solutions. *Preventing Chronic Disease*, 10:130097. doi:http://dx.doi.org/10.5888/pcd10.130097

Eberhardt, M. S., & Pamuk, E. R. (2004). The importance of place of residence: Examining health in rural and nonrural areas. *Americana Journal of Public Health, 94*(10), 1682–1686.

Ergin, N., Bayram, N., Alper, Z., Selimoglu, K., & Bilgel, N. (2005). Domestic violence: A tragedy behind the doors. *Women & Health, 42*(2), 35–51.

Foster, J., Chiang, F., Hillard, R. C., Hall, P., & Heath, A. (2010). Team process in community-based participatory research on maternity care in the Dominican Republic. *Nursing Inquiry, 17*(4), 309–316.

Gaskin, D. J., Thorpe, J., Jr., McGinty, E. E., Bower, K., Rohde, C., Young, J. H., . . . Dubay, L. (2014). Disparities in diabetes: The nexus of race, Poverty, and place. *American Journal of Public Health, 104*(11): 2147–2155.

Giger, J. N. (2012). *Transcultural nursing: Assessment and interventions* (6th ed.). St. Louis, MO: Elsevier.

González-Guarda, R. M., McCabe, B. E., Leblanc, N., De Santis, J. P., & Provencio-Vasquez, E. (2016). The contribution of stress, cultural factors, and sexual identity on the substance abuse, violence, HIV, and depression syndemic among Hispanic Men. *Cultural Diversity and Ethnic Minority Psychology.* doi:10.1037/cdp0000077

Grigoriadis, S., Robinson, G., Fung, K., Ross, L., Chee, C., Dennis, C., & Romans, S. (2009). Traditional postpartum practices and rituals: Clinical Implications. *La Revue Canadienne Psychiatrie, 54*(12), 834–840.

Hartley, D. (2004). Rural health disparities, population health, and rural culture. *American Journal of Public Health, 94*(10), 1675–1678.

Holmes, S. M. (2006). An ethnographic study of the social context of migrant health in the United States. *PLoS Medicine, 3*(10), e448.

Hopson, L. M., & Steiker, K. H. (2008). Methodology for evaluating an adaptation of evidence-based drug abuse prevention in alternative schools. *Children & Schools, 30*(2), 116–127.

Hossain, K. T., & Rashid Sumon, Md. S. (2013). Violence against women: Nature, causes & Dimensions in contemporary Bangladesh. *Bangladesh e-Journal of Sociology, 10*(1), 79–91.

Jeffreys, M. R. (2015). *Teaching cultural competence in nursing and health care: Inquiry, action, and innovation* (3rd ed.). New York, NY: Springer Publishing Company.

Jensen, G. M., & Royeen, C. B. (2002). Improved rural access to care: Dimensions of best practice. *Journal of Interprofessional Care, 16*(2), 117–128.

Keeling, A. W. (2015). Migrant nursing in the great depression: Floods, flies, and the Farm Security Administration. In J. C. Kirchgessner & A. W. Keeling (Eds.), *Nursing in rural America: Perspective from the early 20th century* (pp. 103–120). New York, NY: Springer Publishing Company.

Keeling, A. W., Lusk, B., & Kulbok, P. (2017). Culturally sensitive primary health care interventions: Three exemplars. In S. B. Lewenson & M. Truglio-Londrigan (Eds.), *Practicing primary health care in nursing: Caring for populations* (pp. 161–176). Burlington, MA: Jones & Bartlett Learning.

Kim-Godwin, Y. S., Clarke, P., & Barton, L. (2001). A model for delivery of culturally competent care. *Journal of Advanced Nursing, 35*(6), 918–926.

Koffman, J., Morgan, M., Edmonds, P., Speck, P., & Higginson, I. J. (2008). Cultural meanings of pain: A qualitative study of black Caribbean and white British patients with advanced cancer. *Palliative Medicine, 22,* 350–359.

Kulis, S., Marsiglia, F. F., Elek, E., Dustman, P., Wagstaff, D. A., & Hecht, M. L. (2005). Mexican/ Mexican American adolescents and keeping it REAL: An evidence-based substance use prevention program. *Children & Schools, 27*(3), 133–145.

Lange, B. (2007). The prescriptive power of caring for self: Women in recovery from substance use disorders. *International Journal for Human Caring, 11*(2), 74–80.

Larson, K., Ott, M., & Miles, J. (2010). International cultural immersion: En vivo reflections on cultural competence. *Journal of Cultural Diversity, 17*(2), 44–50.

Leininger, M. M., & McFarland, M. R. (2006). *Culture care diversity and universality: A worldwide nursing theory* (2nd ed.). Boston, MA: Jones and Bartlett Publishers.

Lin, Y.-P., Furze, G., Spilsbury, K., & Lewin, R. J. P. (2008). Misconceived and maladaptive beliefs about heart disease: A comparison between Taiwan and Britain. *Journal of Clinical Nursing, 18,* 46–55.

Lucas Breda, K. (2015). Participatory action research. In M. De Chesnay (Ed.), *Nursing research using participatory action research: Qualitative designs and methods in nursing* (pp. 1–11). New York, NY: Springer Publishing Company.

Maupin, J., & Ross, N. (2012). Expectations of similarity and cultural difference in conceptual models of illness: Comparison of medical staff and Mexican migrants. *Human Organization, 71*(3), 306–316.

Merli, C. (2010). Male and female cutting among Southern Thailand's Muslims: Rituals, biomedical practice and local discourses. *Culture, Health, & Sexuality, 12*(7), 725–738.

Mulongo, P., McAndrew, S., & Hollins Martin, C. (2014). Crossing borders: Discussing the evidence relating to the mental health needs of women exposed to female genital mutilation. *International Journal of Mental Health Nursing, 23,* 296–305.

Muteshi, J. K., Miller, S., & Belizan, J. M. (n.d.). The ongoing violence against women: Female genital mutilation/cutting. *Reproductive Health, 13*(44). doi:10.1186/s12978-016-0159-3

National Rural Health Association. (2016). *What's different about rural health care?* Retrieved from http:// www.ruralhealthweb.org/go/left/about-rural-health /what-s-different-about-rural-health-care

Nauright, L. (2005). Preparing nursing professionals for advocacy: Service-learning. In M. de Chesnay (Ed.), *Caring for the vulnerable* (pp. 357–362). Sudbury, MA: Jones and Bartlett Publishers.

Nauright, L., & Wilson, A. (2012). Preparing nursing professionals to be advocates: Service learning. In M. de Chesnay & B. Anderson (Eds.), *Caring for the vulnerable* (pp. 465–474). Burlington, MA: Jones & Bartlett Learning.

Ndiwane, A. (2008). Laying down the knife may decrease risk of HIV transmission: Cultural practices in Cameroon with implications for public health and policy. *Journal of Cultural Diversity, 15*(2), 2004–2008.

Nichols, M., Stein, A. D., & Wold, J. L. (2014). Health status of children of migrant farm workers: Farm worker family health program, Moultrie, GA. *American Journal of Public Health, 104*(2), 365–370.

Ogunsiji, O. (2015). Understanding the dilemma of de-infibulation for women living with female genital mutilation. *Australian Nursing & Midwifery Journal. 27*(9), 51.

Pandey, K. P., & Shrestha, G. (2014). Assessing current situation of domestic violence against women: A study in Hasandaha, Morang. *Himalayan Journal of Sociology & Anthropology, 6,* 64–85.

Patchell, B. A., Robbins, L. K., Lowe, J. A., & Hoke, M. M. (2015). The effect of a culturally tailored substance abuse prevention intervention with Plains Indian adolescents. *Journal of Cultural Diversity, 22*(1), 3–8.

Pearson, L. (2003). Understanding the culture of poverty. *Nurse Practitioner, 28*(4), 6.

Pecora, P. J., Chahine, Z., & Graham, J. C. (2013). Safety and risk assessment frameworks: Overview and implications for child maltreatment fatalities. *Child Welfare, 92*(2), 143–160.

Purnell, L. (2000). A description of the Purnell model for cultural competence. *Journal of Transcultural Nursing, 11*(1), 40–46.

Purnell, L. (2002). The Purnell model for cultural competence. *Journal of Transcultural Nursing, 13*(3), 193–196.

Purnell, L. (2014). *Guide to culturally competent health care* (3rd ed.). Philadelphia, PA: F. A. Davis.

Purnell, L., & Paulanka, B. (2008). *Transcultural health care: A culturally competent approach* (3rd ed.). Philadelphia, PA: F. A. Davis.

Pyrah, R., & Fellerer, J. (2015). Redefining "sub-culture": A new lens for understanding hybrid cultural identities in East-Central Europe with a case study from early 20th century Lviv-Lwów-Lemberg. *Journal of the Association for the Study of Ethnicity and Nationalism, 21*(4), 700–720.

Roye, C., & Truglio-Londrigan, M. (2017). Community-based participatory research and primary health care: Working with the people. In S. B. Lewenson & M. Truglio-Londrigan (Eds.), *Practicing primary health care in nursing: Caring for populations* (pp. 181–193). Burlington, MA: Jones & Bartlett Learning.

Savage, C. L., Xu, Y., Lee, R., Rose, B. L., Kappesser, M., & Anthony, J. S. (2006). A case study in the use of community-based participatory research in public health nursing. *Public Health Nursing, 23*(5), 472–478.

Scozzaro, C., & Janikowski, T. P. (2015). Mental health diagnosis, medication, treatment and placement milieu of children in foster care. *Journal of Child Family Studies, 24,* 2560–2567. doi:10.1007/s10826-014-0058-6

Stevens, C. A. (2006). Being healthy: Voices of adolescent women who are parenting. *Journal for Specialists in Pediatric Nursing, 11*(1), 28–41.

Streubert Speziale, H. J., & Rinaldi Carpenter, D. (2007). *Qualitative research in nursing: Advancing the humanistic imperative* (5th ed.). Philadelphia, PA: Wolters Kluwer, Lippincott Williams & Wilkins.

Tenkorang, E. Y., Owusu, A. Y., Yeboah, E. H., & Bannerman, R. (2013). Factors influencing domestic and marital violence against women in Ghana. *Journal of Family Violence, 28,* 771–781.

Truglio-Londrigan, M. (2015). Participatory action research: One researcher's reflection. In M. De Chesnay (Ed.), *Nursing research using participatory action, research: Qualitative designs and methods in nursing* (pp. 117–135). New York, NY: Springer Publishing Company.

Tsai, J. H. (2006). Xenophobia, ethnic community, and immigrant youths' friendship network formation. *Adolescence, 41*(162), 285–299.

U.S. Department of Health and Human Services (2008). *Addressing rural health care needs.* Retrieved from http://www.hhs.gov/asl/testify/2008/07/t20080723a.html

U.S. Department of Health and Human Services, Administration for Children and Families. (2010). *The AFCARS report (Adoption and Foster Care Analysis and Reporting System).* Atlanta, GA: Author.

van Zalk, M., Kerr, M., van Zalk, N., & Stattin, H. (2013). Xenophobia and tolerance toward immigrants in adolescence: Cross-influence processes within friendships. *Journal of Abnormal Child Psychology, 41,* 627–639.

Venhorst, C. (2013). Islamic death rituals in a small town context in the Netherlands: Exploration of a common praxis for professionals. *Journal of Death and Dying, 65*(1), 1–10.

Vogus, T. J., Cull, M. J., Hengelbrok, N. E., Modell, S. J., & Epstein, R. A. (2016). Assessing safety culture I child welfare: Evidence from Tennessee. *Children and Youth Services, 65,* 94–103.

Wald, L. D. (1913, December 5). The foreign vote. Speech at meeting of Equal Suffrage League of the City of New York, at the Hotel Astor. Lillian Wald Papers, Writings & Speeches, Voters & Voting, 1913, Reel 25, Box 36, Folder 6, pp. 1–13. New York City Public Library, New York, NY.

Walle, A. H. (2004). Native Americans and alcoholism therapy: The example of Handsome Lake as a tool of recovery. *Journal of Ethnicity in Substance Abuse,* *3*(2), 55–79.

Wood, D. (2003). Effect of child and family poverty on child health in the United States. *Pediatrics, 112*(3), 707–711.

World Health Organization. (2008). *Eliminating female genital mutilation: An interagency statement.* Geneva, Switzerland: Author.

World Health Organization. (2016). *Female genital mutilation.* Retrieved from http://www.who.int /mediacentre/factsheets/fs241/en/

Zhao, M., & Yingchun, J. (2014). Challenges of Introducing participant observation in community health research. *ISRN Nursing.* Retrieved from http:// dx.doi.org/10.1155/2014/802490

For a full suite of assignments and additional learning activities, use the access code located in the front of your book to visit this exclusive website: **http://go.jblearning.com/londrigan**. If you do not have an access code, you can obtain one at the site.

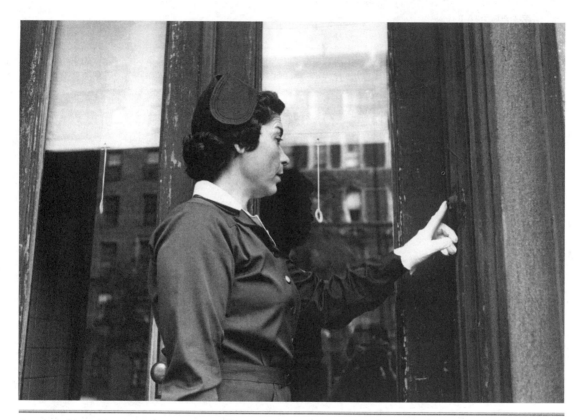

Courtesy of the Visiting Nurse Service of New York.

CHAPTER 9

Healthcare Policy and Politics: The Risk and Rewards for Public Health Nurses

Donna M. Nickitas
Barbara Rome

In addition to what seems to me the advisability of completing and perfecting the government by making men and women share its responsibility, the inevitability of the extension of the suffrage makes objection seem futile. The whole force of evolution is behind it. Women are going into public life whether they wish to or not. They have gone into factories, the professions, they are serving on public committees, they are proposing and even framing legislation. The movement is far greater than the demand for the ballot, and seems to be a force irresistible, one that cannot be swept back. (Wald, 1914, p. 3)

LEARNING OBJECTIVES

At the completion of this chapter, the reader will be able to:

- Describe the expanding role of public health nurses to provide leadership in healthcare advocacy, research, analysis, and policy development.
- Identify ways in which public health nurses analyze laws, regulations, and policies at the institutional, local, state, and national levels.
- Analyze the economic, ethical, and social implications of healthcare policy for population-based care and effectively advocate for policy change.

KEY TERMS

- Advocacy
- Affordable Care Act (ACA)
- Economic policy
- Healthcare access
- Healthcare costs
- Health disparities

- Influence
- Politics
- Public policy
- Social determinants of health
- Social policy

Why Does Federal Healthcare Policy Matter?

Although this question may seem rhetorical, perceptions of and experiences with the U.S. healthcare system can create the belief that to care about or try to understand federal policies on health care is fruitless. At least three issues contribute to this perspective. One prominent issue is the long-standing and interconnected problems the current system is unable to address: the rise in cost of health care, the reduction in employer-based healthcare benefits, the issues of social justice and equity for health access, and an inadequate supply of health providers. A second issue is that the U.S. healthcare system is a vast and multipart healthcare complex that is rigidly hierarchical and not well coordinated or unified in purpose, scope, or values. Moreover, third, but interdependent with the previous issues, is that the politics and the policies that shape the relationship between these inputs and outputs can seem extremely remote and hard to address. This chapter attempts to demonstrate that the linkages among these problems can be understood and that this knowledge is imperative for influencing and practicing public health nursing.

Public Health Nurses as a Political Force

Public health nurses have a professional obligation to articulate how intellectually demanding and complex public health nursing care is and to demonstrate the ways in which they have developed and implemented innovative models of care that promote health: expanding access, enhancing care coordination, improving quality and safety, and reducing costs. Once public health nurses fully appreciate their political force, they are poised to influence healthcare policy. According to the Kaiser Family Foundation (2016), there are 3,963,844 total professionally active nurses in the United States, and of these, 3.1 million are registered professional nurses. As the largest segment of the healthcare workforce, nurses need to be full partners with other health professionals to achieve significant improvements at the local, state, national, and international levels in both the delivery and health policy arenas. As a professional partner, nurses have the expertise in care delivery, as well as the financial, technical, and political savvy to close clinical and financial gaps within a healthcare delivery system (Nickitas, 2011). Despite the large number of nurses in the workforce, they have not fully leveraged their strength to lead change, influence policy, and advance the health of the nation.

It is time for nurses to leverage their numbers and make a difference in policy and politics. For example, nurses have ranked high in public opinion polls, and the public believes that the endorsement by nurses for candidates for political office demonstrates a candidate's integrity. When divided by 435 congressional districts nationally, there are approximately 5,000 registered nurses per congressional district who can mobilize voters.

Lois Capps, congresswoman from California, uses her expertise as a school nurse in her political role.

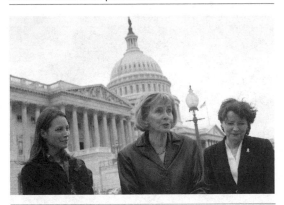

© Kris Connor/Getty Images

The power of the nursing numbers is that 1 in every 45 registered voters is a registered nurse. Nurses can convert votes that make the difference in electing officials who support and endorse nursing's core values and issues. When they exercise their right to vote at any level, from local to federal, nurses are engaged in the political process (Smith, 2016). "Voting is the most fundamental form of advocacy. It is a way nurses' voice their positions on healthcare policy and support policymakers who act on these positions" (Nickitas, 2016, p. 213).

Political Influence: A Call to Action

The Institute of Medicine/Robert Wood Johnson Foundation (IOM/RWJF) *The Future of Nursing: Leading Change, Advancing Health* strongly recommends that nurses become fully engaged in healthcare reform and policy by becoming involved with, speaking out about, and participating in the future of health care (IOM, 2011). Today's public health nurses are pivotal in addressing the health of populations and health equity while building a culture of health that empowers everyone to live the healthiest lives they can, even when they are dealing with chronic illness or the constraints of poverty, housing, education, and income inequality. In fact,

the Robert Wood Johnson Foundation (RWJF) has endorsed creating healthier and more equitable communities through a national initiative called the "culture of health" (RWJF, 2015). Public health nurses are a valuable resource between the patients they serve and community services required to address the **social determinants of health** to impact health outcomes.

Although population health has long been a role for public health nurses, all nurses bear some responsibility for assuring the health of the community, including how focusing on social determinants of health can influence individuals and communities to live healthier lives and change their health outcomes and health equity. Throughout history, public health nurses have played a crucial role in improving the total health of populations by attending to the social determinants of health. The Centers for Medicaid and Medicare Services (CMS, 2016) has a specific goal that addresses the social determinants of health defined as "the conditions in which people are born, grow, work, live, and age, and the wider set of forces and systems shaping the conditions of daily life" (CMS, 2016, p. 26). The National Quality Strategy was developed by the Department of Health and Human Services (U.S. DHHS) to promote quality within healthcare environments. CMS is the agency within DHHS that is focused on creating strategies to improve quality and reduce harm, by

- making care safer by reducing harm caused in the delivery of care,
- ensuring that each person and family is engaged as a partner in their care,
- promoting the most effective prevention and treatment practices for the leading causes of mortality, starting with cardiovascular disease,
- working with communities to promote wide use of best practices to enable healthy living,
- making quality care more affordable for individuals, families, employers, and governments by developing and spreading new healthcare delivery models (National Quality Strategy Stakeholder Toolkit, 2015).

The opportunity to improve the health of communities and populations by understanding and influencing policy is a professional imperative. Public health nurses have a responsibility to advocate for health care as a basic human right and ensure access to an affordable package of essential health services. There is a need to assist public health nurses to enhance their role as advocates and understand resources and polices available to them on both the state and national levels. They must use their collective political influence and become involved in the policymaking process. **Influence** is the ability to persuade or sway an individual or group to support or endorse a single issue (Adams, Chisari, Ditomassi, & Erickson, 2011). Learning to use political influence to shape health and public policy effectively is a key determinant in decision-making, securing support and resources (Yukl & Falbe, 1990).

Policy affect all aspects of public health nursing, including promoting and protecting the health of population through health promotion and disease prevention. Public health nurses have had a distinguished history of **advocacy** in shaping health and public policy through the ages. For example, Lillian Wald and Lavinia Dock were early 20th-century nursing leaders and activists who embraced the social issues of their day. Their professional advocacy and activism were centered in the belief that nurses were responsible for initiating and supporting action to meet the health and social needs of the public, in particular, those of vulnerable populations (International Council of Nurses, 2006).

The Institute of Medicine (IOM) and the RWJF landmark report, *The Future of Nursing: Leading Change, Advancing Health* (2011) also calls for nurses to be better prepared with requisite competencies, including leadership and health policy, as well as competency in specific content areas, including community and public health, to deliver high-quality care. An example of nursing's expanded role to increase access and provide healthcare delivery is an essential component of the **Affordable Care Act (ACA)**. It calls for an expanded role for nurses in the design of more

Early 20th-century nursing leader Lavinia Dock advocated woman suffrage, equating the right to vote with better healthcare outcomes.

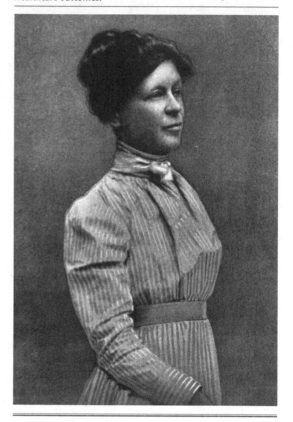

Courtesy of the National Library of Medicine.

efficient and cost-effective models of healthcare delivery (Daley, 2011). The U.S. DHHS has responded to the growing population with chronic conditions through nearly $212 million in grants to prevent chronic diseases, funded in part by the ACA. Funds have focused on preventing tobacco use, obesity, diabetes, heart disease, and stroke (U.S. DHHS, 2014). The focus on prevention and management of chronic disease system is needed to address population-wide health promotion. The Association of Public Health Nurses (APHN) has aligned the professional roles of the nurse to address these system changes including

- Developing partnerships across a variety of disciplines and settings.
- Exploring funding mechanisms to support C/PH nurse roles in chronic disease prevention and control.
- Providing technical support for collection and dissemination of outcome data related to C/PH nurse efforts aimed at the prevention and management of chronic disease.
- Advocating for improved systems of care and public health infrastructure to prevent and manage chronic illness across the lifespan. (Cooper & Shaw, 2016)

The reality is public health nurses will need to attend to the growing U.S. population living with chronic disease and move away from the provision of clinical services to population health. To further develop these roles, APHN proposes that public health nurses position and define their roles in ways that foster the prevention/control of chronic disease within public health and community settings, becoming partners on the chronic health needs of the community where they live, learn, work, play, and pray. This partnership must include building and expanding partnerships with nongovernmental organizations/community partners to develop programs that can reach the population and address the prevalence and prevention of chronic disease. When public health nurses heed the call to political involvement in health and public policy, they not only advance the nursing profession but also improve the public's health (Hall-Long, 2009).

Public health nurses pay a key role in shaping and influencing the delivery of health care. As a member of the healthcare workforce, public health nurses must understand the public policies and political forces creating the context for healthcare delivery in this country. Although policy and politics may seem remote in day-to-day practice, they are the forces that drive the policies within a public health department, provide access to health resources for communities, and even decide who will breathe clean air and who will have lead-free water.

Nurses have been engaged in issues related to environmental health in communities since Florence Nightingale wrote about the effects of clean air and water in her *Notes on Nursing*. To date, a number of nursing organizations actively participate in rallying for clean air and water. Among them are the American Nurses Association (ANA) who advocated for clean air and water in the Global Climate Change Resolution that was introduced to the House of Delegates in 2008 (ANA, 2008). The ANA is a leader in public policies that affect health and exists to promote health of the public and advance the profession of nursing through prevention programs that have an impact on global health (ANA, 2008). Along with the ANA, the White House honored two nurses with Champions of Change awards. Laura Anderko and Therese Smith were awarded for *Changing the Lens: Communicating Public Health Issues and Protecting Human Health in a Changing Climate* (Alliance of Nurses for Healthy Environments, n.d). Nurses have also actively advocated for the Clean Air Act, demonstrating the positive impact it has on the environment and health through testimonies, campaigns, op-eds, and providing testimony to the Environmental Protection Agency (Alliance of Nurses for Healthy Environments, n.d.). These nurses have effectively advocated and influenced public policy, budgets, and laws using the media, facts, and educating government officials and the public on issues related to a healthier environment (Alliance of Nurses for Healthy Environments, n.d.). Nurses are considered the most trusted profession and must advocate for policies that promote health.

When resources are constrained, policy and politics are the levers that continuously influence change at all system levels. To serve communities well, and to influence decision-making that improves access, cost-effective quality, and safety, requires a basic understanding of complex adaptive social systems. Public health nurses are known for their ability to work collaboratively with communities to create environments that promote health and prevent disease. They are activists and use an ecological approach when responding to community needs in program and policy development to enhance the health of populations.

Defining Policy

The word *policy* is Greek in origin and is linked to citizenship (Online Dictionary of Social Sciences, n.d.). Policy represents the manifestations of ideology or belief systems about how the world should work (Rushefsky, 2008). **Public policy** is often used to describe government actions including, for example, economic and social policy. **Economic policy** promotes and regulates markets, whereas **social policy** seeks to improve the conditions of the society and achieve greater social equity (Aries, 2016).

Policy may be implemented through a variety of government systems, including the legislative, executive, or judicial branches of government. Each of these systems has the official capacity to direct or influence the actions, behaviors, or decisions of others (Block, 2008). As distinct systems, each branch of government plays a vital role in the formulation and regulation of health policy. It is important to know, in advance of influencing policy, which branch of government has the authority to legislate and regulate health care. For example, the legislative branch and executive branches of government had key roles in the formation and passage of the landmark policy of 2010 ACA.

Policy and Values

Policy always had a moral dimension because it relates to decisions about how to act toward others. Leavitt (2009) described this ethical approach as one that involves the choices a society or organization makes to reach a desired action. These measures reflect the values and the beliefs of those who develop the policies. Furthermore, policy involves how and what resources should be used to achieve those policies. Thus, policies are often expressed as goals, programs, proposals, laws, and regulations that reflect the values and the beliefs of

those who are developing and directing the policies (Milstead, 2013).

Policies developed by nurses have frequently shown a strong belief in the importance of assisting people to care for themselves despite their illness or disability, and this belief has distinguished nursing's caring attribute from other professions. Caring is a value central to nursing. Watson (2008) suggests that to help the current healthcare system retain its most precious resource—competent, caring, professional nurses—a new generation of health professionals must ensure care and healing for the public while learning about the value of serving others. If public health nurses want policies that reflect their nursing values, then they must get involved in the policy process to ensure their values are represented.

The long-standing interdependence of public policy, politics, and public health often makes it difficult to conceptualize or understand them separately. Public policy, like public health, is population based. Policy encompasses the choices that a government makes regarding goals and priorities and the way it allocates resources to attain these aims. Public health is focused on society, seeking collectively to ensure the conditions in which people can be

A public health nurse participates in a community outreach program.

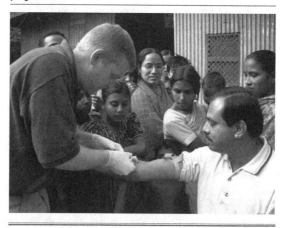

Courtesy of CDC.

healthy. Public health as a discipline is interested in the equitable distribution of social and economic resources because they are such important influences on the health of populations (IOM, 1988). However, unlike public health, public policy reflects a broader array of competing values, beliefs, and attitudes espoused by those designing policy and the stiff competition for limited resources and immediately felt needs. Central to current debates are competing visions between public health and public policy. While the former field is increasingly cognizant of the necessity of a prevention focus, this approach conflicts with demands within the political field because it requires taking a shared long view and investing in the future. Paralleling this tension is a broader national policy debate that pits austerity against investment as the background of policy choices. Within the theoretical framework of the public health nursing practice intervention wheel, federal policy development and implementation are primary components of a public health intervention used at the system level of practice impacting the health of communities (Keller & Strohschein, 2016).

Defining Politics

Politics is often described as the process of who gets to decide what will be done and when it will be done (Milstead, 2013). It involves power and influence for critical decision-making and requires significant investment in social capital. Public health nurses must understand how politics drives policy decisions and have the necessary skills and competencies to care for society and the populations they serve. Kraft and Furlong (2010) suggest that policy involves how conflicts in society are identified and resolved for one set of priorities or values over another. Because resources (money, time, and personnel) are limited or finite, choices must be made. For public health nurses to have the ability to advocate resources for others and actually shape policy, they must have the necessary political skill. This requires the capacity to understand another's values and position and to use that understanding to influence others to act.

Nursing leaders meet with Michelle Obama.

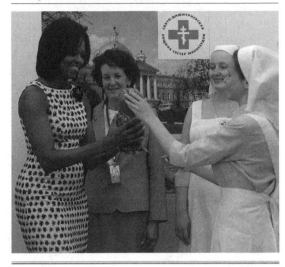

ITAR-TASS Photo Agency / Alamy Stock Photo

The importance of this chapter is that it will assist public health nurses in understanding the interface between new federal health policies that influence the public health of communities as well as public health nursing practices and the economic and political forces that are reciprocally threatening the implementation of these policies. The landmark ACA legislation, enacted by the 111th U.S. Congress, sought to remedy our nation's broken healthcare system. The history and context that are shaping and shaped the fate of this legislation are outlined. The institutional politics at the national and state levels of government are explored. Additionally, the critical need to control **healthcare costs**, to connect prevention with quality care and patient safety, and to integrate technology for improving healthcare coordination will be presented. Regardless of partisan positioning, these areas provide concrete examples of issues that must be addressed in the redesign of a sustainable healthcare system that provides access to quality outcomes for all populations regardless of income, race, or geographic location (Gostin, 2002).

The Current U.S. Healthcare System, Post–ACA 2010

In the current healthcare system, much has been said or written about whether or not the healthcare reform has worked, what it has cost, and the impact it has on each one of us as individuals. It has also been suggested from those who have great faith in our current system that it should have been left alone. It may work well for some people, but on the whole, our healthcare system ranks 37th out of 191 world health systems in the *World Health Report 2000* (World Health Organization, 2010), and our nation has the highest rate of preventable deaths among 19 industrialized nations (Cohen, 2009). The number of nonelderly Americans uninsured has decreased from 49.1 million in 2010 to 32 million today, reflecting the gains made because of the ACA's major coverage provisions that went into effect in January 2014 (The Henry J. Kaiser Family Foundation, 2016). Low-income workers are at the greatest risk to be uninsured because job-based coverage is often not offered; even when it is, these workers are less able to afford the premiums. The lack of health insurance affects access to health care as well as increases costs. The uninsured delay or forgo needed care, making them more likely to be hospitalized for avoidable conditions. Overall, the uninsured are less likely to receive preventive care. Cost barriers to health care have been growing in the past decade, making the uninsured more likely than the insured to be unable pay for necessities because of their medical bills (The Henry J. Kaiser Family Foundation, 2011).

Many people have little or no access to basic health care, living in fear that they will become sick or injured and not be able to afford care. For example, a Tennessee-based organization provides free health care to underserved communities, providing medical, dental, vision, preventative care, and education to isolated and impoverished communities throughout the United States (Remote Area Medical, 2016). Utilizing fairgrounds, arenas, and schools, they create mobile clinics to help alleviate suffering. Because services are free and limited, they are only able to provide care to those that are physically able to come to the clinic. The parking lot opens at midnight, and often people arrive several hours before to get online. They start handing out numbers at 3 o'clock in the morning and volunteer, and patient populations determine how many numbers are given. People wait outside for extended periods of time just to get a number to be seen in the clinic. All patients are offered either dental or vision care and medical care (Remote Area Medical, 2016). Stan Brock founded the organization after a personal injury he sustained in a remote area in South America. He saw firsthand the devastating effects of lack of access to basic medical care and vowed to find a way to deliver care to the most remote communities around the world. However, most of the work the organization does today is in the United States (Remote Area Medical, 2016).

Arguably, one of the greatest strengths of the American healthcare system has been its strong private sector orientation, which facilitates ready access to all manner of services for those with stable coverage and strongly encourages ongoing medical innovation by product manufacturers. Our healthcare system has some of the finest medical facilities, technologies, innovations, treatments, and human talent. Many of the world's best health practitioners are here. Health care generates more new job opportunities than any other sector of our economy. The rapid advance of medical technology over the past 50 years has unquestionably improved the health status of millions of Americans. Employer-sponsored insurance has played a crucial role in retaining this strong private sector presence in the U.S. health industry. However, employer-based coverage is also the Achilles' heel of American health care. As employer-based health insurance costs continue to rise, those increases are being passed on to the employee through increased insurance premiums. Finally, today's open-ended federal tax exemption for some employer-paid premiums encourages broad coverage, which further escalates cost (Capretta, 2009).

Despite its significant strengths, the U.S. healthcare system has long suffered from unequal access, disorganization, and waste; for example, the value it provides does not match its enormous cost. Research conducted over many decades documents significant disparities in the use of health care and in its cost from one location to another. These differences cannot be explained by contrasting rates or varying severity of illness among population groups. Furthermore, it is increasingly apparent that higher rates of health care use do not necessarily lead to better care; in fact, they sometimes lead to worse outcomes (Mechanic, 2011). Former White House advisor and bioethicist on health care, Ezekiel Emmanuel, notes that both political parties do agree that our economy and our nation will not succeed if healthcare costs continue to rise. The fact that few people understand how much is spent on health care versus how much needs to be paid to provide quality care and the difference between the two undermines the importance for needing to implement healthcare reform. He points out that in 2014 the United States spent $3 trillion on health care, averaging over $9,523 per American, according to the Centers for Medicare & Medicaid. In comparing these costs with France, which has roughly a total gross domestic product of $2.806 trillion in 2013, the United States spent on health care what the 65 million people of France spent on everything including health care. The other important problem is growth. If healthcare costs continue to grow faster than the economy (present rate of 2% a year), it will be roughly one-third of the entire economy by 2035 (Emmanuel, 2011).

U.S. Health System and the ACA

The IOM's Quality Initiative, launched in 1996, was a tipping point in collective learning about and acknowledging how poorly the U.S. healthcare system was functioning. Documenting the gravity and high costs of hospital errors on human health and safety became the foundation for clinical practice reform. For example, the IOM publication *To Err Is Human: Building a Safer Health System* found that medical errors caused nearly 100,000 deaths and annually incurred an estimated $28 to $33 million in excess health costs. The reality that costs and

quality were not aligned and that a serious chasm existed between what was known at that time to be quality care and what actually occurred in practice had a collective impact that has led to quality goals becoming institutionalized expectations (IOM, 2000).

On March 23, 2010, President Barack Obama signed into law H.R. 3590, the Patient Protection and Affordable Care Act (P.L. 111-148) and seven days later signed H.R. 4872, the Health Care and Education Reconciliation Act of 2010 (P.L. 1101-152). The goals of healthcare reform created a system that provides healthcare coverage for all and would no longer produce personal bankruptcy. In other words, it was designed to help avoid economic disaster for employers and to hold all parties—doctors, nurses, hospitals, drug companies, and insurers—collectively responsible for making health care better, safer, and less costly (Gawande, 2009). The ACA put in place comprehensive health insurance reforms to increase access, guarantee more healthcare choices, invest in creating a new infrastructure that holds the potential to improve care quality, and contain costs for all Americans. Indeed, the sheer scope and complexity of the nation's healthcare system, as part of a larger political and global economic context, make the implementation of this healthcare legislation a formidable endeavor.

Fortunately, provisions of the ACA have increased access and have been positively felt by the public. These include extending coverage for young adults to stay on their parents insurance until age 26; providing free preventive screenings to seniors on Medicare; filling in the Medicare part D donut hole, which allows millions of seniors to receive checks for $250 (a first phase in closing the gap in drug costs thresholds), and making it illegal for insurance companies to impose lifetime limits on anyone or deny children insurance coverage for preexisting conditions. In 2014, the ACA expanded **healthcare access** for more Americans by preventing insurance companies from discriminating based on preexisting conditions, a clause particularly critical for the 13 million nonelderly adults previously denied coverage because of their medical conditions. Another step to increase access is the provision that employers with more than 50 employees are expected to cover their employees' healthcare costs, with steep per-employee fines for violations. This legislation requires most Americans to have health insurance coverage and added 16 million people to the Medicaid rolls. The combined legislation has extended coverage to an estimated 30 million uninsured Americans (The White House, 2011).

As of 2015, the ACA was projected to cost $1.207 trillion dollars over 10 years, according to the nonpartisan Congressional Budget Office (CBO, 2010). This same office has estimated that it will reduce the deficit by $143 billion over a decade and by $1 trillion over the next 20 years by cutting government overspending and reining in waste, fraud, and abuse in Medicare, Medicaid, and Children's Health Insurance Program (CHIP). Efforts to combat fraud have returned more than $27.8 billion to the Medicare Trust Fund since the inception of the Health Care Fraud and Abuse Control (HCFAC) Program, recovering $3.3 billion in Fiscal Year (FY) 2014 alone (HHS, 2015). The new law invests new resources and requires different screening procedures for healthcare providers to boost these efforts (CBO, 2010).

For states to have a quality healthcare system requires a three-pronged approach: information, infrastructure, and incentives (Fuchs, 2007). In line with Fuchs's three quality areas, the ACA focused on creating an infrastructure to learn what works for continuous quality improvement and to identify cost containment strategies. New institutions are in place to develop these efforts: The Patient-Centered Outcomes Research Institute (PCORI), the Center for Medicare and Medicaid Innovation (CMI), and the Independent Payment Advisory Board (IPAB). The success of this healthcare legislation in achieving quality care delivery and being affordable is critically dependent on these centers working as intended in concert.

The PCORI, with the help of computerized records, determine the comparative effectiveness of treatments. This strengthens evidence-based practice at a national level. As noted earlier, more health care does not necessarily equate to better

health outcomes. Cost savings without compromising quality is the intention driving the strengthening of comparative effectiveness efforts. Similarly, the ACA calls for empowering an independent federal panel, the IPAB, to set Medicare rates free of pressure from providers and other interest groups. The Center for Medicare and Medicaid Innovation is providing funding to test payment models that emphasize the quality of care instead of the quantity of treatments delivered. Demonstration projects will be funded to develop models of care that are effective in the delivery of patient-centered care that is well coordinated and improves patient outcomes. One example of a new delivery system of care being developed is the Accountable Care Organization (ACO). Patient populations/communities would be provided a full spectrum of care services and proactively tracked from acute to home care experiences, but these steps may not be enough to bring about the change that many experts urge: to move away from a system in which we pay for every MRI or drug infusion on a case-by-case basis and toward one in which salaried medical professionals are paid to do what it takes to keep the public healthy (Orszag, 2011).

The debate, however, over performance measures continues as stakeholders argue whether the current standards are sufficient or not, on whether they are valid and how to improve on them (Pronovost et al., 2016). It is suggested that measurement of performance can be enhanced in some ways; transparency, coordinated policies, setting standards, and supporting research and innovation in measuring performance in health care. By implementing feedback loops, we can better understand how to make better use of measures (Pronovost et al., 2016). When these feedback loops occur at all levels (local, regional, and national), they can be used as a tool for improvement as well as better communication with patients, raising their awareness of differences in quality and costs for health care. Despite current steps in reporting of performance for healthcare systems, healthcare performance measures have not yet reach the desired goal of quality care at lower costs. According to Pronovost et al. (2016), the key recommendations for future directions include creating a health measurement and data standard-setting body, building the science of performance measures, and improving the communication of data to patients.

One important theme of the health reform legislation is that of transforming our current medical care system into a coordinated national healthcare system. While the ACA is about insurance coverage and costs, population health is a theme that runs through many aspects of the ACA. Among public health programs, for example, the ACA emphasizes community-based prevention. A population orientation pervades even the coverage provisions, with no copay being required for evidence-based prevention service. In order to make health care available to all, we would do well to remember the history of the first great expansion of coordinated public healthcare coverage when President Lyndon Johnson drove Medicare and Medicaid through Congress in 1965: "the only sure way to bend the curve and curb the rate of increase in healthcare costs is to keep people out of the sick care system, to put as much profit in prevention as there is in acute care, and to put financial gain and pain into how individuals take (or don't take) care of themselves" (Califano, 2009).

Six months after the ACA was signed into law, the U.S. DHHS highlighted the importance of evidence-based preventive medicine by announcing nearly $100 million in grants made possible primarily by the new law's prevention and public health fund. These grants support a variety of critical public health programs in states' and local communities' efforts to fight obesity, increase HIV testing, promote tobacco cessation assistance, expand mental health and substance abuse programs, and track, monitor, and respond to disease outbreaks. The U.S. DHHS justified this effort as follows:

"This investment in prevention and public health will pay enormous dividends both today and in the future," said HHS Secretary Kathleen Sebelius. "To strengthen our health care system, we need to stop just focusing solely on sick care and start focusing more on proven evidence-based ways to keep people healthy in the first place. These grants made possible by the Affordable Care Act will support programs across the country that will make Americans healthier." (U.S. DHHS, 2010)

The prevention and public health fund provides for an expanded and sustained national investment in prevention and public health programs, including wellness and public health activities, prevention research, and health screenings and initiatives such as the Community Transformation Grants (CTG) program. The CTG program focuses on population health, recognizing the priority health needs in communities. To reduce chronic diseases such as heart disease, cancer, stroke, and diabetes, these community programs promote prevention through healthy lifestyle practices. Almost $103 million was awarded to states and communities serving approximately 120 million Americans (CDC, 2010).

As of 2015, $1 billion was made available to the prevention fund, with $885 million transferred to the CDC to help combat heart disease, tobacco use, diabetes, healthcare-associated infections, and other public health problems (American Public Health Association, 2015). The ACA also created a council within U.S. DHHS to provide coordination and leadership at the federal level and among government departments and agencies to develop a national prevention strategy. This council sets goals and objectives for improving health through federally supported prevention, health promotion, and public health programs, in addition to making recommendations that can integrate healthcare practices.

The ACA also provides coverage for preventive health services. Cost sharing is one strategy being used to control healthcare costs. The premise is that by having consumers pay a portion of their medical expenses, such costs will be lowered by discouraging consumers from using care they do not need.

However, any copay for some would prohibit their purchasing care they did need such as not filling prescriptions and/or postponing visits to healthcare providers. As a result, basic evidence-based prevention practices will not require copayments to ensure these are available to all. For example, Medicare Part B coverage offers a personalized prevention plan with no copayment or deductible and includes a health risk assessment and other elements, such as updating family history, listing providers that regularly provide medical care to the individual, body mass index measurement, and other screenings for risk factors. The prevention plan would take into account the findings of the risk assessment and be completed before or as part of a visit to a health professional. Advice and referrals would be offered and might include community-based lifestyle interventions to reduce health risks and promote self-management and wellness, as well as screening schedules related to identified health risks. The new healthcare legislation also improves access to preventive services for eligible adults in Medicaid—for example, increasing access to immunizations and awarding grants to states to provide incentives to Medicaid beneficiaries with chronic illnesses who participate in healthy lifestyle programs and demonstrate changes in health risk and outcomes. The programs are currently funded for five years.

Other provisions in the ACA enhance funding for community health centers; the National Health Service Corp, which provides care to underserved areas and populations; education and outreach campaigns regarding preventive benefits including birth control; and the operation of school-based health centers, with an emphasis on communities with barriers to accessing healthcare services. From improved nutritional labeling for standard menu items in chain restaurants to ensuring employers provide reasonable break times for nursing mothers and funding for the Childhood Obesity Demonstration Project, the new healthcare legislation is strongly focused on prevention and public health needs. The benefits for public health nursing practice are enormous (Trust for America's Health, 2010).

A note of caution: There are vulnerabilities and challenges regarding public health programs. Although the ACA has given historically high attention to prevention and public health, legislative history also shows the field's weaknesses, especially in funding. Historically, population-oriented public health programs have often lost out to other priorities. Efforts have been made to eliminate healthcare disparities, and yet they continue to exist in the United States with certain groups at higher risk of limited or no access to care, poor-quality care, and poorer health outcomes (The Henry Kaiser Family Foundation, 2016). Public health nurses will have to work intelligently to be sure that this history is not repeated. As a nation we move forward with a new administration following the 2016 presidential election. At the time this chapter was being written, the direction we take as a nation with regard to our healthcare system was still unknown. With the new administration calling for repeal of the ACA and no viable replacement plan identified, nursing, in all specialties, need to be at the decision-making table.

Is Health Care a Right?

The ACA has been in the eye of a political storm since its inception. Claims that health reform will fail continue to be spoken, just as threats of repeal were voiced even while President Obama was signing both acts into law. Republicans and conservatives have continued to level criticism against the law since it was passed in March 2010, while President Obama has been vigorous in defending its objectives and future benefits. The public has heard these attacks on the reform loud and clear. According to a Gallup poll on healthcare reform taken in August 2016, 51% of Americans favored repealing the 2010 Patient Protection and Affordable Care Act, whereas 48% still favor keeping it (Gallup Poll, 2016). These numbers have fluctuated since the inception of the ACA, and although the majority of Americans disapprove, the gap is narrowing. Views on this issue are highly polarized and highly partisan, with Republicans strongly for repeal and the large majority of Democrats wanting the law retained and even expanded. Americans' views on repealing the healthcare law mirror their reactions to its passage. Apparently, the public sentiment over the ACA reflects a deep polarization as well (Gallup Poll, 2011b).

Beyond public opinion, ongoing obstacles are facing the implementation of the healthcare bill, especially around the implementation of state exchanges. Exchanges are state-oriented health insurance markets that allow individuals and small businesses access to competitive insurance rates and offer a streamlined way to shop for insurance. In states that have chosen not to set exchanges, the federal government will set them up. To compromise between regulatory/public program advocates and advocates for private/market-driven programs, Medicaid and state health insurance exchanges are the strategies used to increase healthcare coverage, each of which is projected to cover approximately 16 million uninsured Americans (Jacobi, Watson, & Restuccia, 2011). The House of Representatives has continued to vote to repeal the ACA and has compromised the funding necessary to administer it. In short, the obstacles appear to be expanding.

Debate over the ACA before it was even passed and ever since has focused largely on its implications for the role of the federal government in American society. Americans remain divided on whether it is the federal government's responsibility to make sure all Americans have health care: 51% say yes, whereas 47% disagree (Gallup Poll, 2016). Critics of the healthcare law argue that it is an example of too much government control over things that should be left to individuals and private businesses. A majority of Americans agree that a private healthcare system is better than a government-run system, although proponents of the law can point out that it falls short of mandating a government-run healthcare system such as those in Canada or European countries. As of 2014, approximately 36% of Americans have government-provided health insurance, making it clear that the issue going forward is the degree to which government should be involved in health care

in the years ahead, rather than whether the government should get out of the healthcare business altogether (Smith & Medalia, 2015).

State Shared-Power Relationship with the Federal Government

The Commonwealth Fund Scorecard on local health system performances examine how states compare on 38 key indicators of **healthcare** access, quality, **costs**, and health outcomes. The 2016 report of the Commonwealth Fund's *Scorecard on Local Health System Performance*, shows improvements: fewer people uninsured, better quality of care, better efficiency in use of hospitals, and fewer deaths from cancers that are treatable. These gains were made between 2011 and 2014 when the ACA was being implemented, capturing the early effects of healthcare reform in the United States (The Commonwealth Fund, 2016). States have an extensive and complicated shared-power relationship with the federal government in regulating various aspects of the health insurance market and in enacting health reforms. The passage of the ACA health insurance reform legislation was met with immediate and hostile state resistance. Members of 39 state legislatures proposed to limit, alter, or oppose selected state or federal actions, primarily targeted at single-payer provisions and mandates that require purchase of insurance (Cauchi, 2012). There is no doubt that the ACA's sprawling provisions raise a wealth of implementation challenges for states. The ACA also creates a host of opportunities for states to expand access to care, improve quality, and achieve greater efficiency in their healthcare systems. A major challenge for state leaders is to find the resources necessary to pursue these opportunities in this current economic environment. However, many states are moving forward with delivery system reform. For example, over 30 states have engaged in efforts to implement programs to advance medical homes in Medicaid/CHIP programs (RWJF, 2011). These patient-centered medical homes is an approach to deliver high-quality, cost-effective care to people with chronic health conditions. There are now 37 states that have public, private, or both patient-centered medical homes.

Many states are considering what potential role public health can play in a transformed health system. Leveraging the public health system with the ACA to efficiently and strategically partner with the healthcare system will improve access to quality, affordable, and integrated care while also promoting chronic disease prevention. Colorado and Washington are examples of two states that are redesigning their public health efforts using a more systemic perspective. Washington has developed a state strategic roadmap showing how various agencies within the Department of Health will connect to local, state, federal, and private sector partners. Additional elements guiding new ways in which the department conducts business include retraining the public health workforce, modifying and modernizing business practices, and developing long-term strategies for predictable and appropriate levels of financing (Washington Department of Health, 2010). Colorado is one of four states across the country testing a chronic disease prevention integration model under a demonstration project through the Centers for Disease Control and Prevention. One significant strategy that the state is implementing in its Department of Health and Environment is to restructure its prevention services division to move from disease categories (such as tobacco and HIV) to functions, allowing greater flexibility to respond to emerging public health issues that cross categorical program boundaries. Additionally, a new unit was also developed to identify the public health role in the new environment of health reform, taking a comprehensive approach to health outcomes (RWJF, 2011).

A considerable amount of energy and resources are focused on health information technology (HIT) and health information exchange (HIE) at both the state and federal level. The Health Information Technology for Economic and Clinical Health Act within ARRA provides states with substantial funding to support health information technology investment. Some states, such as Massachusetts, Oregon, and Rhode Island, already had legislation or strategic plans in place to support the adoption of HIT and

HIE before the passage of these federal provisions. While these states started early, all states are in the process of undertaking such work, and the federal government has awarded funding to all 50 states, the District of Columbia, and eligible territories through the State HIE Cooperative Agreement Program. This program is designed to support states as they develop the capacity necessary to exchange information within their state and across states (Office of the National Coordinator for Health Information Technology, 2010).

Although other viable health delivery models continue to emerge at the state level, early attempts from such states as Colorado, Washington, Oregon, and Ohio demonstrate the promise of innovative state reform efforts that are trying to improve access while actively evaluating cost-effectiveness and quality changes.

Understanding Policy Making and Public Health Nursing

Using the ACA as an example, we can see how a problem is identified and put on a policy agenda, where a plan to address said problem is developed, adopted, implemented, evaluated, and extended or modified (Hanley & Falk, 2007). This policy process is much like the nursing process: assess, plan, implement, evaluate, and assess again. Again, using the IOM (2011) report, nurses are considered the agent who will transform the healthcare system, ensuring care is patient centered, effective, safe, and affordable. This vision calls upon the entire nursing community to embrace this report as a blueprint for action and requires each and every nurse to use evidence-based research and collaboration to improve health care.

Public health nurses are well positioned because their access to the community and consumer groups helps to raise public awareness about **health disparities**, the quality of care, or lack of access to care for the communities they serve. Public health nurses and consumers collectively can develop ideas and propose policies to solve problems of healthcare access, health disparities, safety, or quality of care.

Public Health Nurses and Political Engagement

Public health nurses' engagement in policy and politics must rise to the level of influence whereby changes in healthcare reform are fully realized. Political participation is viewed as a continuum that extends from no engagement in politics to that of extreme activism. Individuals may choose how much they wish to engage politically throughout their lives in response to their intrinsic and external motivators, time and energy, and resources.

For the public health nurse, time is a valuable resource; therefore, investing one's time in political engagement may vary from nurse as citizen to nurse as activist. The excellent description of the various levels of political activism comes from the work of Kalisch and Kalisch (1982). They have described individual political participation along the continuum ranging from spectator activities to transitional activities to gladiatorial activities (p. 316). For example, nurses who wonder what's happening vote occasionally or not at all; they are not involved in improving their workplace or their community. Nurses who watch things happen are spectators. They expose themselves to political stimuli. They are members of their union. They vote, sometimes they wear buttons or put bumper stickers on cars, and they participate in community activities that are important. It is essential for public health nurses to become involved in political action activities, especially to be involved in their professional or membership organizations. Numbers count, and organizations that represent nurses, especially those with political action committees (PACs) and contribute to political campaigns, are valuable. Because money talks and buys influence, contributing to candidates who promote nursing's agenda to advance the nation's health through healthcare reform is necessary. It is unfortunate that campaigns are expensive, but it costs money to buy television ad time and mail literature to people's homes.

Public health nurses must participate in the political process and not stand on the sidelines waiting for things to happen. There are many ways to participate in the political process, including becoming active members of a political party; attending political meetings, forums, and rallies; helping register people to vote; or contributing and raising money for causes and campaigns through PACs; the American Nurses Association Political Action Committee (ANA-PAC) has grown over the years through nurse contributions. Song (2011) states, "ANA does not use dues dollars to support candidates. Rather, ANA-PAC raises money through the voluntary donations from member nurses across the country. ANA-PAC donates to candidates who work to implement healthy public policy for our profession" (p. 15).

Using Data to Leverage Gaps in Healthcare Quality

Public health nurses know that there are persistent quality and access gaps for minority and low-income groups. These groups have greater health disparities around specific services, including cancer screening, management of diabetes, and access to care. To better assist public health nurses to address the gaps in quality and access, publicly reported sources of county and state data can inform populations, settings, and potential strategies to promote population health. These data provide information about the significant problems confronting communities and compare them to other states and counties. Public health nurses then can use the data to evaluate organizational processes and outcomes to determine if there is an opportunity to improve the health of populations they serve. Using evidence to leverage interventions and actions to improve the health care of populations is how public nurses increase their influence in the public policy arena. The authors of this chapter recommend that the reader examine Chapter 15 to explore further public health nurses' intervention strategies.

Public health nurses must ensure their voices and interests are represented in the legislature at the state and federal levels. For example, professional nursing interest groups have seized on the public's frustration with rising healthcare costs and promoted policies that emphasize the cost-effectiveness of advanced practice nurses. It is up to the public health nurses themselves to inform and educate society about the ways in which nursing contributes to society.

Conclusion

Health and public policy continue to experience turbulent change as a result of the ACA. Public health nurses must use effective strategies to achieve policy goals to promote population health at the state and local levels. To accomplish these goals, public health nurses must understand policy and be familiar with sources of policy at all levels of government. Real successes for political influence and policy implementation occur when public health nurses are prepared, engaged, and respond to or lead change to advance the health of the nation by building coalitions and partnerships with public health officials at state and local levels to address the prevention and management of chronic diseases as well as other environmental and infectious diseases that arise. Advocating for improved systems of care and public health infrastructure is indeed the risk and reward of being public health nurse. The work of the public health nurse continues regardless of political party in office and, as such, public health nurses must also be vigilant in guarding the health of the public.

Additional Resources

American Nurse Association Policy and Advocacy at: http://www.nursingworld.org/MainMenuCategories/Policy-Advocacy

American Nurse Association Politics & Advocacy Congress and Federal Agencies at: http://www.nursingworld.org/MainMenuCategories/Policy-Advocacy/Federal.American Nurse

Association of Nurse Practitioners Political Action Committee at: https://www.aanp.org/legislation-regulation/federal-legislation/pac

American Nurse Association Nursing Legislative Issues and Trends at: http://www.nursingworld.org/StateLegislativeAgendaReports.aspx

Reflections on Nursing Leadership at: http://www.reflectionsonnursingleadership.org/Pages/Vol42_2_Burke_Policy.aspx

U.S. Congress Bills Supported and Opposed by Nurses at: http://maplight.org/us-congress/interest/H1710/bills.

References

Adams, J. M. (2009). The Adams Influence Model (AIM): *Understanding the factors, attributes and process of achieving influence.* Saarbrucken, Germany: VDM Verlag.

Adams, J. M., Chisari, G., Ditomassi, M., & Erickson, J. I. (2011). Understanding and influencing policy: An imperative to the contemporary nurse leader. *Voice of Nursing Leadership, 9*(4), 4–7.

Alliance of Nurses for Healthy Environments. (n.d.). *Advancing clean air, climate, & health: Opportunities for nurses.* Retrieved from https://www.tn.gov/assets/entities/health/attachments/Nurses_Climate_Change_042214.pdf

American Nurses Association. (2008). *Resolution: Global climate change.* Retrieved from http://www.nursingworld.org/MainMenuCategories/WorkplaceSafety/Healthy-Work-Environment/Environmental-Health/GlobalClimateChangeandHumanHealth.pdf

American Public Health Association. (2015). *Get the facts: Prevention and public health fund* [Fact sheet]. Retrieved from http://www.apha.org/~/media/files/pdf/topics/aca/2015_pphf_fact_sheet.ashx

Aries, N. (2016). To engage or not engage: Choices confronting nurses and other health professionals. In D. Nickitas, D. Middaugh, & N. Aries (Eds.),

Policy and politics for nurses and other health professionals. Sudbury, MA: Jones & Bartlett Learning.

Barnes, R. (2011, November). Court to review health overhaul. *The Washington Post*, pp. A1, A16.

Block, L. E. (2008). Health policy: What it is and how it works. In C. Harrington & C. L. Estes (Eds.), *Health policy: Crisis and reform in the U.S. health delivery system* (pp. 4–14). Sudbury, MA: Jones & Bartlett Publishers.

Califano, J. (2009). Bending the curve requires healthcare reform, not just sick care reform: A history lesson. *Kaiser Health News.* Retrieved from http://www.kaiserhealthnews.org/Columns/2009/August/081009Califano.aspx

Capretta, J. (2009). *Healthcare in the United States: Strengths, weaknesses & the way forward.* Plenary Address from CBHD's 15th Annual Conference: *Healthcare and the Common Good.* Retrieved from http://cbhd.org/content/healthcare-united-states-strengths-weaknesses-way-forward

Cauchi, R. (2012). *State legislation challenging certain health reforms.* National Conference of State Legislatures. Retrieved from http://www.ncsl.org/default.aspx?tabid=18906

Center on Budget and Policy Priorities. (2010). *Policy basics: Introduction to the federal budget process.* Retrieved from http://www.cbpp.org/files/3-7-03bud.pdf

Centers for Disease Control and Prevention. (2010). *Community transformation grants: States and communities program descriptions.* Retrieved from http://www.cdc.gov/communitytransformation/funds/-programs.htm

Centers for Medicare & Medicaid Services. (2016). *CMS quality strategy.* Retrieved from https://www.cms.gov/Medicare/Quality-Initiatives-Patient-Assessment-Instruments/QualityInitiativesGenInfo/CMS-Quality-Strategy.html

Cohen, P. (2009). *How health care reform can improve public health.* Retrieved from http://www.kevinmd.com/blog/2009/10/health-care-reform-improve-public-health.html

Commonwealth Fund Initiative Congressional Budget Office. (2010). *How is the Patient Protection and Affordable Care Act (ACA) funded?* Retrieved from http://www.acponline.org/advocacy/where_we_stand/access/internists_guide/i2-how-is-the-aca-funded.pdf

Commonwealth Fund. (2016). *Rising to the challenge: The Commonwealth Fund Scorecard on local health system performance, 2016 Edition.* Retrieved from: http://www.commonwealthfund.org/interactives/2016/jul/local-scorecard/

Cooper, J., & Shaw, K. (2016). *Supporting Community/Public Health Nursing Involvement in the Prevention and Management of Chronic Disease* (APHN Public Health Policy 2015-2016 Position Paper). Columbus, OH: Association of Public Health Nurses.

Daley, K. (2011). From Your ANA President: Nurses lead the way. *American Nurse Today, 6*(5), 18.

Emmanuel, E. (2011). Spending more doesn't make us healthier. *The New York Times Opinionator.* Retrieved from http://opinionator.blogs.nytimes.com/2011/10/27/spending-more-doesnt-make-us-healthier/

Foundation, T. H. (2009, March). *Kaiser Commission on Medicaid Facts.* Retrieved from The Henry J. Kaiser Family Foundation website: http://www.kff.org/medicaid/upload/7872.pdf

Fuchs, V. R. (2007). What are the prospects for enduring comprehensive healthcare reform? *Health Affairs, 26*(6), 1542–1544. Retrieved from http://content.healthaffairs.org/content/26/6/1542.full

Gallup Poll. (2011a). *Public rate nursing on most honest & ethical profession.* Retrieved from http://www.gallup.com/poll/9823/public-rates-nursing-most-honest-ethical-profession.aspx

Gallup Poll. (2011b). *Americans tilt toward favoring repeal of healthcare law.* Retrieved from http://www.gallup.com/poll/150773/Americans-Tilt-Toward-Favoring-Repeal-Healthcare-Law.aspx

Gallup Poll. (2016). *Majority in U.S. support idea of Fed-funded healthcare system.* Retrieved from http://www.gallup.com/poll/191504/majority-support-idea-fed-funded-healthcare-system.aspxpage21

Gawande, A. (2009, January 26). Getting there from here: How should Obama reform health care? *The New Yorker*, pp. 26–33. Retrieved from The New Yorker website: http://www.newyorker.com/reporting/2009/01/26/090126fa_fact_gawande

Gostin, L. (2002). Public health law, ethics, and human rights: Mapping the issues. *Public health law and ethics: A reader.* Retrieved from http://www.publichealthlaw.net/Reader/ch1/ch1.htm

Hall-Long, B. (2009). Nursing and public policy: A tool for excellence in education, practice, and research. *Nursing Outlook, 57*(2), 78–83.

Hanley, B., & Falk, N. L. (2007). Policy development and analysis: Understanding the process. In D. J. Mason, J. K. Leavitt, & M. W. Chaffee (Eds.), *Policy and politics in nursing and health care* (5th ed., pp. 75–93). St. Louis, MO: Saunders/Elsevier.

Health Resources and Services Administration. (2008). *National Sample Survey of Registered Nurses.* Retrieved from http://datawarehouse.hrsa.gov /-nursingsurvey.aspx

The Henry J. Kaiser Family Foundation. (2011). *The uninsured and the difference health insurance makes.* Retrieved from www.kff.org/uninsured /upload/1420-13.pdf

The Henry J. Kaiser Family Foundation. (2016). *Key facts about the uninsured population.* Retrieved from http://kff.org/uninsured/fact-sheet /key-facts-about-the-uninsured-population/

Institute of Medicine. (1988). *The future of public health.* Retrieved from http://iom.edu /Reports/1988/The-Future-of-Public-Health.aspx

Institute of Medicine. (2000). *To err is human: Building a safer health system.* Retrieved from http://www.nap.edu/openbook.php?record_id =9728&page=1

Institute of Medicine. (2011). *The future of nursing: leading change, advancing health.* Washington, DC: National Academies Press.

International Council of Nurses. (2006). *Code of ethics.* Retrieved from http://www.icn.ch/ethics.htm

Jacobi, J., Watson, S., & Restuccia, R. (2011). Implementing health reform at the state level: Access and care for vulnerable populations. *Using law, policy, and research to improve the public's health.* Retrieved from http://www.aslme.org/media /downloadable/files/links/1/5/15.Jacobi.pdf

Kaiser Family Foundation. (2016). *Total number of professionally active nurses.* Retrieved from http://kff. org/other/state-indicator/total-registered-nurses/?cu rrentTimeframe=0&sortModel=%7B%22colId%22: %22Location%22,%22sort%22:%22asc%22%7D

Kalisch, B., & Kalisch, P. (1982). *Politics of nursing.* Philadelphia, PA: Lippincott.

Keller, L., & Strohschein, S. (2016). Population-based public health nursing practice: The intervention wheel. In M. Stanhope & J. Lancaster (Eds.), *Public health nursing: Population-centered health care in the community* (9th ed., pp. 190–216). St. Louis: MO: Elsevier.

Klein, E. (2011, May 6). Medicaid, no Medicare, at most risk. *The Washington Post,* A19.

Kraft, M., & Furlong, S. (2010). *Public policy: Politics, analysis, and alternatives* (3rd ed.). Washington, DC: CQ Press.

Leavitt, J. (2009). Leaders in health policy: A critical role for nursing. *Nursing Outlook, 57*(2), 73–77.

McCarthy, D., How, S., Sabrina K., Schoen, C., Cantor, J., & Belloff, D. (2009, October). *Aiming higher: Results from a state scorecard on health system performance, 2009.* Commonwealth Fund. Retrieved from http://www.-commonwealthfund.org/Publica tions/Fund-Reports/2009/Oct/2009-State-Scorecard .aspx

Mechanic, D. (2011). The brilliant, persistent pursuit of health care as a complex social system: A book review. *Health Affairs, 30*(2), 362–363.

Milstead, J. (2013). *Health policy and politics: A nurse's guide* (4th ed.). Burlington, MA: Jones & Bartlett Learning.

National Quality Forum. (2016). *MAP 2016 considerations for implementing measures in federal programs: Clinicians.* Retrieved from file:///C:/Users /bb2509/Downloads/map_clinicians_2016_final_ report.pdf

Nickitas, D. (2011). Nurses. In D. Nickitas, D. Middaugh, & N. Aries (Eds.), *Policy and politics for nurses and other health professionals* (pp. 75–102). Sudbury, MA: Jones & Bartlett Learning.

Nickitas, D. (2016). Policy, politics, and the presidential campaign: What's at stake for nursing. *Nursing Economics, 34*(5), 213.

Office of the National Coordinator for Health Information Technology. (2010). *State Health Information Exchange Cooperative Agreement Program.* Retrieved from https://www.healthit .gov/policy-researchers-implementers/state -health-information-exchange

Online Dictionary of Social Sciences. (n.d.). *Politics.* Retrieved from http://bitbucket.icaap.org/dict.pl?alpha=P

Orszag, P. (2011). How health care can save or sink America: The case for reform and fiscal sustainability. *Foreign Affairs, 90*(4), 42–56.

Pronovost, P. J., Austin, M. J., Cassel, C. K., Delbanco, S. F., Jha, A. K., Chan, T. H., . . . Santa, J. (2016, September 19). *Fostering transparency in outcomes, quality, safety, and costs a vital direction for health and health care.* Washington, DC: National Academy of Medicine.

Remote Area Medical. (2016). Retrieved from https://ramusa.org/

Robert Wood Johnson Foundation. (2011). *Chapter 8: State efforts improve quality, contain costs and improve health. State of the States initiatives.* Retrieved from http://www.statecoverage.org/stateofthestates2011

Robert Wood Johnson Foundation. (2015). *From vision to action: Measures to mobilize a culture of health.* Princeton, NJ: Author.

Rushefsky, M. (2008). *Public policy in the United States: At the dawn of the 21st century* (4th ed.). Armonk, NY: M. E. Sharpe.

Samuelson, R. (2011, November 7). Busting the budget myths. *The Washington Post*, A19.

Smith, M. (2016). *Time for RNs to get out the vote. The American Nurse.* Retrieved from http://www.theamericannurse.org/ index.php/2014/10/22/time-for-nurses-to-get-out-the-vote/

Smith, J., & Medalia, C. (2015). *Health insurance coverage in the United States: 2014: Current Population Reports* (060-253). Washington, DC: Government Printing Office. Retrieved from https://www.census.gov/content/dam/Census/library/publications/2015/demo/p60-253.pdf

Song, A. (2011). Defining ANA-PAC's role in the political process. *American Nurse, 43*(3), 15.

Stolberg, S. G., & Pear, R. (2010). Obama signs health care overhaul bill, with a flourish. *The New York Times Online.* Retrieved from http://www.nytimes.com/2010/03/24/health/policy/24health.html

Trust for America's Health. (2010). *Patient Protection and Affordable Care Act (HR 3590) selected prevention, public health & workforce provisions.* Retrieved from http://healthyamericans.org/assets/files/Summary.pdf

U.S. Department of Health and Human Services. (2010). *HHS awards nearly $100 million in grants for public health and prevention priorities. News Release.* Retrieved from http://www.hhs.gov/news/press/2010pres/09/20100924a.html

U.S. Department of Health and Human Services. (2014). *News release: HHS announces nearly $212 million in grants to prevent chronic diseases.* Retrieved from http://www.hhs.gov/news/press/2014pres/09/20140925a.html

U.S. Department of Health and Human Services. (2015). *Departments of Justice and Health and Human Services announce over $27.8 billion in returns from joint efforts to combat health care fraud.* Retrieved from http://www.hhs.gov/about/news/2015/03/19/departments-of-justice-and-health-and-human-services-announce-over-27-point-8-billion-in-returns-from-joint-efforts-to-combat-health-care-fraud.html

U.S. Health Care. (n.d.). Retrieved from http://politicscentral.com/us-health-care/

Wald, L. D. (1914, February). Suffrage. Lillian Wald Papers, Writings & Speeches, Suffrage, 1914. Reel 25, Box 36, Folder 3, pp. 1–3. New York Public Library, Humanities and Social Sciences Library, Manuscripts and Archives Division, New York, NY.

Washingtonsblog. (2010, February 23). *Naked capitalism.* Retrieved from Guestpost http://www.nakedcapitalism.com/2010/02/guest-post-greenspan-says-greenspan-worst-financial-crisis-ever-including-the-great-depression.html

Washington Department of Health. (2010). *An agenda for change.* Retrieved from http://www.doh.wa.gov/PHSD/doc/AgendaForChange.pdf

Watson, J. (2008). Social justice and human caring: A model of caring science as a hopeful paradigm for moral justice and humanity. *Creative Nursing, 14*, 54–61.

The White House. (2011). Get the facts straight on health reform. *Health Reform in Action.* Retrieved from http://www.whitehouse.gov/healthreform/myths-and-facts#healthcare-menu

World Health Organization. (2000). *World Health Organization assesses the world's health systems.* Retrieved from http://www.who.int/whr/2000/media_centre/press_release/en/

Yukl, G., & Falbe, C. M. (1990). Influence tactics in upward, downward, and lateral influence attempts. *Journal of Applied Psychology, 75*, 132–140.

For a full suite of assignments and additional learning activities, use the access code located in the front of your book to visit this exclusive website: http://go.jblearning.com/londrigan. If you do not have an access code, you can obtain one at the site.

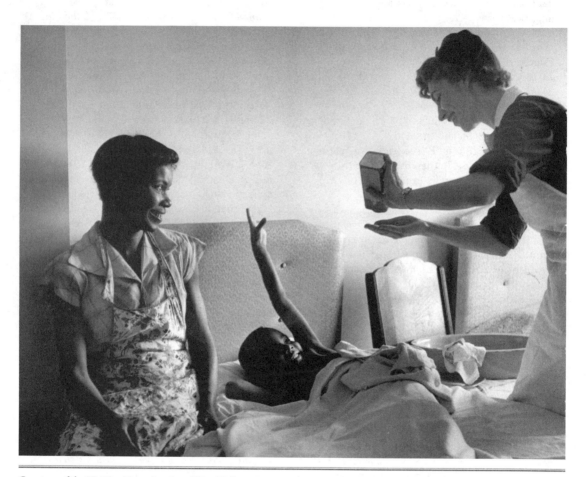

Courtesy of the Visiting Nurse Service of New York.

CHAPTER 10

Social Justice and the Ethics of Public Health Practice

Selina A. Mohammed
Jamie L. Shirley
Dan Bustillos

I have had on my desk at the Settlement an interesting analysis of the last presidential campaign written in English by a young Russian factory girl. She has most intelligently studied the struggle, as it appeared to her through the newspapers, and she concludes "the common people in the United States are discontented, they believe they are entitled to a greater share in the wealth of the nations. They believe that they must have a greater say. Therefore their sudden response to the call of Theodore Roosevelt for 'Social Justice.'" (Wald, 1913, pp. 8–9)

LEARNING OBJECTIVES

At the completion of this chapter, the reader will be able to:

- Describe the role of nurses in social justice and public health ethics;
- Examine the function of social justice and public health ethics in addressing health inequities;
- Analyze how the fundamental tensions in public health influence public decision-making; and
- Apply a framework of ethical analysis to social justice/public health ethics case studies.

KEY TERMS

- ❏ Effectiveness
- ❏ Health inequities
- ❏ Least infringement
- ❏ Necessity
- ❏ Proportionality
- ❏ Public health ethics
- ❏ Public justification
- ❏ Social justice

Introduction

In recent years, as **health inequities** worldwide have escalated, social justice and public health ethics within nursing have reemerged as professional imperatives. This reemergence is evidenced by flourishing national and international taskforce initiatives, organizational position statements, and scholarly literature that center on social justice, ethics, and health equity. In recognition of the unequal distribution of health within and among countries, the World Health Organization (WHO) issued the 1978 Declaration of Alma-Ata that hailed primary health care as the solution for achieving health for all (Reutter & Kushner, 2010). Since that time, the WHO has called attention to the need for healthcare professionals to address social determinants of health and healthcare rights as ways to achieve goals of health equity (Robert Wood Johnson Foundation, 2015; WHO, 2008). Within the nursing profession, the American Nurses Association (ANA), the International Council of Nurses (ICN), and the American Association of Colleges of Nursing (AACN) have also charged that nurses develop a continuum of competencies in social justice, ethics, advocacy, and human rights, in accordance with their level of academic achievement (AACN, 2006, 2008, 2011; ANA, 2015; ICN, 2012).

In this chapter, we explore social justice and the responsibility of nurses to engage in practices that foster health equity. Specifically, we will provide a framework for ethical decision-making that helps to address the tensions that arise in public health nursing. Critical thinking exercises are provided at the end of the chapter to facilitate the application of knowledge and concepts covered in this chapter.

Social Justice in Nursing

Social justice has historically served as the moral foundation for public health nursing. Early nurse-leaders in the field, such as Lillian D. Wald, Lavinia Dock, Florence Nightingale, and Margaret Sanger, emphasized the responsibility of nurses to address social conditions that engender health problems and engaged in various forms of social activism to address health outcomes resulting from income, labor, gender, and race/ethnicity inequities (Bekemeier & Butterfield, 2005; Drevdahl, Kneipp, Canales, & Dorcy, 2001; Lewenson, 2017; Reimer Kirkham & Browne, 2006; Thurman & Pfitzinger-Lippe, 2016). Instead of focusing solely on individuals, these nurse innovators focused on the collective nature of health and populations. They underscored social justice, broad system change, and political action as requisites for enhancing the health of populations (Bekemeier & Butterfield, 2005; Braveman, Egerton, & Williams, 2011; Buettner-Schmidt & Lobo, 2012; Mohammed, Stevens, Ezeonwu, & Cooke, 2017).

Although early public health nursing leaders grounded their practices in social justice, in more recent years, social justice has held more prominence within the nursing profession as discourse rather than direct action (Anderson et al., 2009; Buettner-Schmidt & Lobo, 2012). This shift away from social activism in nursing is due to the influence of liberal and neoliberal ideologies of individualism, fostered by imperialism and capitalist market economies (Reimer Kirkham & Browne, 2006; Thompson, 2014). Concomitantly, the adoption of reductionist and individualistic views of health by biomedicine, which is the predominant medical system and model of health and healthcare delivery in the United States, has also had a heavy influence on nursing. In the biomedical model, health is narrowly defined as the absence of disease (Baum & Fisher, 2014), based on genetics, lifestyle/behavior, or culture. By ascribing responsibility for health to the individual, broader contexts of health are omitted. As a result, downstream health care and health promotion intervention strategies that target individual lifestyle factors are privileged over upstream policies that target social determinants of health (Baum & Fisher, 2014). Furthermore, when health is viewed as individually versus socially based, misconceptions regarding why some groups of people bear a disproportionate burden of disease can foster discriminatory practices and the racialization of health (Mohammed, 2014). Group differences in health come to be seen as the cumulative result of individual group member's poor choices (Levinson, 1998).

In addition to the focus on individualism and its dominant influence on the nursing profession, social justice has waned in nursing as a result of its obscurity in nursing pedagogy around praxis (Mohammed, Stevens, Ezeonwu, & Cooke, 2016). Although many nurse educators present social justice theoretically, they are less likely to teach strategies for implementation and offer opportunities for social justice practice. In addition, social justice is typically regarded in education and practice settings as being pertinent only to public health nurses as opposed to other nurse specialties (Thompson, 2014). This is frequently noted in nursing students themselves who at times consider public health nursing as not relevant to nursing. This, by extension, broaches the question: Is social justice therefore not valuable?

At the professional level, a critical review of three national ANA documents revealed ambiguous and inconsistent conceptions of social justice and a lack of nursing models that address social determinants of health (Bekemeier & Butterfield, 2005). Several articles in nursing literature (Boutain, 2004; Buettner-Schmidt & Lobo, 2012; Grace & Willis, 2012; Matwick & Woodgate, 2016; Pauly, MacKinnon, & Varcoe, 2009; Reimer Kirkham & Browne, 2006; Thompson, 2014) have also noted the lack of consistent conceptualizations and deconstructed how discourses of social justice vary across and within disciplines. A public health nursing practice of social justice requires that these ambiguities and lack of direction be addressed.

Defining Social Justice, Health Disparities, and Health Inequities

Social justice can be characterized as a means to an end (methods, actions, and practices for achieving health equity) and as an end goal itself (as a state of health equity). Through an analysis of the meanings of social justice within nursing literature, Thompson (2014) created the following collective definition:

> *(a) Interventions focused on social, political, economic, and environmental factors that systematically disadvantage individuals and groups; and (b) intervening in the effects of power, race, gender, and class where these and other structural relations intersect to create avoidable disparities and inequities in health for individuals, groups, or communities. (p. E18)*

In another analysis, Matwick and Woodgate (2016) proposed the following operational definition:

> *Social justice in nursing is a state of health equity characterized by both the equitable distribution of services affecting health and helping relationships. Social justice is achieved through the recognition and acknowledgement of social oppression and inequity and nurses' caring actions toward social reform. (p. 7)*

The first definition underscores that social justice involves challenging the status quo and rectifying injustices for vulnerable groups to achieve equitable burdens and benefits (Boutain, 2004; Mohammed, Cooke, Ezeonwu, & Stevens, 2014). The second definition represents social justice as a state of health equity, in which individually and collectively, nurses are agents of change. Although the duality of these definitions—as an action and a result—complicate the landscape of social justice, both of the above definitions call for nurses to think concretely about societal issues of power and hierarchy and to engage in action and practices that reduce socially driven health inequities.

Further complicating the landscape of social justice is the language of health disparities versus health inequities and how they are used in health literature. Health disparities are descriptive indicators of health equity and describe health differences that adversely affect socially disadvantaged groups (Braveman, 2014; Braveman, Egerton, & Williams, 2011). Furthermore, *Healthy People 2020* notes that health disparities include more than race and ethnicity and, in fact, represent many dimensions that are influenced by the social determinant of health (U.S. Department of Health and Human Services [USDHHS], 2016). Analyses of health disparities have established that many of the primary drivers of health stem from the social contexts of our everyday lives (Carey & Crammond, 2015; USDHHS, 2016) leading to health inequities or the absence of equity (USDHHS, 2016). These contexts are often demonstrative of social injustices that affect health status. As a result, the term health inequities has been increasingly used to signify a moral judgment of causality and explicitly link health differences to social, political, and economic injustices that are deep rooted in our society (Braveman et al., 2011; Falk-Rafael & Betker, 2012). Bassett (2015) spoke compellingly about the devastating long-term effect of racism on the poor healthcare outcomes of African Americans in her TED talk *Why Your Doctor Should Care About Social Justice*. Bassett explicitly addresses race, health inequities, and social justice in her role as New York City Commissioner of Health and Mental Hygiene.

A Call to Social Justice Action

Reducing health inequities requires that nurses address the social determinants of health. These determinants of health include the social and material conditions in which people live, work, learn, and play, as well as access to quality health care (Robert Wood Johnson Foundation, 2014). Although addressing social factors may be more arduous than addressing individual behaviors, research has shown that they may have a greater and longer lasting impact on health (Galea, Tracy, Hoggatt, DiMaggio, & Karpati, 2011). All nurses are in a prime position to engage in social justice initiatives and advocate for appropriate programs and policies that target multilevel social change in order to be responsive to the diverse health needs of the people and populations they serve. Working for social justice is an essential and fundamental part

of the moral and ethical obligation of a profession grounded in the context of caring (Mohammed et al., 2017). Only by engaging in this work will we truly be able to curtail the rise of social inequities among different groups of people and achieve health equity.

Public Health Ethics

Public health ethics builds on the foundation of social justice. As the discussion of social justice implies, the moral interests of public health are broad and global. The grand questions of public health include: How can we best achieve social justice in health? How can working toward a broad vision of public health and facilitate social justice? These questions suggest the need for an ambitious reformation of not only our healthcare system but also of society in general.

Public health nursing, however, tends to be practical and focused. The daily questions, although located in the broad sweep of social justice, are narrow and need specific answers. Consider the following questions that public health nurses may face daily: How much coercion is acceptable when encouraging an individual to adopt a new health practice for the good of the community? Does this education program create more stigma than health promotion? Can we justify this level of surveillance of a community in order to preserve its health?

The discussion of ethical decision-making that follows will suggest a strategy for addressing and resolving the practice questions of public health nursing. Throughout, however, we will return to the fundamentally radical claim of social justice—that as healthcare professionals, we have not only the ability but also the moral obligation to reform oppressive structures of power and to be cognizant of the ways our interventions either reinforce or disrupt economic, political, and social systems that prevent all persons from enjoying the benefits of good health. We began this chapter with a discussion of social justice precisely because we should not forget that the most fundamental ethical goal of public health nursing is social justice.

Fundamental Tensions

Within public health ethics, there are three fundamental tensions: 1) the tension between the individual and the community, 2) the tension between the knowledge of the community and the expertise of professionals, and 3) the tension between the competing conceptions of the common good. These three tensions underlie most of the questions in public health. Although in any instance, we have to decide which consideration outweighs the other in order to resolve the particular situation. Ultimately, there is no final resolution to these tensions. Both concepts in each pair represent culturally important values that must be acknowledged. The work of ethical analysis is to argue for why, in a specific case, we choose to act in a way that upholds one more than the other.

Individual versus Community Interests

Most often discussed is the tension between individual and community interests. In public health, we are often asking individuals to do something—or refrain from doing something—in order to benefit the larger community. This tension can be simplistically framed as a competition between two independent entities, the rights of individuals pitted against the common good of the community. It is more helpful and more accurate to understand that neither of these entities are independent of the other. People and communities are intrinsically interrelated. Both people and communities are better off when we honor the liberty rights and autonomy of individuals and when we acknowledge the obligations that they have to their communities (Coggon, 2012).

As implied in its name, public health has a fundamental commitment to the common good of the public at large. Many of the goals of health can only be achieved through communal action to address the social determinants of health. The conditions of our lives are inevitably interconnected in a complicated network of obligations and dependencies. All of us are at one time or another dependent on others in our lives; we need systems in place to assure and ensure that everyone can get the help needed when it is necessary.

At the same time, we have a deep cultural commitment to respect for the autonomy of the individual. Autonomy is primarily understood as self-determination—our right and our ability to make choices for ourselves about the path our lives will take (Beauchamp & Childress, 2012). In Western society, autonomy is understood to be limited primarily by obligation not to interfere with the autonomy of others; our autonomy ends where the autonomy of the next person begins (Mill, 1863). In many healthcare contexts, respect for autonomy is a paramount principle that drives medical decision-making (Beauchamp & Childress, 2012); we provide patients with the widest possible range of options and then allow them to choose for themselves the best course of action.

In the public health context, however, autonomy's limitations are more obvious. As a negative right, autonomy is not a guarantee of the availability of choices. It is merely the right to freely choose among those that are available. Through the lens of social justice, we know that different people have access to different resources. When there are disparities in access to resources based on social location, there is also a disparity in access to autonomy. If options are limited, then it is morally problematic to attribute to those persons the responsibility for their choices (Dawson, 2011). Recognizing that people's autonomy is already constrained as a feature of their membership in a community does not resolve the tension, but it can help us see that this tension is already present even before the public health question is asked.

Knowledge of Community versus Expertise of Professionals

A second tension in ethical discussions of public health concerns the relative importance of and reliance on the expertise of professionals versus the local knowledge of the community. Public health providers have often been criticized for attempting to intervene in communities without adequately understanding the needs, values, and culture of the community. Not only are these interventions disrespectful, but they are also often ineffective because nearly all public health interventions require the collaboration of the community.

At the same time, providers can bring needed expertise and knowledge to a community. Society may have health goals that are not considered important or of which a particular community is not aware. In these situations, public health nurses may be appropriately using their authority to facilitate the agenda. Public health nurses must always be aware of and resist, however, the temptation to frame every situation through this lens of beneficent paternalism.

When we intervene in a community, we are inevitably bringing with us a particular conception of health—and by extension a particular vision of the good life. We need to be thoughtful about the extent to which our well-intentioned interventions are an imposition of cultural values, not merely a neutral improvement in health (Dawson, 2011).

Prioritization of Minority Interests versus the Common Good

The third tension is between minority interests in a community and the larger common good. Related to the tension between individual and community interests, it is primarily a question of how political power is deployed in public health decision-making. Many public health decisions are rooted in a basic utilitarian greatest-good-for-the-greatest-number conception of the common good. The risk in these sorts of calculations, however, is that the interests of a minority may be disregarded (the interests of those who do not fall into the greatest number category). We have a responsibility to notice whether that minority is a group who is already oppressed or vulnerable in society and, if so, to reconsider our calculus to avoid further institutionalized oppression.

This may not be possible in every instance, but if the same group bears the burden consistently over time, the legitimacy of the public health enterprise will be undermined.

Criteria for Public Health Action

A commonly used framework for analyzing public health questions is one outlined by Childress et al. (2002). In their model, they identify five justificatory conditions that must be evaluated for an intervention to be considered ethically acceptable. These are necessity, effectiveness, proportionality, least infringement, and public justification. We will refer to these as the criteria for public health action. The goal of this process of analysis is to maximize each of these criteria. It would be unrealistic to think that all can be fully addressed. In the complexity of practice, compromises may have to be made. The framework, however, helps public health nurses consider all aspects of a situation before moving forward to implementation of an intervention.

Necessity. The criterion of necessity brings up two interrelated groups of questions. First, have we properly identified the goal we are trying to achieve? Is this goal necessary for the health of the community? Are there other, more important goals that we should be pursuing instead? Assuming an affirmative answer to the first two question, there is a second group of interrelated questions: Is the proposed intervention necessary to achieve the identified health goal? Is this the only route to achieving the desired goal? In the inevitably political arena in which public health decisions are made, it is not uncommon to become invested in the means and activities of practice and lose sight of the fundamental intentions.

Effectiveness. The criterion of effectiveness is the degree to which we are sure that the intervention we are proposing will achieve our stated goal. Key to this evaluation is an assessment of the reach of the intervention. Will it achieve the goal for a sufficiently broad spectrum of the community—and in particular—for those most in need?

Proportionality. Few public health interventions are wholly without moral harms that must be considered. Before proceeding with a course of action, we need to identify those potential and foreseeable harms and make sure the good that is intended and expected outweighs those negative considerations.

Least Infringement. The criterion of least infringement is primarily an acknowledgement of the importance of being mindful of individual and minority interests. As previously discussed, there are unresolvable tensions between the common good and the interests of individuals and minority groups. Because most of the goals of public health nursing are collective, this criterion reminds us to avoid unnecessarily abridging their rights and interests.

Public justification. Finally, any intervention needs to be justified to the public. This requires public engagement in as many stages of assessment, planning, implementation, and evaluation as possible. The justification needs to be provided in terms that are consistent with the values and the discourses of the community.

These five justificatory conditions may be applied to assist public health providers and nurses as they engage in their practice and are faced with difficult questions. The following box offers a case study as a way to apply these five justificatory conditions.

CASE STUDY | Case Study and Application of Reflective Questions and the Five Justificatory Conditions

The Chehokia Tribe

You were recently hired as the director of public health nursing for the Port Chehokia Health Clinic (PCHC), a modern multiuse clinic that specializes in preventive, primary and acute care, which is the only healthcare facility in the remote town. The first thing you notice upon your arrival at PCHC is the huge totem pole that greets visitors outside. Rough in places and in others rubbed smooth by scores of hands, the totem pole stands in stark contrast to the modern, sterile façade of the clinic.

Located in the remote northwest region of the Olympic peninsula in Washington State, Port Chehokia is a small, seaside, close-knit community that also serves as the tribal home of the Chehokia Nation. For generations, the same families have cared for each other communally, going back even earlier than the French fur traders who gave them their Christian names. Port Chehokia, which long ago was a vibrant fishing village for the once numerous tribe, today has less than 1,000 people, most of them members of the Chehokia Nation. The community has become financially dependent on the ocean-freight Keystone company. Keystone itself has fallen on hard times since being purchased by the international conglomerate, DCI. There has even been talk of DCI closing some of its smaller port operations altogether, and rumors are that Port Chehokia is among those being considered for closure.

PCHC is part of the Indian Health Service, which receives partial funding from the U.S. government. However, because of federal assistance cuts and the poor economic health of the region, the town's economy relies on direct and indirect funding from Keystone and DCI. Keystone employs much of the town, and about 300 of its employees are Chehokia tribespeople. Through community outreach and philanthropy, Keystone supports much of the town's infrastructure, education, and PCHC. In return, Keystone enjoys generous tax incentives and legal leniency by the local government.

Port Chehokia is geographically isolated in its beautiful and rural location. The community has high rates of Huntington's disease (HD). Its growing incidence is straining resources and affecting the community's ability to collectively care for each other. HD, a genetic disorder that appears without warning between the ages of 30 and 60, causes irreversible mental and motor deterioration and invariably leads to death after several years of anxiety and suffering for both patient and family. There is currently no known treatment or cure for this Mendelian dominant disorder. Everyone who has inherited the gene will develop the disease and also transmit it to approximately half of their children. People who have this disease require extensive ongoing nursing care, which in this location is primarily provided by family and other community members.

Although at this time it does not provide a cure, genetic testing for the disease recently became available. However, the cost is not covered by most insurers, and PCHC does not have the capacity to do these tests. In addition to HD, the community's other major health issue is its high burden of type 2 diabetes, fueled by inequities in social determinants of health.

In an effort to help your clinic's staff learn how to better diagnose, assist, and counsel those affected by the disease, you attend an HD research conference in Seattle. While there, you meet an HD genetic researcher who describes the importance of compiling a genetic database of HD carriers and sufferers in order to better understand the disease. Data from a cluster of HD represents the best hope for a future cure, though the chance of finding such a cure remains remote. The biotech-funded researcher plans to conduct such a study as soon as he finds an HD cluster. This study will provide free genetic testing to research subjects and a consultation with a genetic counselor. Excited, you tell the researcher that you have access to just this kind of cluster back home.

The genetic researcher arrives in Port Chehokia with a proposal approved by an institutional review board (IRB). He plans to call for volunteers from the clinic's patients and deploy a small army of outside recruiters and study personnel in your community. The research forms he provides mention that the study is funded by Helix, a wholly owned subsidiary of DCI, the international conglomerate that owns Keystone. Although at first you were excited about the potential of an HD research study in Port Chehokia, you begin to worry that community members might resist participating in a trial that risks publicly portraying them in a negative light and may have little tangible benefit for participants. You are also concerned that the clinic, the port, and the biotech firm conducting the research are all owned or funded by the same parent company. You express your misgivings to the researcher.

To allay your fears, the researcher offers to include other disorders in the study. This way, HD will not seem as prominent on the informed consent documents. In any case, argues the researcher, the genetic information will be de-identified and securely locked in a file cabinet at the clinic. However, you realize that the data will also be on several researcher laptops and the Helix computer server, which is owned and operated by DCI. The genetic database will be kept in the same electronic medical record system that contains the PCHC patient and employee records and billing. The researcher claims that no one but the subjects, if they request it, will be made aware of their HD status, along with information on the probability of transmitting it to their offspring.

The IRB required the researcher to obtain community consent for the study, so they scheduled a town hall meeting to discuss the research and obtain the community's consent. Elders from the tribal council have requested that you recommend what the community should do in this case.

Note: The people, communities, and institutions portrayed in this case study are entirely fictional. Any resemblance to existing entities is unintentional.

Break up into small teams and carry out the following activity. Once you have completed the activity, return and report out to the entire class.

Write a recommendation that addresses the following question: To what extent can the proposed study be justified by the five criteria for public health action? A deficiency in any of the criteria, while not necessarily fatal for the contemplated public health action, imposes a moral duty to ensure that a strong justification remains or that the intervention be revised to address the deficiency. See below for hints on applying the criteria to cases.

Applying the Five Criteria for Public Health Action to the Case Study

The following are hints for applying the five criteria for public health action to the Chehokia Tribe case study:

- **Necessity**: Is the proposed action *necessary* to achieve our health goal(s)? Have the most important health goals been appropriately identified? In this case, the public health nurse is motivated to bring the HD genetic database research to Port Chehokia for various reasons. What are these, and do they exemplify appropriate health goals? How necessary would you say the research study is to achieve these goals? Is a better understanding of HD an important or the most important health goal for this community at this time?
- **Effectiveness**: To what degree do you think the research study will meet the health goals of the community? If there is virtual certainty that the study will achieve the goal, the research can be considered highly effective. If achieving the health goal is speculative at best, then the study is of low effectiveness.
- **Proportionality**: Are the potential foreseeable harms caused by this study clearly outweighed by the expected benefits? If so, then the study's proportionality is favorable. When more harms are likely to accrue than benefits, a public health intervention is considered to bear disproportionate risk. What are the benefits to the community of participating in this study? What weight should you give to harms such as community stigmatization, risks to individual employment and insurance status, and the burden of knowledge that one has the disease but has no recourse?
- **Least Infringement**: Are there alternatives that would achieve comparable results but better protect the target population's rights and preferences? Do you have concerns about the way the study is structured, related to informed consent and collection and storage of data?
- **Public Justification**: Has there been public transparency and involvement from the community throughout planning and implementation? Can a narrative be constructed that makes sense of this intervention for this community at this time? Do you think the community has been or will be adequately involved in this process? What additional information do you think the community needs to decide whether or not to participate in this study? What metaphors or symbolic elements from the community's history might be invoked to make sense of their participation.

Conclusion

A concern for social justice grounds the work of public health nurses. Although public health nursing practice may take many forms in a variety of settings, all interventions should ultimately be oriented toward the elimination of health inequities. Strategies of ethical analysis can help nurses to move beyond merely talking about social justice to developing a practice that addresses the intertwined interests of persons and communities. Using these skills, public health nurses will be able to advocate for heathier, more equitable communities.

Additional Resources

APHA Code of Ethics at: https://www.apha.org/~/media/files/pdf/membergroups/ethics_brochure.ashxANA

Code of Ethics with Interpretive Statements at: http://www.nursingworld.org/MainMenuCategories/EthicsStandards/CodeofEthicsforNurses/Code-of-Ethics-For-Nurses.html

Robert Wood Johnson Foundation Culture of Health at: http://www.rwjf.org/en/culture-of-health/2014/06/the_role_of_primary.html

Robert Wood Johnson Foundation Social Determinants of Health at: http://www.rwjf.org/en/our-focus-areas/topics/social-determinants-of-health.html

Social Justice Links at: https://freechild.org/social-justice-links/

Mary Bassett (2015, November), Why Your Doctor Should Care About Social Justice, TED talk at: https://www.ted.com/talks/mary_bassett_why_your_doctor_should_care_about_social_justice

References

American Association of Collages of Nursing. (2006). *The Essentials of Doctoral Education for Advanced Nursing Practice.* Retrieved from http://www.aacn.nche.edu/education-resources/essential-series

American Association of Collages of Nursing. (2008). *The Essentials of Baccalaureate for Professional _Nursing Practice.* Retrieved from http://www.aacn.nche.edu/education-resources/essential-series

American Association of Colleges of Nursing. (2011). *The Essentials of Master's Education in Nursing.* Retrieved from http://www.aacn.nche.edu/education-resources/essential-series

American Nurses Association. (2015). Code of ethics for nurses: With interpretive statements. Silver Spring, MD: Author.

Anderson, J. M., Rodney, P., Reimer Kirkham, S., Browne, A. J., Khan, K. B., & Lynam, M. J. (2009). Inequities in health and healthcare viewed through the ethical lens of critical social justice: Contextual knowledge for the global priorities ahead. *Advances in Nursing Science, 2009*(4), 282–294.

Bassett, M. (2015, November). Why your doctor should care about social justice. *TED talks.* Retrieved from https://www.ted.com/talks/mary_bassett_why_your_doctor_should_care_about_social_justice

Baum, F., & Fisher, M. (2014). Why behavioral health promotion endures despite its failure to reduce health inequities. *Sociology of Health and Illness, 36*(2), 213–225.

Beauchamp, T. L., & Childress, J. F. (2012). *Principles of biomedical ethics* (7th ed.). New York, NY: Oxford University Press.

Bekemeier, B., & Butterfield, P. (2005). Unreconciled inconsistencies: A critical review of the concept of social justice in three national nursing documents. *Advances in Nursing Science, 28*(2), 152–162.

Boutain, D. M. (2004). Social justice in nursing: A review of literature. In M. de Chesnay (Ed.), *Caring for the Vulnerable* (pp. 21–29). Sudbury, MA: Jones and Bartlett Publishers.

Braveman, P. A., Kumanyika, S., Fielding, J., Laveist, T., Borrell, L. N., Manderscheid, R., & Troutman, A. (2011). Health disparities and health equity: The issue is justice. *American Journal of Public Health, 101*(Suppl. 1), S149–S155.

Braveman, P. (2014). What are health disparities and health equity? We need to be clear. *Public Health Reports, 129*(S2), 5–8.

Buettner-Schmidt, K., & Lobo, M. L. (2012). Social justice: A concept analysis. *Journal of Advanced Nursing, 68*(4), 948–958.

Childress, J. F., Faden, R. R., Gaare, R. D., Gostin, L. O., Kahn, J., Bonnie, R. J., . . . Nieburg, P. (2002). Public health ethics: Mapping the terrain. *Journal of Law, Medicine & Ethics, 30*(2), 170–178.

Coggon, J. (2012). *What makes health public? A critical evaluation of moral, legal, and political claims in public health.* Cambridge, England: Cambridge University Press.

Dawson, A. (2011). *Public health ethics*. Cambridge, England: Cambridge University Press.

Drevdahl, D., Kneipp, S. M., Canales, M. K., & Shannon Dorcy, K. (2001). Reinvesting in social capital: A capital idea for public health nursing. *Advances in Nursing Science, 24*(2), 19–31.

Falk-Rafael, A., & Betker, C. (2012). Witnessing social injustice downstream and advocating for health equity upstream: "The trombone slide" of nursing. *Advances in Nursing Science, 35*(2), 98–112.

Galea, S., Tracy, M., Hoggatt, K. J., DiMaggio, C., & Karpati, A. (2011). Estimated deaths attributable to social factors in the United States. *American Journal of Public Health, 101*(8), 1456–1465.

Grace, P. J., & Willis, D. G. (2012). Nursing responsibilities and social justice: An analysis in support of disciplinary goals. *Nursing Outlook, 60*(4), 198–207.

International Council of Nurses. (2012). *The ICN code of ethics for nurses*. Retrieved from http://www.icn.ch/who-we-are/code-of-ethics-for-nurses/

Levinson, R. (1998). Issues at the interface of medical sociology and public health. In G. Scambler & P. Higgs (Eds.), *Modernity, medicine, and health: Medical sociology towards 2000* (pp. 65–80). London: Routledge.

Lewenson, S. B. (2017). Historical exemplars in nursing. In S. B. Lewenson & M. Truglio-Londrigan (Eds.), *Practicing primary health care in nursing* (pp. 1–16). Burlington, MA: Jones & Bartlett Learning.

Matwick, A. L., & Woodgate, R. L. (2016). Social justice: A concept analysis. *Public Health Nursing*. Advance online publication. doi:10.1111/phn.12288

Mill, J. S. (1863). *Utilitarianism*. New York, NY: Oxford University Press.

Mohammed, S. A. (2014). Social justice in nursing pedagogy: A postcolonial approach to American Indian health. In P. N. Kagan, M. C. Smith, & P. L. Chinn (Eds.), *Philosophies and practices of emancipatory nursing: Social justice as praxis* (pp. 205–217). New York, NY: Routledge.

Mohammed, S. A., Cooke, C. L., Ezeonwu, M., & Stevens, C. A. (2014). Sowing the seeds of change: Social justice as praxis in undergraduate nursing education. *Journal of Nursing Education, 53*(9), 488–493.

Mohammed, S. A., Stevens, C. A., Ezeonwu, M., & Cooke, C. L. (2017). Social justice, nursing advocacy, and health inequities: A primary health care perspective. In S. B. Lewenson & M. Truglio-Londrigan (Eds.), *Practicing primary health care in nursing* (pp. 61–74). Burlington, MA: Jones & Bartlett Learning.

Pauly, B. M., MacKinnon, K., & Varcoe, C. (2009). Revisiting "who gets care?" Health equity as an arena for nursing action. *Advances in Nursing Science, 32*(2),118–127.

Reimer Kirkham, S., & Browne, A. J. (2006). Toward a critical theoretical interpretation of social justice discourses in nursing. *Advances in Nursing Science, 29*(4), 324–339.

Reutter, L., & Kushner, K. E. (2010). "Health equity through action on the social determinants of health": Taking up the challenge in nursing. *Nursing Inquiry, 17*(3), 269–280.

Robert Wood Johnson Foundation. (2014). *Social determinants of health*. Retrieved from http://www.rwjf.org/en/our-topics/topics/social-determinants-of-health.html

Robert Wood Johnson Foundation. (2015). *Building a culture of health*. Retrieved from http://www.rwjf.org/en/how-we-work/building-a-culture-of-health.html

Thurman, W., & Pfitzinger-Lippe, M. (2016). Returning to the profession's roots: Social justice in nursing education for the 21st century. *Advances in Nursing Science*. Advanced online publication. doi:10.1097/ANS.0000000000000140

Thompson, J. L. (2014). Discourses of social justice: Examining the ethics of democratic professionalism in nursing. *Advances in Nursing Science, 37*(3), E17–E34.

U. S. Department of Health and Human Services. (2016). *Disparities*. Retrieved from https://www.healthypeople.gov/2020/about/foundation-health-measures/Disparities

Wald, L. D. (1913, December 5). The foreign vote. Speech at meeting of Equal Suffrage League of the City of New York, at the Hotel Astor. Lillian Wald Papers, Writings & Speeches, Voters & Voting, 1913. Reel 25, Box 36, Folder 6, pp. 1–13. New York City Public Library. New York, NY.

World Health Organization. (2008). *Primary health care: Now more than ever*. Retrieved from http://www.who.int/whr/2008/en/

For a full suite of assignments and additional learning activities, use the access code located in the front of your book to visit this exclusive website: **http://go.jblearning.com/londrigan**. If you do not have an access code, you can obtain one at the site.

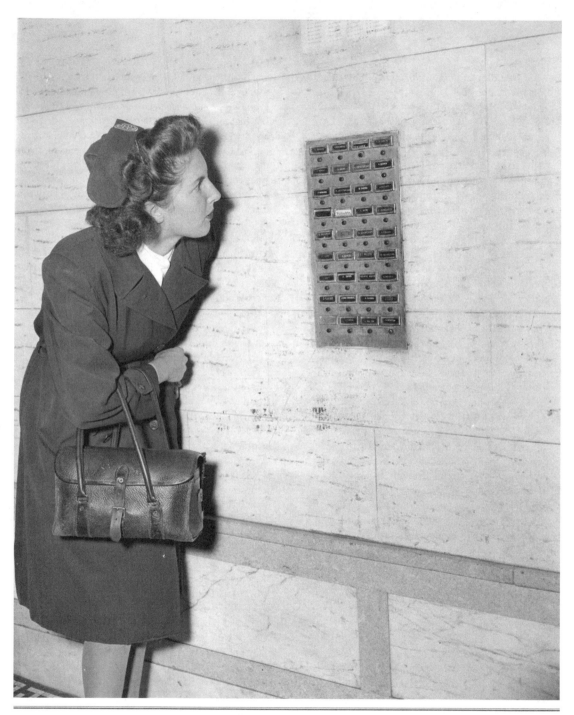

Courtesy of the Visiting Nurse Service of New York.

CHAPTER 11

Hitting the Pavement: Intervention of Case-Finding: Outreach, Screening, Surveillance, and Disease and Health Event Investigation

Margaret Macali
Marie Truglio-Londrigan

The National Red Cross has taken up placing the nurse in the town and country regions and very often the nurse has to do almost everything for the sick people, and also instruct the well people, acting as health officer for the little villages, in the sparsely settled countries. [sic] (Wald, 1917, p. 3)

LEARNING OBJECTIVES

At the completion of this chapter, the reader will be able to:

- Describe the red wedge of the intervention wheel, which includes case-finding, outreach, screening, surveillance, and disease and health investigation.
- Verbalize culturally appropriate and congruent ways to initiate these intervention strategies.
- Explore the various ways that public health nurses apply and perform the strategies of case-finding, outreach, screening, surveillance, and disease and health investigation.

KEY TERMS

❑ Case-finding
❑ Disease and health event investigation
❑ Outreach
❑ Screening

❑ Surveillance
  ○ Directly observed therapy
  ○ Index case

The strength of the intervention wheel (Keller & Strohschein, 2016; Minnesota Department of Health, 2001) is in the identification of specific intervention strategies and the level of practice (systems, community, and individual/family) that are applied by public health nurses who are charged with protecting the public's health. This chapter presents the red section of the intervention wheel, which includes case-finding, outreach, screening, surveillance, and disease and health event investigation. This chapter first describes each of these key intervention strategies. It then demonstrates how to apply them to specific public health case studies, showing the relationship that exists between local, state, and the federal government. Finally, the chapter applies these strategies to case studies so that readers may understand the process of these interventions.

The Intervention Wheel

Case-Finding

Case-finding, as an intervention strategy, takes place at the individual/family level of practice.

Case-finding is exactly what the words imply: to find new cases for early identification of a client with a particular disease or to find cases where particular contact person(s) may be at risk for developing a certain disease. Liebman, Lamberti, and Altice (2002) noted that case-finding is important from several points of view. First, by identifying individuals with a particular disease, treatment may be provided in a timely way, thus resulting in reduced morbidity. Second, the identification of individual(s) prevents further transmission of the disease. Finally, in addition to the early identification of individual(s) with a disease through case-finding, the process of case-finding is also significant in the identification of high-risk individual(s) and "serves as an important opportunity for health education and teaching to promote primary prevention of disease, even among those found not to be infected" (Liebman, Lamberti, & Altice, 2002, p. 345).

Case-finding is important to identify individuals at risk for disease and for the early diagnosis of those with infectious and noninfectious disease(s), including foodborne and waterborne illnesses. For example, Khan et al. (2010) evaluated the effectiveness of a case-finding clinic-based partner notification program for syphilis identification in Madagascar. Index cases were asked to provide sexual contact information. The index case is the first case or instance of a patient coming to the attention of health authorities (Centers for Disease Control and Prevention [CDC], 2014). The index case (individual) or the clinic staff contacted the partner to notify them of potential exposure with a request to come to clinic for testing. Partner notification resulted in case-finding and early identification leading to treatment. In recent years, the process of case-finding has also been instrumental in the identification of individuals experiencing noninfectious disease(s), including chronic illness; mental health issues such as anxiety and depression; and social, spiritual, emotional, or environmental issues, including abuse, violence, and addictions. Skjerve et al. (2007), for example, studied the use of a cognitive case-finding instrument known as the seven-minute screen in a population of older adults for the identification of dementia. Puddifoot et al. (2007) looked at anxiety as a condition that frequently goes untreated because it is not diagnosed; the key question here is how to find the unidentified case. These researchers studied whether two simple written questions would aid in the identification of anxiety in a person, thus facilitating case-finding and ultimately treatment. Similarly, Damush et al. (2008) noted how poststroke depression is often undiagnosed and ultimately untreated, resulting in an increase in morbidity and mortality. The purpose of this study was to determine if detecting patients with poststroke depression using a case-finding algorithm among veteran stroke survivors would be possible. Finally, Tsai et al. (2014) also recognized depression during pregnancy as a highly prevalent undiagnosed issue in South Africa. These authors sought to expand the human capital of community health workers through the use of screening tools that were programmed into mobile phones—mHealth technology—thereby facilitating case-finding of depression in this population.

The essence of case-finding in these particular situations is that this process identifies individuals in need and connects those individuals to resources such as treatments, support groups, agencies, counseling, and other support services. This echoes the words of Keller and Strohschein (2016), who stated, "case-finding locates individuals and families with identified risk and connects them with resources" (p. 206). There are various strategies that the public health nurse may use that facilitate and sustain this case-finding process. One needs only to ask how to find these cases. The answer is outreach, screening, surveillance, and disease and health event investigation.

Outreach

The public health nurse may use various strategies to engage in case-finding. One of these strategies is outreach. The word **outreach** creates a vision for us in which the public health nurse or other public health practitioner actually reaches out into the community and connects with and helps those in need. Keller and Strohschein (2016) noted that "outreach

locates populations of interest or populations at risk and provides information about the nature of the concern, what can be done about it, and how services can be obtained" (p. 200). Rajabiun et al. (2007) described a qualitative study in which they investigated the process of engagement in HIV medical care. Analysis of the data demonstrated that the participants frequently cycled in and out of care based on a number of influences. The researchers identified that those individuals who had cycled out of care must be found so that care could be reestablished. Outreach, therefore, is an intervention that plays a significant role in connecting participants back to the needed care, thus enhancing care of the individual and in the process protecting the public.

Steps of Outreach

The process of outreach is not simple, requiring a number of steps that include the identification of the issue or concern, the population and key characteristics of the population, the plan of action, the methods to implement and monitor the plan, and the evaluation of outcomes, as well as the facilitators and potential barriers to the plan (Minnesota Department of Health, 2001). The public health nurse must also consider where the population lives, the resources available to that population, how they live in the world, and whether or not they want to be found. Proceeding through the steps, a public health nurse can raise the following questions:

1. How will the outreach be carried out?
2. Who will be carrying out the outreach?
3. How will the outreach message be delivered?
4. Where will the final point of contact be?

The first question deals with the how of outreach. How will outreach be conducted so that the public health nurse can gain access to the population and find those in need? Is it via mobile van, motorcycle, walking in the community, telephone calls, knocking on doors, or any other method of connecting with the population of interest? In a school-based community health course, Truglio-Londrigan et al. (2000) worked with community health nursing students in a senior housing project. To gain access to the population of older adults to identify their individual needs, the students knocked on the 99 doors of the building. The students in this course believed that the doors in the apartment buildings were there for protection by keeping people out, but they were actually a barrier to care and services. Their answer to this was to knock on every single door and meet every single person living in the apartment complex. Nandi et al. (2008) assessed access to and use of health services in Mexican-born, undocumented individuals in New York City. To gain access to this population, recruitment took place in communities with large populations of Mexican immigrants. Areas were selected in two phases. In the first, the U.S. Census data were used to identify neighborhoods with the highest numbers of the targeted population. The second step in the process was a walk-through of the key identified neighborhoods to conduct interviews. The idea of walking in the streets where the targeted population reside is also captured in the concepts of street outreach explored by Holger-Ambrose, Langmadé, Edinburgh, and Saewyc (2013) as a means to gain access to sexually exploited youths. In their article about the outbreak of Ebola in a remote region of Liberia, Hagan et al. (2014) discussed the idea of walking down well-worn paths to gain access to their population. The authors in this article noted that one of the primary barriers was the lack of cellphone capability and the rural nature of the land. Many of the villages were only reachable via footpaths in forests. The need to establish village-to-village communication relays was essential for outreach to be achieved (Hagan et al., 2014, p. 183). Finally, the use of the mobile van is also seen as a way to engage in the process of outreach. The mobile van is described as a way for professionals to move out into communities and gain access to hard-to-reach populations and high-risk populations such as drug users who may not come into traditional health clinics (Zucker, Choi, & Gallagher, 2011).

The second question that refers to who will be doing the outreach needs to be addressed by the public health nurse. Will the person be a lay worker who lives in the community and is a member of the population of interest? Mock et al. (2007) wanted to promote cervical cancer screening among Vietnamese American women and noted that the person doing the outreach may have a significant impact on whether or not individuals in need will be found and ultimately connected with the needed resources and care. To this end, Vietnamese women acted in the role of lay outreach coordinator and lay health workers. Another example of this can be seen in the work by Toole et al. (2007) who wanted to conduct a survey of homeless individuals to determine their needs. The difficulty with this process was how to find these homeless individuals. To address this, researchers enlisted formerly homeless individuals and educated them to be research assistants to aid in the process. Finally, rural communities experience limited availability and access to services. How to reach out to these communities and who will do the outreach, therefore, is a consistent concern that public health practitioners and public health nurses must continually be mindful of when developing outreach models. An example of this is an outreach model developed for diabetic retinopathy screening in a remote Australian community. How to reach these communities who have limited or no availability of services and providers was questioned. Glasson, Crossland, and Larkins (2016) evaluated a remote outreach diabetic retinopathy screening model using nonophthalmologist graders to assure diabetic retinopathy screening. Such a model illustrates the necessary connections between outreach, screening, case-finding, and access to needed care and resources.

The third outreach question concerns how the message will be delivered to the population once the connection is established. Is it via the newspaper, flyers, booklets, television ads, songs, radio announcements, Internet advertisement, text messaging, or some other technological advancement not yet discovered? For example, telephone outreach carried out by both staff and patient navigators increases colorectal cancer screening (Basch et al., 2006; Dietrich et al., 2013). In order to determine how the message will be delivered, it is important to know the target population. The public health nurse may have a plan for an outreach process that is well developed, and the population is identified and accessible, but if the message is developed in a way that is not congruent with the population, the message will miss its mark. For example, several years ago, community health nursing students identified a need in conjunction with a county department of health and the office on aging in a local county. That need was to deliver nutritional education to the population of older adults living in a particular community. The community students went to the nutrition center and spoke with the older adults, and indeed, these older adults concurred that programs on nutrition would be very beneficial for those who used the nutrition center. The community students spent a great deal of time in the development of the program. On the day in which the program was delivered, this author was conducting an observation and noted that students arrived in costumes of the Fruit of the Loom guys traditionally seen on the television undergarment commercials. The costumes were great, and the older adults loved them. When the students progressed up to the stage to deliver the message, it was very clear that although their presentation was intriguing to the older adults, the minute they began to deliver their message, they lost the attention of their population. The community students had developed a rap song about the food groups. In the audience, the older adults began to look confused, many asking, "What are they saying?" The message was lost because the connection was lost. The message that the students developed was not congruent with the population they were targeting. This is similar to concepts pertaining to health teaching and educational programming, covered later in this book.

Finally, the fourth question for consideration is where the final point of contact or service in the outreach process is being rendered. The example given concerning the presentation of a nutritional program for older adults in a community nutrition site is an example of the final point of contact for the program delivery. Toole et al. (2007) discussed the dilemma of the homeless and raised the question of where they may go when they first become homeless. The lack of access to services creates a situation where the homeless person will increasingly be more likely to experience poor health. The investigators of this research had to think about how they could access this population to hear the voices of these vulnerable people. The researchers knew if they were going to be successful in gaining access to this population and to find individuals, they must go to where they were. These areas included "(i) unsheltered enclaves (including abandoned buildings, cars, and outdoors) and congregate eating facilities without sleeping quarters; (ii) emergency shelters; and (iii) transitional housing or single room occupancy (SRO) dwellings" (p. 448). It is not unheard of for public health nurses to ride city buses day and night into neighborhoods where they know their clients travel in an attempt to find them and give the care they may need. **Table 11-1** provides examples of points-of-contact for targeted populations.

Screening

Another strategy that public health nurses uses in the process of case finding is **screening**. Keller Strohschein (2016) stated that "screening identifies individuals with unrecognized health risk factors or asymptomatic disease conditions in populations" (p. 200). The seminal work of Leavell and Clark (1965) describes the concept of screening as an intervention strategy that is beneficial in its ability to engage in case-finding for individual(s); it can provide early identification of a disease, thus facilitating prompt treatment. Early identification is a secondary level of prevention during the early pathogenesis period when the person is asymptomatic. The benefits of

---

Table 11-1 **Points-of-Contact for Targeted Populations**

Targeted Populations	Mechanism of Outreach, Access, and Points-of-Contact
Mothers and caretakers of preschool-age children.	Health promotion safety educational programs in park settings as children engage in play.
Heads of households responsible for purchasing food and cooking.	Health promotion educational programs on nutrition outside food stores and accompanying the person as they shop up and down the food aisle.
Older adults who are questioning medications they may be taking.	Health promotion and educational programs on medications delivered at senior citizen nutrition sites.
Day workers waiting to begin their day.	Health promotion programs on immunizations at job pick-up sites.
Adolescents engaging in extreme sports.	Health promotion programs on use of safety pads at a skate park.

---

screening and early identification of disease are numerous:

- Early detection and diagnosis leads to early treatment.
- It breaks the chain of transmission and development of new cases.
- It leads to a decrease in morbidity and mortality.
- It lead to lower costs pertaining to treatments.
- It protects the community and/or the targeted population.

The improvement in health and well-being is documented in the literature. Hartge and Berg (2007) noted that "women can improve their prospects for long-term health by being screened for several cancers with tests proved to decrease morbidity and mortality from colorectal, breast, and cervical cancer" (p. 66). Screening initiatives, developed with community input, results in an increase in the understanding of the targeted population along with an enhanced understanding of potential barriers that must be addressed. The Referral Education Assistance & Prevention (REAP) program, developed and implemented in New Hampshire, is a community program to assist older adults who have an undiagnosed mental health disorder and/or substance misuse or who may be at risk. For example, REAP provides counseling as well as support and referral services that include screening for depression and alcohol abuse (Pepin, Hoyt, Kaaratzas, & Bartels, 2014). Exploring alternative ways of carrying out screening programs and the location of those programs may provide new insight about program delivery resulting in positive outcomes. Vandeburg, Wright, Boston, and Zimmerman (2010) described how the merging of the Routine Universal Comprehensive Screening (RUCS), early identification of woman abuse, with the Ministry of Child and Youth, Early Childhood Development Initiatives (HBHC), a program that involved home visiting component, resulted in improvements in the public health nurse's early identification and disclosure of women experiencing abuse in their home settings.

Liebman and coworkers (2002) identified that case-finding via screening not only is significant because it breaks the chain of further transmission, but also may identify individuals who present with high-risk behavior. This knowledge, therefore, provides opportunities for education that focuses on primary prevention and health promotion. This identification of individuals at risk for a disease through screening presents with the same benefits listed above and also includes the following:

- Early detection of high-risk behaviors and modifiable risk factors, leading to prevention of disease.
- Early detection leading to empowerment of the person or the population being targeted.
- Early detection leading to improvement in lifestyle and quality of life.

The application of screening to identify individuals at risk for developing disease takes us closer to health promotion and disease prevention. Wimbush and Peters (2000) described the implementation of a cardiovascular-specific genogram that may be used to identify persons at risk for cerebrovascular disease within families. These authors further described the complex array of risk factors associated with cerebrovascular disease and noted the differences between modifiable risk factors, such as lack of exercise, high-fat and high-sodium diets, high blood cholesterol, obesity, smoking, high blood pressure, and stress, as compared with nonmodifiable risk factors, such as age, gender, and genetic predisposition. The application of the genogram, a tool used to illustrate family health and relationship patterns over generations, facilitates the public health nurse's understanding of risks present in a family and which of those risks are modifiable. The use of the genogram in this way demonstrated promise as a tool to obtain data to inform the public health nurse as to individuals at risk for cerebrovascular disease. Again, the overall goal is to increase awareness and target risky behavior in others, facilitating prevention and health promotion. Another example is screening older adults 80 years of age and over living independently in the community for the expressed purpose of predicting the risk of nutritional decline, ultimately providing information for public health nurses as they develop targeted interventions (Callen & Wells, 2005). Developing screening tools to identify those at risk, therefore, has the potential for significant health impact.

Screening may take place for an individual, as well as for populations, that include mass screening models and programs. Screening for the individual involves working with one person and performing a screening test such as taking a blood pressure. Conversely, a mass screening may be a situation where a particular population is targeted for a specific screening program pertaining to one or even multiple diseases. The reason a population may be targeted has to do with information derived either from an assessment or surveillance data providing that informs the nurses' decision-making. The data may indicate that the target population is at greater risk for the development of a particular disease. In this case, the public health nurse may engage the population in the development of a mass screening initiative to identify new cases of this disease. Key to the success of the program mandates engaging the population in the early stages of decision-making about the screening choice and how the screening will be initiated (Tembreull & Schaffer, 2005).

The benefits of screening are well documented; however, there are limitations as well. One such limitation is what happens to the individual once he or she is informed that the screening test is positive. For example, in the mass screening, what happens to an individual who is told that his or her blood sugar is elevated? What type of follow-up is provided? What good is this type of mass screening if the public health nurse finds a case, but there is no mechanism to ensure that the individual has access to care for diagnosis, treatment, and follow-up? The University of Medicine and Dentistry of New Jersey's Mobile Health Care Project addressed this issue. They established a collaborative, joint partnership initiative with the Children's Health Fund where a faculty-managed mobile healthcare unit provided care to the underserved population of Newark, New Jersey. One of the goals of this initiative was to provide health promotion services in the form of screenings. Individuals with positive findings were referred to the University of Medicine and Dentistry of New Jersey hospitals and affiliates for treatment and additional referrals (McNeal, 2008), thus making sure people had access to the care they needed. A similar example of collaborative practice addressing the limitation of screening is noted in the multidisciplinary team-based model of care in a rural area of Australia. The model portrays a partnership that facilitates shared work and shared decisions between the visiting specialists from the tertiary care facility who work with collaboratively local health teams (Simm et al., 2014).

The public health nurse and other public health practitioners must engage in continual dialogue in terms of deciding if a disease is, in fact, screenable. The U.K. National Screening Committee (2008) offers advice and recommendations about screening based on evidence: "In any screening program, there is an irreducible minimum of false-positive results (wrongly reported as having the condition) and false-negative results (wrongly reported as not having the condition)" (n.p.). This concern is further defined by others when they speak to the concepts of sensitivity and specificity to address this issue. "Sensitivity quantifies how accurately the test identifies those with the condition or trait . . . . Specificity indicates how accurately the test identifies those without the condition or trait" (McKeown & Hilfinger Messias, 2008, p. 261). For more detailed information about screening tests involving sensitivity and specificity, the following website provides valuable information: https://www.gov.uk/guidance/nhs-population-screening-explained. In addition, a PDF document—*Making Sense of Screening* (2015)—published by Sense about Science also offers valuable information http://www.senseaboutscience.org/resources.php/7/making-sense-of-screening.

With screening comes ethical and economic considerations. For example, the public health nurse and other public health practitioners need to consider the following questions. How ethical is it to conduct screening tests that may inform people they have a disease when they do not? Will these individuals engage in unnecessary testing? Who will pay for the cost of this unnecessary testing? Are there any adverse effects of this unnecessary

testing? What is the emotional trauma that the individual will experience, and is this important to consider? How ethical is it to conduct screening tests that may inform people that they do not have a disease when in fact they do? What will happen to these individuals? How much later will they be diagnosed, and will the diagnosis be too late for any effective treatment modality? What is the emotional trauma that this individual will experience? Will the screening produce positive health outcomes, that is a healthier population? The Public Health Action Support Team (2011) posted an online tutorial entitled *Health Knowledge—Screening*, which addresses many of these questions and speaks about screening not as a singular test but as a process and a program. This tutorial discusses the importance of commissioning high-quality screening programs that are efficient, coordinated, and of good value. Taking the time to access this work will provide you with a comprehensive understanding of screening that also considers cultural nuances.

Public health nurses and other public health practitioners may also refer to the work of the U.S. Preventive Services Task Force (USPSTF) for practice decisions with regard to the above. The USPSTF, sponsored by the Agency for Healthcare Research and Quality, is a panel of experts in prevention and primary care evidence-based medicine. The USPSTF conducts rigorous systematic reviews of peer-reviewed evidence for the effectiveness of preventive services such as screening, counseling, and preventive medications. Based upon these reviews, recommendations are then assigned one of five letter grades to each of its recommendations (A, B, C, D, or I). **Box 11-1** provides an explanation of this grading system and its application for practice.

Various published screening guidelines may be viewed at the USPSTF website. For example, as of October 2008, there were new screening guidelines for colorectal cancer. The USPSTF recommends screening for colorectal cancer using fecal occult blood testing, sigmoidoscopy, or colonoscopy in adults beginning at age 50 years and continuing

---

Box 11-1 USPSTF Grade Definitions

The USPSTF grades its recommendations according to one of five classifications (A, B, C, D, and I), reflecting the strength of evidence and magnitude of net benefit (benefits minus harms).

A: The USPSTF recommends the service. There is high certainty that the net benefit is substantial.
   Suggestion for Practice: Offer or provide this service.
B: The USPSTF recommends the service. There is high certainty that the net benefit is moderate, or there is moderate certainty that the net benefit is moderate to substantial.
   Suggestion for Practice: Offer or provide this service.
C: The USPSTF recommends selectively offering or providing this service to individual patients based on professional judgment and patient preferences. There is at least moderate certainty that the net benefit is small.
   Suggestion for Practice: Offer or provide this service for selected patients depending on individual circumstances.
D: The USPSTF recommends against the service. There is moderate or high certainty that the service has no net benefit or that the harms outweigh the benefits.
   Suggestion for Practice: Discourage the use of this service.
I: The USPSTF concludes that the current evidence is insufficient to assess the balance of benefits and harms of the service. Evidence is lacking, of poor quality, or conflicting, and the balance of benefits and harms cannot be determined.
   Suggestions for Practice: Read the clinical considerations section of USPSTF recommendation statement. If the service is offered, patients should understand the uncertainty about the balance of benefits and harms.

Reproduced from U.S. Preventive Services Task Force. (2013). Grade definitions. Retrieved from http://www.uspreventiveservicestaskforce.org/Page/Name/grade-definitions.

---

until age 75 years. This guideline was given a grade A recommendation. As seen in Box 11-1, the grade A designation means that the USPSTF strongly recommends that clinicians routinely provide the service to eligible patients, thus providing guidance to healthcare providers in the clinical practice setting. The guidelines for this particular situation are listed as grade A recommendations for the age group 50 to 75 years but not for those ages 76 to 85 years. The USPSTF recommends against routine screening for colorectal cancer in adults ages 76 to 85 years; however, there may be considerations that support colorectal cancer screening in an individual patient. In this situation, the grade of C recommendation means the USPSTF may offer this service for selected patients depending on individual circumstances. Finally,

the USPSTF recommends against screening for colorectal cancer in adults older than age 85 years. This recommendation was given a grade of D, meaning that the evidence is insufficient to assess the benefits and harms (USPSTF, 2015). Again, these recommendations provide guidance to the healthcare provider in the clinical practice setting. The USPSTF also concludes that the evidence is insufficient to assess the benefits and harms of computed tomographic colonography and fecal DNA testing as screening modalities for colorectal cancer.

Screening is an important strategy for case finding; however, there are numerous questions and challenges that must be addressed. Wald (2007) addressed these challenges in an editorial noting that quantitative information is needed on screening performance to answer these questions, hence the need for ongoing systemic, evidenced-based reviews.

SURVEILLANCE

One of the oldest surveillance systems date back to centuries. John Snow's work with cholera in London in 1854 is an example of public health surveillance and disease and health investigation, discussed later in this chapter. These past **surveillance** processes focused on communicable diseases, leading to interventions such as quarantine. Today, public health surveillance includes the monitoring of infectious disease, noninfectious conditions, and outbreaks (Fairchild & Bayer, 2016).

Klaucke et al. (1988) stated, "Epidemiologic surveillance is the ongoing and systematic collection, analysis, and interpretation of health data in the process of describing and monitoring a health event" (p. 1). The application of public health surveillance data is noted by the U.S. Department of Health and Human Services and the CDC (U.S. DHHS/CDC, 2006) as data that can be "useful in setting priorities, planning, and conducting disease control programs and in assessing the effectiveness of control efforts" (p. 337). The process of surveillance provides data that inform the public health professional about patterns of disease occurrence and the potential for disease in a population. Surveillance is the "radar of public health" (Fairchild & Bayer, 2016, p. 119). The term *public health surveillance* is presently used in reference to the monitoring of health events in populations, as opposed to *medical surveillance*, which describes the monitoring of individuals (U.S. DHHS/CDC, 1992, 2006). A review of the definition of public health surveillance informs the public health nurse of the exact nature of the process. This process may be viewed in **Box 11-2**.

The first step in the systematic public health surveillance process is that of data collection. Each state has a system of reporting that guides those in practice as to the disease and/or conditions that must be reported, who is responsible for reporting,

---

Box 11-2 Systematic Public Health Surveillance Process

Collection of data
Analysis of data
Interpretation of data
Dissemination of data
Public health action

Modified from U.S. Department of Health and Human Services, Centers for Disease Control and Prevention. (2006). *Principles of epidemiology in public health practice: An introduction to applied epidemiology and biostatistics* (3rd ed.). Washington, DC: American Public Health Association.

---

what information is reported, and to whom and how quickly the information must be reported (U.S. DHHS/CDC, 1992, 2006). Diseases and/or conditions that are reported are known as notifiable. These diseases and/or conditions are revised periodically, with additions to the list, whereas others are deleted depending on trends, patterns that are being manifested by the data, and the health of the public. **Box 11-3** gives examples of notifiable infectious diseases, noninfectious conditions, and outbreaks.

Those responsible for reporting notifiable diseases generally include nurses, physicians, dentists, medical examiners, and administrators of hospitals, clinics, nursing homes, schools, and nurseries, to name a few. These individuals generally submit a case report. The case report is usually sent to the local department of health, which then forwards the case report to the state department of health. In some cases, information may then be sent to the CDC and the World Health Organization (WHO). When the healthcare provider sends the case report to the department of health, this is called *passive surveillance*. If a member of the department of health goes out into the community to obtain information, it is known as *active surveillance*.

The second step in the surveillance process is the analysis of data. As data are collected, they are continually being monitored and analyzed. Sources of data that may be analyzed include those listed in **Box 11-4**.

Box 11-3 Nationally Notifiable Conditions: United States 2016

Infectious Diseases 2016

A

Acanthamoeba disease (excluding keratitis)
Acanthamoeba keratitis
Acquired immunodeficiency syndrome (AIDS)
Amebiasis
Anaplasma phagocytophilum infection
Anthrax
Arboviral diseases, neuroinvasive
    and non-neuroinvasive
Arboviral encephalitis
Arboviral encephalitis or meningitis

B

Babesiosis
Balamuthia mandrillaris disease
Botulism/*C. botulinum*
Botulism, foodborne
Botulism, infant
Botulism, other
Botulism, wound
Brucellosis

C

California serogroup encephalitis
California serogroup encephalitis/meningitis
California serogroup virus diseases
Campylobacteriosis
Cancer
Carbon monoxide poisoning
Chancroid
Chikungunya virus disease
Chlamydia trachomatis infection
Chlamydia trachomatis, genital infections
Cholera
Coccidioidomycosis/valley fever
Congenital syphilis
Crimean-Congo hemorrhagic fever virus
Cryptococcus gattii infection
Cryptosporidiosis
Cyclosporiasis

D

Dengue
Dengue fever (DF)

Dengue hemorrhagic fever (DHF)
Dengue shock syndrome (DSS)
Dengue virus infections
Dengue-like illness
Diphtheria

E

Eastern equine encephalitis
Eastern equine encephalitis virus disease
Eastern equine encephalitis/meningitis
Ebola virus
Ehrlichia chaffeensis infection
Ehrlichia ewingii infection
Ehrlichiosis
Ehrlichiosis and anaplasmosis
Encephalitis
Encephalitis, arboviral
Encephalitis, postinfectious (or parainfectious)
Encephalitis, primary
Enterohemorrhagic *Escherichia coli* (EHEC)
Escherichia coli O157:H7/*E. coli* O157:H7

F

Foodborne disease outbreak
Free-living amebae infections

G

Genital herpes
Genital warts
Giardiasis
Gonorrhea
Granuloma inguinale

H

Haemophilus influenzae, invasive disease
Hansen's disease/leprosy
Hantavirus infection, non-Hantavirus
    pulmonary syndrome
Hantavirus pulmonary syndrome (HPS)
Hemolytic uremic syndrome, post-diarrheal
    (HUS)
Hepatitis A, acute
Hepatitis B, acute
Hepatitis B, chronic
Hepatitis B, perinatal infection
Hepatitis C, acute

(continues)

Box 11-3 *(continued)*

Hepatitis C, chronic
Hepatitis, viral, acute
HIV Infection (AIDS has been reclassified as
    HIV Stage III) (AIDS/HIV)
Human granulocytic ehrlichiosis (HGE)
Human monocytic ehrlichiosis (HME)

I
Influenza-associated hospitalizations
Influenza-associated pediatric mortality
Invasive pneumococcal disease (IPD)/
    Streptococcus pneumoniae, invasive disease

K
Kawasaki syndrome

L
Lassa virus
Lead, elevated blood levels
Lead, elevated blood levels, adult (≥16 years)
Lead, elevated blood levels, children (<16 years)
Legionellosis/Legionnaire's disease or Pontiac
    fever
Leptospirosis
Listeriosis
Lujo virus
Lyme disease
Lymphogranuloma venereum

M
Malaria
Marburg virus
Measles/rubeola
Melioidosis
Meningitis, aseptic/viral meningitis
Meningitis, other bacterial
Meningococcal disease
Mucopurulent cervicitis (MPC)
Mumps

N
Naegleria fowleri causing primary amebic
    meningoencephalitis (PAM)
Neurosyphilis
New World arenavirus–Guanarito virus
New World arenavirus–Junin virus
New World arenavirus–Machupo virus

New World arenavirus–Sabia virus
Nongonococcal urethritis (NGU)
Novel influenza A virus infections

O
Other or unspecified human ehrlichiosis

P
Pelvic inflammatory disease (PID)
Pertussis/whooping cough
Pesticide-related illness and injury, acute
Plague
Poliomyelitis, paralytic
Poliovirus infection, nonparalytic
Powassan encephalitis/meningitis
Powassan virus disease
Psittacosis/ornithosis

Q
Q fever
Q fever, acute
Q fever, chronic

R
Rabies, animal
Rabies, human
Reye syndrome
Rheumatic fever
Rocky Mountain spotted fever (RMSF)
Rubella/German measles
Rubella, congenital syndrome (CRS)

S
Salmonellosis
Severe acute respiratory syndrome-associated
    coronavirus disease (SARS)
Severe dengue
Shiga toxin-producing *Escherichia
    coli* (STEC)
Shigellosis
Silicosis
Smallpox/variola
Spinal cord injury
Spotted fever rickettsiosis
St. Louis encephalitis
St. Louis encephalitis virus disease
St. Louis encephalitis/meningitis

Box 11-3 *(continued)*

Streptococcal toxic shock syndrome (STSS)
Streptococcus disease, invasive,
    group A (GAS)
Streptococcus pneumoniae, drug-resistant
    invasive disease (DRSP)
Streptococcus pneumoniae, invasive disease
    (child, <5 years)
Streptococcus pneumoniae, invasive disease
    nondrug resistant (child, <5 years)
Syphilis
Syphilis, early latent
Syphilis, late latent
Syphilis, late with clinical manifestations (in-
    cluding late benign syphilis and cardiovas-
    cular syphilis)
Syphilis, late, with clinical manifestations other
    than neurosyphilis
Syphilis, latent
Syphilis, latent unknown duration
Syphilis, primary
Syphilis, secondary
Syphilitic stillbirth

T
Tetanus/*C. tetani*
Toxic shock syndrome (other than
    Streptococcal) (TSS)
Trichinellosis/trichinosis
Tuberculosis (TB)
Tularemia
Typhoid fever

U
Undetermined human ehrlichiosis/
    anaplasmosis

V
Vancomycin-intermediate *Staphylococcus
    aureus* and vancomycin-resistant
    Staphylococcus aureus (VISA/VRSA)
Varicella/chickenpox
Varicella deaths
Vibriosis
Viral hemorrhagic fever (VHF)

W
Waterborne disease outbreak
West Nile encephalitis/meningitis
West Nile virus disease
Western equine encephalitis
Western equine encephalitis virus disease
Western equine encephalitis/meningitis

Y
Yellow fever

Z
Zika virus disease
Zika virus disease and Zika virus, congenital
    infection
Zika virus, congenital infection

Adapted from Centers for Disease Control and Prevention. (2016a). Retrieved from https://www.cdc.gov
/nndss/conditions/notifiable/2016/infectious-diseases/.

Noninfectious Conditions 2016

Cancer
Carbon monoxide poisoning
Lead, elevated blood levels
Lead, elevated blood levels, adult (≥16 years)
Lead, elevated blood levels, children (<16 years)
Pesticide-related illness and injury, acute
Silicosis

Outbreaks 2016

Foodborne disease outbreak
Waterborne disease outbreak

Data from Centers for Disease Control and Prevention.
(2016a). *2016 Nationally notifiable infectious diseases.*
Retrieved from https://www.cdc.gov/nndss/conditions
/notifiable/2016/infectious-diseases/; Centers for Disease
Control and Prevention (2016b). *2016 Nationally notifiable non-infectious conditions.* Retrieved from https://
www.cdc.gov/nndss/conditions/notifiable/2016/non-
infectious-conditions/; Centers for Disease Control and
Prevention (2016c). *2016 Nationally notifiable outbreaks.*
Retrieved from https://www.cdc.gov/nndss/conditions
/notifiable/2016/outbreaks/

Box 11-4 Examples of Sources of Data and Reports

Mortality reports
Morbidity reports
Vital statistics
Notifiable disease reports
Laboratory data
Specific topics (cancer registry, adverse drug reactions, injury surveillance systems, and occupational illness)
Birth defects monitoring programs
Surveys (National Health Interview Survey, National Health and Nutrition Examination Survey)

Modified from U.S. Department of Health and Human Services Public Health Service, Centers for Disease Control and Prevention. (1992). *Principles of epidemiology: An introduction to applied epidemiology and biostatistics* (2nd ed.). Washington, DC: American Public Health Association; U.S. Department of Health and Human Services, Centers for Disease Control and Prevention. (2006). *Principles of epidemiology in public health practice: An introduction to applied epidemiology and biostatistics* (3rd ed.). Washington, DC: American Public Health Association.

According to the U.S. DHHS/CDC (1992, 2006), the data are first monitored and analyzed for descriptive information such as time, place, and person. In addition, the public health nurse and other public health practitioners, such as the epidemiologist, must monitor and analyze the data and determine if what they are viewing is expected or different. They must also be able to determine what that difference is. One way of doing this is to look at the recently reported data and compare those data to previous years, looking for trends and patterns.

The interpretation of data is the next step in the surveillance process. As the public health nurse and/or the epidemiologist notes a difference in the expected pattern in a particular population, this is a signal to those involved that additional investigation is necessary, and the information must be disseminated to those in practice for action.

The dissemination of this surveillance data, the fourth step, takes place as information is sent to those in the practice setting to inform and motivate (U.S. DHHS/CDC, 2006, p. 367). During an outbreak, epidemic, natural disaster, or potential terror event, interpretation and dissemination of data are both ongoing and circular, thus affecting public health actions.

The final step in the systematic public health surveillance process is that of action. The entire process would be useless if no action was taken. The action signifies the response to the data, and this response is in the form of an intervention for change. These interventions may be in the form of a coalition whose members work together in a partnership to target a particular population and pool their resources for action and change. The action for change may also be in the form of targeting of monies for programming, research, and policy development.

The material presented above signifies that the public health surveillance process is really a circular process. **Figure 11-1** information loop is a pictorial of this process.

What Is Needed?

The WHO (2008, p. vii) identified key factors that are essential if a systematic public health surveillance system is to be effective; the system must be:

1. Useful
2. Efficient
3. Flexible
4. Representative
5. Simple

Resources are essential to ensure that these key factors are in place. The WHO (2010) notes that a fully functional system warrants that a strong structure and operational processes are in place for the collection of data, storage, and management of that data, including "data recording tools, data reporting forms, databases and electronic systems for data-sharing and analysis" (p. 117). Technology is, therefore, essential for surveillance. In addition to technology, a strong public health infrastructure requires strong human capital and as such the need for "investment in building human resource capacity (including epidemiologists, surveillance, and

Figure 11-1 Information loop.

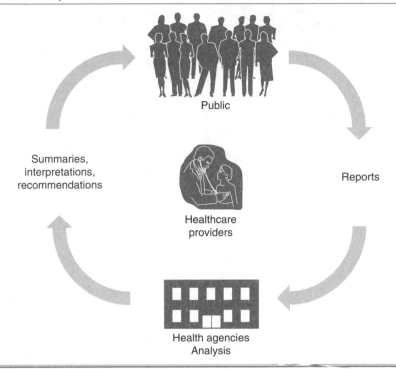

Public

Summaries,
interpretations,
recommendations

Reports

Healthcare
providers

Health agencies
Analysis

Modified from U.S. Department of Health and Human Services Public Health Service, Centers for Disease Control and Prevention. (1992). *Principles of epidemiology: An introduction to applied epidemiology and biostatistics* (2nd ed.). Washington, DC: American Public Health Association; U.S. Department of Health and Human Services, Centers for Disease Control and Prevention. (2006). *Principles of epidemiology in public health practice: An introduction to applied epidemiology and biostatistics* (3rd ed.). Washington, DC: American Public Health Association.

monitoring and evaluation officers, and information technology and management information system specialists) at all levels of the health system through training, mentoring, and supervision" (p. 117). The *Healthy People 2020* (U.S. DHHS, 2016) initiative addresses technology with specific reference to health information technology and health communication. The need to be vigilant in the building and sustaining of this technology is critical to meet the goals and objectives of this national health initiative.

Disease and Health Event Investigation

The final intervention is that of disease and health investigation. Keller and Strohschein (2016) noted

that **disease and health investigation** "systematically gathers and analyzes data regarding threats to the health of populations, ascertains the source of the threat, identifies cases and others at risk, and determines control measures" (p. 200). The entire process may be viewed in **Box 11-5**.

For public health nurses and other public health practitioners, the start of any investigation begins with an event, such as disease, that presents in an individual. This is called the index case. The public health nurse and/or other public health practitioner begin the investigation by asking questions. These questions serve as a reminder to the epidemiological concepts of the agent, host, and the environment discussed earlier in this book. For example, the investigator

> **Box 11-5** Process of Disease and Health Event Investigation
>
> Identifying the source of the threat.
> Identifying cases.
> Identifying the contacts.
> Identifying others at risk.
> Determining control measures.
> Communication with individuals, families, and populations.
>
> Data from Minnesota Department of Health, Division of Community Health Services, Public Health Nursing Section. (2001). *Public health interventions: Application for public health nursing practice.* St. Paul: Minnesota Department of Health.

may ask these questions: Who is affected? Where do they live? Are there any other people affected? Have these people anything in common, or are they connected in any way? Where do the people live? Did they venture into any other locations or venues that they do not commonly go to? Where do they live, work, go to school, and play? Is there a particular time that is presenting as a pattern, for example, during the summer when it is very humid with a lot of rain?

Other data are essential to gather in this systematic process. For example, the public health nurse and other public health practitioners need to go out into the field, conduct direct observation, speak to people in the communities, and develop partnerships. This is critical to the process because subjective information from an individual in the community facilitates trust development and may bring forth information that is important to the success of the investigation. For example, Hagan et al. (2015), which discusses Ebola case-finding in Liberia, demonstrates how working with village chiefs as well as the people in the villages was critical. The partnership established assisted in overcoming resistance and enabled the collection of information, development of culturally sensitive and congruent educational messages, the appropriate transmission of those messages about the disease, and contributed to the design of an appropriate surveillance and investigation. Collecting

specimens is also important in determining what the offending agent is. It is very important to realize that this process is not a one-time deal. In other words, as the public health nurse engages in this investigation, he or she may have to go out into the field not once or twice but multiple times to ensure that the data gathered are reliable and valid. The nurse must share the information with others and confer findings highlighting the importance of team work throughout the investigation.

At the completion of the investigation, the public health nurse will come to know what the problem is and which intervention will correct the issue. Because the public health nurse is dealing with a population, education and communication are generally carried out from a population perspective. Of course, as with any process, once the interventions are initiated, there must be careful monitoring and surveillance to evaluate what the outcome is and if the intervention is a success. One of the most famous examples of this disease and health event investigation took place in the middle of the 19th century, carried out by an anesthesiologist named John Snow. **Box 11-6** describes the disease and health investigation of cholera.

Public Health Issues in Practice

Public health nursing combines nursing practice and public health sciences, focuses on populations even when dealing with individuals, and is always connected with government at a local, county, state, and/or federal level. Public health nursing may start at the population level, working down to the individual index case, defined as "the first case or instance of a patient coming to the attention of health authorities" (CDC, 2014), or it may start with the index case, resulting in an investigation of the source (New Jersey Department of Health and Senior Services [NJDHSS], 2007) and working up to the population at risk. Either way, the population is always the main focus, and the governmental and/or legal relationship is always a part of what guides the practice. Kulbok, Thatcher, Park, and Meszaios (2012) described public health nursing as "population-oriented, preventive health care. . . . having a vital role to achieve

Box 11-6 Disease and Health Investigation of Cholera by John Snow

In 1854, John Snow conducted an investigation of a cholera outbreak in London's Golden Square. Initially, John Snow determined who was afflicted with the signs and symptoms of cholera, and then he identified where they lived. Next, Snow took this information and placed it on a map of Golden Square. By doing so, he had a clear picture of all the cases of cholera in front of him. The picture with all the spots created a visual image that permitted him to see more clearly the patterns and clusters of cases.

Snow believed that the source of the cholera was water, and because of this, he also marked on the map the locations of water pumps used by the population of Golden Square to get their daily water supply. He immediately noted that more cases were around pump A than around pumps B and C.

Snow knew he must talk with the people of Golden Square, so he went out into the community and asked questions. What he found was that the people of Golden Square knew that something was wrong with pump B, and as a result, they stayed away from it and would not use the water. He also found out that pump C was not accessible to the people of Golden Square; thus, they did not use it. At that point, he had an idea. He thought that pump A, known as the Broad Street pump, might be the source for the cholera, but he also noticed that directly east of pump A there were no cholera cases.

This did not make any sense to him, so once again he investigated by asking key questions and making observations. He discovered that the people directly to the east of pump A obtained their water from a very deep well situated in a local brewery. He also found that people who worked in the brewery had a daily allotment of malt liquor. Thus, these people were protected because their source of water was derived from two safe supplies. To further his investigation, Snow then returned to those who were afflicted with cholera or who had lost loved ones and determined that the one item all these individuals had in common was that they obtained their water from pump A. This investigation led to changes in that people who knew that pump A was the contaminated source ceased using this pump and, therefore, halted the cholera outbreak.

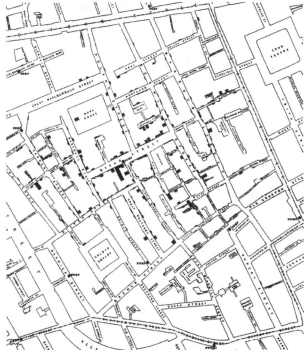

Modified from U.S. Department of Health and Human Services Public Health Service, Centers for Disease Control and Prevention. (1992). *Principles of epidemiology: An introduction to applied epidemiology and biostatistics* (2nd ed.). Washington, DC: American Public Health Association; U.S. Department of Health and Human Services, Centers for Disease Control and Prevention. (2006). *Principles of epidemiology in public health practice: An introduction to applied epidemiology and biostatistics* (3rd ed.). Washington, DC: American Public Health Association.

Reprinted from Snow on cholera being a reprint of two papers by John Snow, M.D., together with a Biographical Memoir by B.W. Richardson, M.D., and an Introduction by Wade Hampton Frost, M.D., Professor of Epidemiology, The Johns Hopkins School of Hygiene and Public Health. New York: The Commonwealth Fund; London: Humphrey Milford, Oxford University Press, pp. 191. © 1936, with permission from Elsevier.

improvements in the health and social conditions of the most vulnerable populations" (para. 2). Much of public health practice, including public health nursing practice, is based on legislation such as sanitary and communicable disease laws. It is because federal, state, and local laws require enforcement that public health nursing can be described as a combination of nursing practice and public health sciences, including the enforcement of federal, state, or local health laws. The U.S. DHHS and the CDC guide public health practice, including public health nursing at the federal level, whereas the State Commissioner of Health and each state's legislated Standards of Performance for Local Boards of Health guide the practice at a local level. As a result, many public health nurses may find they first consult with their state health department rather than the CDC for direction in case-finding, surveillance, outreach, and disease investigation. Because of this, certain examples provided within this chapter relate to the specific state health departments within which the writers function.

Tuberculosis (TB) control, investigation of foodborne illnesses, and rabies prevention, exposure, and follow-up are examples of practice areas guided by the federal regulatory agencies and each state's legislative practice standards. Tuberculosis, foodborne illness, and rabies are all listed as notifiable at the federal level (see Box 11-3), but enforcement of this mandate occurs at the local and state levels. Public health nurses participate in this mandate by ensuring that those individuals already ill receive the appropriate treatment, by checking that contacts to index cases are adequately managed, and by investigating, monitoring, and/or intervening in outbreaks in conjunction with notification or reporting to the state Department of Health and/or CDC. A presentation of these diseases, along with an exploration on the application of the intervention wheel, follows.

Public Health Issue: Tuberculosis

The New Jersey Department of Health and Senior Services (NJDHSS, 2016a) defines *Mycobacterium tuberculosis* as the causative agent for the communicable disease of TB. Tuberculosis is most often a pulmonary disease, but it can also affect other organ systems such as the spine, kidneys, or the brain (NJDHSS, 2016a). In concert with the CDC and the WHO, NJDHSS describes the occurrence of TB as a result of contact with the infectious organism found in droplets from infectious persons when they cough or sneeze (2016a).

Mantoux tuberculin skin testing (TST) continues to be the recommended screening technique to identify exposure to infection by *Mycobacterium tuberculosis* when a significant reaction occurs. If this reaction is combined with a negative chest X-ray and lack of symptoms, the person has latent TB infection (LTBI), is not ill, and is not infectious (NJDHSS, 2016b). An alternate, in vitro blood assay test, QuantiFERON-Gold (QFT-G) is also available and allowed by CDC for identification of LTBI in the same instances in which the TST is used (NJDHSS, 2016b). Tuberculosis disease is considered when *Mycobacterium tuberculosis*, an acid-fast bacilli, is found in a stained smear from a pulmonary or outside, nonpulmonary source (NJDHSS, 2016b). Acute pulmonary TB is a result of reactivation of the latent TB infection or a reinfection.

The NJDHSS, *Standards of Care for Tuberculosis Disease and Latent TB Infection* (2007) provides case definitions of TB as confirmed and presumptive. These standards, still in use, note that confirmed pulmonary TB disease requires a positive sputum/pulmonary culture for *Mycobacterium tuberculosis* and an abnormal chest X-ray along with presenting clinical symptoms of TB disease (NJDHSS, 2007). If cultures are negative or if no specimen could be obtained for culture identification/confirmation, the case is presumptive (NJDHSS, 2007, Standard #3, p. 2). "A presumptive diagnosis of TB must meet the clinical case definition for pulmonary TB to be confirmed" (NJDHSS, 2007, Standard #3, p. 2). A clinical case definition (NJDHSS, 2007) requires the following:

1. Tuberculin skin test reading was significant or positive, indicating latent TB infection.
2. Effective antituberculosis therapy was prescribed and taken.
3. Radiographic change (improvement or worsening) occurred.

Health providers are expected to report to the state department of health any confirmed or probable TB case(s) within 24 hours. This type of reporting is considered passive surveillance because the state receives the report without any specific action on its part. This reporting then initiates a series of activities such as case-finding, outreach, active surveillance, and disease investigation, all located under the banner of TB control.

Tuberculosis control starts with an individual index case; moves to outreaches to family and other close contacts; expands to workplace, school, or other potential exposure sites; and ultimately relates to the population at large. It is the larger population that public health nursing wants to keep safe. In helping specific individuals achieve health, the public health nurse protects the population.

During the case-finding and contact disease investigation stages, population groups are considered at risk based on their exposure to the index case. Each person's closeness to the index case, length of exposure time, and the specific exposure environment are all factored into determination of risk. During the ensuing disease and health event investigation, at-risk populations are interviewed, and skin is tested (screened) to determine their health status. Data information is circular as viewed in Figure 11-1; during this process, surveillance is considered active.

For pulmonary and laryngeal TB cases, treatment is required by law and includes medical management and the potential for **directly observed therapy (DOT)**. DOT is based on standards of care developed from practice-based research. NJDHSS (2007) defined DOT as the "direct observation by a healthcare worker of a patient's ingestion of anti-TB medications at a frequency prescribed by the treating physician" (Standard #6, p. 19). In addition, it "provides the opportunity to identify previously unknown contacts to infectious TB cases, [may help to] identify undisclosed substance abuse [and] allows [for] the healthcare worker to build a therapeutic relationship with the client" (NJDHSS, 2007, Standard #6, p. 19).

Treatment is based on the diagnosis and on the state of resistance exhibited by the bacilli on culture. In addition, the answers to the following questions are important: Is this an active case or a latent TB infection? Is it infectious or noninfectious? Pulmonary or nonpulmonary? Is the person co-infected with HIV? Is the individual pregnant or a child 6 years of age or younger? Goals of treatment are to cure the case and prevent transmission to other individuals, and in doing so, the public health nurse may again need to engage in the process of outreach. Noncompliance by the individual can result in court-ordered confinement until a noninfectious state is achieved.

Public Health Issue: Foodborne Illnesses

Although TB is an example of airborne transmission of disease, foodborne illness is usually transmitted person to person via the fecal–oral route, although vector transmission can occur. Vector transmission takes place, for example, if a fly lands on food after being contaminated by the causative agent. If that food then becomes contaminated, it could become a vehicle for foodborne illnesses such as *Escherichia coli*, *Salmonella*, *Shigella*, or hepatitis A if ingested into the human system.

Foodborne illnesses may be reported as a singular event (one individual) or a family/community event, such as individuals who attended a family picnic, specific restaurant, or day care. Foodborne illness surveillance is passive until a report comes in. Depending on the specific event, surveillance quickly becomes active. The resulting disease and health event investigation begins with the reported event (index case); extends to potential contacts; outreaches to the food supplier, restaurant, day care agency, school, and/or treating hospital; is screened and diagnosed by stool and food samples; and ends with remedial methods to prevent further illness. When commercial food handlers are involved, registered environmental health specialists or sanitarians are also involved. The sanitarian is a state-licensed individual responsible for environmental health inspections and ensuring that compliance is upheld with public health laws. These environmental health specialists work with the food supplier, restaurant, and/or food handler by providing food management education, conducting inspections, and collecting food samples. Legal interventions that may occur include fines, suspension of license, and/or food-handlers course requirements.

The public health nurse works with all public health practitioners throughout the entire process, including the strategies noted in the intervention wheel. To illustrate this involvement, the specifics of shigellosis are examined.

Transmitted by the fecal–oral route and usually person to person, shigellosis is caused by the *Shigella* bacteria (NJDHSS, 2015). Its most common symptoms are diarrhea that can be bloody, nausea, vomiting, stomach cramps, and fever. Although generally self-limiting, the disease can last between one to four or seven days. It is important to note that "asymptomatic infections can also occur" (NJDHSS, 2015, p. 2). Its spread usually occurs among household contacts, children in preschools or day care, persons living in residential facilities, men who have sex with men, and via contact with a contaminated object or food through ingestion or direct contact with an infected person (NJDHSS, 2015). Diagnosis occurs after finding the *Shigella* bacteria in the stool. "A person may continue to transmit the *Shigella* bacteria as long as bacteria are present and excreted in stool" (NJDHSS, 2015, p. 3), which can last approximately four weeks from illness onset. Asymptomatic carriers may be infected for much longer.

As noted in Box 11-3, shigellosis is a reportable illness. Many states, including New Jersey, use the same shigellosis surveillance case definition as the CDC, which is classified as confirmed or probable. Confirmed requires "isolation of *Shigella* from a clinical specimen from any site of the human body, regardless of symptoms" and probable requires a "clinically compatible case that is epidemiologically linked to a confirmed case" (NJDHSS, 2015, p. 4).

When the local health department receives a *Shigella* report, the case finding, outreach, surveillance, and disease investigation processes are initiated. Although the responsibility in this case primarily lies with the health officer, it is often the public health nurse who outreaches to the index case to obtain the history and gather important information pertaining to the signs and symptom. The date when symptoms first appeared is critical because it informs the public health nurse as to the incubation period. For shigellosis, the incubation period may vary from one to four days, but it can also range from 12 to 50 hours and up to one week (NJDHSS, 2015, p. 3). This disease investigation would then need to include specific index case information up to four days before symptom onset. Other important information the public health nurse needs to secure includes a food history such as what foods were eaten, when they were eaten, and where they were eaten; travel history; types and location of outside activity; work history; and inclusion of household contacts. The public health nurse also needs to ask additional questions: Did others eat the same food? Have they also become ill? Did they need to see a doctor? What are the foods common to all who became ill? Are the numbers of reported cases increasing, and are they part of a community group, such as day care or school? Is the index case or subsequent case a person who directly prepares or handles food? The answers to these questions then direct the continued processes of disease investigation, case-finding, outreach, and surveillance. As shown in Figure 11-1, the informational loop is circular. Surveillance continues to be active until all aspects of the disease or outbreak are closed.

Primary prevention is always a first priority in public health practice when it comes to foodborne illness. For example, when an environmental health specialist or sanitarian conducts a restaurant inspection, he or she also provides food handling education. Both practices are meant to prevent any contamination with the management of food. Public health nurses frequently find themselves in situations where the provision of health education is essential for prevention. The following example illustrates this point.

Public health nurses conduct immunization school audits, and at the same time, they may find themselves in the position of providing education in infection control and prevention of communicable diseases. In this one particular circumstance, a public health nurse was provided a table located in the dining area of the preschool to review the infants'/children's immunization records. While conducting this audit, the public health nurse observed one of the child care workers changing a baby's diaper on a changing table located in the same room near the food preparation area. In addition, before-and-after diaper change hand washing was not observed. What educational and prevention opportunities presented themselves with this observation? Besides what the public health nurse should do, what type(s) of referrals could be made to further enhance the infection control interventions for this nursery/preschool?

Public Health Issue: Rabies

Whereas TB and *Shigella* are communicable diseases for which no preventive vaccination exists, rabies can be prevented by vaccination but not by the vaccination of humans; it is the routine vaccination of domestic animals that can help prevent rabies. "Pre-exposure vaccination [for humans] should [only] be offered to persons in high-risk groups, such as veterinarians and their staff, animal handlers, rabies researchers, and certain laboratory workers" (CDC, 2008a, para. 74). It should also be considered for individuals whose work, activities, or travel might cause them to come into contact with potentially rabid animals (CDC, 2008a).

Rabies can be described as a "zoonotic disease caused by the RNA virus in the family Rhabdoviridae genus Lyssavirus" (CDC, 2008a, para. 4) that is typically present in the saliva of clinically ill mammals and is transmitted through a bite. Although all warm-blooded hosts can be susceptible to the virus, in the United States, distinct variants have been found in coyotes, foxes, raccoons, skunks, and several species of bats (CDC, 2011).

The CDC Advisory Committee (2008a) report on human rabies prevention indicated that improved dog vaccination programs, coupled with enhanced stray animal control, has resulted in a considerable decrease of rabies cases in domestic animals since World War II:

In 1946, a total of 8,384 indigenous rabies cases were reported among dogs and 33 cases in humans. In 2006, a total of 79 cases of rabies were reported in domestic dogs, none of which was attributed to enzootic dog-to-dog transmission, and three cases were reported in humans, [none of which] was acquired from indigenous domestic animals. (para. 5)

Even with this decline, rabies still causes concern among public health professionals because confirmed human exposure to the rabies virus is generally always fatal unless appropriate postexposure prophylaxis (PEP) is provided.

The management of potential human exposure requires an accurately assessed risk for infection (CDC, 2008a). Human incubation for rabies may range from days to years but is usually weeks to months. Because of this, the CDC (2008a) considers "administration of rabies post-exposure prophylaxis [as] a medical urgency, not a medical emergency, but [stresses] that decisions must not be delayed" (para. 7). The application of the intervention wheel strategies is presented here to demonstrate the processes that the public health nurse is involved with in cases of human exposure to rabies.

Rabies postexposure follow-up starts with receiving the report of a bite, scratch, or exposure to saliva from a potentially infected animal and extends to outreach and case-finding with the individual(s) exposed. Determination of risk often falls to the public health nurse, especially if the victim did not present to a medical care provider. Other times the assessment may be shared when an emergency room primary care provider reports to the local health department. Containment and quarantine of the domestic animal falls to animal control, with enforcement shared by the licensed environmental specialist or sanitarian. The animal is quarantined and observed for 10 days after a bite (CDC, 2008a, para. 59) to ensure it is not rabid. This quarantine occurs whether the animal was vaccinated or not. Any untoward signs and symptoms compatible with rabies result in the animal being euthanized and the head removed and sent to the state laboratory for testing. Should the exposure be a result of a wild animal, the capture and securing of the head for testing comes under the jurisdiction of animal control and veterinarian services (CDC, 2008a).

The public health nurse's responsibility includes obtaining health/event information, providing post-exposure-related information to the individual(s) involved, and securing, tracking, and documenting the required postexposure treatment for the exposed client. As with foodborne illness, surveillance is passive until the report is received, at which time it becomes active. Recommendations for PEP include the prompt and thorough cleansing of the wound, followed by passive rabies immunization with human rabies immune globulin and vaccination with a cell culture rabies vaccine (CDC, 2008a). Furthermore, the 2010 and still current recommendations included the use of a reduced four-dose vaccine schedule:

These new recommendations reduce the number of vaccine doses to four. The reduction in doses recommended for PEP was based in part on evidence from rabies virus pathogenesis data, experimental animal work, clinical studies, and epidemiologic surveillance. These studies indicated that 4 vaccine doses in combination with rabies immune globulin (RIG) elicited adequate immune responses and that a fifth dose of vaccine did not contribute to more favorable outcomes. For persons previously unvaccinated with rabies vaccine, the reduced regimen of 4 1-ml doses of HDCV or PCECV should be administered intramuscularly. The first dose of the 4-dose course should be administered as soon as possible after exposure (day 0). Additional doses then should be administered on days 3, 7, and 14 after the first vaccination. (CDC, 2010, para. 1)

The disease and health event investigation is shared with health officers, environmental sanitarians, animal control officers, and veterinary professionals who control the animal-related sequence of events. It may also be shared with the state departments of health and the CDC. A classic example of this occurrence happened in July 2007, during the South Atlantic Summer Showdown softball tournament held in Spartanburg County, North Carolina. The CDC (2008b) provided a report regarding this interstate public health response to a rabid kitten. A summation of that report is as follows.

Between July 13 and 15, 2007, approximately 60 teams, with 12 players each, from multiple states participated in the South Atlantic Summer Showdown softball tournament. On July 14, one of the North Carolina coaches, upon finding "an apparently healthy and alert kitten" (CDC, 2008b, para. 3) in a garbage bin, placed the kitten in a box, brought it to six or more different games at two different facilities, and at the end of the day took the kitten to her home. On July 15, the coach's housemate took the kitten to an emergency animal hospital because it had become increasingly lethargic, was behaving abnormally, and had bitten her. When the housemate presented the kitten to the attending veterinarian, however, she reported the kitten had not bitten anyone during the preceding 10 days and released the kitten for care (CDC, 2008b, para. 3). Because the kitten was severely ill, this release allowed for the kitten to be euthanized, with cremation scheduled for July 18.

On July 18, a softball player's mother contacted the emergency animal hospital upon learning the kitten had become sick. Because this mother had also been bitten by the kitten when it was at the tournament, she asked whether the kitten had been tested for rabies. Learning that it had not, she picked up the cat's body and brought it to the local health department, which sent the head to North Carolina's State Laboratory for rabies testing. A positive rabies diagnosis was made. That fact became the starting point for what was eventually a four-state rabies investigation. "Of the approximately 60 teams participating in the tournament, 38 had players and associated family and friends who reported exposure to the rabid kitten" (CDC, 2008b, para. 9). Of that number, 27 individuals were assessed as having exposure that warranted postexposure prophylaxis because they "had reported actual exposure to the kitten's saliva, either through a bite, a lick on the oral or nasal mucosa, or a claw scratch" (CDC, 2008b, para. 9). Cooperation of investigators within the four affected states and the CDC "enabled the expeditious identification and prophylactic treatment of exposed persons while preventing unnecessary administration of PEP" (CDC, 2008b, para. 15).

Case Study 1—TB: When Time Is of Importance

Thus far, this chapter has presented for the reader three different public health issues. The case study described here is a detailed account of one of the issues presented, TB, and the application of the intervention wheel strategies of case finding, surveillance, disease and health event investigation, outreach, and screening.

The Case

On June 14, a 39-year-old woman was admitted to the hospital with complaints of cough, fever, decreased appetite, night sweats, and a weight loss of 23 pounds over the last month. The admission chest X-ray revealed bilateral upper lobe infiltrates. The physician ordered immediate respiratory isolation and a bronchoscope with bronchial wash. The latter took place on June 17 and was positive for acid-fast bacillus. A probable diagnosis of pulmonary *M. tuberculosis* was made; treatment was started on June 19 with first-line anti-TB medications. A report to the local health department occurred on June 21, seven days after the hospital admission, thus initiating an active surveillance. One month later, the final culture was identified as *M. tuberculosis* with pansensitivity to the TB medications that had been prescribed.

Tuberculosis Interview and Plan

On June 22, the public health nurse began the disease and health event investigation when she reached out into the community as she arrived at the hospital to interview the newly reported TB index case. During this communication, she learned the patient had been a part-time volunteer for a local day care center, working approximately two to five hours per week. Reporting that her sister was the center's director, the patient stated her work was mostly secretarial with little exposure to the children. The public health nurse also learned the index case had been coughing for approximately two months, one month longer than noted on admission. Therefore, she may have been infectious longer than previously thought. As a result of this important information, further investigation was needed and in a timely manner.

The state TB nurse manager was called in. Both public health professionals realized that the first steps in the subsequent contact investigation were to identify the infectious period, develop a list of contacts, and then visit the day care center, again signaling the importance of outreach. In talking to the public health nurse and reviewing the health record, the state TB nurse manager determined the infectious period to be February 17 to June 14. This conclusion set the beginning of the infectious period at three months before the cough onset and ended it when the patient was hospitalized in respiratory isolation. The following day both the public health nurse and the TB nurse manager met with the day care director to discuss potential exposure to children and staff, conduct an on-site assessment of environmental factors, identify high-priority contacts during the infectious period, and provide TB education to the key individuals involved.

On-Site Assessment and Identification of Contacts

Because index case confidentiality is always a consideration in work site or congregate setting investigations, the state TB nurse manager obtained a signed written statement from the director of the day care center indicating her obligation to respect the issues of confidentiality as related to the index case and this investigation. The index case also signed a written consent for the health department to conduct the investigation at her work site.

The on-site assessment, which is so important to this disease and health event investigation, again demonstrated the importance of outreach. This assessment revealed a small day care center with low ceilings and only one window, located in the kitchen. The play area room measured 17 by 23 feet; ceiling height was 6 feet 5 inches. There were 35 children, 4 years of age or younger, all born in the United States; there were five staff members. The director reported that the index case had spent most of her time in the play area room.

Given the size of the rooms, poor ventilation, the age of the children, and the infectiousness of the index case, all children and staff were considered high-priority contacts. During the meeting, the director also indicated she had a 6-month-old infant who did not attend the day care but spent approximately five to six hours with the index case on weekends. This infant, also considered a high-priority contact, was available for the public health nurse to plant a TST that same day. When the screening test was read 48 hours later, the reaction was 15 mm, a reaction considered positive. A follow-up chest X-ray revealed infiltrates. The infant was admitted to the hospital with a tentative diagnosis of probable pulmonary TB, and anti-TB medications were started.

Contact Investigation Continues

The disease and health event investigation process continued as the public health professionals collected the names and located information of all identified contacts, in all exposure settings, including household, social, and workplace. Outreach and notification of all contacts were required because they needed TSTs and screening. Educational sessions were also provided to parents of all day care children.

In addition to the 39 children and staff contacts at the day care center, the index case also named nine other high-priority contacts, seven household and two social. Active surveillance and outreach continued as the public health nurse visited the patient's household to verify the contacts, provide education, and conduct TST screening. This visit determined that all household contacts had been identified, and none was immune compromised. The nurse then conducted a home visit to the identified social contacts' residences. There it was discovered that one social contact had a 6-month-old infant not named on the initial index case interview. During this home visit and contact interview, the nurse realized this baby had approximately 70 hours of exposure per week to the index case during the determined infectious period. Furthermore, the infant had been presenting with signs and symptoms of what the mom thought were a cold; she was thinking of calling the baby's doctor. The TB clinic was called, and the infant was referred to the emergency room and then subsequently admitted to the hospital. Probable pulmonary TB was the diagnosis, and treatment was started.

Summary

In the day care center, 14 of 35 children were TST positive; 50%, or seven of these children, were diagnosed with confirmed pulmonary TB disease. All TB cases were treated and later placed on DOT upon hospital discharge. The remaining seven children were placed on treatment for latent TB infection.

Of the household and social contact population, 70% were found to be TST positive; the two infants were diagnosed with confirmed pulmonary TB disease and treated in the same manner as the day care children. The remaining TST-positive adults were placed on treatment for latent TB infection.

As you reflect on this case study, do you see the intervention strategies discussed in this chapter being carried out by the two public health nurses? What exactly did they do, and how did they do it?

Case Study 2—Zika: Anything but Clear

The aforementioned study reflected upon the work involved when the index case is clear, the contacts are local, and the disease is well understood. What about when an outbreak is developing, the disease is still being defined, appropriate interventions and prevention strategies are evolving, and knowledge of long-term consequences is unknown or incomplete? What if this is happening not just locally or even interstate, but spreading from one country to another? The next case described here details the account of case-finding, surveillance, disease and health investigation, outreach, and screening when the picture is anything but clear. The Zika virus outbreak is a recent, ongoing, and classic example of how all segments of healthcare communities deal with such an occurrence. The outbreak timeline here uses information obtained from May 1, 2015, through May 31, 2016.

Initially identified in Uganda in 1947, the first local transmission of the Zika virus in the region of the Americas occurred May 2015 in Brazil, as reported by the WHO (2016). By November 2015, the first Zika virus patient in Puerto Rico was diagnosed (Dirlikov et al., 2016), and by January 20, 2016, Puerto Rico and 19 other countries or American territories were required to report all locally transmitted Zika virus cases to the Pan American Health Organization (Hennessey, Fischer, & Staples, 2016). The WHO, other country public health authorities, the CDC, and local U.S. health departments began to educate healthcare providers and the public to prepare for potential local outbreaks in areas deemed as at-risk locations. In addition, the U.S. Congress and the Senate began debating on legislation to provide monies required to fight the threat.

The Outbreak

It is important for public health nurses to understand the science that informs public health and specifically these intervention strategies. The Zika virus is a mosquito-borne flavivirus (Centron, 2016). Zika is "closely related to dengue, West Nile, and yellow fever viruses. . . . spread is primarily by *Aedes aegypti* mosquitoes, [with] instances of sexual, male-to-female transmission reported" (Hills et al., 2016, para. 1). Intrauterine or intrapartum mother-to-baby transmission, blood transfusion, and laboratory exposure have also been documented (Hennessey, Fischer, & Staples, 2016, para. 3). Though 80% nonsymptomatic, when symptoms do occur, they are usually with "acute onset of fever, maculopapular rash, arthralgia, or conjunctivitis" (Petersen, Staples et al., 2016, para. 1). Zika virus symptoms generally last from several days to one week and are often (80%) nonsymptomatic (Petersen, Staples et al., 2016). As such, without more complete knowledge of the disease's threat to pregnant women and their developing child, there was and is a public health urgency to prevent transmission and fight the outbreak. The urgency becomes clearer when one considers what we do know and all of what we don't yet know about this virus, emerging outbreak, and long-term consequences.

Brazil

The outbreak of the Zika virus was first identified in northeastern Brazil in early May 2015 (Schuler-Faccini, 2016). As the Brazilian outbreak continued, authorities noted an increase in reports of infants born with microcephaly (Petersen, Staples et al., 2016). Because there was no vaccine or medication to prevent infection, treatment consisted of supportive care and, for pregnant women, lab work with monitoring of fetal anatomy and growth every three to four weeks (Petersen, Staples et al., 2016). At the same time, there were no fetal treatment interventions available.

Case-finding, surveillance, disease investigations, and reporting continued. As a result of the disease investigation, data collection, and monitoring, the CDC, via the Morbidity and Mortality Weekly Report (MMWR), soon documented public health implications due to the increased fetal microcephaly suggestive of a possible relationship to Zika (Schuler-Faccinni et al., 2016). This documented report urged the public health community to:

1. Continue with additional studies of the relationship of Zika virus to fetal microcephaly.
2. Remove all potential mosquito breeding areas.
3. Educate and assure that pregnant women in affected areas wear protective clothing, use a U.S. Environmental Protection Agency (EPA)–approved insect repellent, and sleep in a room with screens or under a mosquito net.
4. Continue with risk communication and community mobilization.

Puerto Rico

The first U.S. jurisdiction to report a patient with locally transmitted Zika virus disease was Puerto Rico in December 2015, with the index case indicating symptoms had started the month before in November (Dirlikov et al., 2016). Puerto Rican laboratory surveillance already established for Dengue fever now included the Zika virus, and from November 2015, weekly Zika virus reports gradually increased, whereas Dengue incidence remained low (Dirlikov et al., 2016). Of the 6,157 suspected Zika specimens tested in the lab between November 2015 and April 2016, 683 or 11% tested positive for Zika, including 65 symptomatic pregnant women; 17 (2%) of patients required hospitalization, including five (1%) with suspected Guillain–Barré syndrome" (Dirlikov et al., 2016, para. 1). This triggered a strong epidemiologic and public health response, which included an:

> *increased laboratory capacity to test for Zika virus infection (including blood donor screening), implementation of enhanced surveillance systems, and prevention activities focused on pregnant women. Vector control activities included indoor and outdoor residual spraying and reduction of mosquito breeding environments focused around pregnant women's homes. (Dirlikov et al., 2016, para. 1)*

In addition, blood supply safety was a challenge since it relied on blood donor screening. As a result, Puerto Rico imported all blood products from the United States prior to the availability of a Food and Drug Administration (FDA) detection test on April 2. Furthermore, adverse pregnancy and child health outcomes were monitored through the creation of an active pregnancy surveillance system for Zika virus, with surviving offspring referred to the Special Child Health Services program for coordination and care (Dirlikov et al., 2016).

Meanwhile, eight months after the outbreak identification, the CDC cautioned that anyone with symptoms of Zika virus disease, during or within two weeks of travel (to infected areas), or who have ultrasound findings of fetal microcephaly or intracranial calcifications, should be tested in consultation with state or local health departments (Petersen, Staples et al., 2016, para. 1).

By March 2016, 10 months after outbreak identification, transmission of the Zika virus, through male-to-female sexual contact, by individuals who had traveled to areas of ongoing transmission, were being reported, but at that time, "the length of time that virus might persist in semen [was] unknown" (Hills et al., 2016, para. 9).

As public health officials worried about mosquito control specific to the identified vector (*Aedes* species mosquito), decisions on where and how to effect appropriate control measures were discussed. Insecticide vector control studies yielded considerable geographical differences in vector susceptibility prior to identifying the best source for the control programs (Dirlikov et al., 2016).

Several environmental factors within a country's borders could help define which areas are most likely to be suitable habitats and which areas are not (Cetron, 2016). Factors such as "temperature, precipitation, vegetation, and human population density that define suitable habitat [would vary]; where habitat is unsuitable, the mosquito vector is likely to be absent, and risk is negligible" (Cetron, 2016, para. 3). Because elevation is fixed and comparatively easy to measure, it has historically served as a temperature proxy (Cetron, 2016). Subsequent analysis then focused on "countries and U.S. territories that have ongoing Zika virus transmission" and areas with elevations of 1,500 meters or more (Cetron, 2016, para. 6).

This final analysis concluded that the "*Aedes aegypti* is unlikely to be found at elevations greater than 2,000 m because of unsuitable ecologic factors, including but not limited to low temperature" (Cetron, 2016, para. 6).

This information, published by CDC in March 2016, allowed public health officials greater specificity in providing both at-risk area travel information, as well as where to target mosquito breeding prevention strategies.

By March 23, there were 39 countries and U.S. territories with noted active Zika virus transmission (Petersen, Poles et al., 2016, para. 2) and by April 2016, "increasing epidemiologic, clinical, laboratory, and pathologic evidence [supported] a link between Zika virus infection during pregnancy and adverse pregnancy and birth outcomes, including pregnancy loss, microcephaly, and brain and eye abnormalities" (Petersen, Polen et al., 2016, para. 4). Counseling of women and men, with possible Zika virus exposure and who are interested in conceiving, was recommended by the CDC (Petersen, Polen et al., 2016). It was also documented that females who have Zika virus disease should wait at least eight weeks after symptom onset to attempt conception, and men with Zika virus disease should wait at least six months after symptoms began to attempt conception (Petersen, Polen et al., 2016, para. 1).

The United States

During the aforementioned outbreak timeline, there were 45 states reporting 544 travel-associated Zika virus cases, of which none were locally acquired, and 10 were sexually transmitted (CDC, 2016a). The Zika virus disease and related congenital infections joined the list of those diseases or conditions requiring CDC notification (CDC, 2016a). Because some of the states have mosquito species that could become infected with the Zika virus, the potential

risk for local transmission of the disease existed, causing increased urgency (CDC, 2016b). This occurred with the West Nile virus outbreak where morbidity and mortality continued to increase long after the initial outbreak.

With the Zika virus, the most at-risk population is pregnant women and their unborn babies. Potential long-term consequences could be staggering. Branches of the federal government attempted to agree on funding allocations to fight this disease, while interim guidelines for at-risk employee education and protection were produced by the National Institute for Occupational Safety and Health (CDC, 2016b). Zika virus case-finding, surveillance, outreach, screening, and disease and health investigation *continued* to peak as the country moved into the warmer summer months, and a clearer picture of outbreak consequences will slowly emerge long past the May 1, 2015–May 31, 2016 outbreak timeline of this study.

Summary

How does one summarize an event when the story is incomplete? The answer is that an emerging infectious disease outbreak does not provide the story's ending, even when the initial outbreak is over. This was true of West Nile virus and will also be true of the Zika virus. It can take years to provide the answer to many of our questions.

Since the original study timeline, local Zika virus transmission has occurred in sections of both Florida (CDC, 2016d) and Texas (CDC, 2016e), confirming the fear that a local mosquito species would be able to transmit the virus. The Zika Response Appropriations Act—H.R. 5243, 2016 was passed by the 114th Congress (2016) along with the Continuing Appropriations and Military Construction, Veterans Affairs and Related Agencies Act H. R. 5325 (2017). For further information about these acts, please refer to the reference list and related links listed at the end of this chapter.

The public health challenges on how to provide guidance, effective prevention, and treatment when there are so many unknowns will continue. For example, the level of risk for adverse pregnancy and birth outcomes related to Zika virus infection is not completely known, as is the risk related to Zika virus infection relative to the time of conception (Petersen, Polen et al., 2016, para. 5). We also do not know the "expected duration of a Zika virus outbreak in any particular location" (Petersen, Polen et al., 2016, para. 13); whether mosquito species, already in several other states, will also become infected producing additional local transmission; and the long-term developmental health and financial costs for those infected infants who survive. Because there currently is no vaccine or medication that prevents the virus and no effective treatment to prevent damage to the fetus, the most effective tools are related to the primary prevention strategies of education, environmental, and personal preventive interventions.

As you read the above case study, reflect upon the following. How did the public health community engage in disease investigation? Can you identify the various types of surveillance data the healthcare community is gathering? Is there a place for collaboration between providers and population at risk? What is the role of the government with regard to funding and policy development? How would you as a public health provider use media advocacy to inform the public? These are just some questions you may wish to consider.

Levels of Practice Evident in the Red Wedge

As public health nurses work with their target populations, they must always keep in mind the cultural context of those they serve. With TB, *Shigella*, and rabies, they are concerned about the individual, family, and population's relationship to the index case and how best to reach out to all in the most effective way so that outreach, case-finding, screening, surveillance, and disease intervention may take place. For these interventions to be effective, the nurse must be a part of the community, not in an office behind a desk. The public health nurse must combine nursing practice and public health sciences, including the enforcement of federal, state, or local

laws. The public health nurse must be able to apply and perform the 17 intervention strategies of the intervention wheel and also apply those skills and initiate change at the individual/family, community, and system levels of public health practice. How may the public health nurse apply these 17 strategies at the three various levels of practice? Public health nurses need to examine and explore what ways are best received by the individual/family, population, and community.

Consideration of the case studies above illustrates how public health nurses may practice. On the individual/family level, the public health nurse develops a trusting relationship with each person. Considering the fear that is often associated with a diagnosis of TB, the public health nurse's ability to reach out and connect with the index case, especially in the questioning phase, is critical. The case studies also illustrate the importance of working with each individual, given the sensitivity and the need for confidentiality. This again highlights the importance of trust development in the public health nurse's relationship with each individual contacted during the investigation. Once this relationship is established, the public health nurse may engage in health teaching and counseling, two additional strategies discussed in other chapters, which assist with the disease and health investigation.

On the community level, the public health nurse works with multiple community organizations in partnership and even in the development of coalitions. For example, the emergency department, hospital, day care center, state department of health, and the local department of health were all actively involved in the case-finding, outreach, screening, disease and health investigation, and surveillance. Furthermore, the development of educational programs, counseling, support services, referral, and advocacy initiatives are essential to any public health scenario. The public health nurse also recognizes that the strategies may be different for TB compared with that of the Zika virus. The community in partnership endeavors to serve as a way to enhance the social, human, and economic capital of the community, resulting in positive outcomes.

On the systems level, policy and law sustain and may even scale up the public health process and initiative by ensuring and assuring the health of the people. For example, TB and now Zika are two of the many diseases presented on the Nationally Notifiable Infectious Diseases list. This system-level strategy ensures that newly diagnosed cases are sent to the departments of health, local and state, for follow-up and case-finding via disease event investigation. This ensures and assures the identification of others at risk or active cases yet to be diagnosed, thus protecting the public.

Conclusion

This chapter presents the red sections of the intervention wheel. The section discussed is that of case-finding, outreach, screening, surveillance, and disease and health event investigation. The chapter was divided in a way that permitted the reader to first learn about these four particular public health nursing interventions. The second section presented various public health issues and relationships between public health practice with local, state, and the federal levels of government. The third section offered case studies for review along with considerations of the public health nurse interventions, as applied to various levels of practice. Public health nursing is not a linear practice. It is a challenging practice that requires the public health nurse to think, apply, and do on multiple levels. It is forever changing and challenging.

Additional Resources

Centers for Disease Control and Prevention: National Notifiable Disease Surveillance System at: https://www.cdc.gov/nndss/downloads.html

U.S. Preventative Task Force Screening at: http://www.uspreventiveservicestaskforce.org/BrowseRec/Search?s=screening

World Health Organization Public Health Surveillance at: http://www.who.int/topics/public_health_surveillance/en/

World Health Disease Surveillance and Response Systems at: http://www.who.int/csr/resources/publications/surveillance/WHO_CDS_EPR_LYO_2006_2/en/

United Nations Creative Community Outreach Initiatives at: http://outreach.un.org/ccoi/

United Kingdom National Screening Committee at: NHS population screening explained at: https://www.gov.uk/guidance/nhs-population-screening-explained

---

Lessons from History

The purpose of this section in this intervention chapter is to demonstrate for the reader how history does inform our contemporary practice, and the take-away messages are varied and many.

The history of the American Red Cross Town and Country was adapted from Lewenson, 2017.
Take the time to read the following and see what your take-away is.

Hitting the Pavement: Intervention of Case Finding: Outreach, Screening, Surveillance, and Disease and Health Event Investigation

Long before the determinants of health or *Healthy People 2020* were developed, communities recognized that identifying the health needs of its communities were essential to providing adequate public health nursing care. In 1917, a local town in upstate New York State started the Red Hook Nursing Association, hiring an American Red Cross Town and Country rural public health nurse.

Town & Country Rural Public Health Nurse

Community leaders sought affiliation with the Town and Country in order to start the town's nursing service. Margaret Chanler Aldrich, a wealthy community activist and friend of early-20th-century nursing, advocated the start of a nursing service as a result of the findings of a 1915 report titled, *Sickness in Dutchess County New York: Its Extent, Care, and Prevention.*

Sickness in Dutchess Report

This community assessment examined the kinds of diseases that were prevalent in the rural community, the adequacy of care families received both in the home and hospitals, and the environmental factors that influenced both.

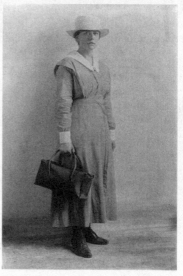

> *It was important to have more exact knowledge of the sickness which had occurred in the county in order to draw trustworthy conclusions as to how adequately or inadequately the existing public and private facilities were meeting the needs of the community. (State Charities Aid Association, 1915, p. 6)*

Courtesy of American Red Cross

No. 136

SICKNESS
IN
DUTCHESS COUNTY
NEW YORK
ITS EXTENT, CARE AND PREVENTION

PART I

A STATEMENT OF FINDINGS

PART II

RECOMMENDATIONS

REPORT MADE BY THE
COMMITTEE ON HOSPITALS
OF THE
STATE CHARITIES AID ASSOCIATION
AT THE REQUEST OF THE
THOMAS THOMPSON TRUST
60 STATE STREET
BOSTON, MASS.

NEW YORK
SEPTEMBER
1915

Reproduced from State Charities Aid Association. (1915). *Sickness in Dutchess County, New York: Its extent, care, and prevention* (Book No. 136) (pp. 1–119). New York, NY: State Charities Aid Association (p. 2). Retrieved from https://babel .hathitrust.org/shcgi/pt?id=mdp.39015068561045;view=1up;seq=1

Districts within Dutchess County Canvassed

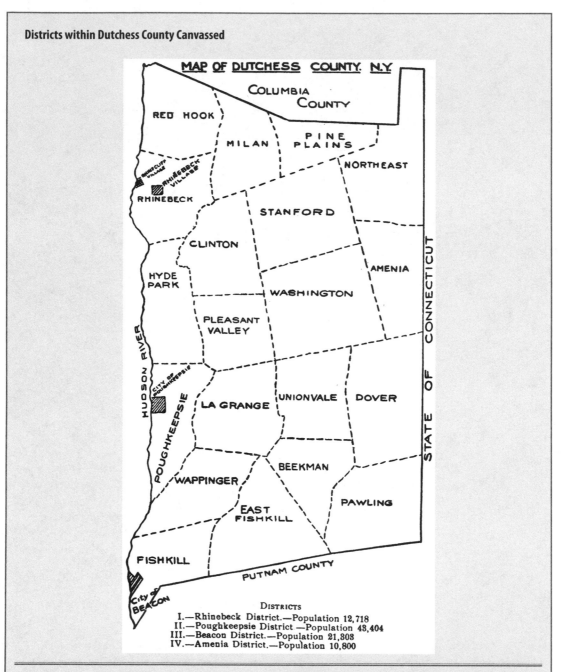

MAP OF DUTCHESS COUNTY, N.Y.

DISTRICTS
I.—Rhinebeck District.—Population 12,718
II.—Poughkeepsie District.—Population 43,404
III.—Beacon District.—Population 21,308
IV.—Amenia District.—Population 10,800

Reproduced from Weber, J. J. (1917). *A county at work at its health problems: A statement of accomplishment by the Dutchess County Health Association during the sixteen months August 1916 to December 1917*. New York, NY: State Charities Aid Association. Retrieved from https://babel.hathitrust.org/shcgi/pt?id=mdp.39015014861580;view=1up;seq=1 p.32.

Between 1912 and 1913, families within five districts in upstate New York rural Dutchess County were queried about illnesses they experienced that year during a door-to-door survey. The adequacy of public health nurses was determined based on the reported illnesses and the environmental barriers to care. Over 53 diseases were reported, including measles, mumps, influenza, pneumonia to alcoholism, cancer, diseases of the digestive track, cardiac, and others. Barriers to care included poor sanitary conditions, overcrowded housing, poverty, lack of education, and inadequacy of public health nurses. The relationship of these barriers as well as the lack of access to a sufficient number of healthcare providers, in particular, nursing, led the town of Red Hook to value the need for a public health nurse.

Table 1. Population, Percentage Covered, Total Cases, and Sickness Rate per 1,000 of Population in Selected Districts*

	4th Ward, Poughkeepsie	Rhinebeck Town	Milan and Clinton	Total
Population	4580	3532	2171	10283
Total number of families	1065	855	463	2383
Number of families not at home	30	57	15	102
Percentage of families covered	97.1	93.3	96.7	95.7
Population covered	4451	3306	2096	9853
Percentage of population covered‡	97.1	93.3	96.5	95.9
Total cases of sickness*	487	774	272	1533
1912 cases of sickness	355	533	139	1027
Total cases per 1000 population, 1912.†	80	161	663	104

*69 cases in the Town of Stanford omitted, as the data obtained was for 12 months only.

†Cases Per 1000 of Population indicated only for purposes of comparison between localities, as data do not include all cases of sickness occurring in district covered. See context under "Sickness Recorded," Page 15.

‡For comment on these figures see Page 12.

Reproduced from State Charities Aid Association. (1915). *Sickness in Dutchess County, New York: Its extent, care, and prevention* (Book No. 136) (p. 87). New York, NY: State Charities Aid Association. Retrieved from https://babel.hathitrust .org/shcgi/pt?id=mdp.39015068561045;view=1up;seq=1

Questions to Consider

1. Access on line the State Charities Aid Association. (1915). *Sickness in Dutchess County, New York: Its extent, care, and prevention* (Book No. 136) (pp. 1–119). New York, NY: State Charities Aid Association. Retrieved from https://babel.hathitrust.org/shcgi/pt?id=mdp.39015068561045;view=1up;seq=1
2. Reflect upon the historical case study above and consider how the 1915 *Sickness in Dutchess County* report illustrates the disease and health event investigation aspect of the intervention wheel.
3. Compare and contrast the use of the 1915 study with the use of large data sets used in clinical decision-making in public health nursing today.

Adapted from Lewenson, S. B. (2017). Historical exemplars in nursing. In S. B. Lewenson & M. Truglio-Londrigan (Eds.), *Practicing primary health care in nursing: Caring for populations* (pp. 1–17). Burlington, MA: Jones & Bartlett Learning.

CASE STUDY AND CRITICAL QUESTIONS	When Care Is not There: The Importance of Public Health Nursing Interventions Marty Hucks, MN, APRN-BC, CNE Tracy P. George, DNP, APRN-BC, CNE Francis Marion University

A 42-year-old woman who lived in a rural, high-poverty county of the South discovered a left breast mass. She worked part-time as a cashier and had no health insurance. The state she lived in did not expand Medicaid, and she could not afford coverage through the Affordable Care Act. Because she had no health insurance, she could not seek health care for her breast mass, and it remained there for two years, gradually getting larger. She just kept hoping that it would go away.

Her children were eligible for Medicaid, so they were able to receive care. When she was at her child's appointment at a family practice office, she mentioned her breast mass to the physician. The family physician referred her to the free clinic in the county, and she immediately made an appointment.

The faith-based free clinic is open just one evening per week, but there are always 15 to 20 patients seen each evening because the need for health care is so great in this area. Some of the clinic patients are homeless, and many have transportation issues, so they walk miles to come to the clinic to be seen.

I was the nurse practitioner seeing her that evening, and this patient told me about her breast mass that had been present two years. Upon exam, there was a hard, egg-sized mass in her left breast, with axillary lymphadenopathy. She told me that she was a single mother and could not afford to be sick. She always put her children's needs above her own, but she realized that this mass needed to be evaluated.

Luckily, the other provider at the free clinic that evening was a surgeon. He reexamined the patient, and he arranged for her to be seen in his office the next day. He agreed to do her surgery and see her for all follow-up care free of charge.

A few months later, I saw the surgeon again. He told me that this patient had stage IV breast cancer. The patient had a lumpectomy and was set up for chemotherapy through a charity care program at a regional medical center. She was doing well.

Since that time, the free clinic has become a provider through the Breast and Cervical Early Detection Program, which benefits low-income, uninsured women. Through this program, the clinic hopes to provide more cervical and breast cancer screening services to this rural, underserved population.

Public health nursing is about caring for the individual, family, community, and the population. The above case is a story about one woman, but this one woman does represent many other woman who may present with determinants of health such as poverty and lack of access to services or services that are limited in availability. Public health issues, however, are varied and complex. Given this complexity, one can also see how the public health nursing interventions of outreach, screening, and case-finding as well as disease and health investigation are essential but limited considered alone. Given the above case study, answer the following questions:

1. Describe what you see to be the barriers for care with regard to access and availability in the case study?
2. If you were a public health nurse, what types of initiatives would you develop to improve outreach, screening, and case-finding? Who would you partner with in terms of community organizations, whether they are governmental or nongovernmental?
3. How would you engage in the process of surveillance, and what large data sets would you monitor for trends about breast cancer in specific populations? What would you do with this information?

Other interventions are also warranted. These interventions may include the development of an infrastructure to serve the needs of this rural and vulnerable population. Strategies such as advocacy, policy change, partnership development, collaboration, and coalition building between the various community organizations with a specific vision and mission targeted to specific populations are needed. Consider how one may begin such a process, and describe in detail.

References

Basch, C. E., Wolf, R. L., Brouse, C. H., Shmukler, C., Neugut, A., DeCarlo, L. T., & Shea, S. (2006). Telephone outreach to increase colorectal cancer screening in an urban minority population. *American Journal of Public Health, 96*(12), 2246–2253.

Callen, B. L., & Wells, T. J. (2005). Screening for nutritional risk in community-dwelling old-old. *Public Health Nursing, 22*(2), 138–146.

Centers for Disease Control and Prevention. (2008a). Human rabies prevention—United States. *Morbidity and Mortality Weekly Report, 57*(RR03), 1–26, 28. Retrieved from http://www.cdc.gov/mmwr/preview/mmwrhtml/rr5703al.htm

Centers for Disease Control and Prevention. (2008b). Public health response to a rabid kitten—four states. *Morbidity and Mortality Weekly Report, 56*(51), 1337–1340. Retrieved from http://www.cdc.gov/mmwr/preview/mmwrhtml/mm5651a1.htm

Centers for Disease Control and Prevention. (2010). Use of a reduced (4-dose) vaccine schedule for post-exposure prophylaxis to prevent human rabies. *Morbidity and Mortality Weekly Report, 59* (RR-20), 1–9.

Centers for Disease Control and Prevention. (2011). Rabies homepage; transmission. Retrieved from http://www.cdc.gov/rabies/tranmission/index.html

Centers for Disease Control and Prevention. (2014). *CDC Glossary.* Retrieved from http://www.cdc.gov/OPHSS/CSELS/DSEPD/SS1978/glossary

Centers for Disease Control and Prevention. (2016a). *2016 Nationally notifiable infectious diseases.* Retrieved from https://www.cdc.gov/nndss/conditions/notifiable/2016/infectious-diseases/

Centers for Disease Control and Prevention. (2016b). *2016 Nationally notifiable non-infectious conditions.* Retrieved from https://www.cdc.gov/nndss/conditions/notifiable/2016/non-infectious-conditions/

Centers for Disease Control and Prevention. (2016c). *2016 Nationally notifiable outbreaks.* Retrieved from https://www.cdc.gov/nndss/conditions/notifiable/2016/outbreaks/

Centers for Disease Control and Prevention. (2016d). *Advice for people living in or traveling to South Florida.* Retrieved from https://www.cdc.gov/zika/intheus/florida-update.html

Centers for Disease Control Control and Prevention. (2016e). *Advice for people living in or traveling to Brownsville, Texas.* Retrieved from https://www.cdc.gov/zika/intheus/texas-update.html

Centers for Disease Control and Prevention. (2016f). Interim guidelines for protecting workers from occupational exposure to Zika virus. *Occupational Safety and Health Administration Fact Sheet.* Retrieved from http://www.cdc.gov/zika/he-providers/index.html

Centers for Disease Control and Prevention. (2016g). *Zika virus disease in the United States, 2015-2016.* Retrieved from http://www.cdc.gov/zika/geo/united-states.html

Cetron, M. (2016). Revision to CDC's Zika travel notices: Minimal likelihood for mosquito-borne Zika virus transmission at elevations higher than 2,000 meters. *Morbidity And Mortal Weekly Reports (MMWR), 65*(10), 267–268. Retrieved from http://www.cdc.gov/mmwr/volumes/65/wr/mm6510e1.htm

Continuing Appropriations and Military Construction, Veterans Affairs and Related Agencies and Zika Response and Preparedness Act. (2017). *114th Congress H.R. 5325 Title 1—Department of Health and Human Services.* Retrieved from https://www.congress.gov/bill/114th-congress/house-bill/5325

Damush, T. M., Huanguang, J., Ried, L. D., Quin, H., Cameon, R., Plue, L., & Williams, L. S. (2008). Case-finding algorithm for post-stroke depression in veterans health administration. *International Journal of Geriatric Psychiatry, 23,* 517–522.

Dietrich, A. J., Tobin, J. N., Robinson, C. M., Cassells, A., Greene, M. A., Dunn, V. H.. . . Beach, M. (2013). Telephone outreach to increase colon cancer screening in Medicaid-managed care organizations: A randomized controlled trial. *Annals of Family Medicine. 11*(4), 335–343.

Dirlikov, E., Ryff, K. R., & Torres-Aponte, J., Thomas, D. L., Perez-Padilla, J., Munoz-Jordan, J., ... Rivera-Garcia, B. (2016). *Update: Ongoing Zika virus transmission—Puerto Rico, November 1, 2015–April 14, 2016.* MMWR Morb Mortal Wkly Rep (MMRW), *65*(17), 451–455. Retrieved from http://www.cdc.gov /mmwr/volumes/65/wr/mm6517e2.htm

Fairchild, A. L., & Bayer, R. (2016). In the name of population well-being: The case for public health surveillance. *Journal of Health Politics, Policy and Law, 41*(1), 119–128.

Fedder, D., Desai, H., & Maciunskaite, M. (2006). Putting a public health face on clinical practice: Potential for using an infectious disease management model for chronic disease prevention. *Disease Management Health Outcome, 14*(6), 329–333.

Findley, S. E., Irigoyen, M., Sanchez, M., Stockwell, M. S., Mejia, M., Guzman, L., . . . Andres-Martinez, R. (2008). Effectiveness of a community coalition for improving child vaccination rates in New York City. *American Journal of Public Health, 98*(11), 1959–1962.

Glasson, N. M., Crossland, L. J., & Larakins, S. L. (2016). An innovative Australian outreach model of diabetic retinopathy screening in remote communities. *Journal of Diabetes Research*. Retrieved from http://dx.doi.org/10.1155/2016/1267215

Hagan, J. E., Smith, W., Pillai, S. K., Yeoman, K., Gupta, S., Neatherlin, J., . . . Nyenswah, T. (2015). Implementation of Ebola case-finding using a village chieftaincy taskforce in a remote outbreak—Liberia, 2014. *Morbidity and Mortality Weekly Report* (MMWR), *64*(7), 183–185.

Hartge, P., & Berg, C. (2007). Improving uptake of cancer screening in women. *Journal of Women's Health, 16*(1), 66–67.

Hennessey, M., Fischer, M., & Staples, J. E. (2016). Zika virus spreads to new areas-region of the Americas, May 2015–January 2016. *Morbidity Mortality Weekly Report (MMWR), 65*(3), 55–58. Retrieved from http://www.cdc.gov/mmwr/volumes/65/wr /mm6503e1.htm

Hills, S. L., Russell, K., Hennessey, M., Williams, C., Oster, A. M., Fischer, M., & Mead, P. (2016). Transmission of Zika virus through sexual contact with travelers to areas of ongoing transmission in continental United States, 2016. *Morbidity Mortality Weekly Report (MMWR), 65*(8), 215–216. Retrieved from http://www.cdc.gov/mmwr/volumes/65/wr /mm6508e2.htm

Holger-Ambrose, B., Langmade, C., Edinburgh, L. D., & Saewyc, E. (2013). The illusions and juxtapositions of commercial sexual exploitation among youth: Identifying effective street outreach strategies. *Journal of Child Sexual Abuse, 22*(3), 326–340.

Jack, S. M., Jamuson, E., Wathen, C. N., & MacMillan, H. L. (2008). The feasibility of screening for intimate partner violence during postpartum home visits. *Canadian Journal of Nursing Research, 40*(2), 150–170.

Khan, M. R., Ravelomanana, N., Van Damme, K., Randrianasolo, B. S., Ramaniraka, V., Ranaivo, N., . . . Behets, F. (2010). Notifying partners of patients with early syphilis in Madagascar: Case-finding effectiveness and public health implications. *Tropical Medicine and International Health, 15*(9), 1090–1098.

Keller, L., & Strohschein, S. (2016). Population-based public health nursing practice: The intervention wheel. In M. Stanhope & J. Lancaster (Eds.), *Public health nursing: Population-centered health care in the community* (8th ed., pp. 190–216). St. Louis, MO: Mosby Elsevier.

Klaucke, D. N., Buehler, J. W., Thacker, S. B., Parrish, R. G., Trowbridge, F. L., Berkelman, R. L., & the Surveillance Coordination Group. (1988). Guidelines for evaluation surveillance systems. *Morbidity and Mortality Weekly Report, Supplements, 37*(S-5), 1–18.

Kulbok, P. A., Thatcher, E., Park, E., & Meszaros, P. S. (2012). Evolving public health nursing roles; focus on community participatory health promotion and prevention. *The Online Journal of Issues in Nursing, 17* (2), para. 3. Retrieved from http://www.nursingworld .org/MainMenuCategories/ANAMarketplace /ANAPeriodicals/OJIN/TableofContents/Vol-17-2012 /No2-May-2012/Evolving-Public-Health-Nursing -Roles.html

Leavell, H., & Clark, E. (1965). *Preventive medicine for the doctor in his community: An epidemiologic approach.* New York, NY: McGraw-Hill.

Lewenson, S. B. (2017). Historical exemplars in nursing. In S. B. Lewenson & M. Truglio-Londrigan (Eds.), *Practicing primary health care in nursing: Caring for populations* (pp. 1–17). Sudbury, MA: Jones & Bartlett Learning.

Liebman, J., Lamberti, M. P., & Altice, F. (2002). Effectiveness of a mobile medical van in providing screening in services for STDs and HIV. *Public Health Nursing, 19*(5), 345–353.

McKeown, R., & Hilfinger Messias, D. K. (2008). Epidemiology. In M. Stanhope & J. Lancaster (Eds.), *Public health nursing: Population-centered health care in the community* (7th ed., pp. 241–277). St. Louis, MO: Mosby Elsevier.

McNeal, G. (2008). UMDNJ School of Nursing mobile healthcare project: A component of The New Jersey Children's Health Project. *The ABNF Journal, Fall,* 121–128.

Minnesota Department of Health, Division of Community Health Services, Public Health Nursing Section. (2001). *Public health interventions: Application for public health nursing practice.* St: Paul: Minnesota Department of Health.

Mock, J., McPhee, S., Nguyen, T., Wong, C., Doan, H., Lai, K. Q., . . . Bui-Tong, N. (2007). Effective lay health worker outreach and media-based education for promoting cervical cancer screening among Vietnamese American women. *American Journal of Public Health, 97*(9), 1693–1700.

Nandi, A., Galea, S., Lopez, G., Nandi, V., Strongarone, S., & Ompad, D. C. (2008). Access to and use of health services among undocumented Mexican immigrants in a U.S. urban area. *American Journal of Public Health, 98*(11), 2011–2020.

New Jersey Department of Health and Senior Services. (2007). *Standards of care for tuberculosis disease and latent TB infection.* Retrieved from http://www.state.nj.us/health/tb/documents/complete_standards_of_care.pdf

New Jersey Department of Health and Senior Services. (2015). *Shigellosis.* Retrieved from http://www.state.nj.us/health/cd/documents/chapters/shigellosis_ch.pdf

New Jersey Department of Health and Senior Services. (2016a). *Tuberculosis: Frequently asked questions.* Retrieved from http://www.state.nj.us/health/tb/tbqa.shtml

New Jersey Department of Health and Senior Services. (2016b). *New Jersey Administrative Code Department of Health and Senior Services Title 8, Chapter 57, Communicable Disease.* Retrieved from http://www.state.nj.us/health/tb/documents/njac8-57_tb_regulation

Pepin, R., Hoyt, J., Karatzas, L., & Bartels, S. I. (2014). New Hampshire REAPs Results: Tailored outreach program assists older adults at risk for mental health conditions and substance misuse. *Journal of American Society of Aging, 38*(3), 68–74.

Petersen, E. E., Poles, K. N., Meaney, D., Ellington, S. R., Oduyebo, T., Cohn, A., . . . Rasmussen, S. A. (2016). Interim guidance for healthcare providers caring for women of reproductive age with possible Zika virus exposure—United States 2016. *Morbidity and Mortality Weekly Report (MMWR), 65*(12), 315–322. Retrieved from http://www.cdc.gov/mmwr/volumes/65/wr/mm6512e2.htm

Petersen, E. E., Staples, J. E., Meaney-Delmon, D., Fischer, M., Ellington, S. R., Callaghan, W. M., & Jamieson, D. J. (2016). Interim guidelines for pregnant women during a Zika virus outbreak—United States, 2016. *Morbidity Mortality Weekly Report (MMWR), 65*(2), 30–33. Retrieved from http://www.cdc.gov/mmwr/volumes/65/wr/mm6502e1.htm

Public Health Action Support Team. (2011). *Health knowledge: Screening* [online tutorial]. Retrieved from http://www.healthknowledge.org.uk/interactive-learning/screening

Puddifoot, S., Arroll, B., Goodyear-Smith, F. A., Kerse, N. M., Fishman, T. G., & Gunn, J. M. (2007). A new case-finding tool for anxiety: A pragmatic diagnostic validity study in primary care. *International Journal of Psychiatry in Medicine, 37*(4), 371–381.

Rajabiun, S., Mallinson, R. K., McCoy, K., Coleman, S., Drainoni, M., Rebholz, C., & Holbert, T. (2007). The public health approach to eliminating disparities in health. *American Journal of Public Health, 98*(3), 400–403.

Schuler-Faccini, L., Ribeiro, E. M., Feitosa, I. M., Horovitz, D. D., Cavalcanti, D. P., Pessoa, A., . . . Brazilian Medical Genetics Society–Zika Embryopathy Task Force. (2016). Possible association between Zika virus infection and microcephaly—Brazil,2015. *Morbidity Mortality Weekly Report (MMWR), 65*(3), 59–62. Retrieved from http://www.cdc.gov/mmwr/volumes/65/wr/mm6503e2.htm

Simm, P. J., Wong, N., Fraser, L., Kearney, J., Fenton, J., Jachno, K., & Cameron, F. J. (2014). Geography does not limit optimal diabetes care: Use of a tertiary center model of care in an outreach service for type 1 diabetes mellitus. *Journal of Paediatrics and Child Health, 50*(6), 471–475.

Skjerve, A., Nordhus, I. H., Engedal, K., Pallesen, S., Braekhus, A., & Nygoord, H. A. (2007). The seven-minute screen (7MS). *International Journal of Geriatric Psychiatry, 8,* 764–769.

Tembreull, C. L., & Schaffer, M. A. (2005). The intervention of outreach: Best practices. *Public Health Nursing, 22*(4), 347–353.

Toole, T., Conde-Martel, A., Gibbon, J., Hanusa, B., Freyder, P., & Fine, M. (2007). Where do people go when they first become homeless? A survey of homeless adults in the USA. *Health and Social Care in the Community, 15*(5), 446–453.

Truglio-Londrigan, M., Arnold, J., Santiao, M., De Sevo, M., Higgins Donius, M. A., & Valencia Go, G. (2000). "Knocking on 99 doors": The experience of The College of New Rochelle (New York). In P. S. Matteson (Ed.), *Community-based nursing education: The experience of eight schools of nursing* (pp. 57–75). New York, NY: Springer.

Tsai, A. C., Tomlinson, M., Dewing, S., le Roux, I. M., Harwood, J. M., Chopra, M., & Rotheram-Borus. (2014). Antenatal depression case finding by community health workers in South Africa: Feasibility of a mobile phone application. *Archives of Women's Mental Health, 17*(5), 423–431.

U.K. National Screening Committee. (2008). *What is screening?* Retrieved from http://www.nsc.nhs.uk/whatscreening/whatscreen_ind.htm

U.S. Department of Health and Human Services Public Health Service, Centers for Disease Control and Prevention. (1992). *Principles of epidemiology: An introduction to applied epidemiology and biostatistics* (2nd ed.). Washington, DC: American Public Health Association.

U.S. Department of Health and Human Services, Centers for Disease Control and Prevention. (2006). *Principles of epidemiology: An introduction to applied epidemiology and biostatistics* (3rd ed.). Washington, DC: American Public Health Association.

U.S. Department of Health and Human Services. (2016). *Healthy People 2020.* Health Communication and Health Information Technology. Retrieved from https://www.healthypeople.gov/2020/topics-objectives/topic/health-communication-and-health-information-technology

U.S. Preventive Services Task Force. (2013). *Grade definitions.* Retrieved from http://www.uspreventiveservicestaskforce.org/Page/Name/grade-definitions

U.S. Preventive Services Task Force. (2015). *Screening for colorectal cancer.* Retrieved from http://www.uspreventiveservicestaskforce.org/Page/Document/UpdateSummaryFinal/colorectal-cancer-screening

Vanderburg, S., Wright, L., Boston, S., & Zimmerman, G. (2010). Maternal child home visiting program improves nursing practice for screening of woman abuse. *Public Health Nursing, 27*(4), 347–352.

Venes, D. (2005). *Taber's cyclopedic medical dictionary* (20th ed.). Philadelphia, PA: F. A. Davis.

Wald, N. J. (2007). Screening: A step too far. A matter of concern. *Journal of Medical Screening, 14*(4), 163–164.

Wald, L. D. (1917, November). The visiting nurse in public health work. Speech delivered at the Chapter for Red Cross Junior League Board. Lillian Wald Papers. Writings & Speeches, Nurses & Nursing, Reel 25, Box 37 , Folder 3, pp. 1–4. New York Public Library, Humanities and Social Sciences Library, Manuscripts and Archives Division, New York.

Wimbush, F., & Peters, R. (2000). Identification of cardiovascular risk: Use of a cardiovascular-specific genogram. *Public Health Nursing, 17*(3), 148–154.

World Health Organization. (2008). *WHO-recommended standards for surveillance of selected vaccine-preventable diseases.* Geneva, Switzerland: Author.

World Health Organization. (2010). *Priority interventions: HIV/AIDS prevention, treatment and care in the health sector.* Geneva, Switzerland: Author.

World Health Organization. (2016). *Time line of emergence of Zika virus in the Americas.* Retrieved from http://www.paho.org/hq/index.php?option=com _content&view=article&id=11959&Itemid=41711 &lang=en

Zika Response Appropriations Act. (2016). *114th Congress, 2016. H.R. 5243.* Retrieved from https://www.congress.gov/bill/114th-congress /house-bill/5243

Zucker, D. M., Choi, J., & Gallagher, E. (2011). Mobile outreach strategies for screening hepatitis and HIV in high-risk populations. *Public Health Nursing, 29*(1), 27–35.

For a full suite of assignments and additional learning activities, use the access code located in the front of your book to visit this exclusive website: **http://go.jblearning.com/londrigan**. If you do not have an access code, you can obtain one at the site.

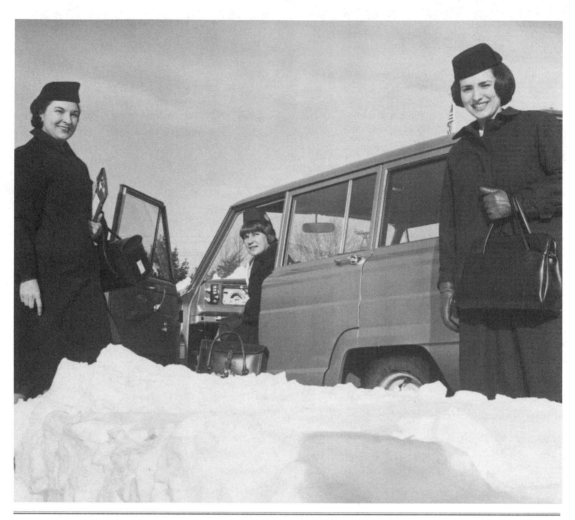

Courtesy of Charlottesville-Albemarle Public Health Nursing, Imogene Bunn Collection: University of Virginia.

CHAPTER 12

Running the Show: Referral and Follow-up, Case Management, and Delegated Functions

Janna L. Dieckmann

The presence of the mother is of great value, and while giving technical nursing care the nurse has exceptional opportunity to demonstrate object lessons in health and sanitation. The daily bath, the antiseptic care of mouth, nasal passage, eyes and excretory organs, the application of hydrotherapy, the careful recording of symptoms, the regularity of visits, the preparing of diet, the skill in making the best use of the surroundings—all these are impressive and achieve results that those without experience might scarcely think credible. (Wald, 1918, p. 8)

LEARNING OBJECTIVES

At the completion of this chapter, the reader will be able to:

- Describe the steps of the referral and follow-up process.
- Describe the case management process.
- Examine the public health nurses' intervention strategy, delegation.

- Discuss how the green wedge intervention strategies may be implemented at the individual/family, community, population, and system levels.

KEY TERMS

- ❏ Case management
- ❏ Delegation

- ❏ Referral and follow-up

The public health nurse designs and implements interventions within a complex network of health, social welfare, housing, and other services. Maximizing nursing services requires nurses' comprehensive knowledge and effective interface with a complex and well-functioning system of services that are available and accessible while offering culturally competent and congruent care. Public health nurses have understood that the determinants of health and the multiple causation of disease mean that individual and population-based change must have multiple foci. Public health nursing services work best by collaborating with other community-based caring and helping systems. Patients, families, populations of interest, systems, and communities—require more than public health nurses can directly provide. Public health nurses are experts in identifying individual, family, and population needs all the while collaborating and making the essential connections to community service providers and services systems.

This chapter addresses three important public health interventions in the green wedge of the intervention wheel: referral and follow-up, case management, and delegated functions. These interventions have similarities, may overlap, and address similar objectives. All three interventions draw the public health nurse to working beyond the nurse–individual dyad, as the nurse seeks to add the contributions of other community services and health providers to improve the health system for the individual, family, population, and the community. At the community practice level, this means public health nurse participation in initiating services or expanding availability and access to meet an identified need. At the systems practice level, the public health nurse strives to provide the evidence to modify organizations and policies that shape systems of care. At the individual/family practice level, this includes interventions to change knowledge, attitudes, beliefs, practices, and behaviors (Keller & Strohschein, 2016).

The first of the three public health interventions addressed in this chapter, referral and follow-up,

"assists individuals, families, groups, organizations, and/or communities to identify and access necessary resources in order to prevent or resolve problems or concerns" (Keller & Strohschein, 2016, p. 206). Case management "optimizes self-care capabilities of individuals and families and the capacity of systems and communities to coordinate and provide services" (Keller & Strohschein, 2016, p. 206). Delegated functions, the third intervention, "are direct care tasks a registered professional nurse carries out under the authority of a healthcare practitioner as allowed by law. Delegated functions also include any direct care tasks a registered professional nurse entrusts to other appropriate personnel to perform" (Keller & Strohschein, 2016, p. 206).

The Intervention Wheel Strategies and Levels of Practice

Referral and Follow-Up

Referral and follow-up interventions are hallmarks of public health nursing. The referral process is defined as "a systematic problem-solving approach involving a series of actions that help individuals use resources for the purpose of resolving needs" (Clemen-Stone, McGuire, & Eigsti, 2002, p. 316). Many studies have analyzed the referral process used as a strategy for varying populations and health/illness experiences. For example, studies have dealt with cancer screening and the referral process in rural regions (Ristevski et al., 2015); sexually active vulnerable adolescent females (Chernick et al., 2015); smoking cessation (Suen et al., 2016); and intimate partner violence (Muench et al., 2013).

As a practice expectation and as an ongoing intervention, the public health nurse seeks to link individuals/families, populations, communities, and systems to resources. New public health nurses quickly gain knowledge of the interfaces between target populations and assistive resources. Experienced public health nurses have extensive information, experiences, and facility in establishing linkages between and among community members, groups, and organizations. Individuals/families, populations, communities, and systems often seek the knowledge and advice of public health nurses when they want to know where to go for help or when they want to improve systems and services that provide resources (Rippke et al., 2001, p. 81).

Referral and follow-up interventions are related to other public health nurse interventions and generally occur in the context of ongoing nursing service. For example, health teaching for weight reduction provided by the public health nurse to a group of adults at a community center may encourage group members' interest in increasing their physical activity and muscle strength. Based on group members' expressed need, the public health nurse would seek and explore appropriate resources and provide group members with a tailored recommendations and referrals of relevant resources. At a later point, the public health nurse would evaluate or follow up on the referrals to determine the extent and the character of the contacts between group members and the resources to which they were referred. In this example, referral and follow-up interventions further the goals of the health teaching intervention but remain a separate intervention characterized by unique guidelines, practices, and values. The referral process is most effective when it is linked to other public health nurse interventions.

Referral and follow-up interventions may be applied with counseling or consultation interventions to link the individual/family, population, community, or system to a resource to prevent or resolve a problem or concern. The more information the public health nurse has about the expressed concern and the targeted intervention, the better and more sustainable the referral and follow-up is likely to be. Referral and follow-up is also used after screening and case-finding (related to surveillance, disease investigation, and/or outreach) to address a need identified by this particular public health nurse intervention. The ethics of both screening and case-finding direct the public health nurse to make formal plans to respond to newly identified needs. For example, when the individual or family has a positive screening result or a case is identified, linkage to a relevant resource is required. Advocacy interventions also generally demand linkage(s) to services and resources to address aspirations and needs at any practice level.

The two other intervention approaches addressed in this chapter, case management and delegated functions, are also interrelated with the referral and follow-up intervention. Case management is a goal-oriented process that uses available resources to achieve case management objectives. Referral and follow-up interventions occur jointly with the case management plan. Delegated function interventions shift care responsibility to an eligible resource or provider of care. The interface with this resource requires the public health nurse to apply referral and follow-up strategies. Additional elements of case management and delegated functions interventions are described in later sections of this chapter.

PUBLIC HEALTH NURSES AS SENDERS AND RECEIVERS OF REFERRALS

Public health nurses make and receive referrals. They may send or initiate a referral on behalf of an individual, or they may receive a referral for a new or already known individual. The process of receiving referrals at a public health nursing organization is generally formal to accommodate the frequency of requests and provide a means to track data and referral outcomes. Referrals—both formal referrals from organizations and professionals and informal referrals from the individual or the individual's network—are received as part of an intake process at the public health nurse organization. In some agencies, public health nurses are permanently assigned to receive referrals, and in some agencies, the intake function rotates among nurses. For cost or effectiveness reasons, intake may be alternatively delegated to skilled non-nurse staff members under the direction of a public health nurse. Once a referral is received, it is weighed, and a plan to respond is established. The referral may be accepted for services from the public health nurse organization, or it may be determined that the needed resources or services are not available from the public health nurse organization. In this situation, the referral may be declined, and the referring agency or person is promptly notified by intake public health nurses. The intake public health nurse, however, may also make recommendations for more appropriate, alternate agencies to receive the referral. Most communities have organized systems of information and referral. These systems request specific information about the individual and the need to closely match the request with an appropriate resource.

The intake function of public health nurse agencies provides nurses and organizations with information about community needs and about gaps in resource availability, affordability, and appropriateness. Even when a public health nurse organization is unable to respond to an intake request, each request helps build a description of current community needs. When a mismatch between community need and existing resources is found, public health nurses and public health nurse organizations will seek to meet emerging or newly defined needs by developing new resources or by modifying or improving existing resources. Analysis of the needs may also suggest that resources exist but that there is a barrier to access. For example, a community organization providing HIV/AIDS prevention and care services has historically targeted a defined geographic area. Now, a neighboring area requires resources because it has experienced increased HIV incidence and AIDS prevalence. One solution would be to expand the existing HIV/AIDS service area into the neighboring community.

GAINING KNOWLEDGE ABOUT AVAILABLE FORMAL RESOURCES

Public health nurses must gain a working knowledge of available community resources to make effective referrals and must develop working relationships with resource organizations to fulfill follow-up obligations. How does a public health nurse build knowledge of community agencies and resources? Descriptive and contact information about community agencies and resources should be included in the public health agency orientation and public health staff development programs. Information can be shared in print or electronic formats, especially when there are changes in eligibility or availability of services. Many public health nurses maintain contact lists or active files of potential community resources. Public health nurse agencies may also develop relationships with specific resources, which may include formal strategies for interagency contact, referral, and follow-up. Consultations with public health nurse supervisors or agency social workers can assist public health nurses to identify relevant resources.

In addition to formal structures for gaining information about community agencies, organizations, and resources, public health nurses learn about agencies through their informal networks. Informal networking with other public health nurses is often the most fruitful source of resource identification. Individuals, families, and other health professionals can provide information about resources, which is especially helpful when it is from the resource user's viewpoint. Observing the presence and activities of other agencies and organizations in a community also suggests who is operating in an area and the types of services offered. For example, home-delivered meals are a strategic service for homebound elders and the chronically ill. Before referring an individual, a public health nurse would pose questions about the service to colleagues and individuals. Perhaps a home-delivered meal program provides excellent meals at the promised time at an inexpensive cost. On the other hand, perhaps the service's waiting list is 10 months, meals are too salty for many recipients, and delivery drivers get lost and miss deliveries. Knowing what to expect from a potential resource, as well as whether the individual can accept the pros and cons of resource operations, enables the public health nurse to weigh the value of the actual referral.

Identifying Referral Needs: When and Who?

A referral must have merit. Merit takes into consideration whether a referral is the right referral at the right time for the right individual. Determining the merit of a referral is heavily influenced by (1) an individual's values as well as the community values and expectations, (2) whether or not referrals are an effective strategy, (3) the timing of a referral, (4) whether the referral is to prevent a problem or address an existing problem, and (5) the nature of the match between the referral resource and the individual.

The important point to be made here is that the *when* and the *who* of the referral process becomes evident as the public health nurse carries out a detailed assessment of the individual and family along with a detailed assessment of the community and the organizational systems within that community. Based upon these assessments and the partnership with individuals and families, public health nurses provide information and make recommendations about potential referrals in order to prevent problems and potential crisis. The actual timing of making referrals may vary among public health nurses and across public health nurse organizations. Some public health nurses wrap referrals into case closure activities, whereas others ensure that referrals are made early enough in the nurse–individual/family relationship. Early referrals ensures that the new community service begins before the public health nurse service terminates, thereby, enabling the public health nurse to both observe the impact of the community resource's contacts with the individual and directly ask the individual about the use and the success of the referral agency's services.

Steps to Conducting Referral and Follow-Up

Implementing the steps of the referral and follow-up intervention assumes active individual participation and control. Assistance in planning is offered to the individual, and the public health nurse collaborates and works with the individual. Because the referral process is individual centered, the public health nurse avoids making decisions for the individual but seeks to establish a working partnership that uses a problem-solving approach involving shared decision-making to achieve shared goals (Truglio-Londrigan, 2013, 2015; Truglio-Londrigan, Slyer, Singleton, & Worral, 2014).

An individual/family, population, community, and system may vary across a continuum as to their ability to contribute to the referral process. Some individuals are dependent on the public health nurse for gathering information, weighing options, and requesting the referral. In these situations, public health nurses use referral planning and implementation for educational purposes and to build relevant skills and independence in individuals. Other individuals are more autonomous in considering and implementing referrals, placing the public health nurse in almost a consultative role. Here, the public health nurse validates and extends the individual's independent problem-solving behaviors. The public health nurse provides these individuals with the opportunity to learn and adopt new behaviors to achieve their next steps to full independence.

The steps to conduct referral and follow-up are sequential; these steps are based on the outline provided by Clemen-Stone, McGuire, and Eigsti (2002) and McGuire, Gerber, and Clemen-Stone (1996). If a need or a resource cannot be identified, or if the individual declines referral, it may be useful to revisit earlier steps. These steps are appropriate for individuals/families, populations, communities, and systems. Additional comments about the implications of the referral and follow-up intervention for communities and systems are found at the end of this section (see Referrals and Follow-Up at Systems and Community Practice Levels later in this chapter).

Step 1: Establish a nursing relationship with the individual. Nursing interventions begin with establishing a respectful working relationship with the individual, which serves as a basis for individualizing or targeting care. The referral and follow-up intervention are often used with existing individuals for whom the public health nurse has provided other public health interventions. Here, the professional relationship has already been established. On the other hand, a public health nurse may initiate a professional relationship with a new individual solely to develop and implement a referral and a follow-up. Whether based in an ongoing collaborative intervention or in a brief encounter, the public health nurse must similarly establish trust and gain the individual's agreement to engage in the referral process. Public health nurses may quickly assess and develop working hypotheses about the individual that may later be confirmed, but the nurse should not establish fixed assumptions in the initial step (Hupcey, Penrod, Morse, & Mitcham, 2001; John, 1996; Matthias, Salyers, & Frankel, 2013; Truglio-Londrigan, 2013).

Step 2: Identify individual need and set objectives for referral. Based on a caring, professional relationship with the individual, the public health nurse gathers information about the individual, their family, and the individual's context. Listening to the individual's perspective on his or her current situation and larger context is crucial (Wolfe, 1962). What is it that the individual sees as his or her need, and what are the parameters of the need? Individuals may benefit from a thorough discussion of the need. Allowing the individual to review and describe a need provides essential information for the nurse, but the process of verbally articulating needs also enhances comprehension of the need, investment in the referral process, and self-efficacy in securing a solution. Because one intention of the referral process is to increase individual autonomy and independence, incorporating strategies that facilitate empowerment is beneficial to strengthening current decisions for self-care and later self-determination (Gallant, Beaulieu, & Carnevale, 2002; Hain & Sandy, 2013).

When the public health nurse has secured an apparent understanding of the needs, the nurse reflects a synthesis of the need back to the individual to confirm that what has been heard is what the individual meant to convey. Probing for further information or perspective may be helpful.

After brief consideration, the public health nurse presents his or her summary of the individual's expressed need and proposes options for addressing this need. Critically important at this point is the nurse's determination whether the need is in actuality one need or several. If several, then the public health nurse proposes at least two ways of posing the need and gains agreement with one interpretive approach. Given a favored approach, the nurse and the individual work collaboratively to establish objectives for the referral.

This give-and-take process may be quite brief, or it may be lengthy, especially in the event of conflict and negotiation (Coulter & Collins, 2011; Roberts & Krouse, 1988; Segal & Smith, 2013). If the referral and follow-up intervention is conducted with an individual/family, organization, community, or system, more than one well-organized meeting may be required to share information, make decisions, and gain a working consensus about objectives. As the process of making a referral proceeds, the nurse and the individual may choose to return to this step for further clarification of need(s) and redetermination of objectives.

Step 3: Search for resources and explore resource availability. A systematic search for resources to meet the need and the identified referral objectives is conducted by the nurse, sometimes with participation of the individual. Public health nurses familiar with meeting needs similar to the individual's may quickly establish a group of options, either from personal experience or from consulting personal or agency resource files. Addressing more complex individual needs may require consultation with professional colleagues or with information and referral specialists. Although the principles of making a good referral can guide the public health nurse, a nurse's experience and confidence in making referrals contributes to a prompt and personalized outcome. A nurse's ability to apply the art of nursing is especially relevant in the selection of potential referral resources. The individual and the resource must fit together in both tangible and intangible ways if the individual is to take advantage of the referral so that the identified goals are achieved. Just because a referral is made does not mean that the individual will access the available referral. There are many factors that may prohibit the individual from engaging in the referral or be a no-show, as described by Lyratzopoulos, Vedsted, and Singh (2015). These authors suggest that throughout the provider encounters there are many missed opportunities when working with patients in timely ways. For example, there are missed opportunities during the initial diagnostic assessments, test performance, and interpretation as well as coordination, referral, and follow-up. There are a wide variety of factors that facilitate these missed opportunities such as language barriers, complexity of the healthcare system, as well as accessing needed services. Much of these missed opportunities are facilitated because of the complex interplay between these factors (Lyratzopoulos et al., 2015). Furthermore, these authors suggest that to develop fail-safe systems, follow-up is essential (p. S89), which will be discussed later in this chapter.

Step 4: Individual decides whether to agree to referral. Information about potential referral resources is presented and discussed with the individual. The individual may select a resource(s), may wish to consider the resource(s), or may decline to agree to any referral. It can be helpful to provide written information to allow a later review of potential resources or later communication with the resource by the individual. Application of the referral and follow-up intervention is based on ethical principles of self-determination that places decision-making in the hands of the individual (McGuire et al., 1996; Moser, Houtepen, van der Bruggen, Spreeuwenberg, & Widdershoven, 2009; Moulton & King, 2010). When an individual is uncertain or declines a referral, the public health nurse may explore the individual's feelings and reasons, identify factors that might facilitate or deter resource use, negotiate use of identified resources, propose a wider variety of referral resources, and/or reassess the individual's needs and objectives for service. If an individual declines a referral at any point, no referral is made.

The nurse must balance encouragement with an open ear that the individual does not wish a referral.

Step 5: Public health nurse matches the individual with resource and makes the referral. The individual and the nurse select a resource or resources that best match the individual's needs and preferences. Does the individual believe the resource will work for him or her? The public health nurse's knowledge of the individual and his or her needs is important in making the referral to the identified resource and in explaining the individual to the agency. If the individual is a population, community, or a system, a referral might be a grant application or similar application to secure program funding. When individuals are more experienced or skilled, they may make the referral themselves; this increased skill in self-managing care is a factor in individual empowerment. Others may lack experience, be self-doubting, or be overwhelmed and emotionally fragile. As the nurse makes the referral, he or she asks questions and gains more information to assist the individual to maximize interactions with the resource. The public health nurse also provides the individual with tailored information about the resource and with anticipatory guidance on using the agency's resources.

Some agencies require detailed application information; the nurse gathers information and confirms with the individual what information should be shared. Some communities use written interagency referral forms that have been developed to address system and resource needs for sharing information. Although patient privacy laws now prevent their use, in the past, the agency that received a written referral would respond in writing to the referral source, describing initial contacts and plans for the referred individual or family (Cady, 1952; Kraus, 1944).

Step 6: Follow-up to facilitate client utilization of resource. Nursing interventions at this step, alternatively called following along, can ease the individual's experience with the resource. Soon after the individual follows through and contacts the resource, the public health nurse contacts the individual to determine the progress and engagement with the resource. Is the individual using the resource as planned? Is the resource agency engaged with the individual? The public health nurse can reemphasize the purpose of the referral, interpret the resource to the individual and the individual to the resource, and promote linkages between the two. If signs of a weak linkage and connection are found, the nurse may advocate for the individual with the resource. The public health nurse can also directly address any barriers to seeking or using the resource.

Step 7: Evaluation of referral process and outcome. Did the individual access and receive services, and what was provided by the resource? Was the individual satisfied by the service? In what way(s) did the individual's status change as a result of working with the resource? Obtaining adequate information and data for evaluation can be challenging, but it is an essential element in the ongoing process of making referrals. Whether the recipient of the referral and follow-up process is an individual/family, population, community, or system, evaluation of the referral and its outcomes has system-level implications. Lack of resources or poor service from resources in the community suggests gaps that public health nurses should address. Because the referral and follow-up intervention is a continuous process, public health nurses learn from each referral and provide feedback to improve the system itself and nurses' utilization of system resources.

Barriers to Successful Referral and Follow-up

Successful follow-through on any referral frequently depends on the resources of individuals and is based on several factors. Wolfe's (1962) classic analysis identified the central role of individual motivation in initiating resource utilization: To what extent does the individual see the referral and resource use as important? Does the referral appear to be practical and relevant to the situation? Individualizing the referral for the individual or the family and tailoring the referral to the expressed preferences enhance referral utilization.

The concepts of perceived benefits and perceived barriers in the health belief model can assist in facilitating follow-through for resource use (Simons-Morton, McLeroy, & Wendel, 2012). Individuals accept a recommended referral only when they expect a benefit that is greater than the perceived barriers. Public health nurse interventions are designed to enhance perceived benefits by clarifying the expected positive impact of accepting the referral and by explaining specific actions to engage with the referral resource. At the same time, public health nurse interventions are directed toward reducing perceived tangible and psychological costs of accepting the referral by identifying perceived barriers and reducing their impact through clarifying misinformation and applying reassurance, incentives, and concrete assistance to use the resource (Champion & Skinner, 2008, pp. 47–49). For example, in a study of women who presented with an abnormal mammogram, improvement with referral follow-through was noted when barriers were addressed via comprehensive education along with support in addressing barriers such as assistance with scheduling appointments, arrangement of transportation, and resolving insurance issues (Perdac-Lima, Ashburner, McCarthy, Piawah, & Steven, 2015).

Public health nurse interventions at the system and community practice levels seek to reduce institutional and systemic barriers; for example, providing care that is respectful and responsive to the cultural ideas values and beliefs of the population being served, enhancing the availability of services by offering evening and weekend service hours, further expanding communication and language assistance, and ensuring that those providing this assistance have the necessary knowledge, skills, and competency, as well as recruiting and promoting diverse leadership (Federal Register, 2013; Office of Minority Health, 2001).

A wide variety of factors may delay or obstruct participation in the referral process or in using the referred resource, despite initial agreement with the significance of the problem, plans for solution, and selection of and referral to the resource. From an individual or family viewpoint, differences in religious/spiritual/cultural beliefs or practices can increase uncertainty and reduce trust of a new resource. Individuals may become uncertain about why they were referred to a resource or doubt that it is a priority and so postpone or forget to engage with services. Structural barriers, such as geographic barriers, may make certain resources unusable, or resources may simply be unavailable. Appointment times may be inconvenient or require a long wait. Financial barriers may place needed resources out of reach or may delay the resource's acceptance by the individual so long that they lose the motivation to make the change.

These barriers may also suggest ineffective or flawed systems or a failure of the system's capacity (Lyratzopoulos et al., 2015) due to the lack of financial or professional resources or a lack of consensus to address individual/family or community problems or concerns. Public health nurses may need to advocate at the community or system levels; for example, this advocacy may include screening services or enhancing existing services to improve utilization, such as translation or handicap accessibility.

Strategies for Follow-up

Several effective strategies are helpful to use in following up on referrals. If resources are limited, public health nurses may establish priorities for whom to contact on the basis of complexity of need or family situation, or on frequency or intensity of individual contacts during the referral process. On the other hand, it may be helpful to invest in following up on all referrals. For example, until 1937, public health nurses in New York City delivered infants' birth certificates directly to the family home because this provided an opportunity to refer newborns for prompt health supervision (Bokhaut & Mahoney, 1960).

Follow-up postcards or letters can be sent to individuals, but responding to mailed forms can require significant effort. Electronic mail or text messaging may provide easier communication

exchanges, but this technique may not be available to all or an acceptable strategy by all. Telephone calls provide a framework for effective follow-up intervention, which may facilitate a review of the referral and its outcomes, supportive listening, additional teaching, or identifying/making additional referrals (Cave, 1989). This additional contact can reconfirm the appropriateness of the referral and the resource for the individual, and it allows for an additional assessment of the individual and context. Follow-up home visits can be extremely useful. One teen pregnancy program found that home visiting led to significant increases in the proportion of prenatal adolescents who identified and kept prenatal appointments; enrolled in the Women, Infants, and Children program; and applied for Medicaid (Flynn, Budd, & Modelski, 2008). Furthermore, the use of patient navigators as a strategy has demonstrated successful outcomes, many also incorporating other strategies such as telephone calls. Luckett, Pena, Vitonis, Bernstein, and Feldman (2015) demonstrated that patient navigators were successful in their work with vulnerable individuals who continually were no-shows for referral to a colonoscopy clinic. These patient navigators were responsible for initially meeting the individual face-to-face; providing language-appropriate materials and resources; discussing potential barriers to referral and follow-up; co-developing solutions; and arranging for transportation, child care, scheduling of appointments, and coordinating of services. In addition, these patient navigators received a list of weekly no-shows and reached out to these individuals via telephone call. The outcome of this work was a decline in the no-shows from 49.7% to 29.5%. A similar program using patient navigators as a follow-up strategy was presented by Percac-Lima, Ashburner, McCarthy, Piawah, and Atlas (2015). In this initiative, patient navigators worked with disadvantaged women with abnormal mammograms to identify potential barriers to their care. These navigators incorporated similar strategies as the former study, also with positive outcomes. These authors found that individuals with patient navigators presented with an improved follow-up by 15% compared with those who did not have patient navigators. Additionally, the technological advancements of today's healthcare environment provide additional evidence of how this technology may be put to use with regard to follow-up (Lillibridge & Hanna, 2008).

Ethics of Referral and Follow-Up

Public health nurses must also navigate several ethical conflicts or challenges embedded in referral and follow-up intervention at any practice level. The first conflict lies in the potential gap between what the individual wishes and wants and the public health nurse's professional determination of need. Should the individual's view or the nurse's view prevail? Some conflicts may arise from a lack of communication or a misunderstanding. In this situation, the public health nurse may have to revisit the process of determining need and selecting objectives to meet the need. Perhaps the individual's need has become more complex or multifaceted than originally determined, or perhaps as a result of the referral process, the individual has become more sophisticated in self-identifying his or her need and has now become more assertive in directing criteria for a reasonable solution. Individuals may also be surprised at the lack of actual resources to meet their need or feel a right to their share out of a belief that others with similar needs have received more assistance.

A second type of ethical conflict in referral and follow-up is determining whether society can or should provide the resources or services that individuals want. Many resources have eligibility criteria that can seem arcane. Is the individual's selected option a need or a want? Differentiating between needs and wants is often a matter of perspective of our needs contrasted against their wants, but public health nurses may have ethical obligations to both the individual and the wider societal system. On what basis do public health nurses make judgments about resource access and distribution? Balancing individual rights to resources against ensuring the wider public good is difficult. The public health nurse must recognize when to protect limited resources and when to strongly advocate for meeting individual needs.

Mandated or legally required referrals are a third type of ethical conflict for the public health nurse. In contrast to a voluntary referral where individuals themselves decide whether to accept or reject, public health nurses must make legal reports or referrals to protect society from certain diseases and health conditions or from violence, abuse, or neglect; for example, parents may neglect immunizations or physically abuse their child, an individual may receive a positive screen for a reportable disease, or a frail older adult may have money stolen by a relative. When referral is mandated, it may be better to directly discuss the mandated referral with the individual/family. If a threat to the nurse is a concern, the discussion may take the form of notification through telephone or written formats. The nurse–individual relationship can survive a mandated referral, thus allowing the public health nurse to be in an excellent position to contribute to and support a solution.

The last ethical conflict occurs when individuals firmly decline a referral. Based on the ethic of self-determination, the solution is extremely clear: the individual always and at any time maintains a right to decline referral. Coercive referrals, or referrals based on subterfuge, have no place in an ethical nursing practice. On the practical side, if individuals oppose a referral, they are very unlikely to engage with or use a resource effectively. Unwelcome referrals are more likely to waste the referral agency's staff time and financial resources. Certainly, public health nurses may provide these individuals with written information about a referral or may call back to check on their subsequent status, but individual refusals of referral are clear and must be respected. Nursing does not practice alone in isolation, and having access to consultation services and working in interprofessional teams only strengthens our practice and certainly a practice where an ethical dilemma is emerging.

REFERRALS AND FOLLOW-UP AT SYSTEMS AND COMMUNITY PRACTICE LEVELS

The principles of referral and follow-up for the individual/family level of practice have been discussed previously in this book. Referral and follow-up, however, also have implications for public health nursing interventions at the systems and community levels. Public health nurse engagement at the community and systems practice levels is often based on direct knowledge gained from individuals/families, of the strengths and weaknesses of the referral process and system, and of follow-up practices in a particular geographic area. Experienced public health nurses often identify weak areas that have the potential to be strengthened through community and systems changes.

Public health nurses must move outside familiar programs and agencies to build linkages with both health and nonhealth resources that seek to monitor and address neighborhood and community needs at the systems level. Thinking broadly and creatively can increase the potential for problem solution through modification of organizations, policies, laws, and/or power relationships. Public health nurse participation and leadership in these initiatives can lead to solutions that can be sustained over time. Perhaps new resources and services will be established in the community, or perhaps nursing organizations will seek support and broaden their existing services. The search for effective and appropriate resources to meet local, contemporary needs is ongoing; evaluation of existing programs and systems is a useful first step.

Acknowledging a need for additional resources and/or greater coordination and linkages among existing agencies may result from careful assessment but also from events that capture community concern. Our daily news often includes tragic reports; one community responded to the murder of a 7-year-old girl by her 12-year-old sister by first gathering and reflecting on the events and on how this might have been prevented. Several agencies had known and worked with this family, but breakdowns in referral and follow-up resulted in inadequate assistance. As a short-term system response, the community nursing service coordinated monthly interagency conferences to discuss cases, problems, and linkages. As a long-term system change, community agencies agreed to work toward improving county mental health services, as well as improve insurance coverage for mental health issues.

The public health nurse also has a role in shaping community norms, attitudes, awareness, practices, and behaviors for referral and follow-up. Are referral systems working well enough that individuals, families, and populations who require assistance are able to locate and use the appropriate resources? Public and private health insurance may not address this expense, but do communities acknowledge these needs? Voluntary charitable groups, such as United Way, provide funding for information and referral services, but many community residents are unfamiliar with this resource and its use. Economic retrenchment in healthcare facilities and agencies may discourage building and maintaining referral and follow-up systems, even when there is evidence that the costs of care can be reduced. Individuals, families, and populations who require referral are often those who least know how to navigate our complex healthcare system. Public health nurses have a role in raising their awareness and in reflecting the deficits of the current referral and follow-up system to the widest community audience. Individuals do need help—and want help—to change, although community attitudes may frame this positive, optimistic quality as overburdening services. Community attitudes and community willingness to make financial commitments are key to improving linkages between those needing resources and existing resources.

Case Management

Case management "optimizes self-care capabilities of individuals and families and the capacity of systems and communities to coordinate and provide services" (Keller & Strohschein, 2016, p. 206). Careful reflection upon the definition of case management provides a detailed accounting of the roles and the responsibilities of the public health nurse who is a case manager. Remember, case management takes place in a variety of settings. Some of these settings may include acute care, school-based programs, public health such as departments of health and/or visiting nurse practices, long-term care, and independent practices. Additionally, the individuals, families, and populations served generally present with complex needs and are vulnerable in their ability to access needed services. As such, a model of case management where there is a care manager who advocates for the individual and family serves the system as well as individuals, families, and populations (Brennan-Ing et al., 2016; Case Management Society of America, 2014; Stergiopoulos et al., 2015).

Case management is often conducted in conjunction with other public health nursing interventions, including both the referral and follow-up intervention and the delegated functions intervention. Depending on individual/family need, a public health nurse using the case management intervention may apply the delegated functions intervention to shift care provision to achieve improved quality or reduced costs or perhaps to secure more culturally relevant care providers fluent in the family's preferred language who are knowledgeable of their cultural practices.

Case management intervention shares some aspects with the referral and follow-up intervention; some have suggested that referral is a component of case management, and others see case management as a more intensive application of referral that involves coordination of that care as well (Brennan-Ing et al., 2016). This chapter interprets case management and referral/follow-up as separate practices that share some elements. For example, the timeline of nurse–individual interactions is quite different between the two as well as the intensity of the work that takes place. In referral, the public health nurse may have limited contacts with the individual/family; after implementing the referral plan, the public health nurse conducts follow-up to facilitate and ensure referral resource utilization and to conduct

evaluation. Case management, in contrast, suggests frequent and more intense interactions over a long period. Ongoing nurse individual/family interactions permit case managers to shadow the individual/family as they use resources to work toward their goal; this approach can be conceptualized as *following along* with the family to facilitate individual/family change. For example, the case management intervention is a systematic approach to care based upon the ongoing work with the individual and family. The work includes a detailed assessment to identify needs. Based upon the needs identified, the public health nurse utilizes his or her knowledge of community resources to link and connect the individual and family to resources. The public health nurse must ensure that connections are strong and that the individual's transition into the new organizational system is seamless. This means the public health nurse will need to provide continual education, teaching the individual and family how to work through and negotiate the healthcare system to obtain their needed resource. Throughout the entire process, communication, collaboration, and ongoing evaluation and management of the utilization of resources is essential (American Case Management Association, 2013).

Case management relates to several other public health nursing interventions. Outreach or case-finding interventions may precede case management to identify individuals/families in need of services; case-finding may also follow case management. Can you think of a situation when this may occur? Case management implementation may include the public health interventions of advocacy, collaboration, consultation, counseling, and health teaching (Rippke et al., 2001).

Framing Case Management

The characteristics of case management can be seen through two contrasting frames. One approach to framing case management relies on its objective, financial outcomes, and cost to relieve a major health system pressure (Stokes et al., 2015). The second contrasting frame for case management relies on meeting the needs and enhancing quality of life for individuals, families, populations, and communities; increasing service quality across the continuum and developing new services when needs are revealed; and developing the capacity of systems and communities to coordinate and provide services (Brennan-Ing, 2016; Hudon, Diadiou, Lambert, & Bouliane, 2015; Rippke et al., 2001; Stergiopoulos, 2015; Stokes et al., 2015). This approach to case management reflects public health nursing values in that it is relationship based—but may yet be a vision rather than a working model.

Case Management at the Individual/Family Practice Level

Case management is a process that is frequently directed toward an individual/family or particular population, especially populations with multiple needs, such as the acute and chronically ill, frail elderly, people living with HIV/AIDS, or homelessness (Brennan-Ing et al., 2016; Hudon, 2015; Maijala, Tossavainen, & Turunen, 2015; Stergiopoulos et al., 2015). As such, the first step in case management at the individual/family practice level is to conduct outreach and case finding to all individuals/families considered at risk and to offer case management services. As this step unfolds, the public health nurse seeks to develop a trusting professional relationship as a basis for effective case management. With the involvement of individuals and families who respond to outreach and meet priority criteria for the agency's case management services, the nurse assesses their functional level to identify their needs. How and what do individuals and families identify as an adequate quality of life, and what is the gap between these goals and their current status? Note that this step should include a comprehensive assessment, including financial resources, especially to ensure adequate financial support; family assessments, as well as assessment of community resources, especially social supports and networks, and whether or not the individual and family have access to these resources.

Using strategies similar to the referral/follow-up intervention, the public health nurse next works with individuals and families to identify helpful resources and design a detailed plan to access these resources. An effective planning process outlines each step to link and connect the individual and family to these services and resources. Because families with multiple needs often require complex resources to meet these needs, the plan should incorporate strategies to form an interprofessional team. Early linkages and connections help professions facilitate coordination and collaboration. The individual/family remains part of the team to assist with troubleshooting to resolve actual or potential barriers to service acquisition and use. Periodic formative evaluations of service organization, coordination, and case management are conducted with providers and the individual/family target of care (Rippke et al., 2001).

Case management by public health nurses has been found to improve health outcomes among women receiving Temporary Assistance for Needy Families (TANF). Kneipp et al. (2011) provided on-site public health nursing case management for women participating in an existing Welfare Transition Program (WTP), a requirement for those receiving TANF. Based on the development of trust with these women, the public health nurse provided case management interventions of "health access or entry into primary care for newly identified symptoms; care coordination; health education; health and social service referrals; obtaining preventive services, screening, and routine care; and assistance in meeting health goals participants had set for themselves" (p. 1761). In combination with the training provided by the WTP, the case management intervention led to improved health status among these women, including improved healthcare visit rates for mental health, reduced symptoms of depression, and improved functional status (Kneipp et al., 2011). Additional research provides evidence that comprehensive case management improves individual engagement with their care and treatment adherence for HIV (Brennan-Inig et al., 2015) and increases stability of housing, reduction in alcohol-related problems, as well as improves community functioning and quality of life in the homeless adults with mental illness (Stergiopoulos et al., 2015). Finally, a qualitative descriptive study by Hudon, Diadiou, Lambert, and Bouliane (2015) reveals that participants demonstrate enhanced satisfaction with case management, noting that the approach facilitates access to care and information as well as ensures coordination among providers. These same participants also identified that improved communication also enhances trust.

CASE MANAGEMENT INTERVENTION AT THE SYSTEM AND COMMUNITY PRACTICE LEVELS

Application of the case management intervention at the system and community practice levels is similar to those for the referral/follow-up intervention. The primary goal is "to create needed resources where resources do not exist or are inadequate" (Rippke et al., 2001, p. 97). The public health nurse intervening at the system or community practice level first identifies a population whose quality of life is at risk and then conducts a resource assessment, similar to a community assessment such as this text's Public Health Nursing Assessment Tool to determine availability, accessibility, acceptability, and cultural competence of existing community resources. Having identified any gaps in community services or in the service system, the nurse collaborates with community organizations and systems to develop policies and plans to address existing gaps. In collaboration with community partners, the public health nurse also ensures and assures that new resources and services are adequate and equitable. Periodic community assessment seeks to determine the "community's capacity to meet the quality-of-life needs of identified populations at risk" (Rippke et al., 2001, p. 97).

Delegation

Delegated functions are direct care tasks that "a registered professional nurse carries out under the authority of a healthcare practitioner as allowed by law. Delegated functions also include any direct care tasks a registered professional nurse entrusts to other appropriate personnel to perform" (Keller & Strohschein, 2016, p. 206). In relation to the delegated function intervention, the public health nurse may initiate **delegation** of functions to others as the delegator or receive delegated function from others as the delegatee.

PUBLIC HEALTH NURSE AS A DELEGATOR

There has been much attention assigned to the strategy of delegation during recent years. The American Nurses Association (ANA) and the National Council of State Boards of Nursing (NCSBN) issued a Joint Statement on Delegation (2006). This joint statement described how delegation is not a singular task but a multifaceted process in which the nurse directs another individual to carry out a nursing task or an activity. The joint statement also noted the importance of supervising the individual to whom the task was delegated. Furthermore, the process of delegation encompasses four phases. These phases include: 1) assessment and planning; 2) communication, both written and verbal; 3) surveillance and supervision; and 4) evaluation and feedback (ANA; NCSBN, 2006). In all matters related to delegation, however, the registered nurse is fully responsible and accountable for the provision of nursing practice, and while they may be delegating one aspect of care, they do not delegate the nursing process itself (ANA; NCSBN, 2006, para. 7). Two expert panels were established by the National Council of State Boards of Nursing (2016) to develop national guidelines that would standardize the nursing delegation process, building upon the previous works. For additional information concerning these national guidelines, the reader may refer to the website box at the end of this chapter. By accessing this link, a more complete listing of the policy considerations and the principles of delegation, including the Five Rights of Delegation, are provided. These five rights include 1) right task, 2) right circumstances,

3) right person, 4) right directions and communication, and 5) right supervision and evaluation (NCSBN, 2016).

When the public health nurse delegates a function to another licensed professional or to unlicensed assistive personnel, the nurse must consider the Five Rights of Delegation. The first right is whether it is the *right task*: Is this a task that may be delegated? Delegatee's Nursing assessment, for example, cannot be delegated under most states' nurse practice acts. In school nursing, the appropriateness of delegating medication administration has received increased attention (ANA-NCSBN, 2006; National Association of School Nurses, 2010, 2011; NCSBN, 2016; Resha, 2010).

The second right is the *right circumstance*, which considers the available resources in order for the task or activity to be delivered safely (ANA-NCSBN, 2006; NCSBN, 2016; Rippke et al., 2001, p. 115). If the nursing assessment reveals stability of the patient and the circumstances, low potential for harm, low task complexity, minimal problem-solving, and predictable task outcomes, a task is more likely to be appropriate to delegate.

In the third right, the nurse considers the characteristics of the delegatee and whether or not they are the *right person*. Does the potential delegatee have "reasonable knowledge, training, and experience to assure consistent and safe performance of the task" (Rippke et al., 2001, p. 115)? A nurse may delegate any nursing functions to another registered nurse, as long as the second nurse has appropriate knowledge, training, and experience for safe and consistent performance of the delegated task. In situations where the nurse delegates to an unlicensed assistive personnel, questions are raised such as the delegatee's education, experience, job description and whether or not there are written policies and procedures for the delegation of the identified activity, just to name a few. Do they have the knowledge and skill to carry out the task, and what does the nurse have to teach to ensure these skills? An important part of this right is the type of validation that needs to take place to ensure of knowledge, skill,

and competency as well as appropriate follow-up (ANA-NCSBN, 2006; NCSBN, 2016).

The fourth right considers whether the task's objectives, directions, and expectations can be clearly communicated (NCSBN, 2016). What is the right *direction and communication*? How will direction and communication take place? What should be the content of that direction and communication? Is the communication two-way? What is it that the nurse needs to know to ensure and assure that care is being delivered with quality and safety in mind? If the task is unfamiliar to the delegatee or requires multiple steps and complex decision-making, the task is less likely to be delegated. For example, maternal outreach workers, who provide postpartum health education and support to women who have delivered a low-birth-weight infants, are selected on the basis of their experiences in working with pregnant and postpartum women and are provided significant additional training. These unlicensed assistive personnel (UAP) provide valuable help and service to the women and to the public health nurse. The UAP and public health nurse establish ongoing communication where the UAP provides the nurse with information about, for example, the mothers' ability to carry out essential activities for their newborn.

Supervision and surveillance by the public health nurse delegator is the fifth right and considers the public health nurse as the responsible party for monitoring the delegated activity (NCSBN, 2016). The delegator must be in communication with the individual carrying out the task; engage in ongoing monitoring, following up and providing feedback; answer questions; and ultimately make the evaluation as to the outcome. In public health nursing, when services are delivered in a variety of locations where the delegator and the delegatee may be in different places, a plan for ensuring opportunities for supervision and evaluation should be concrete. For example, in home healthcare services, the public health nurse supervises a home health aide at regular intervals and is available for questions by telephone or other form of electronic communication. New or emerging patient or home health aide needs can be addressed with supplemental home visits, if needed.

Public Health Nursing as Delegatee

The public health nurse must also consider the implications of these principles when the nurse accepts delegation from other healthcare professionals, including physicians and advanced practice nurses. When the public health nurse accepts delegation from a healthcare professional, and the delegation is allowed by law, the five rights of delegation should be considered to guide the nurse in determining whether or not to accept the delegation. First, is the task to be delegated within a professional nurse's legal scope of practice? Although a nurse may have the knowledge or skill to complete a task, whether or not it is legal may vary according to state nurse practice acts. Second, a public health nurse must consider whether the circumstances are right to implement a task. A hospital-based physician seeking to delegate the task may be unaware or may not appreciate the complexity of the proposed task if it is implemented in an individual's home. The task must also be consistent with the public health nurse's agency policies and procedures, with which the delegator may be unaware or unfamiliar (Rippke et al., 2001).

The third right focuses on the public health nurse's "knowledge, training, and experience to assure safe performance of the task" (Rippke et al., 2001, p. 116). The nurse should not accept responsibility for a task when the nurse lacks or doubts his or her ability to ensure safe and effective care. The nurse must also consider whether the task is appropriate for this individual and whether this individual is stable enough at this time to attempt the proposed task given the public health nurse's knowledge, training, and experience. Fourth, the public health nurse must consider whether the orders, directions, and communications from the physician or nurse practitioner are clear and accurate. The fifth right is ensuring the right supervision is available and determining who is responsible and accountable? The nurse must be clear that the task is within the nurse's legal scope of practice.

Public Health Nursing and Delegation

To be able to delegate and supervise has become a critical intervention strategy for all specialty areas in the professional practice discipline of nursing that requires skill, as well as leadership. Given the complexity of the healthcare system, as well as the complexity of the health needs of the people nurses care for along with limited resources, including limited human capital, delegation has taken center stage. Public health nursing is not immune to any of these challenges, and delegation, as an intervention strategy, has been identified as a way to ensure that care delivery is sustained with care and quality intact (Bystedt, Eriksson, & Wilde-Larsson, 2011; Saccomano & Pinto-Zipp, 2011). Because the focus of delegated functions is generally on direct care tasks, this public health nursing intervention occurs primarily at the individual/family level of practice. However, the community and system level is also operational. For example, the work of the ANA and the NCSBN (2006), as well as the more recent work of the NCSBN (2016) to develop a national guideline to facilitate and standardize the nursing delegation process, are examples of system-level applications. No other public health nursing intervention discussed in this book requires another health professional's authority; all other interventions are nursing functions conducted independently under the local state's nurse practice act (Rippke et al., 2001).

The Intervention Wheel: Application to Practice

Frequently, the frail, elderly population is at increased risk for neglect and abuse. In this population, it is essential to have providers who understand their distinctive needs and clinical presentation of disease. A percentage of the elderly will be found in the nursing home or adult home. Within the walls of these nursing homes is a subpopulation of poor, minority, older adults who present with a complexity of needs.

In caring for the geriatric population, nurse practitioners face numerous challenges, such as clinical presentation of disease, limited access to specialists, and limited access to care. For example, the clinical presentation of a specific disease process in an older adult may be very different from a younger adult, such as in the case of a urinary tract infection. In a younger adult, a urinary tract infection most likely presents with urinary urgency, urinary frequency, and suprapubic tenderness, whereas in an older adult it can present as confusion. The American adult population is growing older, yet the specialists in this field have not kept pace with this growth.

The Case for Case Management

The following is a case study that exemplifies one of the intervention wheel's population-based strategies known as case management. After the case study, there is a discussion as to the process of the case management and an exploration as to the application of case management in relation to the three levels of practice: individual/family, community,

and system. In addition, **Box 12-1** provides questions for further contemplation by the reader after reading the case study.

In the case study, the nurse practitioners are involved in the case management process as they care for their population of older adults and their families. This process not only begins with the assessment that is beyond the individual assessment but also includes the family members with a look into the community from where the individual was admitted. It is evident that the nurse practitioner works together with other members of the healthcare team, but this collaboration also includes the individual and the family members facilitating shared decision-making, which is very much in line with the principles of primary health care (Truglio-Londrigan, 2017). There is a give and take between all members, with the focus being the individual and his wife. The role of the nurse as a care manager is very evident as an educator, communicator, collaborator, and provider of care.

The nurse practitioner, who is working in the role as a case manager in the case study, practices at the individual/family level as evidenced by the education, support, and counseling that is taking place with the individual and his wife. In addition, work at the community level may also be explored as the nurse practitioner case manager reaches out

---

Box 12-1 Exercise Questions to Reflect Upon Post Case Study

- Who is the population of interest in this case?
- Why would this population be considered a vulnerable population?
- What were the major issues for this particular individual and his wife?
- How would you describe the processes of case management that is taking place in the case study?
- What roles did the nurse practitioner exemplify in this case study?
- Can you think of any other healthcare team members who could have been engaged?
- Would there be a situation in which referral and follow-up was necessary? If yes, explain.
- Would there be a situation when delegation would be beneficial? If yes, explain.
- As the nurse practitioner engaged in the process of case management, what other ways could she be engaged at the community and systems levels to enhance the care of the individual and his wife?

CASE STUDY	Nurse Practitioners Enhancing Geriatric Case Management
	Shirley Franco, MSN, FNP

Gericine, a nurse practitioner primary health care group, was created to provide quality care to an underserved population. The nurse practitioners at Gericine care for and manage one of the most vulnerable populations—older adults residing in long-term care. This practice is located in the Northeast, outside of New York City. The Gericine model provides accessible health care while facilitating and planning treatment options that meet the individuals' needs. Nurse practitioners provide a comprehensive and individualized treatment plan and become the case manager for the population they serve.

Case managers are licensed healthcare providers who combine advanced practice nursing care with case management. The case manager becomes the primary care provider, advocate, and facilitator for the individual. He or she is responsible for providing individuals with options and available resources while understanding the individual's status and life-to-death trajectory. Ultimately, the nurse practitioner case manager promotes quality, cost-effective outcomes. A nurse practitioner functioning in the case manager role commonly is faced with providing care for an individual like the situation described in this case study.

An 87-year-old Hispanic man with a history of hypertension, chronic obstructive pulmonary disorder, chronic heart failure, gastroparesis, and recent gastrostomy tube placement for significant weight loss is newly admitted to a long-term care facility. This individual has been seen multiple times by a gastrointestinal specialist, who suggested to the family that a gastrostomy tube may stabilize his weight. Despite the gastrostomy tube, the individual is losing weight and has had a 5-pound weight loss in two weeks. The individual's weight before the gastrostomy tube placement was 112 pounds, but now he is 107 pounds. His wife is Spanish-speaking and does not understand why her husband is still losing weight.

The nurse practitioner is challenged with providing culturally competent care to this man, who is alert and presenting with multiple comorbid conditions, while trying to help his wife understand the disease process and where the patient is in the life-to-death trajectory. The nurse practitioner has carried out a comprehensive assessment, including talking with the individual and his family and assessing the community where he lived the past 50 years of his life. The nurse practitioner notes that both the individual and his wife were active in their community church and that he had been an active member of the green thumb club. In fact, the individual had won many awards for the flowers and vegetables that he has successfully tended over the years.

The nurse practitioner decides that she will need to enlist an interprofessional approach to provide comprehensive care for the man and his wife. The nurse practitioner seeks out the assistance of a social worker to support her need for advance care planning, and she requested that the gastrointestinal specialist be present along with the dietary and nursing staff. Together, the interprofessional team is able to present to the individual and his wife the options and available resources located within the long-term care facility and the local community. They are able to create a plan that changes the current feedings to a higher caloric concentration and a slower infusion rate for easier absorption, and they explain the disease processes of gastroparesis and diabetes so that the individual and his wife understand the current situation and how the diseases progress. The team also establishes a comprehensive advance care plan that encompasses many of the aspects that the individual stated he wanted.

In this case story, the nurse practitioner focused on delivering a collaborative, communicative, and comprehensive plan of care to the individual and his wife. As the nurse practitioner case manager, the focus is on the quality of the care that is delivered while balancing the most cost-effective positive outcome.

to the community and encourages members of their church and the "green thumb" club to come to visit the individual. In fact, the nurse practitioner also encourage the community members to do more than just visit but to be engaged. For example, the members of the green thumb club may consider planting with the individual and the other residents in the long-term care facility on the units or, if possible, work with administration to have a small section of the grounds dedicated to gardening. In this way, the nurse practitioner is attempting to change attitudes of the community to look at the long-term care organization as a building that people can walk into and engage with the individuals rather than walk by the building door. The nurse practitioner may also carry out the intervention of case management on the system level in the following way. From his or her experience, he or she may note that for some individuals in this vulnerable population, the complexity of their problems may warrant more than the already established interprofessional team meetings as directed. The nurse practitioner may request and lobby for a change in the long-term care system. The request may be in the form of a suggestion that, for newly admitted long-term care individuals with multiple needs, weekly meetings take place for the first six months to ensure a smooth transition.

Conclusion

This chapter addresses three public health interventions in the green wedge of the intervention wheel: referral and follow-up, case management, and delegated functions. Each intervention was discussed in detail along with exploration as to how these interventions may be implemented at the individual/family, community, and systems levels of practice. Reflection upon this green wedge informs the reader that there is much overlap between these three intervention strategies, and there are co-existing relationships between all of the other intervention wheel strategies. It is incumbent for the public health nurse to embrace and integrate each of the strategies discussed in this book for populations as well as for individuals and families at all levels of practice.

Additional Resources

Case Management Society of America at: http://www.cmsa.org/

American Case Management Association at: http://www.acmaweb.org/

American Nurse Credentialing Center at: http://www.acmaweb.org/

American Nurses Association Principles at: http://www.nursingworld.org/principles

American Nurses Association and National Council of State Boards of Nursing Position Statement on Delegation at: http://www.nursingworld.org/MainMenuCategories/Policy-Advocacy/Positions-and-Resolutions/ANAPositionStatements/Position-Statements-Alphabetically/Joint-Statement-on-Delegation-American-Nurses-Association-ANA-and-National-Council-of-State-Boards.html

National Council of State Boards of Nursing Delegation at: https://www.ncsbn.org/1625.htm

Lessons from History

The purpose of this section in this intervention chapter is to demonstrate for the reader how history does inform our contemporary practice, and the take-away messages are varied and many. The history of the American Red Cross Town and Country was adapted from Lewenson, 2017. Take the time to read the following, and see what your take-away is.

Running the Show: Referral and Follow-up, Case Management, and Delegated Functions

By the fall of 1916, the town of Red Hook had started the Red Hook Nursing Association and hired the American Red Cross Town and Country nurse, Margaret Ruba. Her work involved doing health assessments of children in the schools within Red Hook, doing home visits to care for the sick, and providing health-related talks throughout various business and civic organizations within the community.

Much of the work involved referrals to healthcare providers, such as physicians and dentists, when problems were found. In the schools, for example, children with problems involving the teeth or poor vision were referred to appropriate providers. Follow-up by the nurse was made to the homes, as in cases of contagious diseases or other problems identified. On December 8, 1916, a few months after arriving in Red Hook, the local newspaper, the *Tivoli Times,* published the following account of Ruba's work, leading to the hiring of a second public health nurse:

A Large Field for Our Red Cross Nurses' Work—December 8, 1916

1. Reflect upon the intervention strategy demonstrated in this historical case study, considering the rural public health nurses' role in the community.
2. Consider the role of the rural public health nurse with that of a public health nurse working in a more urban center.
3. Compare and contrast the role of the public health nurse, whether in a rural or urban center, with that of a public health nurse today.

A Large Field For Our Red Cross Nurse's Work.

The total report of the school examinations of the Madalin, Barrytown, Saulpaugh, Annandale and Fraleigh districts are now in, and out of two hundred and sixty-one children examined, one hundred and eighty-four are defectives. This means either defective teeth or vision, enlarged tonsils, nasal obstruction or deformity. Much of this may be corrected which is one of the aims of the Red Hook Nursing Association.

Miss Ruba has made fifty-three nursing visit last month and forty four visits to the homes of school children, this being in line with the work above mentioned.

She also gave twelve talks to Little Mother's Leagues and four to school children, ten instructive visits and twenty-four business visits making a total of 131 visits and 16 talks.

Minutes of the Red Hook Nursing Association, Box 362.104 R Box Red Hook Nursing Association, Scrapbook, 1916–1917. Adriance Memorial Library, Poughkeepsie, New York.

Modified from Lewenson, S. B. (2017). Historical exemplars in nursing. In S. B. Lewenson & M. Truglio-Londrigan (Eds.), *Practicing primary health care in nursing: Caring for populations* (pp. 1–17). Burlington, MA: Jones & Bartlett Learning.

CASE STUDY AND CRITICAL QUESTIONS	**Rural Health: A Vulnerability and the Older Adult** Marty Hucks, MN, APRN-BC, CNE Tracy P. George, DNP, APRN-BC, CNE Francis Marion University

The patient was a frail, stooped, elderly African American male with balding hair who had been receiving home health services for less than a week. Prior to the recent hospitalization, he had no contact with a medical provider in years, maybe never. His body, spirit, and mind had been ravaged by years of alcoholism, uncontrolled diabetes, and likely other illnesses that had not yet been discerned. His present situation gave testimony to the choices he had made, or that fate had dealt him, years ago. He lived alone and in poverty with no phone service, no central heat or air conditioning, no running water, and no human companionship.

At the initial visit made to his home, the public health nurse (PHN) noticed that ambulation was cumbersome for him, and he walked with an unusual limp. Dislodging a hissing cat, the PHN spread out a sheet of newspaper to cover the surface of a dilapidated and cracked end table and placed her nursing bag on the clean field. After using alcohol gel to clean her hands, she donned the standard home health apron to protect her uniform and brought her equipment out of the bag.

The PHN inquired about his appetite and asked whether he had any food in the house—just some stale peanuts, luncheon meats, and sodas, but his neighbor would bring him some groceries later. The PHN then asked about his bowel and bladder functioning, which are affected by diet, medications, and disease. The nurse had already reviewed his recent lab values, which indicated his renal function was declining to a point where he would require dialysis very soon, but the nurse reflected upon this and was certain this did not register with him. He was focused only on the here and now. Discussion ensured about his medications, what he was able to obtain, and what he had been forced to go without. The PHN recognized that additional assistance would be necessary, not only from other professionals but also possibly from other sectors of the community, many of whom may not be professionals.

The nurse continued and checked his blood pressure and noted that it was mildly elevated. He was afebrile, and his apical pulse was smooth, steady, and ticking along at a healthy rate. His respirations were unlabored and even. His lungs were clear with no sign of pneumonia or heat failure. His belly was nondistended, gurgling, soft, and nontender. He held out a gnarled hand, allowing the nurse to prick the little finger and obtain a drop of blood and then apply it to the reagent strip. After a few moments, the results of his blood sugar reading were available, and they were way too high. His physician would be notified, and his insulin dose would be increased. The PHN began to wrap up the assessment by inspecting his feet, literally the Achilles' heel for a diabetic.

One of the things nurses do is teach diabetics to inspect their feet daily for any sign of trouble, not to go barefoot, to dry thoroughly between their toes, to make sure shoes don't rub, and not to cut their nails too close. The nurse realized that in their experience, little of this advice is ever followed. His feet were cool and dark, and the skin was thickened. The dorsalis pedis pulse, what should have been a familiar tap against the top of the foot and fairly easy to locate in a healthy foot, was absent. Further inspection revealed that the fourth and fifth toes of the right foot were missing altogether; those of the left foot hung in an unnatural position. They were leathery, shriveled, and completely black. It was apparent that there was no life left in them. As the visit came to an end and he walked the PHN to the door, the nurse first heard and then saw that his dead fifth left toe had snapped off close to the ball of the foot. As he proceeded, there was another audible snap and then another.

Auto-amputation is a rare consequence of dry gangrene in the diabetic foot. Thankfully painless at the end, the condition is nonetheless discomforting. In this form of necrosis, the blood supply to distal body parts is slowly cut off due to disease. In contrast to its cousin, wet gangrene, infection is not an issue in this condition because there is literally not enough life left in these oxygen-starved cells for bacteria to be a problem. In time, the body creates a line of demarcation that separates viable from nonviable material, and finally after many months, the body rids itself of the dead tissue.

Together the PHN and the individual gathered the toes in a cellophane cigarette pack and, offering a prayer and a blessing, buried them under a live oak in his back yard. That was the last time this nurse saw him; when she went back the next day, a neighbor told her that he had moved. As she drove away, she thought about that part of the wisdom of nursing, which is learning to live with what cannot be fixed.

I was the nurse in this story above. As I reflect upon this past experience, I have also come to realize that this is one story about one vulnerable individual. How many vulnerable individuals do we not see who ultimately present a picture of a vulnerable population? The importance of surveillance and case-finding is clearly depicted in this case study. Finding the individual and reaching out to the individual are necessary to establish the essential connection, but equally important is what to do when we do once that connection is made?

As you reflect upon the story above that I have shared with you, answer the following questions:

1. Once we as nurses make the essential connection, how can we ensure sustaining that connection? What is the place of case management in sustaining connections?
2. Would delegation play a role as an intervention in this case and in sustaining the connection? If yes, describe the process of delegation that you see.
3. To whom would you refer the individual in this case study, and how would case management facilitate this referral and follow-up?

References

American Case Management Association. (2013). *Standards of practice & scope of services for healthcare delivery system case management and transitions of care (TOC) professionals.* Retrieved from www.acmaweb.org/forms/2013sopbrochure _final_online.pdf

American Nurses Association & the National Council of State Boards of Nursing. (2005). *Joint statement on delegation.* Retrieved from https://www.ncsbn .org/Joint_statement.pdf

Block, D. (2009). Reflections on school nursing and delegation (Editorial). *Public Health Nursing, 26,* 112–113.

Bokhaut, T., & Mahoney, I. E. (1960). A referral plan that serves babies. *American Journal of Nursing, 60,* 824–827.

Brennan-Ing, M., Seidel, L., Rodgers, L., Ernst, J., Wirth, D., Tietz, D., . . . Karpiak, S. E. (2016). The impact of comprehensive case management on HIV individual outcomes. *PLoS ONE, 11(2),* e0148865. doi:10.1371/journal.pone.0148865

Cady, L. L. (1952). Planning referral forms. *American Journal of Nursing, 52,* 175–176.

Case Management Society of America. (2014). *What kind of work does a case manager do?* Retrieved from http://solutions.cmsa.org/acton/fs/blocks /showLandingPage/a/10442/p/p-0005/t/page /fm/0/r/-/s/?sid=TV2:7nNvPURis.

Cave, L. A. (1989). Follow-up phone calls after discharge. *American Journal of Nursing, 89,* 942–943.

Champion, V. L., & Skinner, C. S. (2008). The health belief model. In K. Glanz, B. K. Rimer, & K. Viswanath (Eds.), *Health behavior and health education: Theory, research, and practice* (4th ed., pp. 45–65). San Francisco, CA: Jossey-Bass.

Chernick, L. S., Westhoff, C., Ray, M., Garcia, M., Garth, J., Santelli, J., & Dayan, P. S. (2015). Enhancing referral of sexually active adolescent females from the emergency department to family planning. *Journal of Women's Health, 24(4),* 324–328.

Clemen-Stone, S., McGuire, S. L., & Eigsti, D. G. (2002). *Comprehensive community health nursing:*

Family, aggregate, and community practice (6th ed.). St. Louis, MO: Mosby.

Coulter, A., & Collins, A. (2011). *Making shared decisions- making a reality: No decision about me, without me.* London, England: Foundation for Informed Medical Decision Making.

Federal Register. (2013). National standards for culturally and linguistically appropriate services (CLAS) in health and health care. *The Daily Journal of the United States of America.* Retrieved from https://www.federalregister.gov/documents/2013/09/24/2013-23164/national-standards-for-culturally-and-linguistically-appropriate-services-clas-in-health-and-health

Flynn, L., Budd, M., & Modelski, J. (2008). Enhancing resource utilization among pregnant adolescents. *Public Health Nursing, 25,* 140–148.

Gallant, M. H., Beaulieu, M. C., & Carnevale, F. A. (2002). Partnership: An analysis of the concept within the nurse-individual relationship. *Journal of Advanced Nursing, 40*(2), 149–157.

Hain, D. J., & Sandy, D. (2013). Partners in care: Patient empowerment through shared decision-making. *Nephrology Nursing Journal, 40*(2), 153–157.

Hupcey, J., Penrod, J., Morse, J., & Mitcham, C. (2001). An exploration and advancement of the concept of trust. *Journal of Advanced Nursing, 36*(2), 282–293.

Hudon, C., Chouinard, M. C., Diadiou, F., Lambert, M., & Bouliane, D. (2015). Case management in primary care for frequent users of health care services with chronic diseases: A qualitative study of patient and family experience. *The Annals of Family Medicine, 13*(6), 523–528.

Johns, J. (1996). A concept analysis of trust. *Journal of Advanced Nursing, 24,* 76–83.

Keller, L. O., & Strohschein, S. (2016). Population-based public health nursing practice: The intervention wheel. In M. Stanhope & J. Lancaster (Eds.), *Public health nursing: Population-centered health care in the community* (8th ed., pp. 190–216). St. Louis, MO: Mosby Elsevier.

Kneipp, S. M., Kairalla, J. A., Lutz, B. J., Peneira, D., Hall, A. G., Flocks, H.,… Schwartz, T. (2011). Public health nursing case management for women receiving temporary assistance for needy families: A randomized controlled trial using community-based participatory research. *American Journal of Public Health, 202,* 1759–1768.

Kraus, B. C. (1944). The patient referral system. *American Journal of Nursing, 44,* 387–391.

Lewenson, S. B. (2017). Historical exemplars in nursing. In S. B. Lewenson & M. Truglio-Londrigan (Eds.), *Practicing primary health care in nursing: Caring for populations* (pp. 1–17). Sudbury, MA: Jones & Bartlett Learning.

Lillibridge, J., & Hanna, B. (2008). Using telehealth to deliver nursing case management services to HIV/AIDS individuals. *Online Journal of Issues in Nursing, 14*(1). Retrieved from http://www.nursingworld.org/MainMenuCategories/ANAMarketplace/ANAPeriodicals/OJIN/TableofContents/Vol142009/No1Jan09/ArticlePreviousTopic/TelehealthandHIVAIDSIndivudals.aspx

Luckett, R., Pena, N., Vitonis, A., Bernstein, M. R., Feldman, S. (2015). Effect of patient navigator program on no-show rates at an academic referral colonoscopy clinic. *Journal of Women's Health, 24*(7), 608–615.

Lyratzopoulos, G., Vedsted, P., & Singh, H. (2015). Understanding missed opportunities for more timely diagnosis of cancer in symptomatic patients after presentation. *British Journal of Cancer, 112,* S84–S91.

Maijala, V., Tossavainen, K., & Turunen, H. (2015). Identifying nurse practitioners' required case management competencies in health promotion practice in municipal public primary health care. A two-stage modified Delphi study. *Journal of Clinical Nursing, 24,* 2554–2561.

Matthias, M. S., Salyers, M. P., & Frankel, R. M. (2013). Re-thinking shared decision-making: Context matters. *Patient Education and counseling, 91*(2), 176–179.

McGuire, S., Gerber, D. E., & Clemen-Stone, S. (1996). Meeting the diverse needs of individuals in the community: Effective use of the referral process. *Nursing Outlook, 44*(5), 218–222.

Moser, A., Houtepen, R., van der Bruggen, H., Spreeuwenberg, C., & Widdershoven, G. (2009). Autonomous decision-making & moral capacities. *Ethics Nursing, 16,* 203–218.

Moulton, B., & King, J. S. (2010) Aligning ethics with medical decision-making: The quest for informed patient choice. *Journal of Law Medicine & Ethics, 38,* 85–97.

Muench, J., Jarvis, K., Gray, M., Hayes, M., Vandersloot, D., Hardman, J., . . . Winkle, J. (2013). Implementing a team-based SBIRT model in primary care clinics, *20*(2), 106–112.

National Association of School Nurses. (2010). *Position statement: Delegation* (Rev.). Retrieved from http://www.nasn.org/PolicyAdvocacy/PositionPapersand Reports/NASNPositionStatementsFullView /tabid/462/ArticleId/21/Delegation-Revised-2010

National Association of School Nurses. (2011). *Medication administration in the school setting* (Rev.). Retrieved from http://www.nasn.org /PolicyAdvocacy/PositionPapersandReports /NASNPositionStatementsFullView/tabid/462 /ArticleId/86/Medication-Administration-in-the -School-Setting-Revised-2011

National Council of State Boards of Nursing. (2016). National guidelines for nursing delegation. *Journal of Nursing Regulation, 7*(1), 5–14.

National Council of State Boards of Nursing & American Nurses Association. (2006). *Joint statement on delegation.* Retrieved from https://www.ncsbn .org/Delegation_joint_statement_NCSBN-ANA.pdf

National Council of State Boards of Nursing. (1995). *Delegation concepts and decision-making process: National Council position paper.* Retrieved from https://www.ncsbn.org/323.htm#

National Council of State Boards of Nursing. (2005). *Working with others: A position paper.* Retrieved from https://www.ncsbn.org/Working_with_Others.pdf

Office of Minority Health, U.S. Department of Health and Human Services. (2001). *National standards for culturally and linguistically appropriate service in health care* (Final report). Retrieved from www .omhrc.gov/assets/pdf/checked/finalreport.pdf

Percac-Lima, S., Ashburner, J. M., McCarthy, A. M., Piawah, S., & Atlas, S. J. (2015). Patient navigation to improve follow-up of abnormal mammograms among disadvantaged women. *Journal of Women's Health, 24*(2), 138–143.

Resha, C. (2010). Delegation in the school setting: Is it a safe practice? *Online Journal of Issues in Nursing, 15*(2). Retrieved from http://www.nursingworld .org/MainMenuCategories/ANAMarketplace /ANAPeriodicals/OJIN/TableofContents/Vol152010 /No2May2010/Delegation-in-the-School-Setting.aspx

Rippke, M., Briske, L., Keller, L.O., Strohschein, S., & Simonetti, J. (2001). Public health interventions: Applications for public health nursing practice. *Public Health Nursing Section, Division of Community Health Services, Minnesota Department of Health.* Retrieved from www.health.state.mn.us/divs/opi/cd /phn/docs/0301wheel_manual.pdf

Ristevski, E., Regan, M., Jones, R., Breen, S., Batson, A., & McGrail, M. R. (2015). Cancer patient and clinician acceptability and feasibility of a supportive care screening and referral process. *Health Expectations, 18*(3), 406–418.

Robert, S. J., & Krouse, H. J. (1988). Enhancing self-care through active negotiation. *Nurse Practitioner, 12,* 44–52.

Saccomano, S. J., & Pinto-Zipp, G. (2011). Registered nurse leadership style and confidence in delegation. *Journal of Nursing Management, 19,* 522–533.

Segal, J., & Smith, M. (2013). *Conflict resolution skills.* Retrieved from http://www.helpguide.org/mental /eq8_conflict_resolution.htm

Simons-Morton, B., McLeroy, K., & Wendel, M. (2012). *Behavior theory in health promotion practice and research.* Burlington, MA: Jones & Bartlett Learning.

Stergiopoulos, V., Gozdzik, A., Misir, V., Skosireva, A., Connelly, J., Sarang, A., . . . McKenzie, D. (2015) Effectiveness of housing first with intensive case management in an ethnically diverse sample of homeless adults with mental illness: A randomized controlled trial. *PLoS ONE, 10*(7), e0130281. doi:10.1371/journal.pone.0130281

Stokes, J., Panagioti, M., Alam, R., Checkland, K., Cheraghi-Sohi, S., & Bower, P. (2015). Effectiveness of case management for "'at risk'" patients in primary care: A systematic review and meta-analysis. *PLoS ONE, 10*(7), e0132340. doi:10.1371/journal. pone.0132340

Suen, Y. N., Wang, M. P., Li, W. H. C., Kwong, A. C. S., Lai, V. W. Y., Chan, S. S. C., & Lam, T. H. (2016). Brief advice and active referral for smoking cessation services among community smokers: A study protocol for randomized controlled trial. *BMC Public Health, 16,* 387. doi:http://doi.org/10.1186/ s12889-016-3084-z

Truglio-Londrigan, M. (2017). Coalitions, partnerships, and shared decision-making: A primary health care perspective. In Sandra B. Lewenson & M. Truglio-Londrigan (Eds.), *Primary health care in nursing: Caring for populations* (pp. 89–106). Burlington, MA: Jones & Bartlett Learning.

Truglio-Londrigan, M. (2015). The patient experience with shared decision-making: A qualitative descriptive study. *Journal of Infusion Nursing, 38*(6), 407–418.

Truglio-Londrigan, M., Slyer, J., Singleton, J., & Worral, P. (2014). A qualitative systematic review of internal and external influences on shared decision-making in all healthcare settings. *JBI Database of Systematic Reviews and Implementation Reports, 12*(5), 121–194.

Truglio-Londrigan, M. (2013). *Shared decision-making in home-care from the nurse's perspective: Sitting at the kitchen table—a qualitative descriptive study. Journal of Clinical Nursing, 22*(19–20), 2883–2895. doi: 10.1111/jocn.12075

U.S. Department of Health and Human Services, Task Force on Community Preventive Services. (2011a). *Community preventive services: Interventions to identify HIV-positive people through partner counseling and referral services.* Retrieved from http://www .thecommunityguide.org/hiv/partnercounseling .html

U.S. Department of Health and Human Services. (2011b). Healthy People 2020: *HIV.* Retrieved from http://healthypeople.gov/2020/topicsobjectives2020 /ebr.aspx?topicid=22

Wald, L. D. (1918, December 11). Visiting nursing. Lillian Wald Papers. Writings & Speeches, Nurses & Nursing II, Reel 25, Box 37, Folder 4, pp. 1–9. New York Public Library, Humanities and Social Sciences Library, Manuscripts and Archives Division, New York, NY.

Wolfe, I. (1962). Referral—A process and a skill. *Nursing Outlook, 10*, 253–256.

For a full suite of assignments and additional learning activities, use the access code located in the front of your book to visit this exclusive website: http://go.jblearning.com/londrigan. If you do not have an access code, you can obtain one at the site.

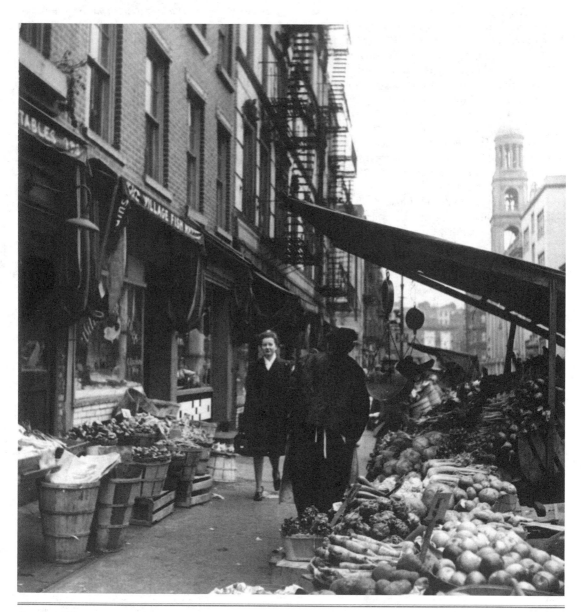

Courtesy of the Visiting Nurse Service of New York.

CHAPTER 13

Working It Out: Consultation, Counseling, and Health Teaching

Lin Drury

Formerly, the mortality among infants and children was heaviest in summer owing to intestinal diseases. The education of the mothers, the establishment of milk stations and the general improvement in community hygiene due to the publicity, the educational campaigns and almost all through education and supervision of the nurses in the homes, has reduced this summer death rate to the point where it is below that of the winter rate. (Wald, 1918, para. 4)

LEARNING OBJECTIVES

At the completion of this chapter, the reader will be able to:

- Describe the public health nursing intervention strategies of counseling, consultation, and health teaching.
- Differentiate between individual/family, community, and system levels of public health practice when applying the public health nursing intervention strategies

of counseling, consultation, and health teaching.
- Discuss the application of the public health nursing interventions of counseling, consultation, and health teaching.

KEY TERMS

- ❏ Consultation
- ❏ Counseling
- ❏ Health teaching
- ❏ Vulnerable populations

The intervention wheel exemplifies how public health nurses work with individuals/families and populations in communities to promote health, prevent disease, and limit the impact of illness. This chapter focuses on the intervention wheel's blue wedge where we find the strategies of counseling, consultation, and health teaching located. It does so by defining and describing these interventions, applying them to an issue in public health nursing practice, and finally demonstrating how to apply and use these interventions via a case study.

This intervention wheel also serves as a tool for conceptualizing public health nursing and facilitating a cognitive and practice shift from individual to population-based nursing. Providers and the general public are more than likely to envision the healthcare system as it is depicted on television—high technology interventions delivered to individuals in life-threatening situations. This vision, however, overlooks the health care that is delivered outside of acute care settings to individuals/families, populations, and the communities within which they live.

Throughout the 20th century, diagnosis and treatment of acute illness have driven reimbursement and shaped unsystematic services focused on sickness rather than health (Institute of Medicine, 2011; Partnership for Prevention, 2007; Schoen, Osborn, How, Doty, & Peugh, 2008; Swider, Levin, & Kulbok, 2015; Wennberg, Fisher, Goodman, & Skinner, 2008). Consequently, it is much more difficult to envision a system focused on promoting and maintaining health and preventing and/or managing chronic illness. Nursing students and registered nurses who are engaged in hospital-based care may wonder how public health nurses design and deliver preventive services for entire populations because their practice is focused on the provision of care to individuals within a circumscribed inpatient unit (Benner, Sutphen, Leonard, & Day, 2010). The very thought may be overwhelming and sometimes confusing. The public, conditioned by prior experience, may wonder why they should see a nurse if they are not sick. The population-based interventions depicted

in the blue wedge of the wheel—counseling, consultation, and health teaching—are critical processes for bridging these gaps and moving providers and the public into preventive care.

The Intervention Wheel

Counseling

The public health nursing intervention of **counseling** begins with professional conversations between the nurse and the individual, family, and/or target population within the context of the community. Counseling "establishes an interpersonal relationship with a community, system, family, or individual intended to increase or enhance their capacity for self-care and coping. Counseling engages the community, a system, family, or individual at an emotional level" (Keller & Strohschein, 2016, p. 206). The counseling relationship helps the population to reflect, clarify views, identify alternatives, examine available resources, and explore options in a supportive context. The public health nurse encourages the individual/family and population to consider the consequences of potential courses of action and formulate their own decisions.

Counseling relationships evolve as the public health nurse earns trust through continuing contact with the population. Deborah Antai-Otong (2007) notes, "Trust is germane to therapeutic and authentic nurse–client relationships.... The client's capacity to trust is governed by early interactions with patients and caregivers.... However, trust evolves through nurse-client relationships that convey acceptance, empathy, caring, and understanding" (p. 29). A study of public health nurses in Canada highlighted the role of trust in client empowerment. Aston, Meagher-Stewart, Edwards, and Young (2009) found that public health nurses fostered trust by shifting the balance of power away from the nurse as expert and instead engaging clients in transparent dialogue through active listening, believing in the client's strengths, and creating an atmosphere of safety and accessibility. Truglio-Londrigan and Barnes (2015) spoke about trust as a process that forms through a connection that unfolds over time, allowing for a working together that further builds the relationship.

Vulnerable populations who have previous negative experiences with the system may require extended time to develop even a tenuous level of trust. Cultural norms and current life stressors may also extend the time required to earn trust (deChesny & Anderson, 2012; Drury, 2008a). In addition, as the sphere of communication widens from individuals/family through community and systems and to populations, the possibility for miscommunication multiplies. Public health nurses as well as other public health practitioners need to be conscious of this as they seek to work with individuals/families and populations, always practicing actions that build trust.

Although public health nurses often deal with sensitive issues such as intimate partner violence, addiction, or homelessness, it is important to keep discussions focused on here-and-now problem solving via counseling. Psychotherapy is not within the scope of practice for public health nurses, and referrals to prescreened sources should be facilitated when needed (Browne, Doane, Reimer, MacLeod, & McLellan, 2010; Keller & Strohschein, 2016). The prescreening process takes place as the public health nurse locates organizations and agencies to serve as partners. These partners may assist the public health nurse in the provision of services such as psychotherapy. The prescreening process clarifies eligibility requirements, fees, and waiting lists, ensuring that those being served will not encounter bureaucratic barriers to treatment. This prescreening process ensures a place where the needs of the individual/family or a population can be addressed. The public health nurse in this situation promotes trust by facilitating access to care and following up on its efficacy.

The literature presents evidence of the importance of counseling as a public health nurse intervention strategy. Edinburgh and Saewyc (2008) studied

a home-visiting intervention that helped young (10- to 14-year-old) sexually assaulted adolescent runaways. The authors noted that the teens in this study refused traditional counseling as an intervention, and traditional counseling was not culturally congruent with the needs of this specific age group. The authors noted "the solution was to offer all teens participation in a therapeutic empowerment group, which met after school weekly under the guidance of a skilled therapist" (p. 45). Other interventions in this home-visiting intervention program included mental health and screening referrals, health education, and daily living skills. Outcomes were positive in terms of reconnecting these young runaways to school and family. Hollenbeck (2008) advocated for universal newborn hearing screening and stressed the importance of providing emotional support, counseling, and education throughout the process, particularly if the screening identified that further examination was needed.

Frank and Grubbs (2008) studied the effectiveness of a faith-based screening and education program focusing on diabetes, cardiovascular disease, and stroke. The study outcomes noted the importance of conducting the programs in small groups that facilitated one-to-one counseling. Huang, Lin, and Li (2008) addressed the vulnerable population of older adults. These authors studied the service needs of residents in community-based long-term care and noted a need for psychological support and counseling pertaining to lifestyle change, role change, and environmental change. The importance of counseling as a population-based intervention is also noted among other public health practitioners. Olshtain-Mann and Auslander (2008) studied parents' stress and perceptions of competence two months after their preterm infant was discharged from a neonatal intensive care unit. These authors noted the importance of emotional support and counseling during the first year after discharge. Although this work comes out of the social work literature, many public health nurses work in early childhood programs supporting families during these first few years after discharge. Counseling is an intervention strategy that public health nurses in all settings apply and do daily in their practice.

Consultation

The complexity of public health practice may require a wide range of expertise. Public health nurses may, therefore, find themselves seeking the **consultation** of others in their practice. These consultation services may include health officers, sanitarians, health educators, area professionals, epidemiologists, environmentalists, and media experts. Public health nurses may consult with a media expert if they need assistance on how to reach out into the community and gain the attention of a targeted population, or the public health nurse may seek consultation services of many different types of professionals or organizations. In this situation, the development of a coalition may be the answer, and the public health nurse may be instrumental in the organization of this coalition and the development of a partnership between and among all involved.

Part of the success of partnerships and coalitions is that every organization involved in the coalition is actively seeking consultation from the other. Working together in these types of partnerships facilitates sharing of ideas and information where everyone's expertise is honored and used in the decision-making process (Butterfoss & Kegler, 2009; Truglio-Londrigan, 2017). The public health nurse works within coalitions to mediate power and ensure that decision-making remains within the target population. Consultation "seeks information and generates optional solutions to perceived problems or issues through interactive problem solving with a community, system, family, or individual. The community, system, family, or individual selects and acts on the option best meeting the circumstances" (Keller & Strohschein, 2016, p. 206). Just as the public health nurses draw upon multiple sources of information to assist populations to meet their needs, they may in turn be sought for consultation purposes to provide nursing expertise within the community at large. Ideally, the coalition includes members of the targeted population.

Hopson and Steiker (2008) demonstrate consultation in adapting the evidence-based drug abuse prevention program called Keepin' It REAL to a variety of schools. The authors noted that schools differ, and each and every school has its own culture and population of students. "Interventions that work well at one school may be a poor fit for others" (p. 116). To address this issue, Hopson and Steiker used a participatory action research (PAR) approach to consult with students and staff to improve the program's "fit within a particular school" (p. 118). "PAR is dialogical and proactive typically focusing on empowerment and with researchers' and participants' values both being central to the planning process" (Kidd & Kral, 2005, p. 187). Kidd and Kral noted that collaboration exists in every phase of a PAR project. The collaborative partnership of the students and staff of the schools is critical so that the researchers may not only collaborate but also engage in consultation and learn from these partners about interventions that are most likely to succeed at each school.

Health Teaching

Health teaching focuses on providing information needed by the individual/family or population so they may become more aware of the promotion of health, the prevention of disease and injury, health screenings, available community services, and how to access those services. Health teaching "communicates facts, ideas, and skills that change knowledge, attitudes, values, beliefs, behaviors, and practices of individuals, families, systems, and/or communities" (Keller & Strohschein, 2016, p. 206). Health teaching engages participants at an intellectual level, whereas counseling engages participants emotionally. In practice, health teaching proceeds from the counseling relationship. For example, if a public health nurse is developing a mammography program for a particular population residing in a particular community, the nurse may first have to provide counseling services to address barriers to participation such as fear. The public health nurse must carefully assess the population and structure information accordingly. Once this assessment is completed, the public health nurse can develop educational programs tailored to the priorities of the individual/family or population. Information must be provided in a user friendly form and offered in measured amounts that can be absorbed easily. The goal for the public health nurse is to facilitate outcomes such as knowledge attainment that will support shared decision-making and behavior change in the individual/family or population (Truglio-Londrigan & Barnes, 2015).

The public health nurse takes a flexible approach that helps the individual/family or population to progress gradually from nonthreatening topics to areas that may be more emotionally or culturally challenging. For example, a public health nurse who offers a support group for battered women may have minimal attendance; however, offering a mothers' group instead may bring women who eventually, once trust is established, reveal abuse. These mothers may explain that if their partner caught them attending a group focused on domestic violence, their risk of battering would increase.

If we are to consider that public health is an interprofessional science, of which nursing is a critical participant, we may see the entire process of the development of educational programs in the following way. For example, multiple organizations in a particular community may form a coalition to promote health. Coalitions, broadly defined, include three essential themes that include partnerships, collaboration, and community need (Truglio-Londrigan, 2017, p. 91). The members of this coalition, in keeping with these three themes, together have agreed to a formal partnership and have identified one of the organizations as the lead agency. Methods of communication, formal and informal, have been developed to reduce miscommunication. The coalition decides to collectively

conduct an assessment of the community to identify issues and organize these issues in order of priority. The coalition also has members of the community involved as key participants. All the data from the community assessment are compiled, and an analysis reveals several issues. One of the issues is obesity in elementary school children. Once the key issue is decided, the members of the coalition must collectively determine who the targeted individual/family or population will be, what content will be delivered, how the content will be delivered, where and when the content will be delivered, and by whom. **Table 13-1** identifies these areas with examples of some of the key questions that the members of the coalition and the public health nurse must ask in the development, implementation, and evaluation of the educational program.

Many of these areas noted in Table 13-1 correspond with the determinants of health noted in the Graphic Model for *Healthy People 2020* (U.S. Department of Health and Human Services [U.S. DHHS], 2010). The determinants of health depicted in this model include physical environment, health services, social environment, individual behavior, and biology and genetic. Policymaking, however, although not depicted in the Graphic Model for *Healthy People 2020*, is described as a determinant of health in the Healthy People website (U.S. DHHS, 2010). Each determinant is considered here as it applies to health teaching and from here forward is referred to as a Systematic Approach to Health Teaching, understanding that there is an overlap of each of these determinants.

Biological/genetic determinants such as age, gender, and ethnicity can influence whether an individual seeks out new information, places relevance on the information, and puts that information to use. For example, Kaye, Crittenden, and Charland (2008) noted that "reaching and properly serving older men can be a challenge for practitioners" (p. 9). Older men may fail to participate in health education programs or actively seek help because "many older men believe that a stigma is attached to seeking

Table 13-1 Questions to Ask in the Development of Health Teaching Programs

Who: Individual/Family/Population	What Is the Issue?	How Is the Program Delivered and by Whom?	When and Where?
Who is the targeted individual/family or population? What do we know about the targeted individual/family or population? What is their age? What is the gender? What are their cultural ideas, values, and beliefs? What is their level of education? What is the primary language spoken? What is their income level? What are past health experiences? What are significant past life experiences? What behaviors or lifestyle characteristics does the individual/family/population exemplify? Are there any physical barriers to participating in the educational program, such as pain, hunger, or illness? Is the individual/family/population ready to learn, or is there an emotional barrier present? Does the individual/family/population not see the issue as a priority at the present time? Are there marital issues or concerns? Child care issues or concerns? Transportation issues or safety issues that must be taken into consideration?	What is the content or the message that must be covered? How detailed is the content or message? Can the content or message be divided into sessions? How will the public health nurse know if the educational program is successful? In other words, what will be the evaluation process? What behavioral change is expected? Did the educational program connect with the individual/family/population and get the message across?	What is the best way to deliver the content given the information pertaining to the individual/family/population? What is the best channel that the message will be delivered given individual/family/population age, gender, and physical and behavioral characteristics? For example, will the educational program be delivered via lecture, one-to-one, small group discussion, demonstration, or media such as billboards, television, or radio? Will the Internet be used as a channel, including text messaging and Facebook? What materials will be used to deliver the message? For example, will there be pamphlets, books, songs, games, or toys? Are the materials appropriate? Is the message clear and to the point? Who is the best person to deliver the message? For example, if the issue involves adolescent boys who are involved in sports, perhaps an athlete is the best person to present the information.	When and where is the best time to conduct the educational program? When and where is the best place to connect with the individual/family/population? For example, if the public health nurse wishes to conduct child car safety seat checks, it may be best to conduct this educational program at parks where young families may bring their children on the weekends.

help" (p. 9). Age is associated with learning styles, sensory capacity, and familiarity with technological developments (Knowles, Holton, & Swanson, 2005). For example, the act of producing a pamphlet requires the public health nurse to be conscious of normal aging changes with regard to vision, requiring the production of pamphlets that have larger print and colors that are easily identifiable.

Working with children also brings challenges. The public health nurse must secure the cooperation of school or organizational officials in addition to obtaining each child's parental consent before any information is presented. Teaching about bodily functions, family life, and sexuality are likely to evoke worry and require extensive preliminary work with organizational officials and parent groups. Detailed consent and opt-out procedures must be agreed on before proceeding. Children's developmental levels are also important—for example, the adolescent's sense of invincibility pairs poorly with information structured to startle or scare participants into compliance. Strategies that emphasize active participation and peer group values are more likely to catch the interest of adolescents. In addition, researchers Borawski et al. (2015) found that school nurses teaching healthy sexual behaviors to high school students contribute to a better understanding of the skills needed in reducing risky sexual health behaviors. Finally, attention to the determinant of genetics suggests that we look at the inherited conditions of particular populations such as sickle-cell anemia, cystic fibrosis, and family history of health disease as a guide to health teaching.

Hassmiller (2017) writes about the *social determinants of health* as where people live, work, and play that influence health care choices people make as a result (p. 35). Providing health education programs that take into consideration where people live, work, and play are part of the role of the public health nurse. For example, the community's level of education and cultural backgrounds are critical considerations in health teaching.

Individuals may be reticent to reveal language, educational, or literacy issues that can interfere with accurate interpretation of health information. Translating written material into the first language of individuals/family or populations may be ineffective if limited education and health literacy are not considered, or if cultural mores render some topics taboo. When the public health nurse is working with an individual or family, discussion of written materials in private to solicit feedback and confirm comprehension while protecting self-esteem is essential. In other situations, enlisting a culturally appropriate licensed medical translator should also be considered.

Economics overlaps heavily with social determinants in terms of educational background, available income, and access to resources (Summers et al., 2009). Nickitas (2017) explains that nurses need to understand how "poverty, economic inequities, stress, social exclusions, and job insecurity" effect those populations who lack access to health care and those who are most vulnerable (p. 77). Individuals/families and populations with limited income may find it difficult to gain access to health education programs, even if they are free. Transportation costs or costs affiliated with babysitting may make participation in these programs impossible. In addition, the implementation of health recommendations such as including fresh fruit and vegetables in the diet may not be an attainable goal. The public health nurse must adapt teaching materials to fit the needs and the economic resources of the target population, providing information on economical substitute sources of fiber, vitamins, and minerals.

Physical environmental determinants such as characteristics of the structural environment may necessitate the tailoring of information or the way in which information is provided. For example, many clinics have environments that are not conducive to teaching given the constant interruptions and the noise, yet many clinic nurses make do with what they have and offer great educational programs.

Box13-1   What To Do When Waiting: Example of Group Health Teaching Diabetes Education

Anny M. Eusebio, RN, MSN, FNP-BC

I practice in an outpatient satellite clinic affiliated to a major hospital in the New York area. The population is about 75% Latino and has limited reading skills in either English or Spanish. There is a high rate of obesity and diabetes in this clinic population. Furthermore, the majority have uncontrolled diabetes despite the best efforts of healthcare providers.

In 2007, we attended an informational session where RNs and NPs were introduced to and taught how to use the U.S. Diabetes Conversation Map Kits created by Healthy Interactions in collaboration with the American Diabetes Association. The concept was intriguing. It uses visually stimulating maps (in five topics) as teaching aides for individuals in group settings. They are appropriate for all educational levels and are available in English and Spanish. These maps provide the data needed for individuals to improve diabetes self-management in a fun and interactive manner. This easy and engaging method facilitates discussion and is appropriate to populations such as ours with limited formal education.

About a year ago, the program was launched in our clinic in an effort to improve education via groups. The education included information such as diet modification and the expected health outcomes, including improved fasting glucose and HbA1c levels. We have one English-speaking diabetes educator who supervises the group meetings. A Spanish-speaking nurse was also educated in the use of the conversation maps.

Over the past four months, this forum was extended to include the family members of the individual participants. This creates a further bond between spouses, children/parents, grandchildren/grandparents, and siblings. In particular, the family members who prepare meals for the individual clients are invited, but all family interested in expanding their knowledge of diabetes are welcome.

These conversation maps are an interesting way to teach about diabetes, not only to individuals but also to groups in a culturally sensitive and congruent way. New studies by Healthy Interactions (2016) show the efficacy of the use of the conversation maps and has become a valuable tool in the diabetic health teaching.

Data from Healthy Interactions, Inc. (Healthyi) in collaboration with the American Diabetes Association. (2008). *U.S. D. conversation map program.* Retrieved from http://healthyinteractions.com/us/en/diabetes/hcp/about/-program; Healthy Interactions, Inc. (2016). *Conversation Map® Programs: A quantitative and qualitative analysis of usage and outcomes.* Retrieved from http://healthyinteractions.com/assets/files/HI_DiabetesAbstract_April_2016.pdf

---

Examples of educational programming in waiting rooms include reading and math corners for young children to enhance literacy while at the same time modeling behavior for families, food corners with varying boxes and cans from grocery stores that can be used as props to teach clients how to read labels, and healthy menu guides that are culturally congruent for the targeted clinic population. **Box 13-1** illustrates this use of clinic waiting time for educational programming.

Individual behavior as a determinant may be viewed in a wide variety of contexts; for example, whether or not a person chooses to engage in cigarette smoking or an exercise program. Yet another example may be the consideration of the psychological status of the target population to determine readiness for learning and behavioral change. Public health nurses frequently encounter individuals and family members in the community who have been discharged from the hospital after an episode of acute illness. Before hospital discharge, these individuals and family members receive volumes of information, typically diet sheets, medication schedules, activity restrictions, and follow-up instructions—all during the stress of illness and compounded by anxiety related to going home. Short hospital stays make this pattern hard to avoid, but nevertheless, the public health nurse must plan accordingly. Expect the newly discharged to be overwhelmed and confused. Allow time during early visits to contact providers, clarify instructions, and adapt the information to fit the client's circumstances (Drury, 2008b). In addition, public health nurses find themselves working with vulnerable populations with complex needs, such as people who are homeless or have mental illnesses compounded by comorbid chronic diseases. These situations must also be accounted for in the development of teaching sessions and/or programs (Drury, 2008c).

Policy as a determinant must also be considered and assessed. In situations where there is a law that has been developed and implemented to protect the public, such as bike helmet laws, the public health nurse must be aware of how the law is implemented and develop health teaching for the population to facilitate compliance. In addition, when developing health teaching, the coalition and its members must constantly ask if the targeted population will be able to access the program they are developing. This question involves discussion pertaining to time of the program, cost of the program, transportation to the program, location of the program, and how the content of the program addresses the targeted populations ideas, values, emotions, and beliefs pertaining to the topic. Similar questions pertain to the determinant of *Health Services* and reflect the seven A's of the Public Health Nursing Assessment Tool as presented in Chapter 3 of this book.

Collective Consideration of Counseling, Consultation, and Health Teaching

What is of interest in the above description of counseling, consultation, and health education is how many of the population-based interventions are closely intertwined with one another. For example, public health nurses find they must carry out counseling first to emotionally support individuals through their decision-making process and at the same time provide education and seek consultation from others. Several well-established and extensively evaluated nurse-managed public health programs demonstrate complete integration of counseling, consultation, and health teaching.

The Transitional Care Model (TCM) (Naylor et al., 2009) provides in-hospital planning and home care support for chronically ill older adults. The nurse-led interdisciplinary team uses hospital visits, consultations with inpatient and outpatient providers, patient and family teaching, home visits, telephone and technology support, and coordination of services to ease patient transitions from hospital to home and prevent readmissions. A randomized clinical trial of the TCM versus standard care for Medicare patients with congestive heart failure demonstrated a savings of $5,000 per TCM patient (Naylor et al., 2004). Multiple clinical trials over the past 20 years have measured the program's success in improving quality of care, preserving physical function, enhancing quality of life, increasing satisfaction with care, and reducing costs (Coalition for Evidence-Based Policy, 2010).

The Nurse–Family Partnership (NFP) (Olds et al., 2010) supports first-time teen and/or unmarried low-income mothers with home visits from public health nurses throughout the pregnancy and for two years after birth. The nurses teach the mothers how to care for themselves and their infants; promote maternal growth through family planning, education, and workforce involvement; and facilitate access to community resources for mother and child. Outcomes for the mothers and their children have been tracked for up to 19 years in randomized controlled trials in at least three different locations. Overarching outcomes compared to controls that are consistent across at least two of the three locations are as follows: child abuse, neglect, and injuries down by 20% to 50%; subsequent births during late teens or early 20s down by 10% to 20%; and child educational attainment up by six percentile points in Grades 1 through 6 for both reading and math. The total cost for the three years of monthly visits is approximately $12,500 per family in 2010 (Coalition for Evidence-Based Policy, 2011).

Insite is North America's first medically supervised injection facility, a place where users of illegal drugs can obtain clean supplies and inject their pre-obtained drugs with less risk of bloodborne disease or death by overdose. Public health nurses in Vancouver, British Columbia, Canada operate the multidisciplinary program that oversees 700 to 1,000 individuals every 18 hours, seven days a week. The program was opened to address a human immunodeficiency virus prevalence of 17% to 30% and hepatitis C virus rates greater than 90% among drug users. The nurses do not supply or administer the drugs, but they observe clients at the injection booths from a centrally located nurses' station. They monitor clients for overdose symptoms, anaphylaxis, or unsafe injection practices. The nurses provide nonjudgmental teaching to reduce harm and offer assistance with any issues or concerns, including primary health care. They work with a network of community partners to help Insite's clients obtain access to basics such as food, clothing, and shelter. Addiction counselors and peer workers are on-site. Intense scrutiny by community and governmental stakeholders has led to rigorous data collection and analysis by external evaluators. Outcomes include a 35% decrease in fatal overdoses in the area and a 30% increase in the use of detoxification services. A 2008 decision by the British Columbia Supreme Court ruled that Insite should remain open and gave the Canadian federal government a year to make necessary changes to laws in order to relieve Insite from the burden of seeking continuous exemptions (Lightfoot et al., 2009).

The Case/Issue

In the other intervention chapters of this book, the authors present issues that public health nurses work with every day. Many of these issues and challenges are disease processes that are communicable, noncommunicable, and chronic illnesses. For this chapter, a community is presented as a system under study with its many issues and challenges. These issues and challenges have a profound effect on the individuals/families and the population that reside within its borders. What follows is a description of this community in need.

Community in Need

The Henry Street Settlement (HSS) is a not-for-profit social service institution located on the Lower East Side of Manhattan in New York City. Since 1893, the settlement has focused on meeting the needs of vulnerable populations and has expanded to include 19 sites serving more than 100,000 clients from around the world and across the life span. Although HSS was founded by the early 20th century nursing leader Lillian Wald and her colleague Mary Brewster to address the health problems of impoverished immigrants, their insights into the determinants of health led to the development of programs encompassing education, recreation, the arts, sociopolitical activism, and economic development in addition to home and agency-based nursing care (Lewenson, Keith, Kelleher, & Polansky, 2001).

Today's HSS programs reach clients in their homes, in day care centers, youth groups, workforce training, homeless shelters, mental health centers, summer camps, senior centers, and in the performing arts. Ironically, nursing did not remain among HSS's core services. As the settlement grew over the decades and professional specialization increased, nurses left HSS and formed the Visiting Nurse Service of New York in 1944. Following this separation, HSS referred clients to outside medical providers (Feld, 2008).

Like their predecessors, current HSS clients are at high risk for a wide range of physical and psychosocial health problems. Substantial populations at HSS today were born in China, Africa, Latin America, or Russia. Disenfranchised by language, culture, and economic barriers, the needs of today's clients are complex and interdependent. Meanwhile, constraints on healthcare spending have reduced providers' incentives to accept such patients. As a result, HSS found its referral sources dwindling and its clients poorly equipped to compete for increasingly scarce public health care.

THE COMMUNITY

In 1893, the Lower East side was a neighborhood of impoverished immigrants who came from countries such as Italy, Ireland, Germany, Hungary, Russia, and other European countries. They found themselves in their adopted city both geographically and socially isolated from the wealthy sections of Manhattan. Wald and Brewster found families doubled and tripled up in small, two-room, deteriorating apartments called tenements. These tenements offered families airless rooms, inadequate plumbing, and vermin. The inadequate housing, coupled with inhuman labor conditions in the many factories that immigrants found themselves working in, fostered the spread of diseases among the population. The same year that Wald and Brewster began HSS, "infants accounted for 25% of all deaths in the community, and children under 5 accounted for 40% of all deaths in the community (Lewenson, 2015, p. 16). Infectious diseases, such as tuberculosis, diphtheria, and pneumonia, contributed to 42% of the mortality rate within that same community (Lewenson, 2015). Poverty and social isolation enforced by language and cultural differences further contributed to despair. Residents in the early 1900s had few options for improvement (Wald, 1915).

Today, the Lower East Side is gentrifying. Luxury housing and business developments are replacing the tenements and attracting upscale residents (National Trust for Historic Preservation, 2008). The shrinking supply of affordable apartments has concentrated the HSS client population into dense blocks of New York City Housing Authority buildings and deteriorating rent-stabilized units. Immigrants still come to the area, and poor families repeat the pattern of previous centuries, doubling

The Lower East Side of New York City, 1893.

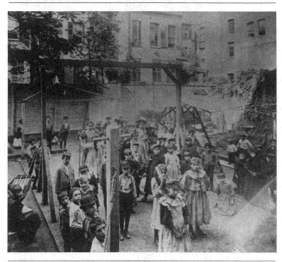

Courtesy of the Visiting Nurse Service of New York.

The Lower East Side of New York City today.

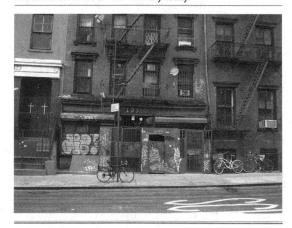

Collection of Lin Drury.

up or taking in boarders to meet rising rents in substandard accommodations. HSS clients share the geography of the Lower East Side but are isolated from their affluent neighbors by an unmarked economic boundary line.

POPULATION AND PROGRAMS

HSS clients range in age from newborns to centenarians. The population is outstandingly diverse, reflecting New York City in terms of race/ethnicity, culture, religion, and education/literacy. Specific programs target selected high-need groups. For example, the Parent Center provides drop-in support, education, and socialization to parents of infants and toddlers. The overwhelming majority of participants are African American or Spanish-speaking women of childbearing age, but there are no restrictions on attendance, and an occasional father or grandparent joins the program. Children in HSS Head Start programs reflect the demographics of families within walking distance of the centers. At one HSS Head Start site, nearly all the children are monolingual Chinese. The Housekeeping program serves more than 2,000 elderly and/or disabled clients throughout the city. On a single day, the caseload of that program includes 62 languages or dialects and an even larger number of cultures.

DETERMINANTS OF HEALTH: ECONOMIC

Clients across HSS programs have one characteristic in common: poverty. In addition, HSS grows its own employees by offering entry-level jobs to successful program participants. Consequently, HSS clients, plus most of the rank-and-file employees, represent vulnerable populations in terms of socioeconomic level, cognitive status, illness or disability, and life circumstances (Aday, 2001; de Chesnay & Anderson, 2012). City demographic data divide Manhattan into 10 clusters by zip code. The HSS area cluster is combined with two more-affluent zip codes in calculating the median household income, but it ranked fourth from the bottom for many years (Thompson, 2007). It is important to note that New York City experiences income inequality that affects the city as a whole (Liu, 2012). This gap has continued for several years, and more recently it was noted that 28% of residents of the Lower East Side live below the poverty level (King et al., 2015). A key finding was the widening gap in illness rates

between rich and poor New Yorkers. Since data collection began in 1990, preventable and manageable chronic disease has risen among low-income residents. For example, hospitalization of people with type 2 diabetes has increased 82% citywide, with poor individuals five times more likely to require hospital care than individuals from the city's wealthiest neighborhoods. The diabetes death rate was 125.2 per 100,000 people in the poorest neighborhoods but only 14.8 per 100,000 people in the richest neighborhoods.

The city comptroller summed up the report by stating that New York needs to do a better job of providing primary and preventive care. He acknowledged that low Medicaid reimbursement rates for routine care and wellness visits contribute to providers' preference for emergency department services for their publicly insured clients (Thompson, 2007).

Low-income New Yorkers are at high risk for a wide range of preventable physical and psychological disorders. They are two to six times more likely to experience serious psychological distress than their counterparts with higher incomes, and they are four times more likely to be hospitalized for substance abuse and/or mental health treatment instead of receiving outpatient care (Karpati et al., 2004; Thompson, 2007), yet the political factors intersecting with the economic factors brings good news to the ability for all New Yorkers to access care. For example, as a result of the passage of the Affordable Care Act, New Yorkers decreased the number of those adults without health insurance, which hovered prior to 2014 at 20% to 14% citywide by 2014 (Community Health Profiles, 2015).

DETERMINANTS OF HEALTH: SOCIAL AND HEALTH SYSTEM

In addition to the economic disparity, many HSS clients are recent immigrants who face documentation issues, language barriers, employment disparity, and cultural distance from healthcare workers. Long-term HSS clients, therefore, not only must deal with poverty but also with social determinants that have an impact on their health. The HHS clients commonly suffer from congestive heart failure, diabetes, hypertension, arthritis, emphysema, cancer, depression, and alcoholism. These individuals would benefit from case management and/or monitoring by a visiting nurse, but most are not eligible for these services under current Medicare or Medicaid regulations. Limited coverage for hearing, vision, and dental care further restricts many clients' functional capacities.

Working-poor clients and HSS front line employees often hold jobs that do not provide paid sick days; thus, they cannot afford to miss work while seeking care. If offered, their health insurance is high in cost and low in coverage; many cannot justify this expense amid conflicting budget priorities. Clients and employees alike seek health care only when they are acutely ill.

For both clients and front line employees at HSS, contact with healthcare providers is often limited to emergency department treatment, and opportunities for preventive care are lacking. Both clients and employees need user-friendly services that are culturally appropriate and available in a context they trust. In response to this burgeoning need for health care, HSS opened an on-site medical office. A multilingual physician and a culturally diverse staff run the office, but appointments during the workday are required. Medicaid and Medicare are accepted, but no free services are available, even for HSS employees. Perhaps as a result, since it opened in 2002 the office has been underutilized (V. Stack, personal communication, 2007). Recent efforts to expand participation in Medicaid-managed care plans and community outreach projects are improving awareness and use of the office.

DETERMINANTS OF HEALTH: ENVIRONMENTAL

The unmarked economic boundary line separating low-income and upscale housing on the Lower East Side also determines the accessibility of shops and services for HSS clients. One subway line runs at the periphery of the area, and taxis do not cruise the streets as they do in middle-class neighborhoods. The blocks within walking distance of HSS are dominated by retailers who aim for low-income customers: currency exchanges, bodegas (gritty urban convenience stores), 99-cent stores, and greasy spoon diners. At the local bodegas, clients on the Supplemental Nutrition Assistance Program (SNAP), commonly referred to as food stamps, find it impossible to spread their entitlement of approximately $5 per day across the entire month. Food pantries draw long lines, but the fruits, vegetables, and whole grains recommended for a healthy diet are not among the available items.

Retailers and professional offices targeting upscale customers have recently opened several blocks away, but they are inaccessible to most HSS clients because of economic disparity, distance, language, and culture. Clients seeking a bank, supermarket, department store, gym, or restaurant must speak English, must have the agility to board a bus or have cash for a gypsy cab (informal and unregulated car service), and then muster up the energy to transport their purchases (and sometimes several children as well) up multiple flights of stairs or unreliable elevators to their apartment. A common refrain among clients is "It's just all too much. . ."

The Intervention Wheel: Applying and Doing

The Intervention

The above presents a picture of a community with needs that have a profound health effect on the individual/families and the population who reside in that community. The proposed answer was to develop a university/community partnership to reintegrate public health nursing in a social service setting through a faculty/student public health nursing clinical practice.

The Partnership: Application of Consultation, Counseling, and Health Teaching

In the mid-1990s, HSS administrators were looking for healthcare resources for their clients, while faculty from Pace University Lienhard School of Nursing sought community health experiences for their nursing students. They discovered a mutual opportunity. Consultations between the school of nursing and HSS led to an AmeriCorps grant in 1995. Ongoing faculty efforts plus internal funding from the school of nursing provided the groundwork for the current partnership between HSS and the school (Lewenson et al., 2001).

In 2004, a Lienhard School of Nursing faculty member, with a specialty in public health nursing, approached HSS with a proposal to develop a faculty practice and student clinical practicum in public health nursing on-site. HSS administrators recognized an opportunity to integrate preventive care, health teaching, and counseling activities into their social service delivery programs. The faculty member initiated the public health nursing practice and began planning for the current partnership.

The purpose of the partnership was to expand the breadth and depth of public health nursing practice at the HSS. The overall goal was to improve the health of an underserved population, HSS clients and employees, by engaging them in the process of community health planning with public health nursing faculty and students from the Lienhard School of Nursing. Thus, the partnership incorporates the public health nursing faculty member, students from the school of nursing, clients and employees from HSS, and community residents and professionals who have interest or expertise on community issues. The partners decide what health issues should be addressed and suggest approaches. All members of the partnership jointly determine what evidence will be collected to assess the outcomes of its work. Members of the partnership continuously discuss where they are going and what process will work best to get them there. This consultation approach is particularly appropriate at HSS, given the facility's history and current pattern of service delivery. The Settlement was founded on the wisdom of listening to its constituency and then acting on the information obtained (Wald, 1915). Most HSS programs go a step further in empowering the population by employing current or former service recipients to mentor new clients. Children are trained as peer counselors, teens run a retail bicycle shop, mental health clients operate a clothing boutique, vocational program graduates gain paid employment within the housekeeping program, formerly homeless people work with shelter residents in preparation for permanent housing, and ambulatory senior citizens visit homebound elderly. The public health nurse faculty member continuously consults with all participants in the partnership to create interventions that provide learning opportunities for the students and positive outcomes for clients and employees. Many of these interventions take the form of health teaching and counseling.

How the Collaborative Partnership Works: Counseling, Consultation, and Education at the Individual/Family, Community, and Systems Levels

Public health nursing practice inclusive of health teaching, counseling, and consultation are often linked, particularly when working with vulnerable populations whose past experiences with the healthcare and social services systems have inspired mistrust. In an attempt to engage a broad range of clients and employees, information, materials, and professional expertise from the school of nursing faculty and students are available at multiple HSS locations. The cultural diversity and life experiences of the school's nursing students make it possible to match the special skills and interests of students with particular populations at HSS. The public health nursing faculty member and students spend time at each location counseling clients and employees and offering nonthreatening health teaching sessions to build trust. As clients and employees share their interests and concerns, the school of nursing faculty member and students respond with information, hands-on interventions, and individualized counseling as needed. The partnership works collectively and collaboratively to design, implement, and evaluate health promotion, early intervention, and disease management programs for the HSS population-at-large. The nursing students perform community health assessments, conduct group health educational programs, organize activity sessions, provide one-on-one health counseling, make home healthcare visits, and provide referrals and follow-up care. The School of Nursing provides loaner and donor equipment and supplies to assist the population in self-monitoring of health or management of chronic illness.

For example, the HSS population is at high risk for a comorbidity pattern of obesity, diabetes, hypertension, and heart disease. A healthy diet is key to interrupting this pattern, but the economic and environmental disparities foster diets high in carbohydrates, sodium, and fat. Students intervene at the systems level by joining with advocacy groups to increase SNAP allocations, contacting the city council to permit the use of food stamps at farmers' markets, and participating in a neighborhood coalition to obtain city-sponsored green carts for the area. At the community level, students canvass local bodegas and more distant grocery stores to counsel managers about the condition and price of perishable foods in an attempt to protect the public. They make reports to the department of health when needed and follow up on results. In addition, students consult with food service administrators on menu planning and provide classes for the cooking staff in the day care and senior centers. They work with the housekeepers and senior companions to select healthy foods when doing grocery shopping and light meal preparation for homebound seniors. On the individual and family levels, students offer

classes and cooking demonstrations throughout HSS that are focused on healthy eating on a budget.

Each counseling and health teaching activity leads to others, sometimes progressing from the individual or group out to a wider audience. Students discovered that homeless clients in a residential shelter program had little experience in meal planning and preparation. They created a series of groups, including grocery shopping field trips, as a way to council and teach this vulnerable population. Shelter clients found they could not stretch their SNAP allotment across the month unless they bought in bulk, but their rooms came with individual-size refrigerators. The students organized their clients to meet with the shelter director and begin a letter-writing campaign requesting larger refrigerators with freezer space. The building has a complex funding stream, multiple layers of management, and subcontracted program operations. It was a challenge just to determine who should receive the letters, but working through the system has united the clients around a common goal. It may be a long time before the Department of Housing and Urban Development responds to the client's request, but they have developed a voice within the shelter program.

Outcomes

The partnership began with eight students during one semester in one HSS program serving one population. After six years, 80 to 100 students deliver year-round care to clients and employees in 12 distinct HSS programs at multiple sites that serve populations across the organization. There is increased participation by clients and employees at each site, as well as an increase in requests for further public health nursing services. Employees are taking an increasingly active role in urging nonparticipating clients and coworkers to obtain services. Public health nurses were hired for HSS programs that had not previously employed them, and recent graduates from the school of nursing with experience in the partnership were hired to provide professional nursing assessments for clients in the housekeeping program. A director of nursing was hired to launch a home healthcare service at HSS.

Lessons Learned

A partnership between two organizations with multiple players is always a work in progress with multiple unknowns. The public health nursing faculty member has made a substantial commitment of time and energy to become a trusted figure within HSS. Changes in clients' circumstances, employee turnover, and school of nursing student rotations are constants that require continuous adjustment and modification. Organizational dynamics, funding issues, and political variables can dramatically alter the climate in which the partnership works. The global economic crisis had an immediate and devastating impact on governmental, corporate, and philanthropic funding to HSS. Budgets have been cut, programs have been trimmed, and some of the new nursing positions have been lost. The number of clients in need of HSS services is rising, while staff and other resources are shrinking.

To address this crisis, the partnership between Lienhard School of Nursing, now part of Pace University's new College of Health Professions, and HSS has expanded and widened its scope to include undergraduate students in computer sciences. A small university grant provides clients in senior services programs at HSS with refurbished wireless computers and mentoring into online social networks. Undergraduate students in nursing and computer sciences work in teams making home visits to homebound low-income older adults who need a virtual social network but who lack the equipment and expertise to gain access. Nursing students assess the client's cognitive and physical capacity to use computers, determining if the client is literate and mentally clear, if a large keyboard is needed because of arthritis, or if an extralarge monitor is required because of visual impairment. Computer science students refurbish donated computers and adapt them to meet the senior's needs. They install these customized computers and

make a series of home visits to provide one-to-one mentoring on how to use email, video chat, and Web searches. Nursing students make continuing contact with the client online and by home visit to reduce social isolation and monitor ongoing health needs. HSS staff members get regular updates on each senior and provide referrals for additional services as needed.

Providing seniors with computers and Internet access brings a virtual community into their homes, fostering mental activity and neighborly monitoring when assistance is needed. Online seniors can stay connected with family and support services without traveling, often forestalling institutional placement. We envision the gradual progression of a virtual senior center for the growing number of HSS clients who can no longer walk to the physical facility. Teaching clients how to use the computer and counseling them in Internet communication strategies will allow thinly stretched HSS case workers to keep in touch with their expanding caseloads online. Virtual home visits will help caseworkers to prioritize when a costly face-to-face visit is required. Cost–benefit data are being collected, and funding is being sought to sustain and expand the program.

The partnership is fluid and ever changing. Participation in all activities and programs is voluntary for all clients and employees who choose to be involved. Data collection is limited to what clients and employees are comfortable in providing. Risks to participants are limited to minor discomfort associated with some screening procedures and potential stress associated with discussing personal issues. Participants benefit, however, by obtaining free and convenient attention for health concerns and by having access to nursing students and a faculty member who provide health teaching and counseling within their own home community. Referrals and follow-up are available for any participant who needs additional care, but still some choose not to take advantage of the services offered. The partnership continues to reach out.

Conclusion

The HSS case study highlights the enormous impact of the determinants of health on the individual/family or population and demonstrates that the nursing interventions of counseling, consultation, and health teaching must address health disparities at the systems level while simultaneously providing direct care to people. The systematic approach to health teaching and the seven A's assist the public health nurse to synthesize information in a complex environment. The PAR ensures that the population guides public health nurses in collaborative practice with the community.

Additional Resources

American Association of Colleges of Nursing at: http://www.aacn.nche.edu/public-health-nursing

American Public Health Association at: https://www.apha.org

Association for Prevention Teaching and Research at: http://www.aptrweb.org/?page=pophealthmodules

Association of Community Health Nurse Educators at: http://www.achne.org/i4a/pages/index.cfm?pageid=1

Centers for Disease Control and Prevention National Health Education Standards at: http://www.cdc.gov/healthyschools/sher/standards/index.htm

World Health Organization—Health Education at: http://www.who.int/topics/health_education/en/

Community Health Profile Manhattan District 3 for Case Study in this Chapter at: https://www1.nyc.gov/assets/doh/downloads/pdf/data/2015chp-mn3.pdf

---

Lessons from History

The purpose of this section in this intervention chapter is to demonstrate for the reader how history does inform our contemporary practice and the take-away messages are varied and many. The history of the American Red Cross Town and Country was adapted from Lewenson (2017). Take the time to read the following, and see what your take-away is.

Working It Out: Consultation, Counseling, and Health Teaching

One of the main goals of all public health nursing was to provide health teaching within the community. The town of Red Hook, where the American Red Cross Town & Country nurse was hired, provided a number of health teaching classes within the community. Ranging from well-baby classes for mothers, care of the sick at home, and classes on maternal child health to nutritional counseling, the public health nurses' role included that of a health teacher. One of the very reasons that Town and Country required of all their rural public health nurses to have an additional postgraduate 3- to 9-month course in public health nursing was their need to be an educator, a communicator, and an advocate in the rural district where they would work. By hiring an educated American Red Cross Town and Country rural public health nurse, the Red Hook Nursing

(continues)

Association addressed one of the main the recommendations of the 1915 Sickness in Dutchess County Report, which was to educate the public about the prevention of diseases and ways to stay healthy.

> *Vastly more can in the end be accomplished by preventative than remedial work. The present exigencies and the acute suffering of the present should not blind us to the necessity of measures whereby a very large portion of existing disease and suffering can be done away with. Not only must personal habits and hygiene often be reformed, but the deep underlying causes of sickness which have their roots in the ignorance of the public as to the causes of disease, and in social and industrial conditions must be removed. It is only in this way we may hope to ultimately to reduce the great economic loss and personal suffering occasioned by sickness, including the expenditures for remedial work. (State Aids Association, 1915, p. 74)*

Miss Margaret Ruba and Other Dutchess County Public Health Nurses (Circa 1916–1917).

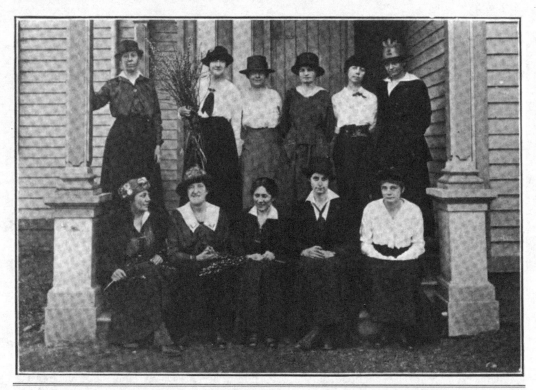

Reproduced from Weber, J. J. (1917). *A county at work at its health problems: A statement of accomplishment by the Dutchess County Health Association during the 16 months August 1916 to December 1917.* New York, NY: State Charities Aid Association. Retrieved from https://babel.hathitrust.org/shcgi/pt?id=mdp.39015014861580;view=1up;seq=1, p. 10 Miss Margaret Ruba standing top row—end on right.

Questions to Consider

1. Search the JSTOR database for early copies of the *American Journal of Nursing,* and search articles about the Town and Country rural public health nurses.
2. Reflect on how the Town and Country rural public health nurses exercised the following three aspects of the intervention wheel: consultation, counseling, and health teaching.
3. Compare and contrast nurses such as Margaret Ruba and other Town and Country rural public health nurses with the consultation, counseling, and health teaching of public health nurses today.

Modified from Lewenson, S. B. (2017). Historical exemplars in nursing. In S. B. Lewenson & M. Truglio-Londrigan (Eds.), *Practicing primary health care in nursing: Caring for populations* (pp. 1–17). Burlington, MA: Jones & Bartlett Learning.

CASE STUDY AND CRITICAL QUESTIONS

A Collaboration Project: Assessing Exercise in African Americans in Church-based Settings

Robin M. White, PhD, MSN, RN
Interim Department Chair/Interim Director of Nursing
Assistant Professor of Nursing
Ohio Northern University

As part of my dissertation project, I collaborated with eight local church ministers of African American churches in a small town in Midwest Ohio. I did so because religion/spirituality is a positive influence in decisions that pertain to health promotion behaviors in the African American population. The church is, therefore, a strong facilitator to access of this population and in the provision of social support and networks that aid in decisions leading to behavior change. The church also serves as a partner in encouraging healthy lifestyles in African Americans in a culturally sensitive way due to long-standing trusting relationships between congregational members and church leaders. In addition, physical spaces needed for activities are generally accessible, and community support often provides spiritual care for its members.

Preliminary research showed that sedentary behavior rates were higher among African American men and women than in other American races and ethnicities, placing them at greater risk for chronic illness. Routine physical activity may reduce the risk of chronic health problems such as overweight and obesity, type 2 diabetes, hypertension, coronary artery disease, stroke, congestive heart failure, and cancers. In the African American population, the disparately high chronic disease burden and lower physical activity rates demonstrated the need to develop effective strategies that increase routine exercise participation.

In this project, I assessed the attitudes of African Americans about exercise in a church-based setting. This provided the information needed to develop effective interventions to improve physical activity in this vulnerable population. Using these interventions, I developed a collaborative project between the church ministers and their congregations. I examined the efficacy of this project using the transtheoretical model (TTM) developed by Prochaska and Velicer. TTM examines stages of change, decisional balance,

(continues)

and self-efficacy for exercise that permits one to assess whether any associations existed between TTM constructs and regular exercise in African Americans. Establishing the collaborative project was important for this population, as strong trusting relationships had already been established between the church and the congregants that potentially facilitated support and buy-in. Participant surveys were used that included information about demographics, stage of change for exercise, decisional balance for exercise, self-efficacy for exercise, and current physical activity.

Data were collected on 200 participants ranging in age from 18 to 85 years ($M = 53.17$), with 69% females and 31% males. The most frequent stage of change was found to be the preparation stage (34%), meaning that people were considering a commitment for changes in the near future (usually within the month), making the initiation of new behavior more likely. Average physical activity in this project was at 105 minutes per week of combined vigorous activity, moderate activity, and walking. Adult physical activity recommendations of the American Cancer Society (2012) included participating in at least 150 minutes of moderate intensity, 75 minutes of vigorous intensity activity each week, or a combination of these spread throughout the week. Statistical outcomes of this study varied, but the findings showed the participants were exercising more, and those who exercised more made comments reflecting better outcomes, such as, "I am in a better mood if I exercise," and "I sleep better if I exercise." However, there were two statistically significant reasons participants gave for not exercising. These included "lack of time" and "too tired."

This research supported the idea that healthcare professionals, especially nurses, when tailoring studies and intervention strategies, are in an optimal position to assess at-risk populations and assist them to initiate and maintain routine physical activity by developing effective interventions when partnering with the population and leaders, thus using the already established trust networks.

Given the above case study, answer the following questions:

1. Select a community and consider the collaborations that would support an effective health promoting exercise.
2. What strategies could you use to ensure the collaboration has an already established foundation of trust?
3. What factors would you consider when you develop an intervention strategy that included consultation, counseling, and health teaching?
4. How would you develop such a program taking into consideration the objectives of *Healthy People 2020*?

References

Aday, L. A. (2001). *At risk in America: The health and healthcare needs of vulnerable populations in the United States.* San Francisco, CA: Jossey-Bass.

Antai-Otong, D. (2007). Nurse–client communication: A life span approach. Sudbury, MA: Jones and Bartlett Publishers.

Aston, M., Meagher-Stewart, D., Edwards, N., & Young, L. M. (2009). Public health nurses' primary care practice: Strategies for fostering citizen participation. *Journal of Community Health Nursing, 26,* 24–34.

Benner, P., Sutphen, M., Leonard, V., & Day, L. (2010). *Educating nurses: A call for radical transformation.* San Francisco, CA: Jossey-Bass.

Borawski, E. A., Adams Tufts, K., Trapl, E. S., Hayman, L. L., Yoder, L. D., & Lovegreen L. S. (2015). Effectiveness of health education teachers and school nurses teaching sexually transmitted infections/human immunodeficiency virus prevention knowledge and skills in high school. *Journal of School Health, 85*(3), 189–196.

Browne, A. J., Doane, G. H., Reimer, J., MacLeod, M. L. P., & McLellan, E. (2010). Public health nursing practice with "'high priority'" families: The significance of contextualizing "'risk.'" *Nursing Inquiry, 17*(1), 26–37.

Butterfoss, F. D., & Kegler, M. C. (2009). The community coalition action theory. In R. J. Di Clemente, R. A. Crosby, & M. C. Kegler (Eds.), *Emerging theories in health promotion practice and research* (pp. 237–276). San Francisco, CA: Jossey-Bass.

Coalition for Evidence-Based Policy. (2010). *Top-tier evidence initiative: Evidence summary for the Transitional Care Model.* Washington, DC: Author.

Coalition for Evidence-Based Policy. (2011). *Top-tier evidence initiative: Evidence summary for the Nurse-Family Partnership.* Washington, DC: Author.

Community Health Profiles. (2015). Health Care. Retrieved from https://www1.nyc.gov/assets/doh/downloads/pdf/data/2015chp-mn3.pdf

de Chesnay, M., & Anderson, B. A. (Eds.). (2012). *Caring for the vulnerable: Perspectives in nursing theory, practice, and research.* Sudbury, MA: Jones & Bartlett Learning.

Drury, L. J. (2008a). From homeless to housed: Caring for people in transition. *Journal of Community Health Nursing, 25*(2), 91–105.

Drury, L. J. (2008b). Increasing competency in the care of homeless patients. *Journal of Continuing Education in Nursing, 39*(4), 153–154.

Drury, L. J. (2008c). Transition from hospital to home care: What gets lost between the discharge plan and the real world? *Journal of Continuing Education in Nursing, 39*(5), 198–199.

Edinburgh, L. D., & Saewyc, E. M. (2008). A novel, intensive home-visiting intervention for runaway, sexually exploited girls. *Journal Compilation, 14*(1), 41–48.

Feld, M. N. (2008). *Lillian Wald: A biography.* Chapel Hill: University of North Carolina Press.

Frank, D., & Grubbs, L. (2008). A faith-based screening/education program for diabetes, CVD, and stroke in rural African Americans. *ABNF Journal, 19*(3), 96–101.

Hassmiller, S. B. (2017). Nursing's role in building a culture of health. In S. B. Lewenson & M. Truglio-Londrigan (Eds.), *Practicing primary health care in nursing: Caring for populations* (pp. 33–60). Burlington, MA: Jones & Bartlett Learning.

Healthy Interactions, Inc. (2016). *Conversation Map® Programs: A quantitative and qualitative analysis of usage and outcomes.* Retrieved from http://healthyinteractions.com/assets/files/HI_DiabetesAbstract_April_2016.pdf

Healthy Interactions, Inc. (2008). *(Healthyi) in collaboration with the American Diabetes Association. U.S. D. conversation map program.* Retrieved from http://healthyinteractions.com/us/en/diabetes/hcp/about/-program

Hollenbeck, L. (2008). Advocating for universal newborn hearing screening. *Creative Nursing, 14*(2), 75–81.

Hopson, L. M., & Steiker, L. K. H. (2008). Methodology for evaluating an adaptation of evidence-based drug abuse prevention in alternative schools. *Children & Schools, 30*(2), 116–127.

Huang, J. J., Lin, K. C., & Li, I. C. (2008). Service needs of residents in community-based long-term care facilities in northern Taiwan. *Journal of Clinical Nursing, 17*(1), 99–108.

Institute of Medicine. (2011). *The future of nursing: Leading change, advancing health.* Washington, DC: National Academies Press.

Karpati, A., Kerker, B., Mostashari, F., Singh, T., Hajat, A., Thorpe, L., ... Frieden, T. (2004). *Health disparities in New York City.* New York, NY: New York City Department of Health and Mental Hygiene.

Kaye, L. W., Crittenden, J. A., & Charland, J. (2008). Invisible older men: What we know about older men's use of healthcare and social service. *Generations, 32*(1), 9–14.

Keller, L. O., & Strohschein, S. (2016). Population-based public health nursing practice: The intervention wheel. In M. Stanhope & J. Lancaster (Eds.), *Public health nursing: Population-centered health care in the community* (9th ed., pp. 190–216). St. Louis, MO: Mosby Elsevier.

Kidd, S. A., & Kral, M. J. (2005). Practicing participatory research. *Journal of Counseling Psychology, 52*(2), 187–195.

King, L., Hinterland, K., Dragan, K. L., Driver, C. R., Harris, T. G., Gwynn, R. C., ... Bassett, M. T. (2015). Community Health Profiles 2015, Manhattan Community District 3. *Lower East Side and Chinatown, 3*(59), 1–16.

Knowles, M. S., Holton, E. F., & Swanson, R. A. (2005). *The adult learner: The definitive classic in adult education and human resource development* (6th ed.). Boston, MA: Elsevier.

Lewenson, S., Keith, K. A., Kelleher, C., & Polansky, E. (2001). Carrying on the legacy of Lillian Wald: Partnership with the Henry Street Settlement and the Lienhard School of Nursing at Pace University. *Nursing Leadership Forum, 5*(4), 116–121.

Lewenson, S. B. (2015). Looking back: History and decision-making in health care. In S. B. Lewenson & M. T. Londrigan (Eds.), *Decision-making in nursing: Thoughtful approaches for leadership* (2nd ed.; pp. 13–32). Sudbury, MA: Jones & Bartlett Learning.

Lewenson, S. B. (2017). Historical exemplars. In S. B. Lewenson & M. Truglio-Londrigan (Eds.), *Practicing primary health care in nursing: Caring for populations* (pp. 1–19). Burlington, MA: Jones & Bartlett.

Lightfoot, B., Panessa, C., Hayden, S., Thumath, M., Goldstone, I., & Pauly, B. (2009). Gaining insight: Harm reduction in nursing practice. *Canadian Nurse, 105*(4), 16–22.

Liu, J. C. (2012, May*). Income inequality in NYC*. New York: NYC Comptroller's Office.

Minnesota Department of Health/Office of Public Health Practice. (2001). *Public health interventions: Applications for public health nursing*. Retrieved from www.health.state.mn.us/divs/cfh/ophp/resources/docs/ph-interventions_manual2001.pdf

National Trust for Historic Preservation. (2008). *National trust for historic preservation names: 2008 list of America's 11 most endangered historic places*. Retrieved from http://www.nationaltrust.org

Naylor, M. D., Brooten, D. A., Campbell, R. L., Maislin, G., McCauley, K. M., & Schwartz, J. S. (2004). Transitional care of older adults hospitalized with heart failure: A randomized, controlled trial. *Journal of the American Geriatric Society, 52*(7), 675–684.

Naylor, M. D., Feldman, P. H., Keating, S., Koren, M. J., Kurtzman, E. T., Maccoy, M. C., & Krakauer, R. (2009). Translating research into practice: Transitional care for older adults. *Journal of Evaluation in Clinical Practice, 15*(6), 1164–1170.

Nickitas, D. (2017). The economics of caring for populations: A primary health care perspective. In S. B. Lewenson & M. Truglio-Londrigan (Eds.), *Practicing primary health care in nursing: Caring for populations* (pp. 75–87). Burlington, MA: Jones & Bartlett Learning.

Olds, D. L., Kitzman, H. J., Cole, R. C., Hanks, C. A., Arcoleo, K. J., Anson, E. A., . . . Stevenson, A. J. (2010). Enduring effects of prenatal and infancy home visiting by nurses on maternal life course and government spending: Follow-up of a randomized trial among children at age 12 years. *Archives of Pediatrics & Adolescent Medicine, 164*(5), 419–424.

Olshtain-Mann, O., & Auslander, G. (2008). Parents of preterm infants two months after discharge from the hospital: Are they still at (parental) risk? *Health & Social Work, 33*(2), 299–308.

Partnership for Prevention. (2007). *Preventative care: A national profile on use, disparities, and health benefits*. Retrieved from http://www.prevent.org/NCPP

Schoen, C., Osborn, R., How, S. K. H., Doty, M. M., & Peugh, J. (2008). *In chronic condition: Experiences of patients with complex health needs in eight countries*. Retrieved from http://www.commonwealthfund.org/publications/publications_show.htm?doc_id=726496

Swider, S. M., Levin, P. F., & Kulbok, P. A. (2015). Creating the future of public health nursing: A call to action. *Public Health Nursing, 32*(2), 91–93. doi:org/10.1111/phn.12193

Summers, C., Cohen, L., Havusha, A., Slinger, F., & Farley, T. (2009). *Take care New York 2012: A policy for a healthier New York City*. New York, NY: City Department of Health and Mental Hygiene.

Thompson, W. C. (2007). *Health and wealth: Assessing and addressing income disparities in the health of New Yorkers*. New York, NY: Office of the New York City Comptroller.

Truglio-Londrigan, M., & Barnes, C. (2015). Working together: Shared decision-making. In S. B. Lewenson & M. T. Londrigan (Eds.), *Decision-making in nursing: Thoughtful approaches for leadership* (2nd ed., pp. 141–162). Sudbury, MA: Jones & Bartlett Learning.

Truglio-Londrigan, M. (2017). Coalitions, partnerships and shared decision-making: A primary healthcare perspective. In S. B. Lewenson & M. Truglio-Londrigan (Eds.), *Practicing primary health care in nursing: Caring for populations* (pp. 89–108). Burlington, MA: Jones & Bartlett Learning.

U. S. Department of Health and Human Services. (2010). *Healthy People 2020.* Washington, DC: U. S. Government Printing Office.

Wald, L. D. (1915). *The house on Henry Street.* New York, NY: Henry Holt & Company.

Wald, L. D. (1918, March 5). The woman voter should realize the relation of the visiting nurse to public health. Lillian Wald Papers, Reel 25, Writings & Speeches, Voters & Voting, New York City Public Library, New York, NY.

Wennberg, J. E., Fisher, E. S., Goodman, D. C., & Skinner, J. S. (2008). *Tracking the care of patients with severe chronic illness.* Retrieved from http://www.-dartmouthatlas.org

U.S. D. conversation map program. (n.d.). Retrieved from http://healthyinteractions.com/us/en/diabetes/hcp/about/-program

For a full suite of assignments and additional learning activities, use the access code located in the front of your book to visit this exclusive website: **http://go.jblearning.com/londrigan**. If you do not have an access code, you can obtain one at the site.

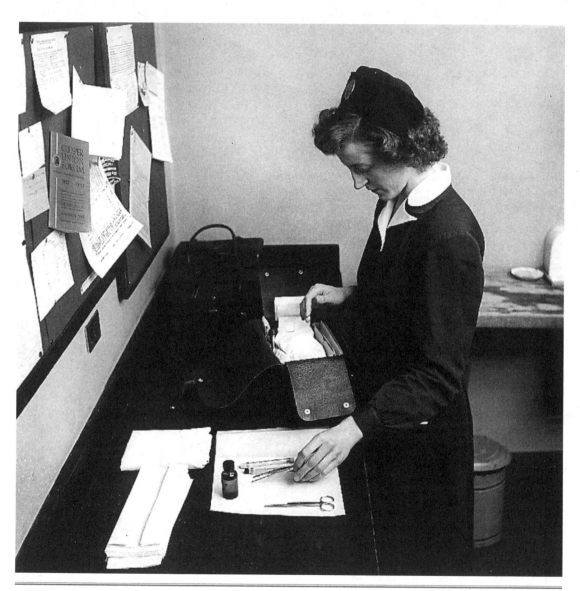

Courtesy of the Visiting Nurse Service of New York.

CHAPTER 14

Working Together: Collaboration, Coalition Building, and Community Organizing

Esther Thatcher
Eunhee Park
Pamela Kulbok

. . . I always consulted the women of our neighborhood before I made a public statement on matters affecting them and their children. Even the least educated had, out of her experience and her devotion to her family, an intelligent contribution to make to the discussions. The foreign mothers and housekeepers must help men to keep the municipal house in order. It is a joint housekeeping affair, and neither element can progress without the other. (Wald, 1913, p. 13)

LEARNING OBJECTIVES

At the completion of this chapter, the reader will be able to:

- Define collaboration, coalition building, and community organizing.
- Apply collaboration, coalition building, and community organizing strategies at appropriate levels of practice.
- Explore evidence-based ways that public health nurses practice collaboration, coalition building, and community organizing to impact public health outcomes.

KEY TERMS

- ❏ Coalition building
- ❏ Collaboration
- ❏ Collective action

- ❏ Community organizing
- ❏ Network

"Every living person has some gift or capacity of value to others. A strong community is a place that recognizes those gifts and ensures that they are given" (Kretzmann & McKnight, 1994, p. 27). This quotation offers a glimpse into the power of collective action. **Collective action** refers to groups of people who organize social or political activities in order to address a shared need (Gilbert, 2006; Siegal, Siegel, & Bonnie, 2009). Different models of collective action can occur, depending on participants' vision, mission, goals, and needs. The intervention wheel strategies covered in this chapter include collaboration, coalition building, and community organizing, all forms of collective action. These collective action—intervention/strategies—are the orange section of the wheel. Bringing together a community through collective action interventions is, by definition, focusing on a specific population who has unique needs. When members of a vulnerable population and community participate in collective action, their experiences of taking leadership and advocating for themselves and their community can lead to enhanced capital and empowerment, along with improved social determinants of health for themselves and other members of the community.

The goals of this chapter are 1) to describe the intervention/strategies of collaboration, coalition building, and community organizing and 2) to provide practical guidance on enacting these three public health interventions. In each main section, collaboration, coalition building, and community organizing are defined and differentiated, highlighting the differences between each. Discussions of practical application of each intervention include its use at each level of public health nursing (PHN) practice

(individual, community, and systems focused), the key principles, and steps of the interventions. Finally, this chapter also provides exemplars where PHN have been involved in collaboration, coalition building, and community organizing.

Frameworks for Collective Action

Paolo Freire had worldwide influence on social justice and education of disadvantaged populations. His goal for education was to liberate people from oppressive circumstances. He engaged students in structured dialogue processes to critically reflect on their own experiences and then to grow through these reflections toward empowerment to take action on behalf of themselves and their communities (Glass, 2001). Freire used the term *praxis* to describe this integration of learning and action to transform one's life. Collective action was at the center of Freire's approach (Campbell, 2014). Freire's work has been highly influential on public and community health practice, education, and research. Community participatory approaches to health practice and research are rooted in Freire's work.

There is continuing emphasis on collective action to achieve better health for all. For example, the Robert Wood Johnson (RWJF) Foundation, one of the largest private health program funders in the United States, recently developed its Building a Culture of Health model (RWJF, 2015; Hassmiller, 2017). This model is a very current and a forward-moving public health framework to address equity and social determinants as foundations of health. The framework's four action areas are: 1) making health a shared value; 2) fostering cross-sector collaboration to improve well-being;

3) creating healthier, more equitable communities; and 4) strengthening integration of health services and systems (Chandra et al., 2016). All four action areas, especially the second area, depend on collective action at the individual, family, community, and/or systems levels to achieve the desired outcome of improved health and well-being.

Undoubtedly, genuine participation is complex and challenging. Promoting successful community participation requires skill, forethought, and insight. Poorly implemented community participation efforts can alienate the very people the program developers intended to benefit and can lead to future community distrust of participation efforts. The orange section of the intervention wheel embodies collective action where it is the people in the community who work together with providers and/or other professionals, nonprofessionals, and organizations to identify needs and develop strategies to address those needs collectively. Given the complexity of today's healthcare environment along with the complex problems, partnerships that exemplify the intervention strategies of collaboration, coalition building, and community organizing are essential (Truglio-Londrigan, 2017).

Collaboration

In this section, collaboration as a public health nursing intervention is examined. Definitions of the term **collaboration** and connections to PHN practice are provided. The context for discussion of collaboration, as an intervention directed toward individuals, communities, and systems, is a community-based participatory research project to prevent adolescent substance use in a rural southern community.

Collaboration, in its simplest form, refers to two or more people who work together toward a shared goal. In today's complex healthcare environment, collaborations are also complex and may include ". . . . healthcare providers, insurers, purchasers, public health departments, community-based organizations, and academic institutions, but also entities that operate outside the traditional sphere of health care, such as faith-based and other non-health community-based organizations, schools, businesses, and other nonhealth governmental agencies" (Varda, Chandra, Stern, & Lurie, 2008, p. E1). Himmelman (2002) described a collaboration approach where each level builds on the other. The lowest level of collaboration is networking, or sharing information in a way that benefits each partner. The next level is coordinating, in which collaborating partners change their practices to help each other and reach a shared goal. The third level is cooperating, which adds the sharing of resources among partners to reach a shared goal. Himmelman (2002) identifies true collaborating as the highest level, in which one partner helps another partner to improve its capacity in addition to the actions in the lower levels. This mutual enhancement helps the collaborating partners to amplify their progress toward their shared goal.

The intervention wheel exemplifies Himmelman's definition of collaboration, emphasizing the resource-intensive approach of enhancing others' capacity (Minnesota Department of Health, 2001). Even though collaborative processes are resource intensive, the ultimate sharing of resources among those collaborating is an enticement to collaborative endeavors (Varda et al., 2008). There are a wide variety of community-based initiatives where collaborative partnerships are informal or formal at varying points of the collaborative endeavor. Individuals or organizations can be partners in collaboration. For example, an individual with expertise in a health issue could collaborate with a public health agency who also needs to address that specific health issue but whose staff may lack the necessary expertise. Collaboration participants might serve in their professional roles, such as PHN collaborating with a spiritual organization. Collaboration participants might also serve in their personal roles, such as residents of a neighborhood or members of a community affected by a health issue.

A **network** is a type of collaboration that usually involves informal or formal relationships where there is cooperation and coordination among partners (Ontario Healthy Communities Coalition, 2016). Networks may form spontaneously when organizations or individuals want to share information, tools, or resources more efficiently. Community health networks might refer clients to each other, use similar documentation practices to facilitate shared information, and provide partner links on their websites. Collaborations may be viewed as a basic building block for the other collective action approaches of coalition building and community organizing. A history of successful collaboration between individuals or agencies can lead to the more complex processes of coalition building or community organizing.

Use of Collaboration

Collaboration is useful in a wide variety of situations where unaffiliated individuals or organizations discover that working together would make their own jobs easier or more successful. Collaboration among different professional or economic sectors has great potential to solve health issues. According to Chandra and colleagues (2016), five benefits of collaboration are to 1) align resources, policies, and activities for more efficiency and effectiveness; 2) improve overall health in groups, communities, and whole nations; 3) improve equity in health outcomes and opportunities for good health; 4) help individual organizations reach their own goals; and 5) develop innovative approaches to more effectively address health problems.

At the individual level, a public health nurse might collaborate with a client after providing other interventions such as case management or health teaching. Through these interactions, the PHN learns about the client's unique perspective on his or her health condition. This helps the PHN to develop a deeper understanding of the condition. The PHN later invites the client to present to a class on his or her health condition. This interaction is considered collaboration because both the nurse and the client have benefitted and have worked together on a shared activity. This interaction, at this point, goes beyond the individual-level public health interventions, such

as health teaching or case management, in which the benefit flows one way to the client.

Collaboration at the community level can occur among individuals or organizations. The aim of the collaboration is to improve health outcomes or health opportunities for members of a community. At the community level, a PHN might collaborate with another professional, such as a school nurse to ensure that all children in the school are fully vaccinated. This partnership might be formal, such as when the public health department and school system have written protocols for coordinating vaccinations. Although the latter is an example of a systems-level approach, the outcomes are positive for the public school community.

Another example of collaboration at the community level involves multiple organizations who collaborate to ensure care for a population with a unique set of needs that exceeds the capacity of any one organization. In the case of newly arrived refugees, organizations might collaborate to ensure that the refugees receive access to health care, housing, schools, employment assistance, and language training. These are all essential services that strengthen the community within which the refugees live and work. The organizations involved in this collaboration might be very diverse, including public health departments, hospitals, schools, housing authorities, refugee-oriented nongovernmental organizations, churches, and volunteer centers.

A collaboration working at a systems level may also be a network of individuals or organizations working toward a policy or other systems-level goal. For example, a PHN might collaborate with drug counselors and law enforcement agencies to advocate for state or local policies that allow needle exchange programs for injection drug abusers.

Factors of Successful Collaboration

A study of the concepts related to collaboration among health organizations found that collaboration is a dynamic process commonly associated with the underlying concepts of sharing, partnership, interdependency, and power (D'Amour, Ferrada-Videla,

CASE STUDY	Community-Based Participatory Research: Preventing Youth Substance Use in a Rural Tobacco Growing County—Examples of Community Organizing, Networking, and Collaboration

The authors were involved in a three-year community-based participatory research (CBPR) project to develop, implement, and evaluate an innovative prevention program with the goal of sustaining effective strategies to prevent youth substance use in a rural tobacco-growing county in the South (Kulbok et al., 2015). CBPR projects are collaborative in nature and engage participants from a target community. This CBPR project focused on prevention of tobacco, alcohol, and other drug use among rural youth, which is critical for healthy youth development. During this CBPR project, the authors (public health nursing researchers) collaborated with investigators from another university and a health system, and with youth, parents, and community leaders from the rural southern county.

We successfully accomplished several project aims. First, we established a community participatory research team (CPRT) in the rural county with youths, parents, and community leaders. Second, we collaborated with the CPRT to complete a community assessment and identify factors influencing local youth substance use by conducting and analyzing community leader interviews and youth and parent focus groups. Third, we evaluated (with the CPRT) the effectiveness of three widely used prevention programs and selected *Health Rocks!*, a national 4-H tobacco, alcohol, and drug use preventive program, as the best fit for this rural tobacco-producing county. Fourth, we pilot tested the *Health Rocks!* program to determine feasibility, acceptability, and preliminary effectiveness data. Youths and adults from the county were trained to lead the *Health Rocks!* program. Two pilot programs were implemented during youth summer camp programs and evaluated positively by the participants and the CPRT.

Our CBPR project demonstrated the six factors of successful collaboration (Mattessich, Murray-Close, & Monsey, 2001). First, the researchers had completed two previous projects in this community on youth tobacco use prevention and were regarded positively as equal partners. We also engaged key community leaders who were respected by local residents. These factors created a favorable social climate for future collaboration. Second, we built a foundation of mutual trust and respect through our prior work together. The researchers and the CPRT, which included youths, parents, community leaders, were racially and socioeconomically diverse. Participation was voluntary and reflected personal interest in and commitment to the project. We used techniques such as nominal group process to allow the voices of all participants to be heard and valued. Third, the CPRT processes and structure allowed for full participation by all members. In particular, the youths' participation was encouraged and valued. Decision-making involved group processes and voting. Members assumed different roles across the three-year project including small group leadership activities. Fourth, lines of communication were open and included face-to-face communication at CPRT meetings, emails, and frequent use of text messaging for CPRT notifications. Fifth, the purpose of the CBPR project was clear to all participants. All CPRT members were committed to the project and involved in all project phases from the community assessment to implementation and evaluation of the youth substance use prevention program. Sixth, the Virginia Foundation for Healthy Youth funded the three-year project. The *Health Rocks!* program materials were available free from the local county cooperative extension agents. While the researchers were the conveners of regular monthly meetings, all CPRT members were engaged in the project activities as full partners.

San Martin, & Beaulieu, 2005). Additional concepts related to the success of a collaboration and the collaborative process include strong leadership, staff who are dedicated, flexible partnership structure, support for building each partner's capacity, identified goals, resources for education, sharing, and the actual launching for projects (Shrimali, Luginbuhl, Malin, Flournoy, & Siegel, 2014). Sharing often refers to collective responsibilities, decision-making, philosophy, values, data, planning, and interventions. Partnership implies two or more people engaged in communication and dialogue, shared decisions with mutual trust and respect, to achieve common goals (Truglio-Londrigan, 2017). Interdependency suggested a mutual dependence, which is necessary to deal with complex healthcare situations and often leads to collective action. Finally, when collaboration is viewed as a true partnership, participants share power equally. Power is a function of knowledge and experience and is the result of interactions between participants. Creating a successful collaboration takes time and effort to build trust among the individual participants, develop effective means of communicating, and an equitable division of labor and benefits. The more complex a collaboration relationship is, the more important it is to create a strong foundation to support an ongoing partnership.

Creating and maintaining a collaborative partnership can be a messy process, and there are many difficulties that can stop or damage the process. Entering into a collaboration can create risk for an individual or organization in terms of financial or labor costs, reputation, or missed opportunities from alternative pathways. Collaborations require time and energy from each partner in order to maintain them. High-level collaborations may yield high-impact solutions, but they can also be frustrating and time-consuming for the members. Potential partners should consider their ability to endure these difficulties and weigh them against the possibility of a successful outcome (Ontario Healthy Communities Coalition, 2016).

The structure and formation of collaboration can vary widely—it can be temporary or long term, informal or formal. For larger or more formal collaborations, factors of success can be grouped into six main categories: 1) environment, 2) membership, 3) process/structure, 4) communications, 5) purpose, and 6) resources (Mattessich, Murray-Close, & Monsey, 2001). **Box 14-1** expands these categories with the positive attributes that contribute to successful collaborations.

Coalition Building

A **coalition** consists of multiple individuals or organizations, often from different sectors, who agree to work together toward a shared goal (Keller & Strohschein, 2016; Minnesota Department of Health, 2001; Truglio-Londrigan, 2017). In community health, these goals are often to develop health-promoting resources in communities, change individuals' health behaviors, or shape public policies (Community Tool Box, 2016a, 2016b). Usually the coalition has a formal leadership and governance structure, and it has a name and other identifying features that distinguish it from its members. A coalition might have paid staff and its own offices, depending on its size and resources. A coalition's resources might come from financial contributions by its members, in-kind donations by its members such as office space or staff time, or external funding such as grants. Coalitions may be permanent or temporary; they can be formed to address a single issue or multiple issues. Typically, a coalition that is well organized and broad based will be more successful in effecting policy change, increasing knowledge of the public, and creating innovative solutions to complex problems of concern (Butterfoss & Kegler, 2009; Truglio-Londrigan, 2017; Wisconsin Clearinghouse for Prevention Resources, 2009).

Coalitions and collaborations can overlap in how they function. Collaborations may have formal policies, staff, and funding that make them identical to coalitions. The words coalition and collaboration are sometimes interchanged. For the purposes of this chapter, the formal structure of coalitions is the focus.

Uses of Coalitions

Coalition building can be beneficial for both addressing health problems directly and for increasing the capacity of the community to address future needs (Keller & Strohschein, 2016). Coalitions can address complex or widespread health issues that go beyond a single organization's scope. Community health problems often have root causes in multiple sectors

Box 14-1 Six Categories of Factors That Influence the Success of Collaboration

1. Environment
   A history of collaboration exists in the community.
   The collaborative group is seen as a community leader in the area in which it is focused.
   There is a favorable political/social climate.
2. Membership
   There is mutual respect, understanding, and trust.
   Cross-section of members in the group is appropriate.
   Collaboration is viewed as being in the self-interest of members.
   There is the ability to compromise.
3. Process/structure
   Members share a stake in both the process and groups.
   There are multiple layers of participation.
   There is flexibility and openness.
   Clear roles and policy guidelines are developed.
   There is adaptability in the face of changing conditions.
4. Communications
   There is open and frequent communication.
   Formal and informal communication links exist.
5. Purpose
   There is a concrete and unique purpose.
   There are clear, realistic, and attainable goals.
   There is a shared vision, with an agreed-on mission, objectives, and strategy.
6. Resources
   Funding is sufficient to support operations.
   The leader, or convener, of the collaborative group is skilled interpersonally and is fair and respected by partners.

Data from Mattessich, P., Murray-Close, M., & Monsey, B. (2001). *Wilder Collaboration Factors Inventory*. St. Paul, MN: Wilder Research. Retrieved from https://www.wilder.org/Wilder-Research/Research-Services/Pages/Wilder-Collaboration-Factors-Inventory.aspx

and levels of society. The socioecological framework is a way to visualize the complex web of interrelated factors that occur at individual, interpersonal, community, and societal levels (Stokols, 1996). For example, asthma is a disease that individuals must manage. However, factors such as housing, air quality, public transportation, and access to high-quality health care all contribute to disparities in asthma prevalence and severity (Bryant-Stephens, 2009). All of these root factors should be addressed in order to improve asthma outcomes. A coalition focused on asthma would bring together representatives from all sectors involved, as well as patients and family members affected by asthma. Coalitions can also have the advantage of size. A coalition, through its collective pooling of resources, can amplify the resources and outreach that any single organization could do. Coalitions can also cover large geographic areas or involve members from multiple localities.

Coalitions can also build community capacity to address future health issues by promoting link-ages and developing leadership among its members (Butterfoss & Kegler, 2009; Truglio-Londrigan, 2017). As described in the collaborations section, it takes time to build trust and communication channels among individuals or organizations. Participating together in a coalition can create these conditions needed for future collaboration between members. Coalitions can provide members with opportunities to develop their leadership skills and experience. These new leaders may assume leadership roles in the coalition or move beyond the coalition to direct other collective actions to promote community health. In either case, the community benefits from its members developing the capacity to become leaders. At the end of this section, there are several examples of coalitions and their specific web links. Take the time to connect to these links to learn more about coalitions.

Factors of Successful Coalition Building

Public health nurses can take a leadership role and initiate or participate in a variety of coalitions (Truglio-Londrigan, 2017). The coalitions might focus on specific topics, such as homelessness or obesity, or a coalition might choose to focus on a geographic area, such as a neighborhood or county. These coalitions tend to have broad long-term goals of improved health for the community and then select several health issues to focus on as short-term or ongoing programs.

Coalitions might work at both the community and the systems-focused levels, or they might focus on just one level. At the systems level, a coalition works to change the root causes of a problem or promote policies that favor a proposed solution. For example, a community health coalition might promote policies to fund drug rehabilitation facilities at systems level, while it also organizes educational programs at the community level.

The success of a coalition depends on how well it meets the unique situation and needs of its members. Six factors associated with successful coalition building were identified in rigorous evaluation studies: 1) create/enact formal procedural rules for governing the coalition, 2) appoint capable

and engaged leaders, 3) promote active participation of members, 4) recruit a diverse membership, 5) encourage member organizations to collaborate with each other, and 6) support group cohesion (Zakocs & Edwards, 2006). Furthermore, success of a coalition is also facilitated if there is respect and trust between and among all coalition members that foster ". . . . shared decision-making, team work and collaboration, and most certainly the willingness to be accountable and responsible toward the coalition's identified vision and mission statements" (Truglio-Londrigan, 2017, p. 101). The factors of coalition success are similar to those of collaborations, as listed in Box 14-1.

According to the Community Coalition Action Theory (Butterfoss & Kegler, 2009), coalitions progress through three key phases, sometimes cycling back to an earlier phase. Tasks during the formation stage are to develop a fully functioning organization and determine the mission and objectives regarding the impact the coalition wants to have in the community. The tasks during the formation stage are to assemble a core group of members with diverse skill sets but who share a strong interest in the coalition's goals. This core group then recruits additional members who represent diverse stakeholder groups. During this phase, the coalition establishes leadership and organizational processes and hires staff if resources allow.

During the maintenance phase, the coalition shifts its focus to planning and implementing its activities in the community. It also works to maintain its membership engagement and resources and increase community awareness of the coalition and the issues it addresses.

Finally, during the institutionalization phase, the coalition reflects on its achievements and assesses its own organizational structure to reassess the best path forward. Some coalitions decide to form their own nonprofit organization that is separate from the member organizations. Other coalitions disband if their usefulness or support has waned.

The unique conditions in a community, or community context, are likely to influence the success of a coalition. Community geography, economics, politics, and history form parts of the context. For example, a history of successful collaboration or previous coalitions makes a new coalition more likely to thrive. The Community Readiness Model is an assessment tool that can identify how ready a community is to take action toward a community health goal (Edwards et al., 2000).

| **CASE STUDY** | Clinch River Valley Initiative: A Rural Southwestern Virginal Coalition |

The Clinch River Valley Initiative (CRVI) is a coalition with the goal of promoting health, economic development, and ecological protection for the river and its nearby communities in rural southwestern Virginia. Coalition members include local businesspeople, community activists, school personnel, public health officials, regional planners, and other government officials. The University of Virginia provides expertise in meeting facilitation, grant writing, and other technical support. During its first six years, the coalition achieved substantial success in creating new recreation facilities for accessing the river, promoting the region as a tourism destination, cleaning up the river, and coordinating downtown revitalization efforts for several towns along the river. At the policy level, CRVI persuaded the state legislature to create a new Clinch River State Park. This multisectoral coalition highlights the ways that community health is embedded in all of these efforts: outdoor recreation opportunities promote physical fitness and stress reduction; economic development generates jobs and improved incomes; and ecological preservation helps protect water quality and wildlife habitat. **Box 14-2** provides additional examples of coalitions in operation across the United States.

Box 14-2 Coalition Examples and Web Links

The Bronx Health REACH Coalition at: http://www.institute.org/bronx-health-reach/about/who-we-are/the-bronx-health-reach-coalition/

Regional Asthma Coalitions in New York State at: https://www.health.ny.gov/diseases/asthma/coalitions.htm

Massachusetts Clubhouse Coalition (CSAC) at: http://www.massclubs.org/

Charlestown Substance Abuse Coalition at: http://www.massgeneral.org/cchi/services/treatmentprograms.aspx?id=1499

Chicago Big Cities Health Coalition at: http://www.bigcitieshealth.org/

Texas Oral Health Coalition at: http://www.txohc.org/

African Communities Public Health Coalition at: http://africancoalition.org/

Washington, DC. Coalition on Long-Term Care at: https://www.iona.org/how-you-can-help/advocacy/dc-coalition-on-long-term-care.html

Childhood Obesity Prevention Coalition Building a Healthier Generation at: http://copcwa.org/

Centers for Disease Control and Prevention—Build Planning Teams and Coalitions at: http://www.cdc.gov/phpr/healthcare/toolbox-build.htm

National Coalition against Diagnostic Violence at: http://www.ncadv.org/

Alaska Workforce Coalition at: https://www.ruralhealthinfo.org/community-health/project-examples/723

Community Organizing

Community organizing is one of the key intervention strategies in the orange wedge of the intervention wheel (Keller & Strohschein, 2016). The definitions of **community organizing** are diverse and evolving, depending on the perspective of the specific community. Community generally refers to a group of people who share a geographic location or other characteristics in common. Communities are groups of individuals who exhibit at least one common characteristic or shared interest; for example, a community of parents of intellectually disabled adults or older adults recently diagnosed with Alzheimer's disease (Brenner & Manice, 2011). Community organizing takes place as communities work together, identify problems, and decide on strategies to implement all for the expressed purpose of reaching a goal together (Keller & Strohschein, 2016; Minkler, 2012). The core element of community organizing is that people in the community come together to discuss community issues and make a collective decision to work together to successfully solve an issue. The assumptions that people are equal, and it is important to have input and participation of the community members underlie the strategy of community. The community, society, and the world can be changed, and people in the community are the agents of change (Walls, 2015).

Neighborhood organizing is a form of community organizing (Rubin & Rubin, 2001). Saul Alinsky, who is considered the founder of community organizing, emphasized collective actions by forming organizations to address immediate issues of community members. Community organizing is focused on solving problems of the community (Alinsky, 1946; Rubin & Rubin; 2001; Walls, 2015). When there is social change, there is a greater need for community organizing and transformative changes in the broader community and society (Pyles, 2013; Rubin & Rubin, 2008; Walls, 2015). An important aspect of community organizing resides in the questions: How does one organize a community and what skills are needed to organize the community toward action? The answer to these questions offer a glimpse into its complexity. Community organizing is, therefore, illustrative of primary health care (Truglio-Londrigan, 2017). With this more progressive point of view, community organizing has evolved to address large social changes for issues including policy changes; democratic changes; social justice; and a combination of social movements, online activism, civic engagement, and political campaigns.

Public health nursing competencies include basic and advanced skills that nurses need for community organizing. The public health nurse's role includes leading community organizing for health issues. Key elements of public health nursing practice include focusing on the health needs of the entire population, assessment of population health, and addressing multiple determinants of health. Successful outcomes in these areas require strategies for community organizing. Given the fact that community organizing has a participatory nature, public health nurses may need to serve as model, mentor, catalysts, teachers, or facilitators and fulfil a linking role in the organizing process (Rubin & Rubin, 2008). Organizers as a catalyst identify ways to facilitate people toward action; for example, by communicating with local leaders about issues and problems in their communities. Organizers as teachers help community members learn the necessary knowledge and skills they need to know in order to participate in the organizing process as well as the planning, implementation, and evaluation. As facilitators, public health nurses lead meetings and group process and do administrative work. Most importantly, as a facilitator, the public health nurse knows when to let go and support the people in the community to lead and use their voices. Throughout the entire process, the public health nurse guides, mentors, models, and above all listens to the people in the communities. Public health nurses can link their communities to outside groups and the broader society.

Uses of Community Organizing

Community organizing is beneficial when public health nurses assess health issues, particularly when there is greater need than an individual's effort can address (Rubin & Rubin, 2001). It is also beneficial when there is a need for community members' input in a systematic way, so that it enhances the capability to solve issues with more resources and social support. One key to community organizing is to identify what the key ingredients are to access the key members of a community and the stakeholders so that these same individuals embrace the notion of being engaged in any organizing efforts (Burton, O'Mara-Eves, & Thomas, 2014, p. 2857). Community organizing embraces the stakeholders and the community members as being equal and to gain equity in society and have shared power for shared decision-making, particularly when they may not have opportunities to express their perspective. In this way, community members will be empowered and the community issues may be solved with self-sufficiency.

Community organizing is a strategy that public health nurses apply to enact community and system-level changes. An example is noted when public health nurses work on diverse community health issues. For example, public health nurses may want to address childhood obesity in their community by increasing healthy eating options in the neighborhoods and regular physical activity programs in town parks. Furthermore, the public health nurse may see the need to address this specific issue in this specific population by seeking broad changes in policies or social structures; for example, working with school systems to alter policies on physical education classes. Other system-level changes may be brought about through community organizing and include health policy changes related to the environmental that may include sanitation, water, and other areas such as disability rights and climate justice.

How is the process of community organizing started? Public health nurses can bring community members together and hold a kickoff meeting. For the kickoff meeting to be successful, the public health nurse needs to have a cultural awareness of the specific community. This is important, for the kickoff meeting needs to be developed with an awareness of the community's cultural ideas, values, and beliefs as well as a historical understanding of how the community has worked in the past. This information serves to assist public health nurses in their endeavors. At the meeting, a task force may be created to begin the process of community organizing, which may later evolve into a more formal coalition to address the identified issue of childhood obesity. In the meetings, public health nurses gather information, identify issues and strategies, and make action plans with the key community members. Strategies could include engaging community partners to raise awareness. For example, in today's technological environment community organizing may be sustained and strengthened through the use of social media. Public health nurses mobilize people and plans, evaluate, adjust, and keep the plan moving with the community. In this way, complicated health issues can be addressed at a community level and find a sustainable solution.

Factors of Successful Community Organizing

There are strategies that may be implemented for successful community organizing (Kahn, 2010; Rubin, & Rubin, 2008). These strategies include:

- Understanding the community: Knowing people's self-interest and finding common interests are key principles for successful results. Understanding characteristics of the community, what is important to the community, and knowing the community culture and strengths are critical elements.
- Vision and shared goal: Creating and emphasizing a shared vision and goal.

- Group dynamics and power: Understanding who the key people are in the community and who holds the formal and informal power.
- Communication: Implementing communication strategies to ensure that messages are clear and everyone has all of the information they need to participate in the organizing process and make informed decision. Effective and efficient communication prevent miscommunication and misunderstandings. The methods and the means of communication must be carefully developed and implemented to meet the needs of the specific members of the community. Use of Facebook, Instagram, Twitter, blogs, email, and text messaging may work for some members of the community, whereas others may wish a simple phone call.
- Flexible and creative: Developing plans for community organizing that are unique to the community but most of all flexible and able to respond to the needs of the specific community over time.
- Empower participants: Supporting the initiative and the ability to lead future initiatives are more likely to occur when community members feel ownership in the initiative.

Stages of the Strategy

The following steps are general guidelines for community organizing. It is critical to think about the process of these strategies and tailor them according to what is most appropriate for each instance of community organizing (Rubin & Rubin, 2008; Walls, 2015).

1. Identifying a community health issue: The first step is defining and assessing a community and identifying the issues of concern by the community.
2. Planning: The planning phase includes goal setting, identifying potential facilitators and barriers, planning purposeful action, and developing an evaluation plan. Shared decision-making is essential during these steps with the community members.
3. Community partners and involving people: Part of the planning step is finding and involving community partners or stakeholders, community organizations, and community members. One method that can be implemented is simply knocking on doors, informing people with an invitation to participate.
4. Resource mobilization and expert availability: This includes knowing the resources and the expertise available and knowing how to generate, obtain, and use these resources and expertise.
5. Community action: Collective behavior will occur during this process. Organizing social action appropriately is important.
6. Evaluation: Community actions will need to be evaluated systematically via formative and summative evaluation according to the purpose and goal of community organizing.

During the whole process, the natural conversation with community members will allow the public health nurse to build a trusting relationship, understand the potential partners' motivation and self-interests, and create clear values. These interactions will be reflected in the public relationship, which indicates the official, accountable relationship between organizations.

Case Study

A public health nurse collaborated with a social worker and a county attorney to organize the Hmong Youth Task Force, aimed at reducing sexual exploitation and truancy among Hmong girls in a U.S. community (Saewyc, Solsvig, & Edinburgh, 2007). They used community organizing strategies to develop a coalition of community leaders and service providers, who identified needs, such as early intervention programs and resources for agencies to provide culturally and linguistically appropriate care. One such strategy of organizing the community included reaching out to Hmong community leaders and professionals. This initial respected group then reached out to the wider Hmong community to raise awareness of the issues, change social norms about girls, and promote use of community services. Some of the accomplishments of these efforts were the development of lasting connections between the Hmong community and mainstream organizations, the statewide dissemination of improved training and guidelines for youth exploitation services, and progress toward change in the local Hmong culture.

Conclusion

This chapter presents the interventions/strategies of the orange section of intervention wheel noted to be a process of collective action (Keller & Strohschein, 2016, p. 195). Collaboration, coalition building, and community organizing are aimed at harnessing the collective energy of more than one person or group.

Perhaps Margaret Mead said it best when describing the power of collective action: "Never doubt that a small group of thoughtful, committed citizens can change the world; indeed, it is the only thing that ever has" (Margaret Mead®, used with permission). Public health nurses can incorporate best practices when engaging in or supporting collective action to address health concerns. The strategies in the orange section of the wheel used in public health nursing maximizes the efforts of each individual or organization toward a mutual goal. Public health nurses are key players in any of these efforts, but they are not the only key players. Working with community members collectively via community organizing, collaboration, and coalition building fosters positive health outcomes along with enhancement of the community's capacity (Truglio-Londrigan & Barnes, 2015).

Additional Resources

County Health Rankings Work Together at: http://www.countyhealthrankings.org/roadmaps/action-center/work-together

Robert Wood Johnson Foundation at: www.rwjf.org

Freire Institute at: http://www.freire.org/

Community Tool Box at: http://ctb.ku.edu/en

Clinch River Initiative Valley Initiative at: www.clinchriverva.com http://coalitionswork.com/resources/tools/

Refugee Services Collaborative of Greater Cleveland at: http://rsccleveland.org/

Transforming Communities at: http://www.transformcommunities.org/

Healthy People in Healthy Communities at: http://www.healthypeople.gov/2010/Publications/Healthy Communities2001/default.htm

---

Lessons from History

The purpose of this section in this intervention chapter is to demonstrate for the reader how history does inform our contemporary practice, and the take-away messages are varied and many. The following history of the American Red Cross Town and Country was adapted from Lewenson (2017). Take the time to read it, and see what your take-away is.

(continues)

Working Together: Collaboration, Coalition Building, and Community Organizing.

Margaret Chanler Aldrich and others in the community based their need to establish the Red Hook Nursing Association on the outcomes of the 1915 *Sickness in Dutchess County* report. The tables published in this report clearly indicated the need for public health nurses to work alongside physicians and other social agencies that existed in the local and statewide arena. Even so, with the collaborative efforts of those serving on the community nursing committee that eventually led to the Red Hook Nursing Association, Aldrich wrote in the local newspaper that everyone needed to participate in making the community healthier. In subsequent letters to the editor, Chanler Aldrich continued to express concern about the study's findings, highlighting the disease found and the inadequate care provided in the county. She urged each person to take part in this community effort by subscribing to the proposed Red Hook Nursing Association.

Photo of news clipping from the Tivoli Times, April 6, 1916.

Located in Adriance Memorial Library, Poughkeepsie, New York, Box 362.104 R Box Red Hook Nursing Association, Scrapbook, 1916–1917.

"Unless everyone takes part . . . by fighting disease, and by keeping an expert on the spot," Chanler Aldrich wrote, "Dutchess County will lag behind . . . Our doctors cannot be our nurses" (Aldrich, April 6, 1916).

The town committee came together on a weekly basis to plan for the nursing association. The various stakeholders included the whole town in its effort to raise funds for this venture. Everyone in the community was invited to purchase subscriptions to be part of the newly formed Red Hook Nursing Association and raise funds to hire the American Red Cross Town and Country nurse.

Subscriptions to the Red Hook Nursing Association

Questions to Consider

1. Reflect on the meaning of *collaboration, coalition building,* and *community organizing* when developing public health nursing initiatives such as the American Red Cross Town and Country.
2. Explore the value public health nurses bring to the strategies of collaboration, coalition building, and community organizing.
3. Explore the kinds of educational background a public health nurse needs to implement the strategies of collaboration, coalition building, and community organizing.

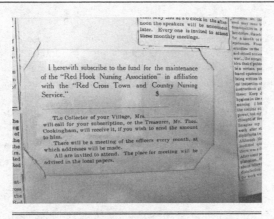

Located in Adriance Memorial Library, Poughkeepsie, New York, Box 362.104 R Box Red Hook Nursing Association, Scrapbook, 1916-1917.

The above case is adapted from Lewenson, S. B. (2017). Historical exemplars in nursing. In S. B. Lewenson & M. Truglio-Londrigan (Eds.), *Practicing primary health care in nursing: Caring for populations* (pp. 1–17). Burlington, MA: Jones & Bartlett Learning.

CASE STUDY AND CRITICAL QUESTIONS	**Collective Action to Address Adolescent Risk Behaviors** Marianne Cockroft, PhD, RN The University of North Carolina at Chapel Hill

Every spring, senior high youth anticipate end-of-school-year activities. Prom and graduation celebrations are milestone events that often bridge the gap between childhood and adult status. All too often, however, youth are unprepared for the peer pressures that accompany these special times. Sexual activity and the use of illegal substances can be dangerous and can turn a joyous celebration into a physical, psychological, and spiritual disaster for teens. This case study describes how collaboration, coalition building, and community organizing were used to develop two innovative intervention programs by the members of a high school PTA in North Carolina. Their mission was to encourage healthy social behaviors, promote safe driving practices, and prevent injury in high school youth on prom night.

(continues)

Collaboration

Parent–Teacher Associations (PTA) are dedicated to the educational success as well as the health and well-being of all students through strong family and community engagement (National PTA, 2016). Schools with active PTAs demonstrate collaborative efforts between students, parents, teachers, administrators, and other members of the community. A common goal of these individual groups is the health and safety of the youth.

With knowledge of the recent deaths of several teens in the area due to motor vehicle accidents and substance abuse, the local PTA identified a critical need to contribute to a solution of this complex problem in the community. The president of the PTA, who had experience in grant writing, and the chair of the health and safety committee, a parent volunteer with experience in public health nursing, led the development and the implementation of an intervention plan and, in addition, secured funding for the programs through a grant from the North Carolina PTA (NCPTA).

Coalition Building

A temporary coalition was formed to address the trifold mission. The alliance of the high school PTA with the local town council, the Safety and Health Council of North Carolina, local police department, and local businesses exemplified a strong commitment from a variety of organizations to address the identified concerns. Prior to prom night, the Safety and Health Council of North Carolina agreed to provide Alive at 25, the National Safety Council defensive driving program, at the high school to educate the students on the conflicts and consequences that arise with high-risk social behaviors. With the grant awarded by the NCPTA and matching funds contributed by the local town council, the PTA created an after-prom party, a supervised alcohol- and drug-free event aimed at reducing the opportunity for teens to engage in the risky behaviors associated with prom night.

Community Organizing

Maximizing the community resources was paramount to the success of the after-prom party. Numerous volunteers from the community participated in the preparations and the delivery of the event. Tasks included the development and analysis of a survey for students, solicitation of door prizes and donations of food from local businesses, securing the party venue, decorating the facility, contracting with professional entertainment, advertising the event, coordinating volunteers, communication with parents, developing student check-in and check-out procedures, set up, clean up, and party monitors. A local police and school resource officer provided parking lot security. All businesses approached provided free or discounted services to support the worthy cause.

The inaugural event was deemed a success by students, parents, school administration, and members of the community, and it has been sustained with additional fundraising efforts. This case study demonstrates how a nurse can contribute valuable knowledge and leadership skills in the development of innovative community-level interventions to promote adolescent health.

Website

http://www.pta.org/about/content.cfm?ItemNumber=944&navItemNumber=552

Given the case story, consider the following questions:

1. How was community organizing initiated?
2. Can you think of any other community organization that could have been valuable to this community organizing?
3. What purpose was the survey of the students?
4. Consider the members of the coalition, and identify other groups or organizations who would have been valuable to the success of the mission of the coalition.
5. Would you consider the student union a potential member of the coalition? If yes, provide a rationale.
6. What strategies would you suggest to strengthen the partnerships and the collaborative process of this initiative?

References

Alinsky, S. D. (1946). *Reveille for radicals.* Chicago, IL: University of Chicago Press.

Alinsky, S. D. (1971). *Rules for radicals.* Chicago, IL: University of Chicago Press.

Arnstein, S. R. (1969). A ladder of citizen participation. *Journal of the American Institute of planners, 35*(4), 216–224.

Berkowitz, B. (2000). Community and neighborhood organization. In J. Rappaport & E. Seidman (Eds.), *Handbook of community psychology* (pp. 331–357). New York, NY: Springer Science+Business Media LLC. doi:10.1007/978-1-4615-4193-6_14

Bobo, K. A., Kendall, J., & Max, S. (1991). *Organizing for social change: A manual for activists in the 1990s.* Minneapolis, MN: Seven Locks.

Brager, G., Specht, H., & Torczyner, J. L. (1987). *Community organizing.* New York, NY: Columbia University Press.

Brenner, B., & Manice, M. (2011). Community engagement in children's environmental health research. *Mount Sinai Journal of Medicine, 78*(1), 85–97.

Brunton, G., O'Mara-Eves, A., & Thomas, J. (2014). The "'active ingredients'" for successful community engagement with disadvantaged expectant and new mothers: A qualitative comparative analysis. *Journal of Advanced Nursing, 70*(12), 2847–2860.

Bryant-Stephens, T. (2009). Asthma disparities in urban environments. *Journal of Allergy and Clinical Immunology, 123*(6), 1199–1206.

Butterfoss, F. D., & Kegler, M. C. (2009). The community coalition action theory. In DiClemente, R. J., Crosby, R. A., & Kegler, M. (Eds.), *Emerging theories in health promotion practice and research* (2nd ed., pp. 237–276). San Francisco, CA: Jossey-Bass.

Campbell, C. (2014). Community mobilisation in the 21st century: Updating our theory of social change? *Journal of Health Psychology, 19*(1), 46–59.

Chandra, A., Acosta, J. D., Carman, K. G., Dubowitz, T., Leviton, L., Martin, L. T., . . . Plough, A. L. (2016). *Building a national culture of health: Background, action framework, measures and next steps.* Santa Monica, CA: Rand Corporation.

Christens, B. D., & Speer, P. W. (2011). Contextual influences on participation in community organizing: A multilevel longitudinal study. *American Journal of Community Psychology, 47*(3–4), 253–263. doi:10.1007/s10464-010-9393-y

Christens, B. D., & Speer, P. W. (2015). Community organizing: Practice, research, and policy implications. *Social Issues and Policy Review, 9*(1) 193–222.

Community Tool Box. (2016a). Chapter 5, Section 5. Coalition Building 1: Starting a Coalition. Retrieved from http://ctb.ku.edu/en/table-of-contents/assessment/promotion-strategies/start-a-coaltion/main

Community Tool Box. (2016b). Section 1. Strategies for community change and improvement: An overview. Retrieved from http://ctb.ku.edu/en/table-of-contents/assessment/promotion-strategies/overview/main

Connery, R. H. (1968). *The politics of mental health: Organizing community mental health in metropolitan areas.* New York, NY: Columbia University Press.

D'Amour, D., Ferrada-Videla, M., San Martin, R. L., & Beaulieu, M. D. (2005). The conceptual basis for interprofessional collaboration: core concepts and theoretical frameworks. *Journal of interprofessional care, 19*, 116.

Edwards, R. W., Jumper-Thurman, P., Plested, B. A., Oetting, E. R., & Swanson, L. (2000). Community readiness: Research to practice. *Journal of community psychology, 28*(3), 291–307.

Gilbert, M. (2006). Rationality in collective action. *Philosophy of the social sciences, 36*(1), 3–17.

Glass, R. D. (2001). On Paulo Freire's philosophy of praxis and the foundations of liberation education. *Educational Researcher, 30*(2), 15–25.

Hassmiller, S. B. (2017). Nursing's role in building a culture of health. In S. B. Lewenson & M. Truglio-Londrigan (Eds.), Practicing primary health care in nursing: Caring for populations (pp. 33–60). Burlington, MA: Jones & Bartlett Learning.

Himmelman, A. (1993). An introduction to community-based collaboration with a collaborative design planning guide. *Communities working collaboratively for change.* Minneapolis: University of Minnesota.

Himmelman, A. T. (2002). Collaboration for a change. *Definitions, models, roles and a guide for collaborative process.* Minneapolis: Hubert Humphrey Institute of Public Affairs, University of Minnesota.

Kahn, S. (2010). Top 20 principles for community organizing. *Social Policy, 40*(2), 23–24. Retrieved from Education Research Complete database.

Kahn, S. (2010, March 19). 20 principles for successful community organizing [Review of the book *Creative community organizing: A guide for rabble-rousers, activists and quiet lovers of justice*]. *Alternet.* Retrieved from http://www.alternet.org/story/145924/20 _principles_for_successful_community_organizing

Kegler, M. C., Rigler, J., & Honeycutt, S. (2010). How does community context influence coalitions in the formation stage? A multiple case study based on the Community Coalition Action Theory. *BMC Public Health, 10*(1), 1.

Keller, L. O., & Strohschein, S. (2016). Population-based public health nursing practice: The intervention wheel. In M. Stanhope & J. Lancaster (Eds.), *Public health nursing: Population-centered health care in the community* (9th ed., pp. 190–216). St. Louis, MO: Mosby Elsevier.

Kretzmann, J. P., & McKnight, J. L. (1994). *Building communities from the inside out: A path toward finding and mobilizing a community's assets.* Chicago, IL: ACTA Publications.

Kulbok, P. A., Meszaros, P. S., Bond, D. C., Thatcher, E., Park, E., Kimbrell, M., & Smith-Gregory, T. (2015). Youths as partners in a community participatory project for substance use prevention. *Family & community health, 38*(1), 3–11.

Lewenson, S. B. (2017). Historical exemplars. In S. B. Lewenson & M. Truglio-Londrigan (Eds.), *Practicing primary health care in nursing: Caring for populations* (pp. 1–19). Burlington, MA: Jones & Bartlett Learning.

Mattessich, P., Murray-Close, M., & Monsey, B. (2001). *Wilder Collaboration Factors Inventory.* St. Paul, MN: Wilder Research. Retrieved from https://www .wilder.org/Wilder-Research/Research-Services /Pages/Wilder-Collaboration-Factors-Inventory .aspx

Merriam-Webster Dictionary. (2015). Retrieved from http://www.merriam-webster.com/dictionary /collaborate

Minkler, M. (2012). *Community organizing and community building for health and welfare* (3rd ed.). New Brunswick, NJ: Rutgers University Press.

Minnesota Department of Health. (2001). *Public health nursing section: Public health interventions— applications for public health nursing practice.* St. Paul, MN. Retrieved from http://www.health .state.mn.us/divs/opi/cd/phn/wheel.html#citation

Olson Keller, L., Strohschein, S., Lia-Hoagberg, B., & Schaffer, M. (1998). Population-based public health nursing interventions: A model from practice. *Public Health Nursing, 15*(3), 207–215.

Ontario Healthy Communities Coalition. (2016). *Types of collaborations.* Retrieved from http://www .ohcc-ccso.ca/en/courses/community-development -for-health-promoters/module-three-community -collaboration/types-of-col

Prochaska, J. O., DiClemente, C. C., & Norcross, J. C. (1992). In search of how people change: Applications to addictive behaviors. *American psychologist, 47*(9), 1102–1114.

Pyles, L. (2013). *Progressive community organizing: Reflective practice in a globalizing world* (2nd ed.). New York, NY: Routledge.

Quad Council of Public Health Nursing Organizations. (1999). *Scope and standards of public health nursing practice.* Washington, DC: American Nurses Association.

Quad Council of Public Health Nursing Organizations. (2011). *Quad Council competencies for public health nurses.* Washington, DC: Author.

Quad Council of Public Health Nursing Organizations. (2011). *Quad council competencies for public health nurses.* Retrieved from http://www.resourcenter.net /images/ACHNE/Files/QuadCouncilCompetencies ForPublicHealthNurses_Summer2011.pdf

Robert Wood Johnson Foundation. (2015*). Building a culture of health.* Retrieved from http://www.rwjf .org/en/how-we-work/building-a-culture-of-health .html

Rothman, J. (1999). *Reflections on community organization: Enduring themes and critical issues.* Itasca, IL: F. E. Peacock Publishers.

Rothman, J., Erlich, J., & Tropman, J. (1995). *Strategies of community intervention* (5th ed.). Itasca, IL: F. E. Peacock Publishers.

Roussos, S. T., & Fawcett, S. B. (2000). A review of collaborative partnerships as a strategy for improving community health. *Annual review of public health, 21*(1), 369–402.

Rubin, H. J., & Rubin, I. (2008). *Community organizing and development* (4th ed.). Boston, MA: Pearson/ Allyn & Bacon.

Saewyc, E. M., & Solsvig, W. (2008). The Hmong youth task force: Evaluation of a coalition to address the sexual exploitation of young runaways. *Public Health Nursing, 25*(1), 69–76.

Schutz, A., & Miller, M. (2015). *People power: The community organizing tradition of Saul Alinsky.* Nashville, TN: Vanderbilt University Press.

Shrimali, B. P., Luginbuhl, J., Malin, C., Flournoy, R., & Siegel. (2014). The building blocks collaborative: Advancing a life course approach to health equity through multisector collaboration. *Maternal and Child Health Journal, 18*(2), 373–379.

Shirley, D. (1997). *Community organizing for urban school reform.* Austin: University of Texas Press.

Siegal, G., Siegal, N., & Bonnie, R. J. (2009). An account of collective actions in public health. *American Journal of Public Health, 99*(9), 1583–1587.

Smock, K. (2004). *Democracy in action: Community organizing and urban change.* New York, NY: Columbia University Press.

Speer, P. W., Tesdahl, E. A., & Ayers, J. F. (2014). Community organizing practices in a globalizing era: Building power for health equity at the community level. *Journal of Health Psychology, 19*(1), 159–169. doi:10.1177/1359105313500255

Stoecker, R., (2009). Community organizing. In R. Hutchison (Ed.), *Encyclopedia of urban studies: Community organizing* (p. 180). Thousand Oaks, CA: SAGE Publications, Inc. doi:http://dx.doi.org/10.4135/9781412971973.n66

Stokols, D. (1996). Translating social ecological theory into guidelines for community health promotion. *American journal of health promotion, 10*(4), 282–298.

Taber, J. (2011). The public health model: Democratic community organizing. *Fourth World Journal,* 10(1), 73–94. Retrieved from Education Research Complete database.

Truglio-Londrigan, M. (2017). Coalitions, partnerships, and shared decision-making: A primary healthcare perspective. In S. B. Lewenson & M. Truglio-Londrigan (Eds.), *Practicing primary health care in nursing: Caring for populations* (pp. 89–108). Burlington, MA: Jones & Bartlett Learning.

Truglio-Londrigan, M., & Barnes, C. (2015). Working together: Shared decision-making. In S. B. Lewenson & M. Truglio-Londrigan (Eds.), *Decision-making in nursing: Thoughtful approaches for leadership* (pp. 141–162). Burlington, MA: Jones & Bartlett Learning.

Varda, D. M., Chandra, A., Stern, S. A., & Lurie, N. (2008). Core dimensions of connectivity in public health collaboratives. *Journal of Public Health Management, 14*(5), E1–E7.

Wald, L. D. (1913, December 5). The foreign vote. Speech at meeting of Equal Suffrage League of the City of New York, at the Hotel Astor. Lillian Wald Papers, Writings & Speeches, Voters & Voting, 1913. Reel 25, Box 36, Folder 6, pp. 1–13. New York City Public Library, New York, NY.

Walls, D. S. (2015). *Community Organizing.* Hoboken, NJ: John Wiley & Sons.

Wisconsin Clearinghouse for Prevention Resources. (2009). *Prevention—Coalition building.* Retrieved from http://wch.uhs.wisc.edu

Zakocs, R. C., & Edwards, E. M. (2006). What explains community coalition effectiveness? A review of the literature. *American Journal of Preventive Medicine, 30*(4), 351–361.

For a full suite of assignments and additional learning activities, use the access code located in the front of your book to visit this exclusive website: http://go.jblearning.com/londrigan. If you do not have an access code, you can obtain one at the site.

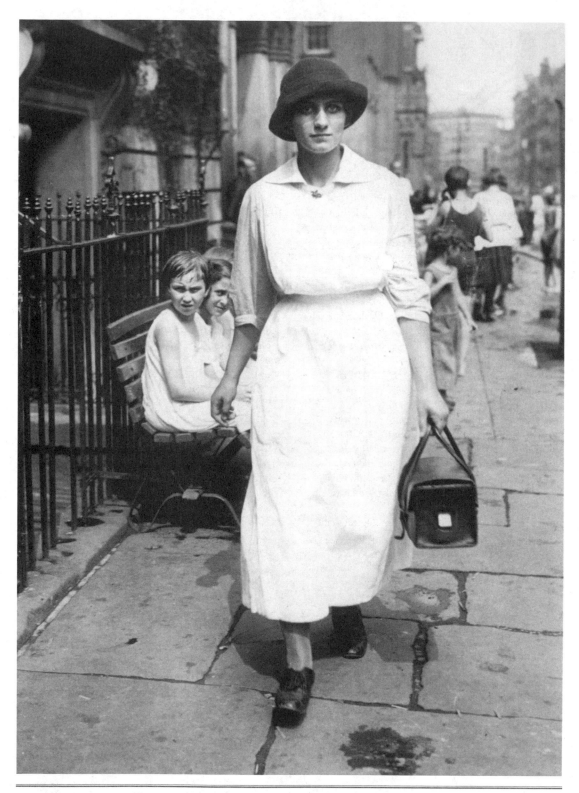

Courtesy of the Visiting Nurse Service of New York.

CHAPTER 15

Getting the Word Out: Advocacy, Social Marketing, and Policy Development and Enforcement

Susan Moscou
Nancy Murphy

Another phase of the social opportunities of the nurse is the occasion so often presented to her to talk frankly and wisely on the subject of Sanitary and Moral Prophylaxis in sexual hygiene. The community is growing out of its false conventional attitude in relation to this most serious question, and no more far-reaching education can be given than intelligent knowledge of the danger that lies in neglecting this subject. The doctors have taken it up and have organized for the purpose of spreading truth among the laity as well as to stir up a sense of obligation among the physicians themselves. Who more than the district nurse has the opportunity of unforced occasions for helping the mothers to deal with knowledge and delicacy with their sons and daughters. (Wald, 1907, p. 2)

LEARNING OBJECTIVES

At the completion of this chapter, the reader will be able to:

- Describe social marketing, advocacy, and policy development and enforcement.
- Apply social marketing, advocacy, and policy development and enforcement to the levels of public health practice.
- Explore the ways that public health nursing may apply and do social marketing, advocacy, and policy development and enforcement.

KEY TERMS

- ❏ Advocacy
- ❏ HIV
- ❏ Policy development
- ❏ Policy enforcement
- ❏ Preexposure prophylaxis (PrEP)
- ❏ Social marketing

The intervention wheel strategies describes public health interventions that are applicable to public health nursing. This chapter presents the yellow section of the intervention wheel, otherwise known as advocacy, social marketing, and policy development and enforcement. Advocacy is considered the precursor to policy development, and social marketing is viewed as a strategy for carrying out advocacy (Minnesota Department of Health, 2001). It is important to remember advocacy and policy can significantly change direction depending on who is elected to Congress and the Presidency as well as who is appointed to the Supreme Court.

This chapter is divided into three sections. The first section provides a discussion about the emerging use of preexposure prophylaxis (PrEP) to reduce HIV infections in adolescent populations because youth in the United States account for approximately 22% of new HIV infections in the age group of 13–24 years (CDC, 2016a). HIV infections in adolescents remain a major public health issue. The second section is a case study that highlights how the prevalence of HIV in adolescents and young adults should be viewed as a public health issue. Finally, the third section depicts how the public health nurse, in the case study, engages in advocacy, social marketing, and policy development and enforcement, which are public health interventions leading to the three levels of public health practice: individual/family, community, and system focused. Please remember that the exemplars in this chapter are time sensitive, and as evidence is gathered there will be ongoing alterations in practice.

The case study in this chapter provides a paradigm of how a public health nurse uses the intervention wheel to implement PrEP at a school-based clinic. The nurse gathers the appropriate facts about the prevalence of HIV infections in adolescents and then compares that data with current guidelines and trends about HIV prevention. Once the public health nurse has the relevant data, the nurse applies public health interventions of advocacy and social marketing to develop policy and enforcement strategies around the implementation of PrEP in the school-based clinic. Advocacy, social marketing, and policy development and enforcement strategies are applied at the population, community, systems, and individual/family levels.

Issue: The Implementation of PrEP within Adolescent School-Based Clinics

There are an estimated 1.2 million persons living with **HIV** infection in the United States. In 2014, approximately 44,000 new HIV infections were diagnosed. Among males, gay and bisexual men accounted for an estimated 83% (29,418) of HIV diagnoses and 67% of all diagnoses. Racial and ethnic data about HIV infections in men who have sex with men (MSM) show that Black/African American MSM accounted for 11,201 of estimated HIV diagnoses, White MSM accounted for 9,008, and Hispanic/Latino MSM accounted for 7,522. Heterosexual contact accounted for approximately 24% of all HIV diagnoses, with women accounting for 19% (8,328). In 2014, young people aged 13–24 accounted for 22% of new HIV infections, even though they comprised 16% of the U.S. population. Young MSM accounted for 92% of all new HIV diagnoses. As the numbers indicate, young MSM are at higher risk for acquiring HIV (CDC, 2016a).

The development of effective antiretroviral treatment (ART) for HIV in 1996 transformed infection with HIV from a life-threatening and terminal condition into a serious but manageable chronic illness for those who are able to access care and maintain continuous ART (Bartlett, 2006). Long-term or sustained HIV viral suppression, where the HIV virus is undetectable in the body, works to repair immune system functions and decrease individual morbidity and mortality. ART has also demonstrated that HIV treatment reduces the risk of transmitting HIV to sexual partners (Bavinton et al., 2015; Cohen et al., 2011). Treatment as prevention has become the mantra in HIV care (Montaner et al., 2014); however, in 2011, only 86% of those living with HIV infection were diagnosed, 40% were engaged in care, 37% were prescribed ART, and 30% achieved viral suppression (Bradley et al., 2014). Therefore, additional HIV prevention efforts are critical.

Preexposure Prophylaxis

Reducing new HIV infections is the number one goal of the National HIV/AIDS Strategy: Updated to 2020, which provides information needed to address the U.S. response to the HIV epidemic (Office of National AIDS Policy [ONAP], 2015). **Preexposure prophylaxis** or PrEP is a prevention strategy for individuals who are HIV negative to prevent new infections. PrEP reduces the risk of acquiring HIV. Current PrEP recommendations are that individuals take oral HIV medication tenofovir and emtricitabine, product name Truvada®, daily to prevent the transmission of HIV when exposed to HIV through unprotected sex or injection drug use. PrEP reduces HIV infection in individuals who are at higher risk for contracting HIV. PrEP, combined with consistent condom use and other prevention strategies, is considered a powerful HIV prevention tool (CDC, 2016b).

The U.S. Public Health Service (2014) released comprehensive clinical practice guidelines for PrEP.

The guidelines state that PrEP should be offered to adults at risk for HIV infection. The guidelines also identify that the completed PrEP clinical trials did not include individuals under the age of 18 (p. 43). Research about the efficacy and the safety of PrEP in adolescents is underway (CDC, 2017), and PrEP may soon be indicated for minor adolescents (Mullins, Lally, Zimet, & Khan, 2015). Truvada® has been used as a part of HIV treatment in adolescents for many years without toxic side effects. Based on the safety profile, off-label use of PrEP medications for adolescents aged 13–18 after high-risk exposure have been recommended by the International Antiviral Society–USA Panel (Marrazo et al., 2014).

Prescribing or dispensing PrEP, testing for sexually transmitted infections (STIs), and education about HIV prevention methods are not prohibited by states. However, laws and regulations that may be relevant for PrEP-related services differ by jurisdiction. "Clinicians considering providing PrEP to a person under age of legal adulthood (a minor) should be aware of local laws, regulations and policies that may apply" (USPHS, 2014, p. 42). Minors can consent to medical care to diagnose and treat STIs in all jurisdictions. Only eight states require consent for preventive or prophylactic services (e.g., condoms or emergency contraception). Minors can consent to HIV services in 34 states, and 17 jurisdictions allow minors to consent to STI testing and treatment but do not have a specific provision in which HIV is classified as an STI or communicable disease (Culp & Caucci, 2013). Recent analysis of law and policy regarding PrEP and youth has been undertaken (Burda, 2016). The present PrEP guidance summary is shown in **Box 15-1**.

The Intervention Wheel Strategies and Levels of Practice

Advocacy

What is **advocacy**, and why is it important to the public health nurse? Advocacy can be defined in several ways, depending on one's perspective.

Box 15-1 PrEP Guidance Summary

1. Substantial risk factors for acquiring HIV infection
   a. Men who have sex with men
   b. Heterosexual men and women
   c. Injection drug users
2. Clinical eligibility for PrEP
   a. Documented negative HIV test
   b. No signs or symptoms of HIV infection
   c. Normal renal function
   d. Not taking contraindicated medications
   e. Documented hepatitis B virus infection and vaccination status
3. Prescription medications (current recommendation)
   a. Daily oral dose of Truvada® (tenofivir and emtricitabine) for 90 days
4. Other required services
   a. Follow-up visits every three months
   b. HIV testing
   c. Adherence counseling
   d. Behavioral risk reduction counseling
   e. Renal function testing at three months, then every six months
   f. STI screening every six months
   g. Assess pregnancy intent and pregnancy test every three months
   h. Access to clean needles
   i. Access to drug treatment programs

Reproduced from U.S. Public Health Service. (2014). *Preexposure prophylaxis for the prevention of HIV infection in the United States—2014; A Clinical Practice Guideline.* Retrieved from https://www.cdc.gov/hiv/pdf/prepguidelines2014.pdf

---

Cohen, de la Vega, and Watson (2001) presented a value-neutral view of advocacy and spoke of this concept as action oriented. They noted how advocacy influenced decisions on the political, economic, and social systems front that affect people. However, nursing advocacy is not value neutral because of the nursing code of ethics. The American Nurses Association (ANA) new *Code of Ethics for Nurses with Interpretive Statements* (2015) delineates the role of nurses in relation to their patients, families, and profession. Nurses are responsible for advocating and promoting the health, safety, and the rights of their patients. Furthermore, the ANA's *Public Health Nursing: Scope & Standards of Practice* (2013) addresses the responsibility of public health nurses to serve and protect the public who cannot address their own concerns.

Nursing advocacy has been a central role of nurses and public health nurses specifically. Ballou (2000) discussed the three ideologies present in the nursing literature. These ideologies included 1) professional nursing as a moral endeavor, 2) advocacy, and 3) caring. The public health nurse is participating in advocacy when he or she ". . . pleads someone's cause or acts on someone's behalf, with a focus on developing the capacity of the community, system, individual, or family to plead their own cause or act on their own behalf" (Keller & Strohschein, 2016, p. 206). This advocacy is not only an intervention or strategy but a process.

CASE STUDY   HIV and Adolescent School-based Clinics

Ms. Jones, a public health nurse, has worked at Greene Junior High School's school-based clinic with a family nurse practitioner (FNP) for 10 years. Ms. Jones and the FNP work collaboratively in which Ms. Jones is responsible for triage, screening, and health education of the students who utilize the clinic. Because the FNP only works part-time, Ms. Jones' primary responsibility is to assist students with their healthcare needs. Students come to the school-based clinic for acute medical problems such as colds, sore throats, STIs, along with HIV testing, pregnancy testing, contraception management, and management of chronic medical conditions such as asthma and diabetes. Last year, a group of students formed a Gay-Straight Alliance (GSA) club. GSA clubs are student-run organizations that bring together lesbian, gay, bisexual, transgendered, and questioning (LGBTQ) and straight students to support each other, provide a safe place to socialize, and create a platform to fight for racial, gender, LGBTQ, and economic justice (GSA Network, 2016). Ms. Jones and the FNP played a major role in supporting the students to form the GSA club. The GSA invited Ms. Jones to discuss PrEP with its members as part of their educational campaign about HIV awareness, prevention strategies, and to incorporate a PrEP program as part of the services offered by the school-based clinic.

In preparation for the PrEP lecture and program development, Ms. Jones, who recently obtained a master's in public health, approached this request using her knowledge about public health, epidemiology, social epidemiology, and health policy. Additionally, as a member of the Society for Adolescent Health Medicine (SAHM), the National Association for School Health Nurses (NASN), and the Association for Public Health Nurses (APHN), Ms. Jones has a network of colleagues who can provide guidance and support in developing a PrEP program in a school-based clinic.

Ms. Jones investigated the prevalence of STIs, HIV infections, and PrEP utilization in adolescent populations as well as consent laws in states about dispensing or prescribing PrEP to adolescents. Additionally, Ms. Jones contacted other school-based clinics in her state and other states to gain information about their policies in dispensing and/or prescribing PrEP to adolescents, and how school-based clinics provide PrEP to students who are uninsured or students who have insurance but PrEP medications are not covered. Further, Ms. Jones examined if local, state, or federal programs existed that assisted school-based clinics in purchasing PrEP medication so PrEP could be dispensed by the school nurse.

Ms. Jones learns that PrEP is considered an emerging public health prevention approach, which reduces HIV infections in adolescents. Based on extensive research and evidence-based practice, Ms. Jones is convinced that PrEP should become part of the healthcare services offered at the school-based clinic. Implementing PrEP will require that Ms. Jones has systems in place to provide education to students, parents, principals, teachers, staff, and the community about:

- Risk factors of acquiring HIV infections.
- Clinically eligible patients.
- Medication prescription or dispensary of Truvada® (emtricitabine/tenofovir) at the school-based clinic.
- Other clinic services such as follow-up visits at 3 months and 6 months for HIV testing, adherence counseling, STI assessment, and laboratory testing (renal function).
- Cost of offering or prescribing PrEP to adolescent students.

The following sections (advocacy, social marketing, and social policy and enforcement) describe the strategies Ms. Jones can use to implement PrEP at the school-based clinic.

as well. Bu and Jezewski (2007) noted that this advocacy process consists of ". . . a series of specific actions for preserving, representing and/or safeguarding patients' rights, best interest and values in the healthcare system" (p. 104). These authors carried out a concept analysis on patient advocacy. Their findings revealed three core attributes: 1) safeguarding patients' autonomy, 2) acting on behalf of patients, and 3) championing social justice in the provision of health care (Bu & Jezewski, 2007). Reflecting upon their findings informs the reader that a nurse is and can be an advocate not only for an individual or family unit but for a group or population as well as a system and even an organization.

Advocates support a particular cause or issue to get individuals and communities involved in influencing the public and policymakers about their particular issue. Using the case study, Ms. Jones identified a burgeoning public health problem in which HIV prevention using PrEP can then lead to lower rates of HIV infections in adolescents.

The first step in advocacy is to introduce the problem to those who assist in supporting the PrEP program. Ms. Jones knows that successful advocacy requires that people are informed and well educated about the issues. After meeting with the GSA, Ms. Jones approaches the principal about their request for a PrEP program. Ms. Jones provides the principal with compelling evidence about the success of PrEP in preventing HIV infections. Ms. Jones then requests that the principal put the PrEP program on the agenda for the upcoming teacher and staff meeting. After the teacher and staff meeting, Ms. Jones meets with the GSA chapter at the high school to discuss the outcome of the meeting and to plan for the upcoming Parent–Teacher Association (PTA) meeting.

In preparation for the PTA meeting, Ms. Jones prepares a fact sheet that contains information about the estimated number of adolescents diagnosed with STIs, HIV, and PrEP. The fact sheet also describes the role of school-based clinics in disseminating information about PrEP and providing PrEP. On the community-focused level, Ms. Jones conducts research about the actual number of students requesting testing for STI, HIV, and pregnancy as well as gathering data about student requests for condoms, contraception, emergency contraception, and educational pamphlets. Additionally, Ms. Jones investigates the consent laws of states about PrEP and if there are specific rules and regulations governing school-based clinics. Ms. Jones collects these data to address questions and possible objections that parents may raise. Ms. Jones knows that when parents and teachers

---

Box 15-2 Advocacy Intervention Applied at the Population, Community, System, and Individual/Family Levels

- Population of interest: GSA students and other students at risk for HIV infection.
- Problem: HIV infections in adolescents.
- Community example: Ms. Jones, RN, MPH, works with the GSA students to understand how the organization wants to develop PrEP program to promote HIV awareness. The GSA is planning a PrEP school rally.
- System examples: Ms. Jones works with the school leadership, teachers, staff, PTA, and GSA to bring them together in the implementation of the PrEP program. Additionally, Ms. Jones works with the local and state Departments of Health to determine how to offer PrEP medication in school-based clinics.
- Individual/family example: Ms. Jones meets with individual parents of children enrolled in the school-based clinic to discuss the importance of PrEP, sexual and health education, and the importance of parental guidance.

have information about the problem, they are more likely to participate in advocacy activities that can influence decision makers to make changes at the high school. **Box 15-2** provides examples of how Ms. Jones uses advocacy interventions at population, community, systems, and individual or family level. Of note, there is quite a bit of strategic overlap in each of these levels. Ms. Jones can use many of the same strategies at the other levels. The examples provided in Box 15-2 demonstrate that Ms. Jones is also an advocate for the GSA students and families. By providing the GSA students, parents, and community with the information about PrEP, participation in the program increases, and these constituencies learn how to use their own voices to speak both individually and collectively.

COMMUNITY-FOCUSED LEVEL

The community-focused level is important to get out the message about HIV prevention strategies, which consist of PrEP, STI, and HIV screening, condom use, and health education. At the community-focused level, Ms. Jones must identify the different community groups that can play an advocacy role in dealing with the problem. Before meeting with the GSA, PTA, Board of Education, and Community School Board, Ms. Jones must have the information needed to educate these groups. Ms. Jones uses epidemiological and social epidemiological approaches to gather information about HIV prevalence in adolescents (community, local, state, and national level) as well as PrEP use in adolescents. Ms. Jones gathers this information by examining student health records in the school-based clinic (looking at STI and HIV screening requests and rates of infection and treatment), observation (looking at the utilization of health education seminars in the school-based clinic), and the health statistics provided in large databases.

Ms. Jones examines the social determinants of health—environmental factors and social factors—that play a role in STI and HIV prevalence in adolescents. Looking at this information, Ms. Jones can identify social factors of health that

the school-based clinic can play a role in through the development of initiatives. An example of this may be the enhancement of social supports and social networks for this specific targeted population of adolescents regarding STIs, which increase the risk for HIV and unintended pregnancies. Environmental factors and social factors can increase or decrease behaviors that lead to STI infections. The school-based clinic is an environmental factor. If the clinic is available to students, Ms. Jones may see a decrease in STIs. Additional examples of social factors contributing to health outcomes are poverty (within the family and neighborhood of the children), socioeconomic status (family and neighborhood), discrimination experienced by children growing up in their particular neighborhood, and stigma.

When Ms. Jones completes the community assessment, she has the information to prepare the fact sheet about the PrEP program for the principals, teachers staff, GSA, and PTA. Ms. Jones then approaches each group about its role in implementing and supporting the PrEP program at the school-based clinic. The GSA has the main responsibility to educate students and plans a PrEP school rally. The purpose of the PrEP rally is to provide the student body with reliable and accurate information about contracting STIs and HIV, and they will hear stories from adolescents taking PrEP to debunk myths and misinformation. After the rally, Ms. Jones will work with the GSA to develop student health liaisons. The student health liaison works closely with Ms. Jones and the family nurse practitioner (FNP) to plan other educational seminars, encourage STI and HIV testing, and provide students with resources. The PTA has the main responsibility to advocate for the PrEP program by educating other parents and working closely with the school-based clinic.

When Ms. Jones receives a commitment from the parents and educational establishment to implement PrEP at the school-based clinic, Ms. Jones recognizes that other organizations outside of the school must be contacted. Ms. Jones informs the GSA and the

PTA they need to advocate for the PrEP program to the Board of Education and the local Community School Board. Ms. Jones, the GSA, and PTA meet with the Board of Education to discuss the PrEP program. The presentation convinces the Board of Education to implement PrEP and sanction the PrEP school rally. Additionally, the Board of Education and the local Community School Board agree that the school-based clinic and the GSA should develop additional strategies and interventions to prevent and reduce the STIs and HIV infections in adolescents.

Ms. Jones contacts the Departments of Health at the local and state levels to find out how the school-based clinic can offer PrEP to adolescents who are uninsured or their insurance does not cover PrEP medications.

System-Focused Level

The system-focused level is important in setting up partnerships, which assure buy-in and ensures strategies that sustain change. At the systems level, Ms. Jones works with the Board of Education, the local Community School Boards, local Departments of Health, and local Community Health Centers who provide care to adolescents from her high school. She engages them to partner with the school-based clinic to implement PrEP, develop surveillance programs, and evaluate the effectiveness of PrEP in adolescents. While this appears to be a community-level approach, there are system-level applications present as well, for example, in the establishment of policies to ensure and assure the safe and diligent application of PrEP process. In addition, Ms. Jones knows that developing policies that both facilitate and sustain the development of PrEP in the school-based clinic needs specific mandates to ensure system-level changes.

Individual/Family-Focused Level

The individual/family-focused level is important to ensure that individuals or families have a stake in the process of reducing the incidence of STIs,

which contribute to HIV exposure. On the individual/family level, Ms. Jones makes arrangements for the GSA to develop educational workshops for students and parents. The workshops will address understanding the role of PrEP, who is eligible for PrEP, the medications used for PrEP, and follow-up services for PrEP. Additionally, these workshops provide a venue for Ms. Jones to work with individual students, GSA students, educators, and families.

The process to implement PrEP started when the GSA, a student organization, approached Ms. Jones about a potential problem affecting adolescents at the high school. Ms. Jones' discussions with the GSA and then subsequent research led to the implementation of PrEP program. The PrEP program could not have been developed and implemented without an understanding of the role of advocacy as outlined in the intervention wheel.

Social Marketing

Social marketing is defined as the utilization of ". . . commercial marketing principles and technologies for programs designed to influence the knowledge, attitudes, values, beliefs, behaviors, and practices of the population-of-interest" (Keller & Strohschein, 2016, p. 206). Social marketing makes use of "commercial marketing strategies to promote public health" (Evans, 2006, p. 1207) on the population level. It is a process that is developed and implemented with a focus on a targeted population (Grier & Bryant, 2005). The key to this intervention is answering the question: How do public health nurses apply the principles of social marketing to practice? Social marketing requires that public health nurses have knowledge, competencies, and skills to develop marketing approaches for the purpose of executing a population-based behavioral change, which is generally directed to a specific population. One way to begin is to understand the role of social marketing in facilitating behavioral changes. According to Daniel, Bernhardt, and Eroglu (2009), there are many activities that a public health professional may develop and implement to influence changes in behavior, but to ensure maximum effect, the best approach needs to be a comprehensive marketing mix. The Four Ps is a model that depicts a comprehensive marketing mix. The Four Ps represent *product, price, place,* and *promotion* (Daniel et al., 2009; Grier & Bryant, 2005; & Storey, Saffitz, & Rimon, 2008).

In social marketing, the *product* is the benefit associated with the behavioral change. This, however, may not be easy to determine, and it is for this reason that those responsible for developing social marketing initiatives must know their target population. "The marketing objective is to discover which benefits have the greatest appeal to the target population and design a product that provides those benefits" (Grier & Bryant, 2005, p. 323). Developing a social marketing strategy for adolescents engaged in sexual activities or becoming sexually active requires a product that facilitates decreasing one's risk for STIs and HIV infection. *Price* refers to the cost, from the target population's perspective, in order to receive or achieve the benefit. The target population will weigh the cost and barriers to the benefits when making decisions to engage in behavior change or not to engage in behavior change. If the school-based clinic can offer PrEP at no cost or a minimal cost to the students, more adolescents will seek care at the school-based clinic. *Place* refers to where the target population may be reached or the point of contact for the delivery of the information. Research may be necessary to identify these locations or the ". . . . life path points—places people visit routinely, times of day, week, or year of visits, and points in the life cycle—where people are likely to act so that products and supportive services or information can be placed there" (Grier & Bryant, 2005, p. 323). An example of place is when public health nursing students who wish to deliver messages about preventing STIs attend school sports events to pass out flyers about PrEP. Finally, *promotion* is the fourth component of the marketing mix. Promotion refers to communication and the messages being delivered to the target population. Components of communication include type of content, extensiveness of content, language used in the delivery of content, who delivers the content, and literacy levels. Additionally, how the content will be delivered (e.g., pamphlets, flyers, email, billboards, television, Instagram, texting, tweeting, songs, and blogs) and who delivers the message determine the success of the marketing mix strategy. The component of promotion must also be designed with the specific population in mind. Ultimately, social marketing is used to influence health behaviors. What follows is Ms. Jones' strategy for social marketing at the individual/family, community, and system practice levels.

Ms. Jones recognizes that using social marketing has the potential to bring about an understanding of preventing HIV infections in adolescents and getting people involved to make changes necessary to understand the HIV risk factors and prevention strategies. Ms. Jones must use a myriad of communication strategies to ensure that the message is developed, delivered, and received in a way that is targeted to the intended population so that behavioral change is possible. One way for Ms. Jones to ensure this is to work with the targeted population to understand what social marketing strategies will have the greatest impact for the targeted population. Before Ms. Jones begins to engage in aspects of social marketing, she must also approach the situation with a working knowledge of the 4-Ps. However, because the population in question is adolescents, the family and the community must also buy into the notion that HIV infections are being seen in epidemic proportions in their communities. The application of the health promotion model, along with the 4-Ps model, may assist Ms. Jones as she makes decisions pertaining to the intervention of social marketing.

Ms. Jones creates a social marketing wheel to visualize the steps needed to develop a PrEP health education campaign around the problem of HIV infections in adolescents (**Figure 15-1**). Social marketing is similar to health teaching because they

Figure 15-1   PrEP campaign social marketing wheel.

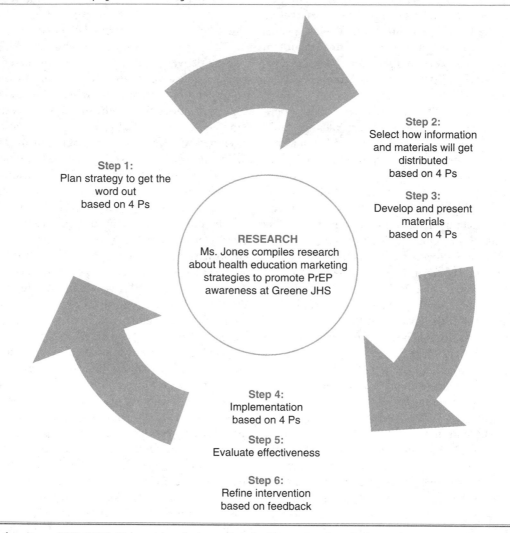

Data from Evans, W. D. (2006). How social marketing works in health care. *British Medical Journal, 332,* 1207–1210.

both call for social campaigns to change public attitudes and behavior to solve a particular problem (Kotler & Roberto, 1989). Social marketing overlaps with advocacy as well as policy development and enforcement.

Effective social marketing begins with research about the targeted population. The information

gathered will assist Ms. Jones as she works with the key individuals, community organizations, and the population in planning, developing, and implementing the social marketing initiative that it is carefully targeted and tailored. During the beginning research phase, Ms. Jones may work with individual key members of the community and/or conduct focus groups to assess the level of knowledge of each targeted group (principal, teachers, staff, GSA, adolescents attending the school-based clinic, as well as students who have not utilized services in the clinic) to gain a wide range of perspectives. Working with key members of the community and/or focus groups also serve to elicit suggestions about crafting a health promotion campaign to implement PrEP at the school-based clinic as well as developing strategies to encourage students to use the school-based health clinic for their sexual health needs. Additionally, Ms. Jones works with each of the focus groups to create a health promotion slogan. Slogans may be different depending on the targeted population. These strategies are needed to ensure that an effective social marketing message will be understood by students, parents, teachers, members of the Board of Education, the Community School Board, and local Departments of Health. Further, Ms. Jones recognizes that by holding several focus groups, she is able to reach out to many different constituents, which are needed to understand each group's unique perspective about approaching and addressing this problem.

Based on interviews with key members of the community and the focus groups, Ms. Jones co-develops a plan with the population about the content of the health message, how the health message will be presented and distributed, and by whom. Specifically, Ms. Jones works with GSA, teachers in the art department, and media services to create posters, brochures, public service announcements, blogs, Facebook entries, and a school-based clinic webpage. The GSA and teachers decide that a PrEP school rally will allow the majority of students to participate. The Board of Education decides to present awards for the most innovative and creative messaging mediums (e.g., poster, brochure, public service announcement, blog, email, tweet). The Community School Board works with the local businesses and community centers to place the media materials in areas that are most visible.

The implementation phase of the social marketing is followed by evaluation. Part of the evaluation process is to determine whether social marketing has been successful. For Ms. Jones, this may mean tracking the intended targeted population of adolescents to see if there are reductions in sexual risk behaviors, increased condom use, and requests for PrEP. Determining the success of the PrEP program requires that Ms. Jones decide on the type of data she will collect and track. In addition, Ms. Jones may also consider if the social marketing was delivered in the way that it was intended. Based on this type of evaluation, Ms. Jones must determine whether the program continues, continues with minor revisions, continues with major revisions, or is discontinued. Evaluation takes place throughout the implementation phase, as Ms. Jones continually engages in an ongoing evaluation process by assessing knowledge, attitudes, and beliefs of the population. Other examples of evaluations on the system-focused level are the board of education developing policy to ensure and assure the population that the program runs effectively and efficiently according to best practice, implementing PrEP at other school-based clinics in their districts, provision of resources, and approving multiple PrEP school rallies. The Board of Education works closely with the Department of Health to bring more health education resources to its schools. Furthermore, examples of successful outcomes on the community-focused level are the Community School Board working in concert with GSA and the PTA to set up health education seminars at the school. Examples demonstrating individuals/family-focused level outcomes are behavioral change as evidenced by attendance of families at health education events at the high school and reductions in STIs. What is important to mention here is that there is much overlap between and among the different levels of public health nursing practice. In fact, take time to review the complex skills that Ms. Jones carries out to successfully initiate the intervention strategy of social marketing.

Policy Development and Enforcement

Policy development is the final resolution of what comes out of advocacy and social marketing. **Policy development**, in fact, is often unsuccessful unless it is carried out in conjunction with advocacy.

> *Policy development places health issues on decision makers' agendas, acquires a plan of resolution, and determines needed resources. Policy development results in laws, rules and regulations, ordinances, and policies. **Policy enforcement** compels others to comply with the laws, rules, regulations, ordinances, and policies created in conjunction with policy development. (Keller & Strohschein, 2016, p. 206)*

Chapter 9 of this book gave a detailed accounting of a population-based intervention, along with particular strategies. The application of these strategies applied to the various levels of Ms. Jones's practice is highlighted below.

Ms. Jones has been successful in bringing together all the stakeholders in the school and the surrounding communities to deal with the problem of adolescent HIV infection. Ms. Jones has seen that the programs addressing adolescent sexual health were developed by partnerships with school leadership, GSA, students, school-based clinic, PTA, Board of Education, local school boards, and Departments of Health. These relationships were formed to ensure that adolescents have access to PrEP and sexual education in a setting that is nonjudgmental, appropriate for their age group, and welcoming. Ms. Jones knows that programs started at the school-based clinic need to be sustainable to ensure that the interested parties such as students, teachers, parents, community partners, the Board of Education, and the Department of Health continue their involvement. Ms. Jones is charged with making sure that decision makers are informed about the problem of HIV infections in

adolescents so that laws, rules, regulations, ordinances, and policies can be enacted to address this issue. Further, Ms. Jones needs to make certain that the programs and interventions developed are effective to address the problem of HIV infections in adolescents, PrEP medications are available, surveillance systems are set in place to monitor health statistics, and school-based clinics become a model for addressing adolescent sexual health at the community-focused, systems-focused, and individual/family-focused levels. The basic steps needed for policy development and enforcement are illustrated in **Figure 15-2**.

Step 1 requires that Ms. Jones identify the issue—the need for PrEP in adolescent school-based clinic—and the relevance of the issue locally and nationally. By identifying the problem and the target population, Ms. Jones decides what can be done about this issue. During this phase, Ms. Jones sets a policy agenda and identifies the local, state, and federal policymakers who would have authority to develop and mandate policies.

Step 2 requires that Ms. Jones begin to formulate policy and establish goals and objectives to resolve this problem. Because Ms. Jones has already started the advocacy and social marketing process earlier, many of the key stakeholders have already been identified and involved in resolving the problem.

Step 3 requires that Ms. Jones draft a policy to address the issue. The policy should consist of a budget and funding for PrEP and arrange for public hearings as necessary to bring this problem to the attention of additional stakeholders.

Step 4 requires that Ms. Jones develop rules and guidelines needed to sustain the suggested programs. Ms. Jones has to also decide how these programs will be monitored and who will be responsible for monitoring these programs.

Step 5 requires that Ms. Jones know how the enforcement of any policy will take place. Strategies for policy enforcement can take many forms such as negotiation, education, and legal repercussions.

Figure 15-2 Policy development process and enforcement.

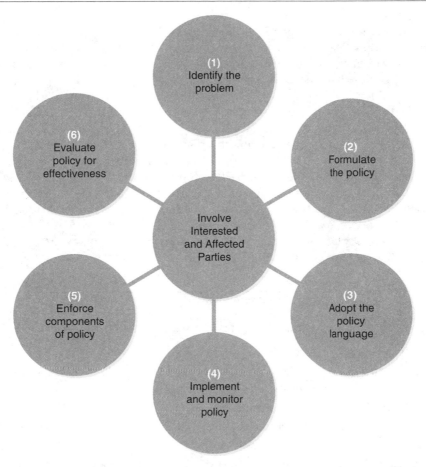

Data from Minnesota Department of Health Division of Community Health Services Public Health Nursing Section, 2001.

Step 6 requires that Ms. Jones evaluate the effectiveness of all policies implemented. This phase is an ongoing process and is necessary to assess the effectiveness of a strategy, intervention, or program. This phase provides policy developers with knowledge about the program and is the basis for improvement.

Ms. Jones knows that policy development and enforcement can also be achieved by legislation or regulation. Legislation provides a legal framework that embodies the principles of a program, and the policy basics are unlikely to change. Enacting policy legislatively requires approval by a governing body such as Congress, the state assembly, and so forth.

The laws are promulgated and passed by a legislative branch and then, after passage, implemented by local, state, or federal administrative agencies. Legislation provides the basis for the regulatory process; therefore, regulations have the force and the effect of the law that are issued by an executive authority of the government (Leavitt & Sonenberg, 2015; Milstead, 2008).

Even though Ms. Jones' advocacy, social marketing, policy development, and enforcement strategies were mostly developed on the local level, many of the interventions put into place can lead to government action. The success of enacting legislation and regulations will largely depend on the involvement of the interested parties and the ongoing evaluation of the programs. Ms. Jones knows that public health nurses have a responsibility to identify health problems that affect the larger community/population and that policy development and enforcement come out of the principles of public health nursing.

Conclusion

This chapter discusses the advocacy, social marketing, and policy development and enforcement sections of the intervention wheel. The growing public health problem of HIV in adolescents was used to discuss how public health nursing could bring this issue to the attention of interested parties. The strategies used by public health nursing consist of advocacy, which then leads to social marketing, and then culminates with policy development and enforcement. Further, this chapter discusses how public health nursing strategies can be applied on the community, systems, and individual/family levels.

Additional Resources

The Advocacy Project at: http://www.advocacynet.org/

World Advocacy at: http://www.worldadvocacy.com/

World Vision at: https://www.worldvision.org/get-involved/advocate

World Relief at: http://www.worldrelief.org/advocate/

How Social Marketing Works in Health Care at: https://www.ncbi.nlm.nih.gov/pmc/articles/PMC1463924/

Social Marketing for Public Health at: samples.jbpub.com/9780763757977/57977_ch01_final.pdf

A Guide to Health Promotion through Social Marketing at: https://www.clearinghouseforsport.gov .au/__data/.../Social_Marketing_Guide.pdf

Using Social Marketing to Manage Population Health Performance at: http://www.rwjf.org/en/library /research/2010/09/using-social-marketing-to-manage-population-health-performance.html

American Public Health Association-Community Health Planning and Policy Development at: https:// www.apha.org/apha-communities/member-sections/community-health-planning-and-policy-development

Centers for Disease Control and Prevention—What is Policy? at: http://www.cdc.gov/policy/analysis /process/definition.html

Influencing Policy Development Community Tool Box at: http://ctb.ku.edu/en/influencing-policy-development

Gay-Straight Alliance at: https://gsanetwork.org/

Society for Adolescent Health at: https://www.adolescenthealth.org/Home.aspx

Lessons from History

The purpose of this section in this intervention chapter is to demonstrate for the reader how history does inform our contemporary practice and the take-away messages are varied and many. (The history of the American Red Cross Town and Country given here was adapted from Lewenson, 2017.) Take the time to read the following and see what your take-away is.

Getting the Word Out: Advocacy, Social Marketing, and Policy Development and Enforcement

Using the example again of the start of the Red Hook Nursing Association in Red Hook, New York, we see how the town mobilized between 1915 and 1917 to advocate the hiring of a public health nurse. Using the *Sickness in Dutchess County* report to highlight the health needs within their rural community, Margaret Chanler Aldrich, one of the community leaders used local media outlets of the day—the newspaper—as a way to promote the town's affiliation with the American Red Cross Town and Country. Along with speaking at community meetings and opening her home to the community for fundraising events, Chanler-Aldrich was a strong advocate for an educated rural public health nurse. In one of her letters to the editor of the local paper, she wrote the following:

> *We have only just begun to realize that much unnecessary time is lost to sickness for want of nursing the moment it is needed. The old-fashioned neighborhood nurse . . . has died; her place has been taken by the nurse trained for three years and who receives proper remuneration for her invaluable services. But this remuneration puts her out of reach unless those who need her are very well off; and they do not send for her in time to prevent illness . . . Our township contains 4,700 souls subject to illness. If one in four will find the dollar, Dutchess County will begin to look less black on the health map of New York State. Our present condition is disgraceful as everyone knows who has a child at the age liable to measles or any other disease which is contagious. Let us subscribe for a Red Cross nurse . . . .* (Aldrich, 1916, March)

In addition, town meetings were held on a regular basis to inform the community of the progress being made in the affiliation with the American Red Cross Town and Country. At these meetings, nurses from the Town and Country would speak to the community, informing them of what they needed to do in order to start the association, as well as what services the public health nurse could provide to the families and populations within the community. In one such meeting in 1916, Miss Harrison, a Town and Country rural public health

Letter to the Editor, March 1916 (exact date unknown).

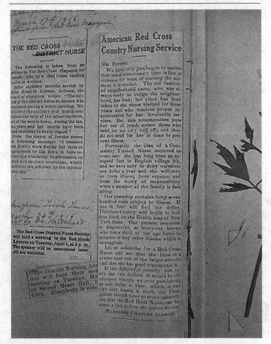

Located in Adriance Memorial Library, Poughkeepsie, NY, Box 362.104 R Box Red Hook Nursing Association, Scrapbook, 1916–1917.

(continues)

nurse from Purchase, New York, in nearby Westchester County, spoke. Her speech about the work she did in her community was also published in the local paper for those unable to attend the mass meeting. Starting the Red Hook Nursing Association was a community effort involving all sectors of the town, and it took the social media of the day to get the word out.

Questions to Consider

1. Reflect on the kinds of technology available to the American Red Cross Town and Country and other public health nurses during the early part of the 20th century.

2. Consider how technology changed over time and how public health nurses harnessed these changes when implementing the intervention strategies of advocacy, social marketing, and policy development and enhancement.

3. Discuss how understanding the historical exemplar presented in this box, and the others throughout the intervention chapters, may influence the way you advocate for populations and communities today.

Modified from Lewenson, S. B. (2017). Historical exemplars in nursing. In S. B. Lewenson & M. Truglio-Londrigan (Eds.), *Practicing primary health care in nursing: Caring for populations* (pp. 1–17). Burlington, MA: Jones & Bartlett Learning.

Local Paper Publication of Address that was Delivered at Red Cross Meeting

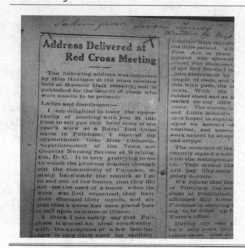

Located in Adriance Memorial Library, Poughkeepsie, NY, Box 362.104 R Box Red Hook Nursing Association, Scrapbook, 1916–1917.

CASE STUDY AND CRITICAL QUESTIONS

Implementing a Public Awareness Campaign on Sleep Hygiene for College Students

Shellene Dietrich, MS, RN, FNP-BC, DNP
Coleen Francis-Jimenez, MS, RN, FNP-BC, DNP
Melida Knibbs, MS, RN, FNP-BC, DNP
Ismael Umali, MS, RN, FNP-BC, DNP
Karen Martin, RN, MSN, FNP-BC
Marie Truglio-Londrigan, PhD, RN, GNP, FNYAM

Sleep health is important for the college student population. Poor sleep behavior practices and the resulting poor sleep may compromise student memory and grades. There are a number of factors that place this population at risk for poor sleep health; these factors include consumption of alcohol, caffeine intake, drug use, lack of a regular relaxing bedtime routine, misuse of lighting, use of technology prior to sleep, and excess environmental noise. These factors are not reflective of healthy sleep practices that facilitate sleep health.

Healthy Campus 2020 is an initiative that reflects the work of higher education professionals representing numerous organizations and disciplines. The vision of *Healthy Campus 2020* is to promote healthy campus communities via the establishment goals and objectives. One of the student objectives pertains to the need to address sleep health.

College students may have limited knowledge about sleep health and healthy sleep behavior practices. Sleep education programs that focus on sleep health may help college students become aware of sleep health, alter behavior that facilitates sleep, and improve sleep health.

To address sleep health on a college campus in the northeastern part of the United States, an interprofessional team on the college campus collaborated to develop a public awareness sleep campaign using Healthy Campuses as the guiding framework. The public awareness campaign was designed and targeted for the specific college population to increase the population's awareness about sleep and healthy sleep health behavior practices. Components of the sleep campaign included:

- Flyers
- Posters
- Electronic messaging boards
- Articles published for students in the student newspaper
- Articles published for faculty and staff in the university paper
- Poster presentation at scholarship day with take-away bookmarks

Evaluation was conducted through the use of Qualtrics web-based survey. The results provided evidence that the students on the campus as follows:

- 73% of students saw the information from the public awareness campaign.
- 79% of students learned something from the public awareness campaign.
- 91% stated that they did change behavior due to the information that they learned.

Furthermore, students offered subjective responses about the specific behavior that was changed.

- I stopped drinking coffee four hours before bed.
- I leave on absent sounds at bedtime but avoid light or TV at bedtime
- I go to sleep earlier.
- Instead of six hours of sleep, I try to get eight hours.
- I am trying to shut off my TV, phone, and computer before I go to bed, but it's difficult.

The collaborative team will be working together to reflect upon the sleep awareness campaign and develop another initiative for the new academic year. One major change will be to identify ways to involve students through all levels of program development and implementation.

Given this case study, answer the following questions:

1. How is this project one of advocacy?
2. What is the importance of partnering with the student population in the development, implementation, and evaluation of future sleep programs?
3. How would the engagement of these students enhance their own empowerment toward self-advocacy?
4. How might social media be of use in getting the word out to this specific population?
5. What are the potential organizational policy changes that may be developed to ensure and assure students of an environment that facilitates sleep?

This may be an interesting project for a public health nursing course or for the nursing student organization. How might a class of nursing students develop initiatives identified as priorities in *Health Campuses 2020*? Check out the following link: https://www.acha.org/healthycampus

References

American Nurses Association. (2013). *Public health nursing: Scope & standards of practice.* Silver Spring, MD: Author. Retrieved from http://nursingworld .org/FunctionalMenuCategories/MediaResources /PressReleases/2013-PR/New-Edition-of-Public -Health-Nursing-Scope-Standards.pdf

American Nurses Association. (2015). *The new code of ethics for nurses with interpretive statements.* Washington, DC: Author.

Ballou, K. (2000). A historical-philosophical analysis of the professional nurse obligation to participate in sociopolitical activities. *Policy, Politics, & Nursing Practice, 1*(3), 172–184. http://dx.doi.org/10.1177 /152715440000100303

Bartlett, J. G. (n.d.). Ten years of HAART: Foundations for the future. *Medscape.* Retrieved from http:// www.medscape.org/viewarticle/523119

Bavinton, B. R., Jin, F., Mao, L., Zablotska, I., Prestage, G. P., & Grulich, A. E. (2015). Homosexual men in HIV serodiscordant relationships: Implications for HIV treatment as prevention research. *Journal of the International AIDS Society, 18,* 19884. http://dx.doi .org/10.7448/IAS.18.1.19884

Bradley, H., Hall, H. I., Wolitski, R. J., Van Handel, M. M., Stone, A. E., LaFlam, M., . . . Valleroy, L. A. (2014). Vital signs: HIV diagnosis, care, and treatment among persons living with HIV—United States, 2011. *Morbidity and Mortality Weekly Report, 63*(47), 1113–1117. Retrieved from https://www.cdc .gov/mmwr/preview/mmwrhtml/mm6347a5.htm

Burda, J. P. (2016). PrEP and our youth: Implications for law and policy. *Columbia Journal of Gender and Law, 30,* 295–263. Retrieved from http:// scholarship.law.umassd.edu/cgi/viewcontent .cgi?article=1139&context=fac_pubs

Bu, X., & Jezewski, M. A. (2007). Developing a mid-range theory of patient advocacy through concept analysis. *Journal of Advanced Nursing, 57*(1), 101–110. http://dx.doi.org/10.1111/j.1365-2648.2006

Centers for Disease Control and Prevention. (2016a). Basic statistics. Retrieved from http://www.cdc.gov /hiv/basics/statistics.html

Centers for Disease Control and Prevention. (2016b). PrEP. Retrieved from http://www.cdc.gov/hiv/basics /prep.html

Centers for Disease Control and Prevention. (2017) Evaluating the acceptability, safety, and use of daily Truvada pre-exposure prophylaxis in healthy, HIV-uninfected adolescents. Retrieved from https:// clinicaltrials.gov/show/NCT02213328

Cohen, D., de la Vega, R., & Watson, G. (2001). *Advocacy for social justice: A global action and reflection guide.* Sterling, VA: Kumarian Press.

Cohen, M. S., Chen, Y. Q., McCauley, M., Gamble, T., Hosseinipour, M. C., Kumarasamy, N., . . . Fleming, T. R. (2011). Prevention of HIV-1 infection with early antiretroviral therapy. *The New England Journal of Medicine, 365*(6), 493–505. http://dx.doi .org/10.1056/NEJMoa1105243

Culp, L., & Caucci, L. (2013). State adolescent con-sent laws and implications for HIV pre-exposure prophylaxis. *American Journal of Preventive Medicine, 44*(1), S119–S124. http://dx.doi.org /10.1016/j.amepre.2012.09.044

Daniel, K. L., Bernhardt, J. M., & Eroglu, D. (2009). Social marketing and health communication: From people to places. *American Journal of Public Health, 99*(12), 2120–2122. http://dx.doi.org/10.2105 /AJPH.2009.182113

Evans, W. D. (2006). How social marketing works in health care. *British Medical Journal, 332,* 1207–1210. http://dx.doi.org/10.1136/bmj .332.7551.1207-a

Grier, S., & Bryant, C. A. (2005). Social marketing in public health. *Annual Review of Public Health, 26*(1), 319–339. http://dx.doi.org/10.1146/annurev .publhealth.26.021304.144610

Keller, L. O., & Strohschein, S. (2016). Population-based public health nursing practice: The interven-tion wheel. In M. Stanhope & J. Lancaster (Eds.), *Public health nursing: Population-centered health care in the community* (9th ed., pp. 190–216). St. Louis, MO: Mosby Elsevier.

Kotler, P., & Roberto, E. L. (1989). *Social marketing: Strategies for changing public behavior.* New York, NY: New York Free Press.

Leavitt, J. K., & Sonenberg, A. (2015). Getting involved: Public policy and influencing outcomes. In S. B. Lewenson & M. Truglio-Londrigan (Eds.), *Decision-making in nursing: Thoughtful approaches for leadership* (2nd ed., pp. 205–221). Burlington, MA: Jones & Bartlett Learning.

Lewenson, S. B. (2017). Historical exemplars. In S. B. Lewenson & M. Truglio-Londrigan (Eds.),

Practicing primary health care in nursing: Caring for populations (pp. 1–19). Burlington, MA: Jones & Bartlett Learning.

Marrazzo, J. M., del Rio, C., Holtgrave, D. R., Cohen, M. S., Kalichman, S. C., Mayer, K. H., . . . International Antiviral Society-USA Panel. (2014). HIV prevention in clinical care settings: 2014 recommendations of the International Antiviral Society–USA Panel. *JAMA, 312*(4), 390–409.

Milstead, J. A. (2008). *Health policy and politics: A nurse's guide* (3rd ed.). Sudbury, MA: Jones and Bartlett Publishers.

Minnesota Department of Health Division of Community Health Services Public Health Nursing Section. (2001). *Public health interventions: Application for public health nursing practice.* St. Paul: Minnesota Department of Health.

Montaner, J. S., Lima, V. D., Harrigan, P. R., Lourenco, L., Yip, B., Nosyk, B., . . . Kendall, P. (2014). Expansion of HAART coverage is associated with sustained decreases in HIV/AIDS morbidity, mortality and HIV transmission: The "HIV treatment as prevention" experience in a Canadian setting. *PloS One, 9*(2), e87872. http://dx.doi.org/10.1371/journal.pone.0087872

Mullins, T. L., Lally, M., Zimet, G., Kahn, J. A., & Adolescent Medicine Trials Network for HIV/AIDS Interventions. (2015). Clinician attitudes toward CDC interim pre-exposure prophylaxis (PrEP) guidance and operationalizing PrEP for adolescents. *AIDS Patient Care and STDs, 29*(4), 193–203. http://dx.doi.org/doi:10.1089/apc.2014.0273

Office of National AIDS Policy. (2015). National HIV /AIDS Strategy for the United States: Updated to 2020. Retrieved from https://www.aids.gov/federal -resources/national-hiv-aids-strategy/nhas-update.pdf

Sakraida, T. (2005). Nola J. Pender: The health promotion model. In T. A. Marriner-Tomey & A. M. Raile-Aligood (Eds.), *Nursing theorists and their work* (5th ed., pp. 624–639). St. Louis, MO: Mosby.

Storey, J. D., Saffitz, G. B., & Rimon, J. G. (2008). Social marketing. In K. Glanz, B. K. Rimer, & K. Viswanath (Eds.), *Health behavior and health education: Theory, research, and practice* (4th ed., pp. 435–464). San Francisco, CA: Jossey-Bass.

U.S. Public Health Service. (2014). *Preexposure prophylaxis for the prevention of HIV infection in the United States—2014 clinical practice guideline.* Retrieved from www.cdc.gov/hiv/pdf/guidelines /PrEPguidelines2014.pdf

U.S. Public Health Service. (2014). *Preexposure prophylaxis for the prevention of HIV infection in the United States—2014* Retrieved from http://www .cdc.gov/hiv/pdf/prepprovidersupplement2014 .pdf

Wald, L. D. (1907). Lillian Wald Papers, Box 35, Folder 6, Reel 24, pp. 1–4. New York Public Library, New York, NY.

For a full suite of assignments and additional learning activities, use the access code located in the front of your book to visit this exclusive website: http://go.jblearning.com/londrigan. If you do not have an access code, you can obtain one at the site.

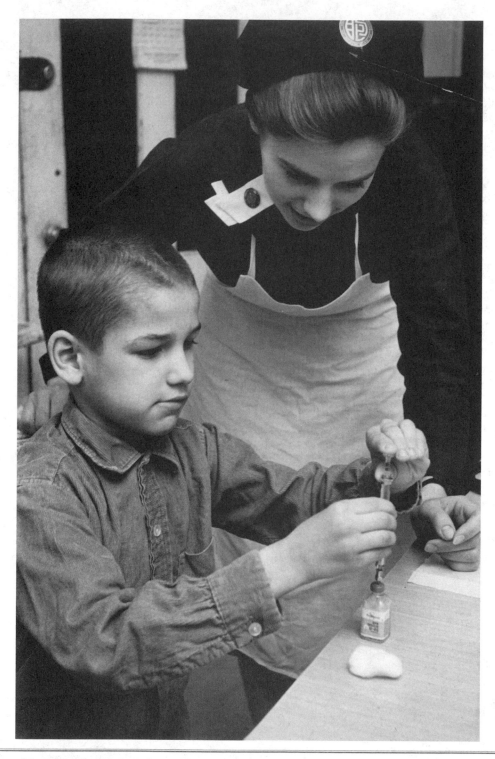

Courtesy of the Visiting Nurse Service of New York.

CHAPTER 16

Protecting, Sustaining, and Empowering: A Historical Perspective on the Control of Epidemics

Christine E. Hallett

The first concrete plans for instructing tuberculosis patients were undertaken by the Henry Street Settlement nurses. From the time we first began our work we realized that the chief danger to the community from this disease lay in ignorance, and began systematic visiting of homes where it was discovered. (Wald, 1918, p. 6)

LEARNING OBJECTIVES

At the completion of this chapter, the reader will be able to:

- Explore the ways in which human societies have attempted to combat global epidemics.
- Appreciate the role of the nurse, working alongside governments, doctors, and scientists, in the prevention of epidemic diseases.
- Explore the role of the nurse in the treatment and care of patients with life-threatening infectious diseases at different historical moments and in different places.

KEY TERMS

- ❏ Epidemic disease
- ❏ Infection control
- ❏ Pandemic

From its beginnings, the human race has shared its habitats with infective microparasites. Harmless—even beneficial—microbes inhabited our planet long before we emerged as a species. They began the long evolutionary process that would enable them to live alongside—often in parasitic or symbiotic relationships with—their neighbors before the antecedents of the human species had even emerged from the primeval ocean. Catalyzing vital processes, such as the decomposition of the planet's toxic organic waste, microbes have long existed in a precarious, yet often positive, relationship with other organic life, yet human beings notice their presence only when they fail to adapt quietly and harmlessly to the changing patterns of human life.

Of the many microparasites that inhabit our environment, it is the most inefficient and the least well adapted that cause recognized infections. A bug that fails to live symbiotically with its host may expect to limit its own lifespan. If it kills its host, it will die. If it keeps the host alive yet in a weakened state, it can expect that its host will eventually find a way to eradicate it. The purpose of this chapter is to trace the means by which humans have attempted to eradicate certain of those bugs they consider harmful: the bacteria and viruses that cause epidemic and endemic infections. The chapter focuses on three case studies of specific diseases appearing at specific historical moments: bubonic plague, as it appeared in the early modern Italian city-states during the 16th and 17th centuries; Spanish influenza as it appeared in the cities of the United States in 1918 and 1919; and AIDS as it appeared in the United Kingdom during the 1980s.

The bubonic plague bacillus and the influenza virus caused **epidemic** diseases that affected such large sections of the world's population that they came to be seen as global epidemics or, more correctly, as **pandemics**. HIV exists on the cusp between endemic and epidemic disease, affecting large numbers of people worldwide; it is often spoken of as an epidemic because of its capacity to spread rapidly in certain populations and geographical areas of the world at certain times.

Humans have taken a range of measures to protect themselves against or to destroy pathogenic microorganisms. Through its case studies, this chapter considers four different approaches to disease: state-sanctioned control measures, medical interventions, nursing care and support, and individual empowerment. It traces the means by which human societies, more or less effectively, learned to protect themselves against, overcome, and survive severe life-threatening infection on a large scale. It focuses, in particular, on how societies mobilized and used nurses as frontline agents in combating infection.

Protecting the People Against God's Wrath: Bubonic Plague in Early Modern Italy

The Black Death, the second recorded pandemic of the disease known as bubonic plague, swept across Europe from Central Asia between 1348 and 1353, causing millions of deaths and devastating entire villages (Alexander, 1980; Hirst, 1953; Preto, 1978; Slack, 1985; Zinsser, 1935). Caused by the bacterium later to be named *Yersinia pestis*, the disease was carried in the body of a particular species of flea known as *Xenopsylla cheopis*, which in turn inhabited a particular species of rat, *Rattus rattus*, also known as the black rat. It may seem extraordinary that a disease carried by one species of microbe in the bloodstream of one species of flea on the back of one species of rat could destroy so many communities, yet the lifestyle of the Middle Ages created an ideal ecological niche for these species. The black rat could live easily in the thatched roofs and grain stores of the largely agrarian communities of the 14th century, and the frequent overcrowding and lack of opportunities for good hygiene practices meant that flea and lice infestations were commonplace. Once the opening up of trade routes to the East transported the plague to Western Europe, it rapidly gained a foothold there.

The first case study considers one small corner of the world two centuries after the plague caused its first great wave of devastation. The case-fatality rate of bubonic plague was probably around 30%, and its associated form, pneumonic plague, was even more lethal, with an 80% case-fatality rate. Having burned itself out by killing a large proportion of its host population, the Black Death remained endemic in the European rodent population, literally hovering at the gates of the towns and cities of early modern Europe. At particular risk were the inhabitants of the Italian city-states such as Venice, Florence, Naples, and Rome that traded with the East, bringing within their borders goods likely to be infested with the black rat. Although they did not realize the disease was carried by rat fleas, the populations of these cities nevertheless recognized that it was somehow imported from outside. These states were the first to introduce systematic measures to protect their populations from plague (Christensen, 2003).

When confronted by plague, the magistrates of the city-states had three aims: to avoid allowing the disease to arise in or to enter the city; to prevent its spread; and to maintain social order while, as much as possible, caring for the sick. Health magistrates, known as *Provveditori alla Sanita*, appeared to have thought in terms of a complex relationship between plague and disorder. Plague was itself a form of physical disorder that could most easily arise in a disorderly environment that exuded disease-forming *miasmas* or *pestilential* states of the air. Once plague had taken hold of a community, the relationship between disease and social disorder was mutually reinforcing. The effect was perceived to be a spiral one in which the health, both physical and moral, of the community grew increasingly out of control. The work of the magistrates was to arrest this process. To properly coordinate their efforts during epidemics, the governments of Italian city-states appointed specialist health boards, known as "Sanita," with wide-reaching powers, which became permanent in many Italian city-states during the course of the 1400s (Campbell, 1931; Carmichael, 1983, 1986; Palmer, 1978).

Arising from a disorder within nature, plague threatened to create chaos within the community. Italian sanitary legislation aimed to prevent such chaos. Many of the measures in force during the Renaissance were introduced by legislation of the early 13th century, which preceded even experience of the Black Death (Carmichael, 1986). There were numerous attempts to legislate for cleanliness within city-states. Unpleasant smells were believed to be particularly dangerous because they were associated with noxious harmful vapors that composed the miasma. By the end of the 14th century, there was already legislation against the keeping of animals such as pigs and ducks in Florence and against the selling of manure inside the city (Carmichael, 1986). The health authorities came to regard it as their responsibility to control the release of offensive smells associated with industrial activities such as tanning, butchery, and the retting of hemp (Cipolla, 1992; Palmer, 1978).

In taking responsibility for the eradication of plague, the patriciates (nobilities) of early modern cities fulfilled their roles as guardians of order and protectors of the state. King (1986) has identified the main preoccupations of Venetian patricians as evident in their humanistic writings. Noblemen such as Gasparo Contarini, Daniele Barbaro, Paolo Paruta, and Nicolo Contarini promoted the myth of a Venetian republic that was ordered and harmonious and in which the nobility conformed to the principle of "unanimitas." The Venetian patriciate presented itself as the personification of order within the state. Furthermore, its members also saw themselves as the state's defense—as "moenia civitatis," or the "walls of the city" (King, 1986; Pastore, 1988; Ulvioni, 1989). The Italian Health Boards were the most effective and efficient organizations for controlling plague in Western Europe, and their measures became models for the establishment of health controls in other states (Cipolla, 1979, 1992).

Calvi (1989) examined the efforts of magistrates to maintain stability in Florence during the epidemic of 1630–1631. Through a close examination of the criminal trial records of the Health Magistracy and a reading of Francesco Rondinelli's contemporary account of the plague, she discovered that the regulations imposed during the "virtual dictatorship" of the public health officials reflected the desire for order and uniformity. Most of the 300 trials she examined dealt with violations against property, crimes committed by public health workers, and the unlawful hiding of the ill (Calvi, 1989).

It had been recognized since the Black Death that some diseases could be transmitted between individuals (Biraben, 1975; Campbell, 1931). An idea of contagion was part of the general stock of knowledge in early modern Europe. In Thomas More's *Utopia* (1516), the hospitals were situated outside the town so that people with diseases "such as be wont by infection to creep from one to another" (p. 35) might be separated from the rest of the population (Ficino, 1989). However, a theory of contagion was not articulated effectively until the mid-16th century, when it formed the basis of a work by Girolamo Fracastoro (1930). His *De Contagione et Contagiosis Morbis et Eorum Curatione, Libri III*, first published in Venice in 1546, has interested historians because its theories bear some superficial resemblance to a germ theory of disease (Fracastoro, 1930; Nutton, 1990).

Fracastoro emphasized that where plague was concerned, the most frequent means of transmission was contagion between individuals. He distinguished between diseases that were merely common to communities and those that were also contagious (Fracastoro, 1930). The dominant theme in his work was the idea that plague was caused by invasion. It could be passed on from person to person rather than simply arising spontaneously from a disordered environment. It could also be carried in fomites—porous objects such as cloth and wood—and thus be transported between one community and the next. These ideas had immense influence in the Italian city-states, where plague came to be seen as an invading force against which siege measures must be adopted.

During the early modern period, as plague came to be identified more as an invasion from outside the state, measures taken by city-state magistrates to preserve order were increasingly reinforced by a range of defensive strategies. Many of these plans were already quite old, dating from the time of the Black Death, but all appear to have been imposed with increasing rigor and determination during the 16th and 17th centuries. In the late 1500s, Gasparo Contarini (1599) commented on the work of the *Provveditori alla Sanita*, the city's health magistrate:

> His chiefest office is to forsee that there come not into the citie an contagious infection, which if at any time it happen to creepe in (as sometimes it chanceth) then to take such diligent and carefull order that in as much as maybe the same come not to spread any further. (n.p.)

Throughout the early modern period, when it became known to its neighbors that a state was affected by plague, it was usual for commerce with that state to be banned. This meant the cessation of all forms of communication, including trade, with the plague-infested region, against whose inhabitants the frontiers were closely guarded (Carmichael, 1983). Banning was controlled by means of a system of health passes that permitted only those who were well or who came from healthy areas to enter a territory. Passes were introduced by Milan during the 15th century and were then used by other states in the first half of the 16th century (Brozzi, 1982; Cipolla, 1973, 1979; Modena, 1988; Palmer, 1978; Petraccone, 1978). Centorio degli Hortensii (1631) described a series of measures introduced by the health deputies of Modena during the plague of 1575–1577: "Besides unpaid officials at the gates, paid officials will be posted at the pass of the Fossa Alta, at the pass of the Marzoia at the high bridge and the low bridge. . . at Buon Porto, on the bank of the River Secchia, at San Marino, on the border with Mirandola" (p. 17). They added that guards at these posts must be able to read and write and must be in possession of an official seal to stamp the passes of those allowed through (Hortensii, 1631). The defensive nature of these measures is striking: They illustrate the extent to which plague came to be associated with invasion.

All ships coming to the early modern state from any area suspected of plague were made to undergo quarantine. Crew members were not permitted to enter the city or unload goods during the quarantine period, which usually lasted 40 days. This measure was originally designed to provide an early warning system for diseases on ships but became one of the most enduring measures against contagion (Campbell, 1931; Carmichael, 1983; Palmer, 1978). It also became a measure for isolating entire communities of people. During a general quarantine, only doctors and members of the government were allowed to leave their homes (Petraccone, 1978; Ulvioni, 1989).

When plague was diagnosed in an Italian city-state, the victims were quickly segregated from the rest of the population. The sick were examined, and persons discovered to be suffering from the plague were taken to the *lazzaretto*, or pest house. The Lazzaretto Vecchio of Venice, founded by decree of the Senate on August 28, 1423, was the first permanent pest house in Europe (Campbell, 1931; Palmer, 1978). It was situated about two miles from the city on a small island off the Lido that had previously been the home of the Eremite Monastery of Santa Maria di Nazareth (Chambers & Pullan, 1992). A decree of the Venetian Senate on April 17, 1464, provided for "two suitable and competent citizens not of noble rank" (Chambers & Pullan, 1992, p. 114) to be appointed for each sestiere of the city to ensure that all infected persons were taken to the Lazzaretto Vecchio and all infected houses evacuated. The notary, Rocco Benedetti, described the horrors of the Venetian Lazzaretto Vecchio, which seemed to him like "Hell itself" (Chambers & Pullan, 1992):

From every side there came foul odors, indeed a stench that none could endure; groans and

sighs were heard without ceasing, and at all hours, clouds of smoke from the burning of corpses were seen to rise far into the air. Some who miraculously returned from that place alive reported, among other things, that at the height of that great influx of infected people there were three or four of them to a bed. Since a great number of servants had died, and there was no one to take care of them, they had to get themselves up to take food and attend to other things. Nobody did anything but lift the dead from the beds and throw them into the pits. . . . And many, driven to frenzy by the disease, especially at night, leapt from their beds, and, shouting with fearful voices of damned souls, went here and there, colliding with one another, and suddenly falling to the ground dead. Some who rushed in frenzy out of the wards threw themselves into the water, or ran madly through the gardens, and were then found dead among the thornbushes, all covered with blood. (pp. 118–119)[1]

A sufferer who died at the pest house was buried there or in a cemetery apart from the city. Survivors were usually sent to a convalescent hospital to undergo a 40-day quarantine before being returned home (Chambers & Pullan, 1992). The *lazzaretti* were also centers for the disinfection of fomites. In the Venetian *lazzaretti*, goods from infected homes and ships were aired for 40 days and, during that time, were constantly turned and moved to release any infection they might have absorbed (Brozzi, 1982; Castellacci, 1897; Pastore, 1988).

The monitoring and the control of the poor were closely associated with the prevention of plague: It was a means of propitiating God, a measure for promoting order, and a defensive strategy. Indeed,

---

[1] Reproduced from Chambers, D., & Pullan, B. (1992). *Venice: A documentary history, 1450-1630*. Oxford, UK: Blackwell. Reproduced with permission of Blackwell Publishing, Inc.

the development of organized systems of poor relief was probably stimulated by the experience of plague, a disease associated with poverty at an early stage in its history (Preto, 1978; Pullan, 1971, 1992). Governments and physicians observed that the poor were affected in greater numbers than the rich. Theorists devised explanations for this pattern: The poor lived disorderly lives, their inadequate diets were a source of corruption that could spread through the community, and they did not dispose of waste properly and hence lived among filth that might create a poisonous miasma (Anselment, 1989; Biraben, 1975; Carmichael, 1986; Grell, 1990).

During the plague of 1575–1577, physicians expressed the view that the poor were a threat to the health of the community. Nicolo Massa and Girolamo Mercuriale both went so far as to argue that the poor should be removed from towns when there was a threat of plague. Mercuriale referred to them as *fomes* for the disease (Palmer, 1978, p. 144). In August 1576, the state, perhaps acting on such advice, decided that the link between poverty and plague was related to poor housing conditions and chose a site at Zaffusina at which to relocate the poor from plague-affected areas. It was said that the site could have accommodated over 10,000 people, and provision was made for the supply of tents and huts, but the plan was never put into effect (Preto, 1978).

Hospitals originated as hostels for the poor rather than as specialist centers for the cure of disease, and as such, they were centers for the isolation of those likely to disrupt the social order (Cartwright, 1977; Pullan, 1992). The poor could be seen as plague in microcosm. The Mendicanti hospitals established in many Italian states from the 1560s onward were designated to remove beggars from public places (Park & Henderson, 1991). By building hospitals, magistrates responded to plague in three ways. First, by caring for its poor, the state obeyed God's commands and might thereby deflect his anger and prevent disease. Second, by housing beggars, the state avoided the problems associated with squalor,

dirt, filth, and bad smells that could give rise to miasma. Third, if the poor were seen as carriers of plague in a contagious sense, the state, by isolating them in hospitals, protected healthy citizens from the disease they carried.

Measures adopted by states from the second half of the 1400s illustrate their recognition that plague could easily be brought into cities by immigrants whose origins were uncertain (Carmichael, 1983). In 1498 in Venice, it was decreed that all lodging housekeepers must have licenses (Pullan, 1971). The tendency to associate plague with invasion through theories of contagion is apparent in the way in which particular individuals were blamed for bringing plague into a city. It was believed, for example, that during October 1629 a soldier from Lecco brought the disease into Milan in a bundle of clothing obtained from German troops (Calvi, 1989; Cipolla, 1973; Galassi, 1966–1970).

A decree of the Venetian Council of Ten and Zonta of September 12, 1539, described how orders had been given to the *Provveditori alla Sanita* (Chambers & Pullan, 1992):

> To bar from this city many poor persons suspected of carrying the plague, who, as we had heard by letters from Milan, had been expelled from the Milanese state and from Piedmont, and it was thought that they were certain to come here. Not only did the Provveditori carry out these orders both wisely and thoroughly, but they also expelled from Venice some 4000–5000 beggars and other kinds of persons who had recently come to live in this city. (p. 126)

The approaches of the Italian city-states to the prevention and control of bubonic plague were thus a mixture of the pragmatic and the ideological. By closing their gates to anyone who might carry the disease and removing from their homes all those who were believed to be infected, states protected their healthy citizens. In holding masses and processions and in establishing hospitals for the poor, they worked to propitiate divine wrath. Most did not, however, have the capacity to provide adequate care and attention to those who succumbed to the disease. Early modern pest houses were places of dread, from which one had a poor chance of emerging alive.

Serving and Sustaining a Desperate Population: Influenza in the Modern United States

Modern sensibilities may identify a degree of ruthlessness in the approaches to plague prevention of the early modern Italian city-states. If the beleaguered *Provveditori alla Sanita* took harsh and desperate measures, this can have been only because of their fundamental sense of helplessness when confronted by infectious disease. They had no cure. Keeping their options open, they worked hard to propitiate God. Epidemics might, after all, as the Bible suggested, be visitations of divine wrath, yet they also directed their energies toward protecting the healthy in their communities. The sick they condemned to the overcrowded pest houses, where desperate and overwhelmed nursing attendants struggled to offer rudimentary support.

Perhaps no greater contrast can therefore be imagined than between the frantic efforts of the early modern pest house attendants and the home care offered by the confident district nurses of modern cities in the early 20th century. The influenza pandemic of 1918–1919 threatened to overwhelm much of Europe, the European colonies, and North America, yet one of the most striking findings of historians is that although medical science stood by helpless before this deadly disease, nursing care seemed effective in reducing death rates. Although no efforts have ever been made to quantify the successes of early 20th-century district nurses (it is impossible to prove definitively that they actually saved lives), the writings of contemporaries indicate that there was a strong belief that good nursing care had made a real difference to survival rates.

This phenomenon of good nursing care appears frequently in the writings of physicians and nurses in the late 1800s, but is rarely accompanied by a definition. It appears to refer to those nursing actions that enabled the patient's physiological system to survive best while his or her immune system fought the infectious disease. Thus, the maintenance of a steady temperature by the judicious use of blankets and the warming of sick rooms; the provision of copious fluids and nourishing food, usually in the form of nutritious soup; and the maintenance of patient hygiene, rest, and sleep acted both to stabilize the system and prevent the development of new complications. Providing these prerequisites for recovery seems deceptively simple. In reality, providing core nursing care for a very ill individual required great artistry, skill, and patience, whereas going into a home to care for a person with a known deadly and incurable disease required more than a little courage.

The so-called Spanish influenza epidemic of 1918–1919 (caused by the virus H_1N_1) is estimated to have caused a global mortality of between 50 and 100 million (Johnson & Mueller, 2002; Quinn, 2008). It developed toward the end of the World War I and probably killed at least twice as many people as the war itself (Crosby, 1989; Johnson, 2006; Patterson & Pyle, 1991; Phillips & Killingray, 2003). Reid (2005) observed that accurate figures are difficult to obtain, partly because influenza was not made a notifiable disease until 1918 and partly because early cases were often labeled as bronchitic pneumonia or just pneumonia. It appears to have originated in China and then may have been spread throughout the United States via the mobilization and movement of troops who were housed in overcrowded barracks. From the American military camps, it spread rapidly to Europe, where war-weary populations succumbed rapidly (Byerly, 2005; Quinn, 2008). Its most puzzling and unusual feature was its tendency to attack young, apparently healthy adults. Its mortality rate was very high within this group and was lower among the elderly (possibly because of acquired immunity) and the very young (Barry, 2005; Reid, 2005).

A devastating disease, Spanish influenza caused severe headache, cough, breathing difficulties, nosebleeds, aching joints, and intense fatigue. A characteristic symptom was the severe cyanosis that could rapidly turn the faces of sufferers blue or even black. The disease was often extremely rapid in its onset. An apparently healthy individual might suddenly collapse in the street, with blood pouring from his nose, and then die before there was time to get him to a hospital. Already severe in its respiratory symptoms, the disease was frequently complicated by acute and severe bronchopneumonic symptoms, and death was frequently from these complications rather than from the more systemic effects of the virus. Victims of this terrifying disease became feverish to the point of delirium, cyanosed until their skin was black, and weak to the point of utter helplessness (Quinn, 2008).

Joyce Sapwell (n.d.), a British volunteer-nurse, wrote the following in her diary:

The terrible flu pneumonia epidemic broke out. About one-third of the staff were down with it, and the hospital was full. We had had one hundred and eight deaths in eight weeks. I was put on night duty in charge of four huts at the bottom of the hospital, the main part was full, each hut had 20 beds. Three of them flu pneumonia and one with convalescent colonials. I had not even one orderly to help. Several patients became delirious, and if they got out of bed, they usually died. (n.d., n.p.)

Quinn (2008) argued that political leaders were slow to respond to the threat of the influenza outbreak, prioritizing the war effort over the fight against the disease. U.S. President Woodrow Wilson, for example, at first ignored the advice of doctors to publicize details of the outbreak and to halt troop movements (Quinn, 2008). Doctors themselves were helpless against the disease. Just as in the Italian city-states there had been no

cure for bubonic plague, similarly, 20th-century medical science was unable to discover a magic bullet that would kill the influenza virus, yet the perspective on disease of North Americans in the 1900s was very different from that of 16th century Italians. The emergence of germ theory in the late 1800s, prompted largely by the research of scientists such as Louis Pasteur and Robert Koch, had revolutionized medicine and given both physicians and the societies they served a sense of mastery over disease (Gradmann, 2001; Latour, 1988). If cures could not be found immediately, they would, nevertheless, eventually become available. The early 20th century's faith in science gave its people a belief that they could, collectively, control their own destiny. In the meantime, a range of remedies was attempted, from the use of opium and quinine to traditional herbal cures and bloodletting. Heroic remedies such as strychnine and steam baths, along with smallpox, diphtheria, and antitetanus serum, were also tried without success (Quinn, 2008).

The nurses of the United States were also very different from the largely untrained sick-room attendants or servants of the Early Modern period. The rapid development of medical science in the second half of the 19th century meant that the character of nursing had changed beyond recognition. Retaining their core functions of the care and nurturing of the sick, nurses were now also carefully trained technicians who administered the new, scientific, and often heroic remedies devised by medical science with dexterity and intelligence. It was their fundamental nursing skills, however, that came to the fore when they nursed thousands of influenza patients from 1918 to 1919. Many of those who died did so from exhaustion and starvation. Nurses could prevent these deaths. They took soup and hot drinks to the houses of sufferers and offered care and comfort that enabled the absolute rest that might help the body more effectively fight the disease (Keen-Payne, 2000). Quinn (2008) cites the Australian nurse in the outback town of Byrock, Australia, who delivered food and medicines single-handedly to a town of 27 families.

Keeling (2009), using New York as a case study, showed that community-based nursing organizations could have a profound effect on both the well-being and probably the survival rates of whole communities of individuals. Keeling focused on the efforts of the Henry Street Settlement, a group of public health nurses founded in 1893 and working under the directorship of Lillian Wald. These nurses had for decades been working with the poorest communities in the city, basing most of their activities in the Lower East Side, where immigrant families lived in destitution. They were no strangers to epidemic disease and had at their disposal an armory of measures to improve the health, hygiene, and nutritional status and to promote the comfort of their severely ill patients (Buhler-Wilkerson, 2001; Keeling, 2007).

Wald and her nurses worked in cooperation with the American Red Cross, the U.S. Public Health Service, volunteer organizations, and city health officials. They used warm blankets, baths, and fresh air to both comfort patients and promote their capacities to fight the infection. Perhaps most importantly, they enabled their patients to obtain complete rest, so enabling their immune systems the best chance of destroying the virus without also overwhelming the body itself. City authorities provided automobiles for their use, and they were able to transport pneumonia jackets and quarts of soup to the homes of the sick, offering warmth and nourishment to patients. They were able to keep large numbers of sufferers at home, thus relieving the desperately overcrowded hospitals, preventing unnecessary journeys for already severely weakened patients, and containing the spread of the disease (Keeling, 2009).

The influenza epidemic of the early 1900s was poorly controlled and contained. It is possible to argue that the governments of Western developed nations had learned nothing from the stringent isolation and quarantine regulations of their forebears in the Early Modern city-states. It can also be argued that the nursing services of the early 20th century were able to ensure that influenza, although just as horrific as bubonic plague in its effects, was not a disease that left its victims totally helpless. Nursing care offered hope, not just to sufferers themselves but to entire societies.

Empowering the Vulnerable: AIDS in Contemporary Britain

The AIDS virus, it can be argued, is a much more efficient microparasite than that which caused Spanish influenza. The reaction of the human body to influenza was rapid and devastating. Death or recovery followed infection within days; both outcomes ultimately destroyed the virus. HIV has a much more hidden effect on the body and can live within its host's cells for several years before the destruction of body systems begins, symptoms emerge, and treatment is sought. This subtle infection has demanded a subtle response—and one, again, in which nurses have been among the active agents in the fight against the spread of the disease.

The third case study focuses on the responses to AIDS within the large cities of the United Kingdom in the 1980s. London, Manchester, Liverpool, Edinburgh, Dundee, and Glasgow were the epicenters of HIV's spread within Britain. It quickly became well known that the AIDS virus thrived within body fluids and was spread by direct contact with those fluids. It was recognized that the virus could live outside the human body only for short periods of time, and it could not survive desiccation or extremes of temperature. Soon after the development of the first cases of HIV, it was recognized that its three main methods of transmission from host to host were via sexual intercourse, through blood transfusion, and through the sharing of hypodermic needles. It was, furthermore, fairly rapidly realized that the virus was spreading through the homosexual communities of large cities throughout the world.

The disease appears to have originated in Africa, where its prevalence was and still remains very high. Speculation as to the origin of the disease in medical experimentation soon gave way to efforts to combat it and find a cure. Scientists achieved some success in developing therapies for **infection control** within a human host and transformed the condition from a rapidly fatal disease to one that can be survived as a long-term, chronic condition. This moderate success of medical science has, however, been more than matched by the efforts of public health professionals, including nurses, to educate and empower populations to collectively control the disease.

The first cases of AIDS probably developed in the mid- to late 1970s. The disease, however, was not recognized as a distinct entity until large numbers of cases of its associated conditions, Kaposi's sarcoma and *Pneumocystis carinii* pneumonia, began to appear in large U.S. cities in 1981 (AVERT, 2009; Hymes, Green, & Mann, 1989). Centers for the control of communicable diseases throughout the developed world began to study what was being recognized as a new disease. The first case of AIDS to be documented in the United Kingdom appeared in December 1981 (Dubois, Braitwaite, Mikhail, & Batten, 1981). Because the earliest recorded symptoms affected gay men and because the disease was, at first, so closely associated with the gay community, some believed it could be transmitted only through homosexual contact. The disease was even, for a time, referred to as gay compromise syndrome (Brennan & Durak, 1981). Then a rapid increase in cases among hemophiliacs, who acquired the virus through blood transfusions, led to a dawning recognition that the disease could be transmitted in body fluids through both sexual contact and transfusion (Bateman, 1994). The recording of the first cases of the disease in women in January 1983 along with a rapid rise in the incidence among hemophiliacs also drew more public attention

to a disease that could no longer be dismissed. Amid widespread fear and uncertainty, the name *acquired immune deficiency syndrome* was coined and the disease clearly defined in September 1982 (Connor & Kingman, 1988). In May 1983, the AIDS virus, at first referred to as the lymphadenopathy-associated virus, was first isolated by scientists at the Pasteur Institute in Paris (Barre-Sinoussi et al., 1983; Harden, 1992).

One of the earliest voluntary organizations for the prevention and control of AIDS was formed in the United Kingdom in 1982 and came to be known as the Terence Higgins Trust, named after one of the disease's earliest victims (Berridge, 1996). Similar organizations developed in other western European countries and in the United States, and it was through these independent, well-organized, and proactive voluntary organizations that AIDS first became a disease that was controlled through individual education and empowerment. By conveying clear messages about how to protect oneself through safe sex, activists within the gay community probably prevented many potential cases of the disease.

By 1985, messages about AIDS prevention were spreading beyond the gay community. Clear statements were being made about which groups were most at risk. These included heroin addicts who shared needles, and the first needle exchanges were established in the Netherlands, soon to be followed by large numbers of other similar projects. In the United Kingdom, general practitioners were operating needle exchanges by the mid-1980s, as indicated by a study conducted in one Edinburgh-based practice (Robertson et al., 1986). The Kaleidoscope needle exchange in London and the Maryland Street needle exchange in Liverpool were established around the same time, and a national campaign was launched, based on the message "don't inject AIDS" (AVERT, 2009).

As data became available from parts of Africa where AIDS was a much more established disease, it became clear that heterosexuals were at serious risk. The disease was clearly spreading through the heterosexual community, and vaginal transmission came to be recognized as an important cause of this spread. The first international conference on AIDS, held in Atlanta, Georgia, in April 1985, recognized that the disease was now a global pandemic (Mann, 1989). Irresponsible media reporting fueled public panic during the mid-1980s. Widespread fear led initially to widespread homophobia and created a scenario of moral panic that damaged the earliest health education campaigns by distorting their message. It also isolated sufferers, limiting the support they obtained (Fowler, 1991; Gronfors & Stalstrom, 1987; Tester, 1994; Wolf & Kielwasswe, 1991). Nevertheless, even amid the mass media-fueled panic of the mid-1980s, clear messages were beginning to reach those at risk, and deliberate actions such as safer sex, the use of clean hypodermic needles, and the abstention of those at risk from blood donation were already beginning to have an effect (Arno & Feiden, 1992).

The history of the containment and control of HIV can be interpreted in part as a history of successful self-help. Voluntary organizations, often established by individuals whose friends or family members had died of AIDS, often led the way in developing campaigns that would both raise awareness of the disease and its transmission and overcome prejudice, thus promoting respect and compassion for sufferers. The Cardiff AIDS helpline grew out of an existing telephone service for gay men, and "body positive" groups throughout the country developed centers and helplines to support sufferers and those anxious about the disease. "Body Positive London" was established in 1985 and provided vital help and support for what was really the epicenter of the AIDS epidemic in the United Kingdom (Berridge, 1996). The charity AVERT was founded in 1986 to campaign against AIDS-related prejudice and injustice, and the National Union of Journalists issued a leaflet advising journalists to offer more positive and respectful reporting of those with HIV (Berridge, 1996). In the same year, the London Lighthouse, a care center for AIDS sufferers, was planned in the face of opposition from

a small faction of hostile local residents and won widespread support (Cantacuzino, 1993).

In September 1986, the recognition that the drug azidothymidine could slow the progress of the disease led to the development of the first successful drug therapies for AIDS sufferers. Eventually, highly active antiretroviral therapy became widely used and dramatically lengthened the lifespans of those who obtained treatment early, yet it was still successful health education that had the greatest impact on bringing the disease under control and preventing the escalation of the pandemic.

In 1987, the British government developed its prevention campaign through the newly formed Health Education Authority, using mass media to promulgate the message "don't die of ignorance." Advertising on prime-time television, using hard-hitting slogans and visually arresting images such as an iceberg and a tombstone, the Authority reached millions of viewers. A televised "AIDS week" was held from February 27 to March 8 in which rival television stations simultaneously showed a film entitled "*AIDS—The Facts*" and advertised an AIDS helpline number. In the same year, the National AIDS Trust was established to coordinate the activities of self-help and voluntary organizations (Berridge, 1996). Also in 1987, Princess Diana opened the first specialist ward for AIDS at the Middlesex Hospital, making the point by shaking hands with HIV-positive patients that the virus could not be transmitted by skin contact. In 1988, health education campaigns gained ground throughout the world, and in that year the first annual World AIDS Day was organized by the World Health Organization (1988).

From the discovery of the first cases of AIDS in 1981 to the launch of successful awareness campaigns in the mid-1980s, rapid progress was made in developing projects that would combat the spread of the disease. Health education campaigns are difficult to evaluate, and some of the early attempts to measure the effectiveness of government campaigns in the mid-1980s produced inconclusive or disappointing results (Baggaley, 1988; Sherr, 1987). Nevertheless, it was possible by the early 21st century to demonstrate that reductions in the incidence of a range of sexually transmitted infections (among them HIV) had followed and were probably the result of these campaigns (Nicholl et al., 2001). Nicholl and Hamers (2002) showed that incidences of a range of sexually transmitted diseases, not just AIDS, reduced significantly after the campaigns of the mid-1980s. They further argued that, as memory of those campaigns faded, there was a resurgence of HIV, gonorrhea, and syphilis throughout Europe (Nicholl & Hamers, 2002).

Furthermore, awareness-raising campaigns have at times had beneficial and unforeseen knock-on effects. The AIDS-awareness campaigns carried benefits on a global scale. Laurie Garrett argued that donations of public and private funds to third-world countries increased dramatically because of the awareness-raising campaigns of HIV activists. Though the effects of this philanthropy have been patchy because of the poor coordination of health promotion programs, the tendency of awareness-raising campaigns to arouse the compassion of individuals in the developed world can be seen as a positive development (Garrett, 2007; Leclerc-Madlala, 2005). These developments should not, however, give rise to complacency. African nations in particular have struggled to obtain the drug therapies they require and develop effective health-promotion strategies in line with the World Health Organization's global program on AIDS (Friedman & Mottiar, 2005; VanderVliet, 2001).

Conclusion

The study of past epidemics offers us perspective on the ways we tackle the threats posed by our own era. It also teaches us that although new threats arise constantly and present new challenges, these threats and challenges are not so different from those faced by our ancestors. What does differ over time are the resources at our disposal to tackle new epidemic diseases. Among the most vital resources at the disposal of modern governments are the skilled workforces that combat epidemics, and among the largest—but least well recognized—of these are the nurses who care for the sick, empower the vulnerable, and undertake much of the work in terms of data collection and treatment implementation. All of this makes it possible for the science and art of health care to destroy the causative organisms of disease.

The three case studies presented here were chosen because each demonstrates a distinct response—or more often, reaction—to an epidemic. All three of the diseases presented—bubonic plague, influenza, and AIDS—took their host populations by surprise. A study of the collective responses of some of those populations can offer insight into how humans perceive and combat disease. In the early modern Italian city-states, magistrates adopted a "protective" approach to outbreaks of bubonic plague. They quarantined their cities, they moved the sick and their belongings to pest houses, and they imposed controls aimed at both preventing the spread of disease within their walls and propitiating "divine wrath." Their approach was a classic containment strategy.

In New York City and other U.S. cities during the early 1900s, the movement of the sick was not controlled, and, in fact, troop movements probably exacerbated the epidemic. Quarantines were not strictly imposed, and, although antisocial and obviously dangerous behaviors, such as spitting in public were outlawed, controls on public behavior were relatively mild. The American and European approach to Spanish influenza was one in which compassion overrode protectionism, and enlightened self-interest ensured both negative consequences (the spread of the disease throughout the world) and ultimately positive outcomes (the support of individual sufferers).

The response to the AIDS epidemic in the United Kingdom was one in which self-help groups, often supported by local health professionals, led the way in offering information and support to vulnerable groups, demonstrating how clear messages could be conveyed to those at risk. The awareness and education campaigns of the mid-1980s in the United Kingdom were interesting and valuable because of their audacity (in the context of their time) and because of the commitment they demonstrated. Against a backdrop of mass media–induced fear and negative stereotypical attitudes to sufferers, self-help groups were able to develop awareness programs that probably saved lives. The government followed swiftly, launching some of the most effective mass media campaigns ever devised for health education purposes. One of the problems with such campaigns was the difficulty of evaluating their effectiveness. It was only in retrospect that researchers were able to demonstrate epidemiological patterns that pointed to their success.

These differences in approach to disease highlight the differences between societies and their cultural norms. In early modern Italy, even though some city-states were nominally republics, the power of state and church was paramount; by contrast, the modern, liberal society of early-20th-century New York was one in which every individual life was considered more important than the power of the state. In the United Kingdom during the 1980s, an open society with a free press and a highly active National Health Service at first distorted and later promoted a health promotion strategy that depended on the conveying of clear messages to vulnerable and often ostracized communities.

In each of these scenarios, nurses, however independently they defined their roles and however determinedly they pursued their health-promoting strategies, were highly dependent on states and local authorities to sanction and enable their work. The pest-house attendants of early modern cities struggled in the face of hopelessness and lack of resources. The nurses of early-20th-century New York, by contrast, supported as they were by local authorities, the Red Cross, and numerous voluntary agencies, were able to move rapidly into effective action. In the British cities of the 1980s, nursing personnel in a range of scenarios, such as genitourinary medicine clinics, specialist AIDS units, community health centers, and public health departments, were, after some initial delay, assisted by effective mass media campaigns to offer clear health-promoting messages to their client groups.

It would be all too easy to present this story as one of progress, one in which governments and societies became increasingly compassionate and effective. Such a perspective would be both complacent and distorting. States and societies have never been capable of doing more than the virulence of disease and the limitations of resources have permitted. As our own societies confront the advent of new and terrifying diseases, such as severe acute respiratory syndrome, Ebola, and Zika, we can learn from the struggles of those past societies that confronted similar terrors and stood and fought then with all the means they had at their disposal, but the lessons are not simple ones. We should also be heartened by the knowledge that states and societies—with nurses among their vanguards—have survived epidemic diseases.

Perhaps, ultimately, societies will completely escape the ravages of epidemics only when they have learned to fully understand the nature of their cohabitants on this planet: the vast range of microorganisms that cause both harm and good to human populations. All too often it seems that the spread of disease can be traced to human behavior: the opening up of trade routes, troop movements, lifestyle changes, and possibly even the direct scientific manipulation of existing microorganisms. Perhaps only when human societies have learned to recognize quickly the consequences of their collective actions and have gained the skills required to launch concerted efforts that override vested interest will they cease to encounter the devastation caused by epidemic disease.

Additional Resources

Centers for Disease Control and Prevention/Bubonic Plague at: http://www.cdc.gov/plague/history/

Centers for Disease Control and Prevention/Ebola at: http://www.cdc.gov/vhf/ebola/outbreaks/history/chronology.html

History Today at: http://www.historytoday.com/ole-j-benedictow/black-death-greatest-catastrophe-ever

The Henry J. Kaiser Family Foundation at: http://kff.org/global-health-policy/timeline/global-hivaids-timeline/

The New York Times/The Ebola Outbreak 2014 at: https://www.youtube.com/watch?v=xUBpoyKxArU

American Experience/The Forgotten Plague—The Deadliest Killer at: https://www.youtube.com/watch?v=gsaBmJjIDpM

U.K. Centre for the History of Nursing at: http://sites.nursing.manchester.ac.uk/ukchnm/aboutus/

University College Dublin—UCD Irish Centre for Nursing and Midwifery History at: http://www.ucd.ie/icnmh/

References

Alexander, J. T. (1980). *Bubonic plague in early modern Russia*. Baltimore, MD: Johns Hopkins University Press.

Anselment, R. A. (1989). Smallpox in seventeenth—century English literature: Reality and the metamorphosis of wit. *Medical History, 33*, 72–95.

Arno, P. S., & Feiden, K. L. (1992). *Against the odds: The story of AIDS development, politics and profits*. London, UK: HarperCollins.

AVERT. (2009). Retrieved from http://www.avert.org

Baggaley, J. P. (1988). Perceived effectiveness of international AIDS campaigns. *Health Education Research, 3*(1), 7–17.

Barre-Sinoussi, F., Chermann, J., Rey, F., Nugeyre, M. T., Chamaret, S., Gruest, J., . . . Montagnier, L. (1983). Isolation of a T-lymphotropic retrovirus from a patient at risk for acquired immune deficiency syndrome (AIDS). *Science, 220*(4599), 868–871.

Barry, J. (2005). *The great influenza: The epic story of the deadliest plague in history*. New York, NY: Viking Press.

Bateman, D. (1994). The good bleed guide: A patient's story. *Social History of Medicine, 7*(1), 115–133.

Berridge, V. (1996). *AIDS in the U.K. The making of a policy, 1981–1994*. Oxford, UK: Oxford University Press.

Biraben, J. (1975). *Les hommes et la peste en France dans les pays europeens et mediterraneens* (Two volumes). Paris, France: Mouton.

Brennan, R. O., & Durak, D. T. (1981). Gay compromise syndrome. *Lancet, 2*, 1338–1339.

Brozzi, M. (Ed.). (1982). *Peste Fede e Sanita in una Cronaca Cividalese del 1598*. Milan, Italy: Giuffre.

Buhler-Wilkerson, K. (2001). *No place like home: A history of nursing and home care in the United States*. Baltimore, MD: Johns Hopkins University Press.

Byerly, C. (2005). *Fever of war: The influenza epidemic in the U.S. Army during World War I*. New York, NY: New York University Press.

Calvi, G. (1989). *Histories of a plague year. The social and the imaginary in baroque Florence* (D. Biocca & B. T. Ragan, Trans.). Berkeley University of California Press.

Campbell, A. (1931). *The Black Death and men of learning.* New York, NY: Columbia University Press.

Cantacuzino, M. (1993). *Till break of day.* London, UK: Heinemann.

Carmichael, A. G. (1983). Legislation in the Italian Renaissance. *Bulletin of the History of Medicine, 57,* 516–536.

Carmichael, A. G. (1986). *Plague and the poor in renaissance Florence.* Cambridge, UK: Cambridge University Press.

Cartwright, F. F. (1977). *A social history of medicine.* London, UK: Longman.

Castellacci, D. (Ed.). (1897). *Curiosi ricordi del Contagio Di Firenze nel 1630. Archivio Storico Italiano* (5th series). Anno XX.

Chambers, D., & Pullan, B. (1992). *Venice. A documentary history.* Oxford, UK: Blackwell.

Christensen, P. (2003). "In these perilous times": Plague and plague policies in early modern Denmark. *Medical History, 47,* 413–450.

Cipolla, C. M. (1973). *Cristofano and the plague.* London, UK: Collins.

Cipolla, C. M. (1979). *Faith, reason and the plague.* Brighton, UK: Harvester Press.

Cipolla, C. M. (1992). *Miasmas and disease.* (E. Potter, Trans.). New Haven, CT: Yale University Press.

Connor, S., & Kingman, S. (1988). *The search for the virus. The scientific discovery of AIDS and the quest for a cure.* London, UK: Penguin Books.

Contarini, G. (1599). *The commonwealth and government of Venice* (L. Lewkenor, Trans.). London, UK: John Windet.

Crosby, A. W. (1989). *America's forgotten pandemic: The influenza of 1918.* Cambridge, UK: Cambridge University Press.

Dubois, R. M., Braitwaite, M. A., Mikhail, J. R., & Batten, J. C. (1981). Primary Pneumocystis carinii and cytomegalovirus infections. *Lancet, ii,* 1339.

Ficino, M. (1989). *Three books on life* (C. V. Kaske & J. R. Clark, Trans.). Binghamton, NY: Medieval and Renaissance Text and Studies.

Fowler, R. (1991). *Language in the news: Discourse and ideology in the press.* London, UK: Routledge.

Fracastoro, H. (1930). *De Contagione et Contagiosis Morbis et Eorum Curatione, Libri III* (W. C. Wright, Ed. & Trans.). New York, NY: G. P. Putnam and Sons.

Friedman, S., & Mottiar, S. (2005). A rewarding engagement? The treatment action campaign and the politics of HIV/AIDS. *Politics and Society, 33*(4), 511–565.

Galassi, N. (1966–1970). *Dieci Secoli di Storia Ospedaleria a Imola* (Vol. II). Imola, Italy: Galeati.

Garrett, L. (2007). The challenge of global health. *Foreign Affairs, 86*(1), 14–38.

Gradmann, C. (2001). Robert Koch and the pressures of scientific research: Tuberculosis and tuberculin. *Medical History, 45,* 1–32.

Grell, O. P. (1990). Plague in Elizabethan and Stuart London: The Dutch response. *Medical History, 34*(4), 424–439.

Gronfors, M., & Stalstrom, O. (1987). Power, prestige, profit: AIDS and the oppression of homosexual people. *Acta Sociological, 30*(1), 53–66.

Harden, V. A. (1992). Koch's postulates and the etiology of AIDS: An historical perspective. *History and Philosophy of the Life Sciences, 14*(2), 249–269.

Hirst, L. F. (1953). *The conquest of plague.* Oxford, UK: Clarendon Press.

Hortensii, C. D. (1631). *I cinque libri de gli avvertimenti, ordini, gride et editti: fatti et osservati in Milano, ne'tempi sospetosi della peste de gli anni MDLXXVI & LXXVII.* Milano, Italy: Bidelli.

Hymes, K. B., Green, J. B., & Mann, J. M. (1989). AIDS: A worldwide pandemic. In M. S. Gottlieb, D. J. Jeffries, D. Mildvan, A. J. Pinching, & T. C. Quinn (Eds.), *Current topics in AIDS* (Vol. 2). London, UK: John Wiley & Sons.

Johnson, N. (2006). *Britain and the 1918–19 influenza pandemic.* London, UK: Routledge.

Johnson, N. P. A. S., & Mueller, J. (2002). Updating the accounts: Global mortality of the 1918–1920 "Spanish influenza" pandemic. *Bulletin of the History of Medicine, 76,* 105–115.

Keeling, A. (2007). *Nursing and the privilege of prescription, 1893–2000.* Columbus: Ohio State University Press.

Keeling, A. (2009). "When the city is a great field hospital": The influenza pandemic of 1918 and the New York City nursing response. *Journal of Clinical Nursing, 18*(19), 2732–2738.

Keen-Payne, R. (2000). "We must have nurses": Spanish influenza in America, 1918–1919. *Nursing History Review, 8,* 143–156.

King, M. L. (1986). *Venetian humanism in an age of patrician dominance.* Princeton, NJ: Princeton University Press.

Latour, B. (1988). *The pasteurization of France* (A. Sheridan & J. Law, Trans.). Cambridge, MA and London, UK: Harvard University Press.

Leclerc-Madlala, S. (2005). Popular responses to HIV/AIDS and policy. *Journal of Southern African Studies, 31*(4), 845–856.

Mann, J. M. (1989). AIDS: A worldwide pandemic. In M. S. Gottlieb, D.J. Jeffries, D. Mildvan, A. J. Pinching, & T. C. Quinn (Eds.), *Current topics in AIDS* (Vol. 2). London, UK: John Wiley & Sons.

Modena, L. (1988). *Life of Judah* (M. R. Cohen, ed. & Trans.). Princeton, NJ: Princeton University Press.

More, T. (1516). *Utopia.* (R. Robinson, Trans.). Aldershot: Ashgate Publishing.

Nicholl, A., & Hamers, F. (2002). Are trends in HIV, gonorrhoea, and syphilis worsening in Western Europe? *British Medical Journal, 324,* 1324–1327.

Nicholl, A., Hughes, G., Donnelly, M., Livingstone, S., De Angelis, D., Fenton, K., . . . Catchpole, M. (2001). Assessing the impact of national anti-HIV sexual health campaigns: Trends in the transmission of HIV and other sexually transmitted infections in England. *Sexually Transmitted Infections, 77,* 242–247.

Nutton, V. (1990). The reception of Fracastoro's theory of contagion: The seed that fell among thorns? *Osiris, Second Series, 6,* 196–234.

Palmer, R. J. (1978). The *control of plague in Venice and Northern Italy, 1348–1600.* Unpublished doctoral dissertation The University of Kent at Canterbury.

Park, K., & Henderson, J. (1991). "The first hospital among Christians": The Ospedale di Santa Maria Nuova in early sixteenth century Florence. *Medical History, 35,* 164–188.

Pastore, A. (1988). Tra Giustizia e Politico: Il Governo della Peste a Genova e Roma nel 1656/7. *Rivista Storica Italiana, Anno 100,* 126–154.

Patterson, D. K., & Pyle, G. F. (1991). The geography and mortality of the 1918 influenza pandemic. *Bulletin of the History of Medicine, 65,* 4–21.

Petraccone, C. (1978). La Difesa Contro la Peste. *Archivio Storico per le Province Napoletane. Third Series, Anno XVI,* 253–280.

Phillips, H., & Killingray, D. (2003). *The Spanish influenza pandemic of 1918–19. New perspectives.* London, UK: Routledge.

Preto, P. (1978). *Peste e Societa a Venezia nel 1576.* Vicenza, Italy: Neri Pozza.

Pullan, B. (1971). *Rich and poor in renaissance Venice.* Oxford, UK: Basil Blackwood.

Pullan, B. (1992). Plague and perceptions of the poor in early modern Italy. In T. Ranger & P. Slack (Eds.), *Epidemics and ideas* (pp. 101–123). Cambridge, UK: Cambridge University Press.

Quinn, T. (2008). *Flu: A social history of influenza.* London, UK: New Holland.

Reid, A. (2005). The effects of the 1918–1919 influenza pandemic on infant and child health in Derbyshire. *Medical History, 49*(1), 29–54.

Robertson, J. R., Bucknall, A. B. V., Welsby, P. D., Roberts, J. J. K., Inglis, J. M., Peutherer, J. F., & Brettle, R. P. (1986). Epidemic of AIDS-related virus (HTLV III/LAV) infection among intravenous drug abusers in Scottish General practice. *British Medical Journal, 292,* 527–530.

Sapwell, J. (n.d.). *The reminiscences of a VAD in two world wars.* London, UK: The Red Cross Archives.

Sherr, L. (1987). An evaluation of the UK government health education campaign on AIDS. *Psychology and Health, 1,* 61–72.

Slack, P. (1985). *The impact of plague in Tudor and Stuart England.* London, UK: Clarendon Press.

Tester, K. (1994). *Media, culture and morality.* London, UK: Routledge.

Ulvioni, P. (1989). *Il Gran Castigo di Dio.* Milan, Italy: F. Angeli.

VanderVliet, V. (2001). AIDS: Losing "the new struggle"? *Daedalus, 130*(1), 151–184.

Wald, L. D. (1918, December 11). Visiting nursing. Written for the Foreign Bureau. Lillian Wald Papers. Writings & Speeches, Nurses & Nursing II, Reel 25, Box 37, Folder 4, pp. 1–9. New York

Public Library, Humanities and Social Sciences Library, Manuscripts and Archives Division, New York, NY.

Wolf, M. A., & Kielwasswe, A. P. (Eds.). (1991). *Gay people, sex and the media*. London, UK: Haworth Press.

World Health Organization. (1988). *AIDS prevention and control: Invited presentations and papers from the World Summit of ministers of health on programmes for AIDS prevention*. London, UK: World Health Organization.

Zinsser, H. (1935). *Rats, lice, and history*. Boston, MA: Little, Brown.

For a full suite of assignments and additional learning activities, use the access code located in the front of your book to visit this exclusive website: **http://go.jblearning.com/londrigan**. If you do not have an access code, you can obtain one at the site.

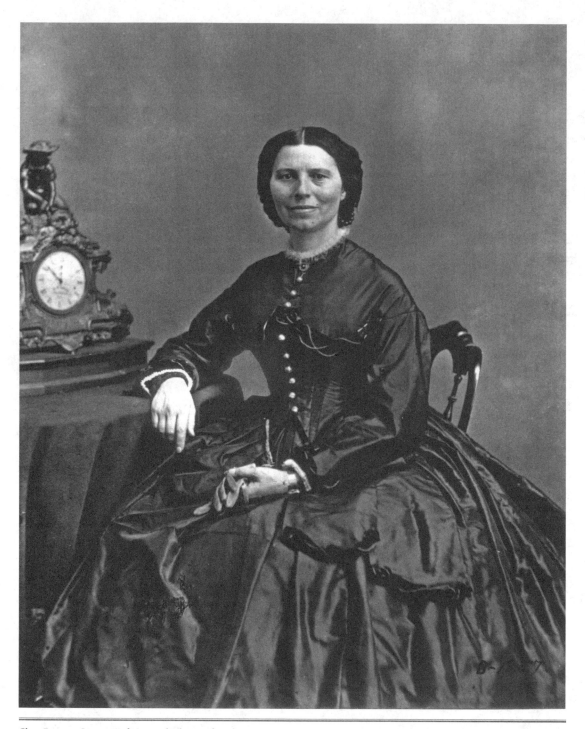

Clara Barton. Courtesy of National Library of Medicine.

CHAPTER 17

Historical Highlights in Disaster Nursing

Barbra Mann Wall
Arlene Keeling

It is not uncommon for physicians and nurses to recognize in a home the results from care and education instilled by a nurse at some previous time. During the siege of influenza here, this was particularly noticeable. While there was a great deal of hysteria and panic all through the city, its evidence was not noticed in homes that had previously known the ministrations of a visiting nurse. (Wald, 1918, p. 9)

LEARNING OBJECTIVES

At the completion of this chapter, the reader will be able to:

- Explore historical roots of disaster nursing through the lens of past disasters in the late 19th and 20th centuries.
- Describe the activities of public health nurses as they responded to past disasters.
- Relate past experiences of disaster nursing to present-day problems.

KEY TERMS

❑ American Red Cross
❑ Disasters

❑ Emergency preparedness
❑ Nursing history

This chapter examines specific instances of disaster nursing through the lens of **nursing history** to illustrate the important role nurses have had in providing prompt, efficient care to the ill or injured. In her classic text, *Disaster Nursing and Emergency Preparedness for Chemical, Biological, and Radiological Terrorism and Other Hazards,* Tener Veenema (2007) argues for the importance of disaster responses that are evidence based. Evidence for practice for disaster management logically comes from history—understanding what worked and what did not work in the past. Although others have recorded the Red Cross and medical responses to disasters, the nursing response and **emergency preparedness** is often overlooked, accepted as routine, or merely as following orders.

Nurses' work is highlighted during three late-19th-century **disasters**: the yellow fever epidemic of 1888, the Johnstown flood of 1889, and the 1900 Galveston hurricane. These disasters are historically significant because they mark the first **American Red Cross** response, resulting in the federal government giving it a formal charter to provide disaster relief. In addition, the chapter focuses on three 20th-century disasters: the 1918 influenza pandemic, the 1947 Texas City ship explosion, and the 1964 Alaska earthquake.

The causes of each disaster varied, and the response was tailored for the problem. In 1888, for example, mosquitoes caused the yellow fever epidemic in Jacksonville, Florida, and in 1889, catastrophic rains caused the Johnstown flood in Pennsylvania. As in Johnstown, the devastation from the 1900 Galveston hurricane—the most deadly hurricane of the 20th century—resulted from a largely uncontrollable force of nature. Death came from drowning or injury, as buildings collapsed, and the unexpected and vicious storm surge devastated the coastal city. By contrast, the flu was a biological event—the rapid and overwhelming spread of a deadly virus. The Texas City disaster related to the consequences of increasing industrialization and the growth of the oil industry in the state, and it demonstrates what happens when hazardous materials are not properly

contained. At that time, it was the worst industrial accident in the country's history, killing over 500 people. The Alaska earthquake demonstrated the problems that can occur from seismic risks. In 1964, it was the second largest earthquake ever recorded, after the 1960 earthquake in Chile.

Although the disasters resulted from different causes, some related to weather, others to industrialization, and others to the spread of disease, in other ways these disasters reveal similarities. They occurred suddenly and without warning, they devastated communities, and they demanded a nursing and medical response. After each disaster, nurses organized and provided care in both hospitals and the community.

Yellow Fever and the Johnstown Flood

Before World War II, there was no permanent program of federal disaster relief in the United States, and private voluntary agencies such as the American National Red Cross and the Salvation Army took primary responsibility for disaster response (Kreps, 1990; Rubin, 2007). The International Committee of the Red Cross was founded in Geneva, Switzerland, in 1863 by Henry Dunant; today, national Red Cross societies exist in nearly every country in the world, with the American National Red Cross, organized in large part by Clara Barton, founded in 1881 (Moorehead, 1998).

During the 1888 yellow fever epidemic in Jacksonville, Florida, the Red Cross recruited nurses to the danger zone. Barton turned to New Orleans for help; there, many people had already had the disease and thus were immune. She recruited 30 nurses, both white and black, to travel with her by train to Jacksonville. On arrival in Jacksonville, however, the train's engineer refused to stop in the epidemic area. Thus, in the midst of a torrential rain, 10 nurses jumped off the moving train so they could assist the sick. Earning $3.00 a day, they worked 72-hour shifts for 79 days. A scandal developed, however, when several men and women refused to work for the $3.00-a-day wage in hospitals and instead went into private nursing where they could make more money. Other nurses were accused of immoral conduct (Kernodle, 1949). Barton provided an explanation. She admitted that many of the volunteers she recruited were untrained, and clashes developed between them and the local boards of health, which employed federal and municipal health officers who used newer scientific methods. In addition, many adventurers responded and called themselves Red Cross nurses even though they were not. Consequently, the local health board deported them (Barton, 1904; Dock & Pickett, 1922). Barton believed it was unfair to judge the status of Red Cross nurses by these latter individuals (Barton, 1904).

Consequently, the director of Sandhills Fever Hospital did not rely on Red Cross nurses. Rather, he recruited trained nurses and students, a new type of nurse that he had witnessed as an intern at the Bellevue Hospital in New York City. At Sandhills, his chief nurse was Jane Delano, a graduate of Bellevue who later became president of the American Nurses Association and director of the Red Cross Nursing Service (D'Antonio & Whelan, 2004; Kernodle, 1949). One of Delano's classmates, Lavinia Dock, followed her there. As a trained public health nurse, Dock and the other nurses brought improved care to patients through their emphasis on order, cleanliness, ventilation, and nutrition, and they demonstrated the critical importance of what this new nursing profession could offer (D'Antonio & Whelan, 2004; Dock & Pickett, 1922).

A year later, the Red Cross was called on to help at the site of the Johnstown Flood. On the afternoon of May 31, 1889, heavy rains had been pouring down on central Pennsylvania when the decaying South Fork Dam broke. Millions of tons of water and debris came crushing down into the valley in what became the worst flood in the nation's history. Within 10 minutes, over 2,200 people were killed, and tens of thousands more were injured or made homeless. Nurses and physicians from Mercy Hospital in Pittsburgh were among the first to respond, both at the scene and in their hospital

(Rafferty, 1974). Clara Barton and her relief team arrived five days later, on June 5. They distributed supplies to thousands of survivors and provided warm meals, medical care, and shelter to many in buildings that became known as Red Cross Hotels (Kernodle, 1949; National Park Service, 2006). Most of the nursing, however, was handled by a branch of the American Red Cross from Philadelphia not associated with Barton. Led by Lavinia Dock, graduate nurses trained in hospitals and public health worked in tent hospitals set up for the ill and the injured. Their nursing proved invaluable as they worked with Barton and other Red Cross relief workers to carry out sanitation measures to prevent disease (Barton, 1904; Dock & Pickett, 1922).

The Galveston Hurricane, 1900

On September 10, 1900, meteorologist and eyewitness John D. Blagden wrote the following to his family (2000):

> There is not a building in town that is uninjured. Hundreds are busy day and night clearing away the debris and recovering the dead. It is awful. Every few minutes a wagon load of corpses passes by on the street . . . The more fortunate are doing all they can to aid the sufferers, but it is impossible to care for all. (pp. 17–18)

Two days before, on September 8, a hurricane had hit Galveston, Texas, leaving approximately 8,000 people dead. The image of death pervaded the accounts of the Galveston storm, and by September 12, newspapers were filled with stories about recovering the dead. Eventually, the bodies had to be burned en masse in bonfires throughout the city. During the storm, both blacks and whites took refuge in two local hospitals, John Sealy and St. Mary's Infirmary. Both suffered damage but were able to take patients again within a few days (Bixel & Turner, 2000).

Clara Barton and her staff arrived on September 17 and found an impromptu local relief committee that was tending to disaster recovery needs and collecting supplies. Barton was 78 years old at the time, and this would be her last trip to the scene of a disaster. She had presided over many disasters, and with each one her fame grew (Barton, 1900; Moorehead, 1998). Her arrival in Galveston was met with great fanfare, as one assistant recalled, "When Miss Barton's train got in, the guards were ready, soldiers at present arms, everything in very martial style; in fact, it was the only spice of the theatrical that there was in the whole business" (Fayling, 2000, p. 91).

Although the Red Cross had recruited nurses during the yellow fever epidemic and the Johnstown Flood in the 1880s, in Galveston it was primarily responsible for obtaining supplies. Rather than assuming total control, Barton and her staff worked with the local relief committee, supplying food, clothing, and shelter. Galveston women had formed a new Red Cross auxiliary, and Barton ensured they would provide greater leadership at the distribution stations. The Red Cross also worked with volunteers from various charitable and patriotic societies, including the Women's Relief Corps, the Women's Christian Temperance Union, and the Grand Army of the Republic. Blacks had formed their own relief committees, and Barton also set up a special fund for them (Barton, 1900). Barton stayed in Texas for two months. In addition to providing help in Galveston, she and her staff distributed supplies to people in towns and villages over a 1,000-square-mile area that had suffered severe damage. Barton had a policy of restarting local work. When the hurricane washed away strawberry plants of farmers in six storm-swept counties and no money was available to buy more, she helped secure over 1 million plants.

After Barton's retirement, the Red Cross reorganized in 1905 and created state and territorial branches. One of the organization's newly assigned responsibilities included nursing during peacetime emergencies such as fire, floods, pestilence, and other national disasters. The state and local committees of enrolled Red Cross nurses served as volunteer recruiters of other nurses when the need arose. The new structure would be critical to the nursing response to the influenza pandemic when it hit the United States in the autumn of 1918.

The Flu Pandemic, 1918–1919

The influenza epidemic of 1918, killing over 40 million people worldwide and causing over 675,000 deaths in the United States (Hilleman, 2002; Johnson & Mueller, 2002), challenged the nation's public health service, the American Red Cross, the medical and nursing professions, and the U.S. federal government in much the same way it challenged other nations around the world. In 1918, the extremely high death rate—particularly among young adults—from a rare and highly contagious form of influenza was mysterious and frightening. According to one historian (Byerly, 2005),

> The influenza and pneumonia of 1918 shocked medical officers and soldiers alike. It rendered strong, healthy men powerless and struggling for breath; it distorted and saturated the lungs of those it killed; it rendered helpless professional physicians of great skill and knowledge; it consumed an enormous amount of army resources; and it killed in such great numbers that images of sick and dead bodies and coffins stayed with the survivors for the rest of their lives. (p. 87)

When the flu hit the cities of the United States and killed citizens, not soldiers, the country was unprepared for the magnitude of the crisis. Reflecting on the events of that year, nurse leader Janet Geister (1957) later wrote: "We weren't ready in plans and resources, nor were we ready in our thinking. A country-wide epidemic was utterly inconceivable" (p. 583). To complicate the situation, the United States had only recently entered the war in Europe, and thousands of physicians and nurses had just been deployed. Few were left to cope with a major epidemic at home.

In the United States, influenza first broke out in Kansas at a crowded military recruit camp. It then traveled with the soldiers to the cities of the East Coast, notably Boston, Philadelphia, and New York, where it also arrived on ships from Europe. Within a matter of days, it raced south and westward across the country along transportation lines (Crosby, 2003; Markel et al., 2007).

On September 6, 1918, the *Boston Globe* reported an outbreak of old-fashioned grippe among the sailors on the Commonwealth Pier (Fayling, 2000). By September 17, influenza reports were front-page news. Within the next 24 hours, health authorities recorded 41 more deaths, and the Boston health commissioner issued a warning against public hysteria. On September 18, only 12 days after the explosion of the epidemic in Boston, the flu spread through Philadelphia, the center of the war industry. Within days hundreds of sailors were ill; civilians were also succumbing to flu. Almost simultaneously, the epidemic erupted in New York City.

Meanwhile in Boston, where they had been dealing with the flu for over two weeks, health officials were alarmed enough to send a telegram to the American Red Cross headquarters in Washington, D.C., to ask for nurses. In Washington, it was becoming increasingly clear that this was no ordinary flu epidemic. Reports were coming to the Red Cross from cities up and down the East Coast. The new strain had devastated Boston and was now sweeping through New York, Philadelphia, and Washington. It was also racing south and west. The Red Cross had to take action. As a result, on September 24 members of the American Red Cross National Committee assembled in Washington to discuss the federal response. Their plan was to implement the decentralized response they had adopted for home defense a year earlier. The U.S. Public Health Service would manage the medical response and distribute posters and pamphlets educating the public about the illness. The Red Cross National Committee would communicate with its local organizations and direct the nursing response. The major response would have to be done at the local level (Fieser, 1941). Thus, immediately after the meeting, Director of the Red Cross Bureau of Nursing Services Clara Noyes telegraphed all Red Cross Divisions with a directive: "Suggest you organize Home Defense nurses . . . to meet present epidemic . . . Provide nurses with masks" (Noyes, 1918, p. 2).

In New York City, Lillian Wald, director of the Henry Street Settlement, did not need to be told to organize the nurses. In fact, she was all too aware of the alarming rapidity with which the flu was affecting the city's residents; her staff had already been working around the clock. In the slums of the Lower East Side, epidemics of infectious diseases were commonplace, and in September 1918, it seemed this was just another bad flu epidemic, only this time the intensity of the disease and the devastation it caused were remarkable. Finally, on October 10, the Atlantic Division of the Red Cross assembled New York City nursing leaders to plan their response. At that meeting, the nurses created the Nurses' Emergency Council to organize a city-wide response. The Red Cross also inserted a "quarter page advertisement in all the Sunday papers, calling for service from the women of the city" (Doty, 1919, p. 951).

In Philadelphia, the situation was becoming increasingly serious, in part because on September 28, despite the fact that 123 civilians had been admitted to hospitals with flu just the day before, the city proceeded with its scheduled Liberty Loan parade to raise money for the war effort. Pandemic then exploded. By October 3, a doctor estimated that the city had seen 75,000 cases since September 11. Finally, the city government allocated $100,000 from its emergency war defense fund to combat the disease (Visiting Nurse Society, 1918, n.p.). It also coordinated all relief organizations under the direction of a central office and notified citizens struck with flu to call "Filbert 100" to obtain "a nurse, a doctor, an ambulance, or an automobile" (Visiting Nurse Society, 1918, n.p.).

Under the direction of Katherine Tucker, RN, the Philadelphia Visiting Nurse Society handled thousands of influenza cases. In many of the families, more than one member was ill; when both parents succumbed, the nurses had to supply food for the entire family. Soup kitchens were set up where the nurses could obtain soup, bread, and milk for such cases. As family after family was affected, the city's social infrastructure crumbled. Thousands of city workers were out sick, including streetcar drivers, telephone receptionists, shopkeepers, and garbage collectors. When the few nurses there also became sick, the situation became critical. There were simply not enough nurses. According to Health Director Kreusen (Visiting Nurse Society, 1918), "If you would ask me the three things Philadelphia most needs to conquer the epidemic, I would tell you 'Nurses, more nurses, and yet more nurses'" (n.p.).

The flu then spread south and west, affecting cities and towns across the nation. Many of the cities suffered extremely high mortality rates, and as the dead piled up, health boards and emergency councils closed theaters, schools, and churches (Barry, 2005). By late November 1918, the virus had made its way around the world. The second wave was over. However, the virus mutated again, and a third wave struck in December and then in January 1919. Of all the major cities hit, San Francisco confronted the wave most efficiently, using both masks and vaccines to prevent its spread (Barry, 2005). Local chapters did their best to cooperate with the American Red Cross. According to one report, "Every chapter in Idaho, Oregon, and Washington has appointed a committee on influenza" (Kilpatrick, 1919, p. 1). The same was true for coal mining camps in Kentucky, logging camps in Michigan, and in small towns across the United States. In every area, nurses were key to the response, and they responded promptly, without regard to race, class, or color.

1947 Texas City Ship Explosion

In 1947, the Dean of the University of Texas School of Nursing at Galveston wrote about healthcare workers' responses after a ship explosion in Texas City, Texas (Bartholf, 1947), "We were proud of the performance of the whole organization, and particularly of the nurses and doctors—they just clicked and came up to par in a wonderful fashion. I had never seen morale quite so high in this institution" (p. 558). Indeed, nurses and other healthcare personnel often experience a sense of camaraderie after working in a disaster, but this event also shows a more complicated story of competition among healthcare personnel.

In the late 19th and early 20th centuries, disasters mainly resulted from natural events such as hurricanes, disease, tornadoes, earthquakes, and floods, but as industry expanded in the 1900s, industrial accidents increased, with similar devastating results. On April 16 and 17, 1947, what was called the worst industrial catastrophe in U.S. history occurred when ammonium nitrate fertilizer on two merchant ships exploded in the Texas City, Texas, docks, killing 405 people, with another 63 unidentified dead (Minutaglio, 2003; Stephens, 1997; Wall, 2008). When the first of the ships, the *Grandcamp*, exploded in the harbor, it caused smoke to rise 2,000 feet in the air and flaming cargo to fly over a one-mile radius. The nearby Monsanto Chemical Plant caught fire from flying steel and burning debris, killing 145 workers. Every fireman who initially responded died, decimating the local fire department. Two planes flying over the docks at the time of the explosion fell from the sky, and windows shattered in Houston, Galveston, and other Texas cities. In addition to the many deaths, 3,000 injuries occurred, one-third of all city dwellings were demolished, and 2,500 people lost their homes ("1200 Feared Dead," 1947; Boyle, 1947; Stephens, 1993).

A major priority after any disaster is the establishment of order out of chaos. With no disaster plan in place, the mayor and the police chief had to recruit volunteers, and the disaster response initially was piecemeal. Without a local hospital, Texas City physicians and nurses organized a clearing station where casualties were triaged and the most serious moved to hospitals in surrounding cities and towns. Texas City clinics were full as well, and physicians and nurses worked with no water or electricity. A nurse's aide at one of the local clinics remembered that men from one of the plants came to help, and they worked like Trojans (Wheaton, 1948, p. 18).

The resources of other healthcare teams quickly organized and converged on the scene. Alerted by smoke columns across Galveston Bay, orthopedic surgeons, residents, senior medical students, nurses, and nursing students from John Sealy Hospital immediately left for Texas City with plasma, blood, and other supplies. Within an hour after the initial explosion, local American Red Cross chapters began mobilizing. Late in the evening of the first explosion, the Director of Nursing Service from the Red Cross Midwestern Area arrived from St. Louis and started recruiting more than 500 nurses from Texas and nearby states. As in every disaster since Clara Barton's day, many untrained women offered their services, so it became necessary to weed them out by checking credentials (Kernodle, 1949).

In all, 3,000 persons required sudden medical assistance, and after emergency first aid was provided, casualties went to 21 area hospitals. Many were hospitalized at the University of Texas Medical Branch (UTMB) facilities. Survivors began arriving within an hour, and all medical and nursing personnel were placed on 24-hour call. A nurse came in from her vacation and worked in a dispensary set up in the jail. Other nurses, both registered nurses and licensed practical nurses, worked at this dispensary and at the morgue. Soon, several busloads of nurses, under motorcycle escort, came to Texas City and eventually went on to Galveston hospitals (Wheaton, 1948).

John Sealy Hospital handled a total of 498 casualties. Within the first five hours, nurses and physicians classified 362 patients in the emergency department, gave them preliminary treatment, and hospitalized them. While physicians performed minor surgery

in hallways, volunteer military medical and nursing personnel enabled 10 rooms to be outfitted for surgery. Doctors and nurses operated nonstop over the next two days. Multiple puncture wounds, contusions, cuts from shards of glass, compound fractures, and head, eye, and ear injuries (especially ruptured eardrums) were common. Sixteen patients died from severe head injuries (Blocker & Blocker, 1949; Leake, 1947).

In 1948, the Sisters of Charity of the Incarnate Word told the story of the response of Galveston's St. Mary's Hospital to the Texas City disaster to a writer for *Hospital Progress*, the official journal of the Catholic Hospital Association. St. Mary's benefited from nurses, and nurse anesthetists flown in from San Antonio. Sixteen operating rooms were set up, and the sisters opened an unfinished wing to take in 96 patients. During that time, 186 patients were detained in the hospital, whereas eight died (McLeod, 1948). The Red Cross provided 2 billion units of penicillin, 5 million units of tetanus antitoxin, large quantities of whole blood and plasma, streptomycin, sulfa drugs, and gas gangrene antitoxin (Girardeau, 1947).

In 1958, a research associate in the Disaster Research Group of the National Academy of Sciences interviewed several nurses after another disaster and found they were apt to feel insecure when physicians were not around. At the time, most nurses were still trained in hospital diploma programs, and they were task oriented. The data from the Texas City explosion both support and refute this conclusion. Although nurses indeed concentrated on tasks, they also developed a sense of pride when they were able to perform new assessments and expand their nursing roles, both dependent and independent of physicians.

As examples, students from the Schools of Nursing at John Sealy and St. Mary's Hospitals, part of UTMB, worked with teams to care for casualties, both at the scene and in hospitals. Stories from two students reveal they did more than merely assist the physician. One, who constructed her story in the *American Journal of Nursing* (Molsbee, 1947), worked on the pediatric ward at John Sealy Hospital and helped transfer children to other sites to make room for 40 injured adults. Patients came in ambulances, private automobiles, trucks, and milk wagons. Many activities of the nurses who suddenly found themselves in the midst of a disaster were improvised. Although it is not standard practice today, this student learned to fill 20-, 30-, and 50-cc syringes with morphine and give it by changing needles between patients. Nurses did not have regular charts, so they pinned tags on patients' clothes with dose and time they gave the medications (Molsbee, 1947).

A year after the explosion, another student from John Sealy composed a memoir of the events. An operating room supervisor had recruited her to Texas City as the student walked down the steps of the hospital. She was still in her nursing uniform, and, in the first part of the narrative, the form of her language conformed to the image of the compliant student she was taught to be. She said she "didn't have permission from the nursing office" (Givin, 1948, n.p.) to go. The supervisor cried, "It doesn't matter. I give you permission!" This group was one of the first from UTMB to arrive on the scene. Nurses' training in organization and carrying out specific tasks helped them maintain order. The student was able to adapt to the situation and administer first aid to severely burned patients, including giving morphine for pain. In fact, she had an "open order to administer hypodermics of pain relievers as I saw the need. . . . In a situation like this," she wrote, "you are oblivious to anything except doing the job at hand. Somehow, everything you have ever learned in this area comes to the surface, and you do the best you can." She worked there for several hours and accompanied a patient back to the hospital in a station wagon, guiding the driver while she held the patient's intravenous infusion. By that time, the hospital grounds were covered with tents, and the Red Cross had arrived (Givin, 1948).

In the above nurse's memoir, her image of a compliant nurse who had to follow orders and adhere to set routines was altered. She wrote, "I later realized there was no way that you could take a holistic view of a patient in a situation like this; it's only the immediate needs that are met. I will never forget that day, from the time I felt the vibrations of the explosion coming down those steps of the main building to now when I realize what a confident twenty-year-old nurse I was." She was amazed at how, when she was at the scene of the disaster, "everything began to fall into place, and regardless of rank or race, we were a team" (Givin, 1948, n.p.). Thus, as the nursing student reconstructed her story, she moved herself from a peripheral position as a student with little power to a central position, where her words and deeds proclaimed her as equal with the other responders. These included those with higher rank such as physicians and people of a different race. Her opportunity to nurse during this disaster led her to repudiate her perceived limitations as a nursing student.

Although the people worked together initially, tensions quickly developed over who would get credit for the rescue work. Regular units of the armed forces arrived on the afternoon of April 16, but they worked independently of the Red Cross. This led the mayor to publicly criticize the Red Cross in the newspaper. He expressed his concern to an official that the Red Cross was "taking credit for everything that is being done in the way of relief" (Givin, 1948, n.p.). For one thing, its workers "went down to the gymnasium morgue and took it over from our people . . . after they had worked there ever since the explosion" (Givin, 1948, n.p.). Furthermore, the Red Cross had called a press conference that featured physicians it had brought in from the outside. "What about 10 of our local doctors that worked night and day?" the mayor retorted. "What is being said about them to those reporters?" (*Houston Chronicle*, 1947, n.p.). No mention was made of the nurses.

African American and Mexican American residents from El Barrio and The Bottom, the neighborhoods closest to the docks, suffered most from the disaster. Many were left homeless after these areas were utterly destroyed. On April 19, the African American newspaper, the *Informer*, described the disaster, provided photographs, and told stories of dramatic escapes and heroic rescues on the part of African Americans. Black physicians and nurses from Houston cared for African American survivors at John Sealy Hospital, and they also rendered aid at the scene. African American morticians and embalmers came to help, and two ministers from local black churches carried the injured and dying in their cars to hospitals in Galveston ("Employee of Texas City," 1947; "Many Negroes killed," 1947).

Red Cross nurses worked at the disaster site and in hospitals, and many stayed for two months until the regular nursing staff could take over. Red Cross and local public health nurses participated in case-finding activities by making home visits to care for the injured, seeing 2,231 patients in their homes (American National Red Cross, 1947). One of the most difficult tasks was to work with grieving families. City officials set up a temporary morgue in the local high school gymnasium, but they had no system for identifying the dead. Trained nurses accompanied families attempting to locate their missing relatives as they pulled back blankets and viewed the bodies, some so mangled they were never identified (Johnston, 1947).

Even though there were problems with communication and transportation, several groups responded quite well to the disaster, including medical and nursing personnel, because they had the skills and discipline needed for emergencies (Stephens, 1997). Writing after the disaster, Chauncey Leake, vice-president and dean of UTMB, noted that the successful responses were a result of the application of military medical principles by a team of skilled specialists in a specialty hospital center. This included first aid by trained rescue personnel; preliminary dressings by general practitioners; rapid diagnosis and sorting by a team of specialty physicians; surgery with careful anesthesia and adequate wound drainage; generous administration of plasma and whole blood; use of penicillin, tetanus, and gas gangrene antitoxins; fluid control; and careful recordkeeping (Leake, 1947). Although this account risks overestimating physicians' importance at the expense of others, nurses no doubt participated in these activities.

Between 1900 and 1947, new research had occurred in blood types, the treatment of gas gangrene, and the use of penicillin and other antibiotics, and Texas City survivors benefited from these discoveries. Emergency medical techniques used in World War II were also put to good use and accounted for a more organized response. At the same time, skill and discipline proved essential to successful disaster relief responses. Particularly for nurses and other healthcare personnel, their jobs required them to deal with emergencies on a day-to-day basis. Although the disaster was new to them, the response process was familiar.

Finally, by 1947 changes were beginning to be seen in nurses' model identities that reflected those of skilled professionals. The writings of nurses who cared for victims in the aftermath of the Texas City disaster revealed self-images of skilled, hard-working, and often exhausted professionals who had opportunities to expand their healthcare roles in new ways. One student nurse chose to remember her experience in the 1947 disaster as a change in how she perceived herself as a nurse, no longer as a novice but as a competent and decisive professional.

After the Texas City disaster, on May 5, 1947, the Central Committee of the American National Red Cross approved a plan for the enrollment of nurses in the Red Cross Nursing for service to local communities through chapter programs. This plan replaced the type of enrollment in operation from 1905 to 1946, which served primarily as a reserve for the Army and the Navy. This would prove beneficial to survivors of disasters in the future.

The Alaska Earthquake of 1964

On March 27, 1964, at 5:36 p.m., the strongest earthquake ever recorded on the North American continent struck Alaska. In Anchorage, the chronicler of Providence Hospital, which became the chief receiving agency of the injured in that city, wrote, "Everyone seemed to sense the need for immediate action and responsibility" (*Chronicles of the Sisters of Providence*, 1964, n.p.).

Known as the Good Friday Earthquake, it had a tremor that lasted approximately 4 minutes, measured 8.6 on the Richter scale, and caused damages estimated at $750 million. It was so powerful that tremors could be felt over a 500,000-square-mile area, with shock waves tearing boats from moorings as far away as the Gulf of Mexico. Tsunamis struck all along the western coast of North America from the Arctic to as far south as Crescent City, California. In addition to Anchorage, a number of Alaskan communities such as Seward, Kodiak, and Valdez were affected, as well as several coastal native villages.

The two-year-old Providence Hospital was the largest private hospital in the state. Owned and operated by the Sisters of Providence, it became the primary medical emergency center for the entire region. The fact that Providence Hospital received minimal damage was extremely important in its response to the disaster. It quickly shifted to emergency power, and its lights drew supplies and personnel from all over the city to its facilities. Two hospitals in the area, the 40-bed Presbyterian and 300-bed U.S. Air Force hospital at Elmendorf, suffered extensive structural damage. Although the Air Force facility evacuated to nearby barracks and the 395-bed U.S. Public Health Service's Alaska Native Hospital, Presbyterian's patients went to Providence Hospital. Because it became obvious that Providence would be the center of medical and nursing attention, there was little need for further coordination of medical care (Haas, 1964).

Hospital staff members mobilized quickly to care for survivors. Sister Barbara Ellen was administrator of Providence, and she and her five sister assistants coordinated the task of keeping the hospital in operation. They had to deal with lack of water and elevator use, no effective sanitation, and no sterilizers. Pharmacy medications had spilled all over the floor, and all phone links were dead (Special Report, 1964). Within a few minutes, an emergency generator restored electricity and heat to vital areas such as the emergency department, surgery areas, nursing stations, and main halls. The U.S. Army provided a generator for the kitchen, and firemen pumped water from a nearby spring into the hospital (*Chronicles of the Sisters of Providence*, 1964).

No nurse left her unit to go to a safer place, and none of the 75 patients in the hospital at the time received injuries from the quake (*Chronicles of the Sisters of Providence*, 1964). Indeed, a survey team of sociologists from the Disaster Research Center, who arrived within 28 hours after the quake, stated, "Few if any persons actually abandoned an ongoing organizational responsibility" (Haas, 1964, p. 26). The physicians responded with their own action plan, and some brought their families. Key people were pulled to the emergency department, and within 30 minutes, the first survivors arrived. Calmness was maintained throughout the hospital, led by Sister Barbara Ellen, who never lost control of the situation (*Chronicles of the Sisters of Providence*, 1964). Indeed, her authority and her maintenance of control in the crisis helped maintain stability throughout the emergency (Fortier, 1964). As the radio broadcasted a need for registered nurses, off-duty Providence personnel came as well as nurses from the evacuated Presbyterian Hospital. Military personnel from Elmendorf Air Force Base and Fort Richardson delivered a 200-bed civil defense hospital to Providence with beds and cots that were set up in the cafeteria, halls, and business office (Langston, 1964; Sister Philias, 1964). Eventually, Providence did not fill to capacity, however, and not all these supplies were needed (Haas, 1964).

The damage to the American Red Cross headquarters in downtown Anchorage delayed its response, but within 24 hours, it had mobilized. Sigrid Bullard from Redwood City, California, the Red Cross Nursing Director for the Alaska disaster, put out a call for volunteers, and 45 registered nurses and 27 trained Red Cross nurses' aides responded. All the aides and many of the nurses cared for survivors at Providence Hospital throughout the emergency period (Office of Public Information, 1964).

At Providence Hospital, nurses and physicians set up a triage system in the emergency department. Admissions personnel registered 108 people the first night, but only a few were critically injured. In the operating suites, flashlights and battery-operated lights were available in addition to the auxiliary power; one doctor delivered a baby by flashlight early Saturday morning when all power briefly failed. Sterilizers were not operational because there was no steam, and nurses washed instruments and sterilized them with Bunsen burners. They had to improvise in other ways, with one using snow as a substitute for hypothermia for a patient undergoing a craniotomy. Others heated water for infant formulas in the doctors' coffee urn, and they used distilled water for drinking purposes (Langston, 1964; Sister Philias, 1964).

Public health nurses' roles in this disaster included investigating home-based cases, seeking out dislocated families, distributing food and clothing, performing health screenings, and helping survivors find shelter. The morning after the earthquake hit, public health nurses first went to Providence Hospital to see if they were needed. When told that the hospital had sufficient personnel, they went to the state's Civil Defense Headquarters, where they assisted in evacuations (Haas, 1964). Nurses also opened clinics in outlying areas where they provided immunizations. Nurses, including volunteers from Juneau and Fairbanks, aided Anchorage school nurses, as did many retired nurses. One opined, "This was a very exciting experience of community cooperation" (Beltz, 1964). Other school nurses who were able to leave their families responded over the next two weeks, caring for more than 300 evacuated Aleuts from Old Harbor and Kaguyak, where a tidal

wave had destroyed their villages. Making formula for babies became a full-time job, and eventually Aleut midwives took over the responsibility from the local school nurses (Scott, 1964). Other nursing care required taking vital signs, dispensing medications, and listening to survivors' problems.

Farther away, a public health nurse from the Prince William Sound area was summoned to Anchorage from her post deep in the interior of the state. The village of Chenega was totally destroyed, 23 people died, and all the survivors were forced to move. This nurse and a team of physicians and sanitation engineers visited potential evacuation sites to evaluate available housing and water supplies for Chenega's residents (Bonehill, 1964).

Red Cross nurses were on the front lines to care for survivors in emergency shelter. Some nurses worked in typhoid immunization clinics and in shelters such as one that housed 166 Aleuts evacuated from Kodiak Island, which had suffered immense structural damage; it was 350 air miles from Anchorage, and it listed 19 dead or missing (Office of Public Information, 1964). This was the area to which Hazel Heywood, then Director of Nursing services for the Red Cross chapter in Milwaukee, Wisconsin, was assigned. Because communications had been knocked out, nurses' only contact with Red Cross headquarters was through the Alaska Communications System, with nurses and others manning the calls as they came through. The disaster teams supplemented the agencies already at the scene. To this end, her first job was to relieve the fatigued nurse at a schoolhouse shelter where 600 to 700 people had congregated. Babies needed formulas and clean diapers, and someone was able to bring a washing machine into the schoolhouse. The Red Cross set up its headquarters in a local church in Kodiak and provided nursing coverage for the schoolhouse shelter until April 7. It dispensed groceries and clothes to the needy, helped with housing, and fed evacuees waiting for stateside naval flights. Nurses checked for survivors, a monumental job because there were no transportation facilities, telephones, newspapers, or roads to reach outlying villages on the island (Farley, 1964).

American Red Cross volunteers went to other badly damaged areas. The greatest death toll was in Valdez, where 32 men, women, and children were killed when huge sections of land slid into the sea. A Red Cross representative from San Antonio, Texas, helped care for hospitalized and sheltered survivors there. Fairbanks experienced only a momentary swaying of buildings, and at St. Joseph's Hospital, the local Red Cross nursing chairwoman helped screen evacuees from Valdez for communicable diseases and other needs for medical and nursing care (Benson, 1964).

Most of the nurses in Seward, which had been severely damaged, were on duty somewhere, "herding children, gathering families together, setting up first aid stations. . . . The nurses did everything, scrubbed, cooked, set up trays, washed dishes, answered lights, comforted the hundreds who swarmed about the Hospital that first night and all the next day" (Blue, 1964, p. 1). A Red Cross nurse from Oregon dealt with disrupted health and sanitation facilities and the dangers of communicable diseases.

Red Cross survey teams made daily trips into the remote, mountainous Alaskan countryside. To obtain information about distant villages, U.S. Public Health Service physicians and Division of Public Health nurses and sanitary engineers also visited sites in Prince William Sound and Kodiak Island. They provided medical and nursing care, preventive measures, health teaching, and further assessments of sanitary conditions. They worked in an advisory role with agencies responsible for the care of refugees, and as they returned to the areas badly damaged or destroyed, they helped in arranging temporary facilities (Office of Public Information, 1964).

Conclusion

Public health nurses' disaster work has a long history. The exemplars presented in this chapter are illustrative of the growing focus on expert emergency preparedness nursing practice. In the late 19th and early 20th centuries, nurses provided care and comfort measures, as well as fluid and nutrition. In fact, during the yellow fever epidemic and the 1918 influenza pandemic, nursing care was usually the only treatment for the illness. As the 20th century progressed, nurses began participating in emergency first aid at the scene. They took vital signs, cared for physical and emotional wounds, administered plasma, and gave medications. Although many carried out traditional tasks of easing fears, they also worked with intravenous infusions, surgery, infection control, and pain relief. Nurses, along with others, worked around the clock, often too busy to eat. They had to work without electricity and sustain adequate communication at all times. The work of nurses during these emergencies reduced the impact of the disaster on the community and decreased morbidity and mortality from communicable diseases. Just as in Galveston in 1900 and Anchorage in 1964, today's disasters witness large numbers of individuals in hospitals and shelters.

Nurses today know that their practice during emergencies is necessary, and it is a practice that they do and do well. They have the knowledge, the skill, and discipline needed to do the work. Disasters, such as the ones discussed in this chapter, demonstrate the need for nurses who are qualified and knowledgeable on how to administer care in states of emergence such as case-finding, referral, advocacy, and ensure that the needs of individuals, families, and the vulnerable are met. As in the past, public health nurses today take charge and apply their leadership skills to facilitate collaborative partnerships with the American Red Cross and numerous other federal, state, and local agencies and organizations in preparation for emergencies, during emergencies, and after emergencies as they collectively engage in evaluation of the emergency response.

Additional Resources

1947 Texas City Explosion Disaster at: http://www.texascity-library.org/disaster/first.php

USGS-1964 Alaska Earthquake and Tsunami at: http://earthquake.usgs.gov/earthquakes/events/alaska1964/

The Yellow Fever Epidemic in Philadelphia 1793 at: http://ocp.hul.harvard.edu/contagion/yellowfever.html

The Johnstown Flood at: https://www.youtube.com/watch?v=WxXGh65IjiY

American Red Cross at: http://www.redcross.org/

References

American National Red Cross. (1947). *A preliminary report on the Texas City explosions.* Texas City file. Rosenberg Library, Galveston, Texas. St. Louis, MO: American National Red Cross, Midwestern Area.

Barry, J. (2005). *The great influenza: The epic story of the deadliest plague in history.* East Rutherford, NJ: Viking Press.

Bartholf, M. (1947). Co-operation. *American Journal of Nursing, 47*(8), 558.

Barton, C. (1900). *To the people of the United States. 1900 Storm online manuscript exhibit* (Red Cross Records, MSS # 05-0007). Retrieved from http://www.gthcenter.org/exhibits/storms/1900/Manuscripts/RecCross_7/index.html

Beltz, A. (1964). Greater Anchorage health district. *Alaska Nurse, XIII*(4), 8.

Benson, R. (1964). Fairbanks reports. *Alaska Nurse, XIII*(4), 11.

Bixel, P. B., & Turner, E. H. (2000). *Galveston and the 1900 storm.* Austin: University of Texas Press.

Blagden, J. D. (2000). Letter to family, September 10, 1900. In C. E. Greene & S. H. Kelly (Eds.), *Through a night of horrors: Voices from the 1900 Galveston storm* (pp. 17–18). College Station: Texas A&M University Press.

Blocker, V., & Blocker, T. G. (1949). The Texas City disaster: A survey of 3,000 casualties. *American Journal of Surgery, LXXVII*(5), 756–771.

Blue, E. (1964). Seward General Hospital. *Alaska Nurse, XIII*(4), 1.

Bonehill, B. A. (1964). Prince William Sound area as seen by a PHN after Alaska's disaster. *Alaska Nurse, XIII*(4), 10.

Boyle, H. (1947, April 18). Monsanto explosion offers foretaste of atom bomb. *The Houston Chronicle*, n.p.

Byerly, C. (2005). *Fever of war: The influenza epidemic in the U.S. Army during World War I.* New York, NY: New York University Press.

Chronicles of the Sisters of Providence. (1964). Seattle, WA: Sisters of Providence Archives.

Crosby, A. (2003). *America's forgotten pandemic: Influenza 1918* (2nd ed.). Boston, MA: Cambridge University Press.

D'Antonio, J., & Whelan, J. (2004). Moments when time stood still: A look at the history of nursing during disasters. *American Journal of Nursing, 104*(11), 66–72.

Dock, L., & Pickett, S. (1922). *History of the American Red Cross.* New York, NY: MacMillan.

Doty, P. M. (1919). A retrospect of the influenza epidemic. *Public Health Nurse, 11*(12), 949–957.

Employee of Texas City café tells of his escape. (1947, April 19). *Informer*, p. 10.

Farley, J. M. (1964, April 26). Alaskan earthquake jolts nurse's schedule. *The Milwaukee Journal*, n.p.

Fayling, L. R. D. (2000). Fear influenza outbreak among sailors may spread. In C. E. Greene & S. H. Kelly (Eds.), *Through a night of horrors: Voices from the 1900 Galveston storm* (p. 91). College Station: Texas A&M University Press.

Fieser, J. (1941). *Report to Mr. Atkinson, January 15, 1941 re: Influenza Epidemic of 1918.* NARA CP Records of the Red Cross, Box 557, 500.2 Influenza.

Fortier, E. J. (1964). *Observations for Sister Philias on Providence Hospital and earthquake.* Seattle, WA: Sisters of Providence Archives.

Geister, J. (1957). The flu epidemic of 1918. *Nursing Outlook, 5*(10), 582–584.

Girardeau, G. (1947). *Annual report, July 1, 1946, to July 1, 1947. Galveston County Chapter.* St. Louis, MO: American National Red Cross.

Givin, L. P. (1948). *Memoir, Texas City disaster.* Austin: University of Texas Medical Branch Library.

Haas, J. E. (1964). Some preliminary observations on the responses of community organizations involved in the emergency period of the Alaskan earthquake. *Disaster Research Center Working Paper #2.* Newark: Disaster Research Center, University of Delaware.

Hilleman, M. R. (2002). Realities and enigmas of human viral influenza: Pathogenesis, epidemiology and control. *Vaccine, 20,* 3068–3087.

Houston Chronicle. (1947, April 21). Retrieved from http://www.redcross.org/services/nursing/0,1082,0_389_,00.html#develope

Johnson, N., & Mueller, J. (2002). Updating the accounts: Global mortality of the 1918–1920 "Spanish" influenza pandemic. *Bulletin of the History of Medicine, 76,* 105–115.

Johnston, M. E. (1947, April 18). Relatives claim dead at morgue. *Houston Post,* p. 20.

Kernodle, P. B. (1949). *The Red Cross nurse in action, 1882–1948.* New York, NY: Harper and Brothers.

Kilpatrick, E. (1919). *Report of the Northwest ARC Division, 1919,* in National Archives Records Administration, College Park (NARACP), 803.11 epidemics, Box 689, folder 1.

Kreps, G. A. (1990). The Federal Emergency Management System in the United States: Past and present. *International Journal of Mass Emergencies and Disasters, 8*(3), 281.

Langston, D. V. (1964, July 27). Report of a hospital in a disaster area. *Journal of the American Medical Association,* 306–307.

Leake, C. D. (October, 1947). *Copy of military medical principles applied to a civilian disaster.* Austin: University of Texas Medical Branch Library.

Many Negroes killed, scores injured in Texas City blast. (1947, April 19). *Informer,* p. 1.

Markel, H., Lipman, H. B., Navarro, J. A., Sloan, A., Michalsen, J. R., Stern, A. M., & Cetron, M. S. (2007). Nonpharmaceutical interventions implemented by U.S. cities during the 1918–1919 influenza pandemic. *Journal of the American Medical Association, 298*(6), 644–653.

McLeod, T. (1948). When disaster strikes. *Hospital Progress, 408,* 411.

Minutaglio, B. (2003). *City on fire: The explosion that devastated a Texas town and ignited a historic legal battle.* New York, NY: HarperCollins.

Molsbee, A. F. (1947). Students give disaster service in Galveston. *American Journal of Nursing, 47*(6), 414.

Moorehead, C. (1998). *Dunant's dream: War, Switzerland, and the history of the Red Cross.* London, UK: HarperCollins.

National Park Service, U.S. Department of Interior. (2006). *Johnstown flood.* Retrieved from http://www.nps.gov/jofl/faqs.htm

Noyes, C. (1918, September 25). *Memo to all division directors.* National Archives Record Administration (NARA). Memo found in CP Box 689 of the influenza epidemic records of 1918, Record Group 803.11.

Office of Public Information, Western Area, American Red Cross. (1964). *Nurses answer call quickly for Alaskan disaster duty.* Anchorage, AK: American Red Cross Office.

Rafferty, J. (1974). *Mercy Hospital, 1947–1972: An historical review.* Pittsburgh, PA: Mercy Hospital.

Rubin, C. B. (Ed.). (2007). *Emergency management: The American experience, 1900–2005.* Fairfax, VA: Public Entity Risk Institute.

Scott, E. (1964). School nurses—Anchorage. *Alaska Nurse, XIII*(4), 6.

Sister Philias. (1964). *Three C's for an operating room in disaster.* Seattle, WA: Sisters of Providence Archives, PMCA, Box 32.

Special Report. (1964). Hospitals and the Alaskan earthquake. *Journal of the American Hospital Association, 38,* 23–24A.

Stephens, H. W. (1993). The Texas City disaster: A re-examination. *Industrial and Environmental Crisis Quarterly, 7*(3), 189–190.

Stephens, H. W. (1997). *The Texas City disaster, 1947.* Austin: University of Texas Press.

1200 Feared dead in Texas blasts. (1947, April 17). *New York Times,* n.p.

U.S. Department of Health and Human Services. (2010). *Healthy People 2020.* Retrieved from http://www.healthypeople.gov/2020/default.aspx

Veenema, T. G. (2007). *Disaster nursing and emergency preparedness for chemical, biological and radiological terrorism and other hazards* (2nd ed.). New York, NY: Springer.

Visiting Nurse Society. (1918). Newspaper clipping from scrapbook. VNS Collection, UPenn CSHN, Barbara Bates Center of the History of Nursing.

Wald, L. D. (1918, December 11). Visiting nursing. Written for the Foreign Bureau. Lillian Wald Papers. Writings & Speeches, Nurses & Nursing II, Reel 25, Box 37, Folder 4, pp. 1–9. New York Public Library, Humanities and Social Sciences Library, Manuscripts and Archives Division, New York, NY.

Wall, B. M. (2008). Healing after disasters in early 20th-century Texas. *Advances in Nursing Science, 31*(3), 211–224. Excerpts reprinted with permission.

Wheaton, E. L. (1948). *Texas City remembers.* San Antonio, TX: Naylor.

For a full suite of assignments and additional learning activities, use the access code located in the front of your book to visit this exclusive website: **http://go.jblearning.com/londrigan**. If you do not have an access code, you can obtain one at the site.

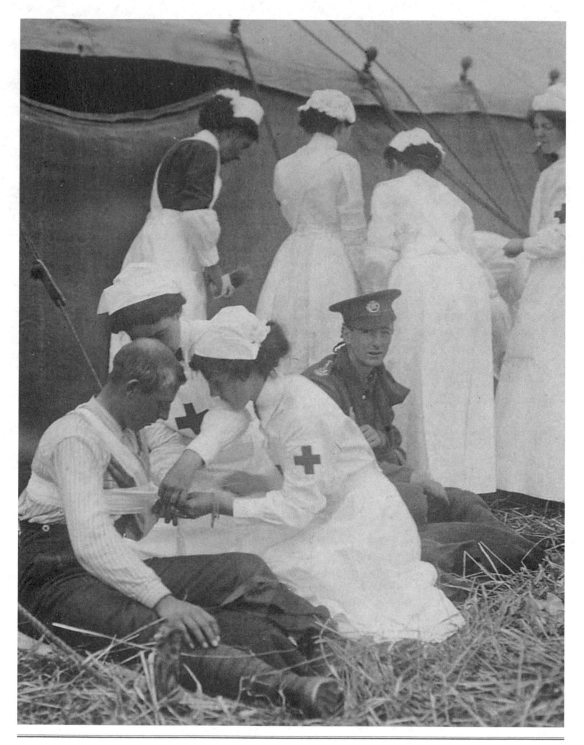

Courtesy of the Keeling Collection, University of Virginia Center for Nursing Historical Inquiry.

CHAPTER 18

Present-Day Disasters and Disaster Management: Social Determinants of Health and Community Collaboration

Sherrie Lee Murray

Humanitarians have always wanted to save the babies for their appeal is irresistible, but at present the importance of saving the babies is also a national concern. Begin early in life to do your share to maintain service for the people. The nurse in her district, whether in town or in country, becomes your representative. (Wald, 1917, p. 4)

LEARNING OBJECTIVES

At the completion of this chapter, the reader will be able to:

- Describe emergency preparedness.
- Reflect on the meaning of emergency preparedness and protecting the public.
- Describe how resiliency of the individual, family, population, and community play a part in recovery and how the burden of reliance is shifting.
- Describe surge capacity as used in disaster preparedness.

KEY TERMS

❏ Preparedness
❏ Resiliency

❏ Surge capacity

Introduction

Knowing history informs nursing practice by helping to gain perspective and learn ways to mitigate future adverse outcomes in an emergency. Past emergencies and the response to those emergencies provide evidence for us on what was effective and what needs to be changed to prevent disasters and to improve response outcomes for individuals, families, populations, and communities, especially for vulnerable populations in the event of a disaster (Mann-Wall & Keeling, 2011; Truglio-Londrigan & Lewenson, 2011). It may also help to diminish the disparities that exist and improve outcomes (Biedrzycki & Koltun, 2012). The preceding two chapters dealt with past epidemics and disasters, providing a foundation on emergency and emergency response. Knowing what has taken place serves to strengthen what is taking place today as we brace for the next hurricane that may strike the coastline of the United States. Retrospective insight can give us the knowledge we need to make the changes that will improve surge capacity within hospitals and facilities as well as increasing resiliency for communities and community members. It is instrumental in allowing us to see the need for community involvement as well the need to address primary health care needs and social determinants within communities to formulate stronger supports necessary to recover (Biedrzycki & Koltun, 2012).

Previously, disaster preparedness had a very narrow focus. Emergency preparedness originates from a military and civil defense perspective of the 1950s in response to nuclear threats during the Cold War. One of the first researchers in disaster planning and management was an Army nurse, Harriet H. Werley (Leifer & Glass, 2008). Even then, Major Werley had a vision that revolved around an interdisciplinary approach to the management of disasters (Leifer & Glass, 2008). She saw the importance of having the nurse involved in emergency management, planning, and research (Leifer & Glass, 2008). The purpose of this chapter is to review the current-day model of emergency management and briefly discuss lessons learned from past emergencies. In addition, this chapter will examine our present emergency management model developed based upon ongoing reflection, with the aim to improve outcomes for communities across the United States.

Disaster and Emergencies

The term *disaster* has been defined as ". . . a sudden, calamitous event that seriously disrupts the functioning of a community or society and causes human, material, and economic or environmental losses that exceed the community's or society's ability to cope using its own resources. Though often caused by nature, disasters can have human origins" (International Federation of Red Cross and Red Crescent Societies, nd, para. 1). The World Health Organization (WHO) as well recognizes that in a disaster there is an upheaval of the functional ability of the society or community, resulting in extensive losses that go beyond the capabilities of the community to manage using its own means (WHO, 2016). Both the WHO as well as the International Federation of Red Cross and the Red Crescent Society go on to describe that although the disaster may be caused by natural means, the impact and the actual failure occurs when the system itself becomes overwhelmed. If the individual, family, population, or community is of poor economic means or they lack the resources to help themselves, the impact of the disaster is often magnified. The social determinants of health, such as poverty, may affect the designation of a catastrophe as stated by the WHO and the Red Cross. The disaster and the corresponding results of the disaster are compounded by the community's inability to cope and limited resources, leading to increased susceptibility furthering the catastrophe (IFRC, 2016). **Figure 18-1** offers an illustration of how the American Red Cross views the role of public health nurses as they implement the intervention wheel while working with communities before, during, and after a disaster.

Federal Emergency Management Agency (FEMA) designates two different types of disasters: an *emergency disaster*, which is managed mainly by the state or tribal government, and a *major disaster*, which is

Figure 18-1 Public Health Interventions & the Red Cross

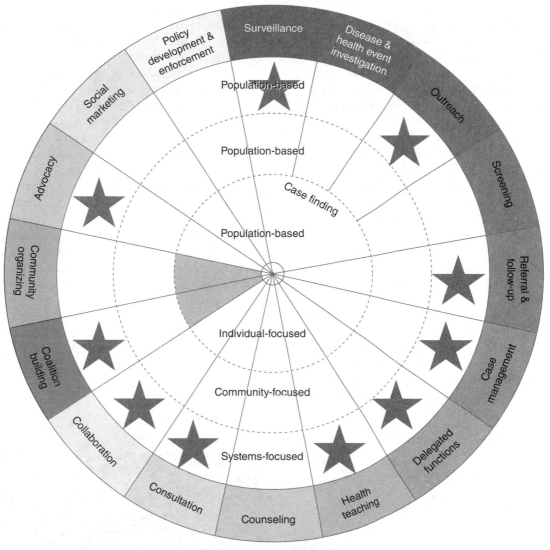

★ Public health interventions & the Red Cross

Modified interventions wheel courtesy of Linda MacIntyre, PhD, RN. Wheel graphic published in Minnesota Department of Health Office of Public Health Practice. (2006). *A collection of "getting behind the wheel" stories*. St. Paul, MN: Author.

primarily the responsibility of the federal government (FEMA, 2016). Based on recommendations from the Institute of Medicine Report (2010), nurses are to be full partners in preparing for and participating in all stages of a disaster. Exploration of the phases of emergency management and the effects of the social determinants of health on the ability to prepare and recover from a catastrophe along with implications for the registered nurse (RN) and the advanced practice registered nurse (APRN) is important to consider.

Four Phases of Emergency Management

The four phases of emergency management portray a systematic process developed to minimize the impact of the emergency by carrying out the actions and the processes of mitigation, **preparedness**, response, and recovery (see Figure 18-2).

Jackman and Beruvides (2013) discuss hazard *mitigation* in the United States. In reality, risk mitigation occurs within all phases of administration and planning. Mitigation includes those acts designed to prevent future emergencies as well as the alleviation and easing of an issue that may occur because of an emergency and to produce improved outcomes for the individuals, families, populations, or community involved. Mitigation includes possible legislation, improved reconstruction, and regular vulnerability risk assessment (Jackman & Beruvides, 2013). Hazard Mitigation Plans (HMPs) are required at all levels of government and all phases of emergency management. HMPs entail an explicit risk assessment. The purpose is to know and recognize the community and population vulnerabilities to improve outcomes for those most who most closely will be affected by the disaster. In evaluating the threats and resources

available to the individuals, families, populations, and communities, the governmental agencies, as well as the community members, can better prepare for the disaster. The rationale is, with planning and intervention, there is alleviation of long-term and more dire effects of a catastrophic event.

In reality, mitigation cannot prevent or eliminate all risks, and, therefore, *preparation* is a critical phase in the disaster management. This means being prepared for any event to take place at any time so that prevention reduces the loss of life and property. According to Jakeway, LaRosa, Cary, and Schoenfisch (2008), preparedness is the ability to "assure capacity to effectively respond to disasters and emergencies" (p. 355). Strategies are developed to effectively ensure and assure this capacity. For example, a public health nurse who works in a community close to the sea and is aware of the vulnerable population of older adults living in marginal housing will work with the community (key informants and organizations) to develop educational programs and establish a continual review process of evacuation routes so that in the event of a natural disaster there will be an effective and efficient response to meet the needs of this vulnerable population.

Response is the ability of healthcare personnel to enter into the community and provide the services

In the event of an emergency in process, the response is triggered.

Figure 18-2 Phases of Disaster Management Model

The four phases of emergency management

Mitigation

Preparedness

Response

Recovery

Reproduced from FEMA. (n.d.). Emergency management in the United States. Retrieved from https://training.fema.gov /emiweb/downloads/is111_unit%204.pdf

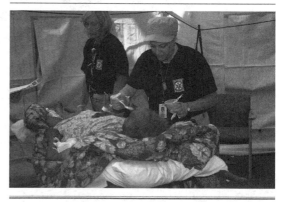

Photo by Win Henderson/FEMA

that are necessary to protect lives and property. The response also moves beyond the immediately felt emergency and includes the needed services after the emergency has occurred (Burkle, 2006; Jakeway et al., 2008). In the example provided above, the public health nurse will be in the affected community during the emergency and works with older adults who may have been evacuated from their homes, providing the physical, emotional, psychological, and crisis care as needed.

Recovery encompasses that which takes place to recover from the event and restore the community so that systems function (Jakeway et al., 2008). For the public health nurses working with older adults in a seaside community, recovery may mean working together to ensure that the safety of the environment and housing have been addressed before the older adults returning to their homes. This may encompass ensuring that Meals on Wheels services are operational so that older adults who rely on these meals are, in fact, available and operational. These actions involve community collaboration beyond just working with professional groups and may require intersectorial collaboration.

These four phases frequently overlap with public health providers, the nurse being one, who collaborate and continually evaluate and reflect upon the emergency management phases, identifying what worked, what did not work, and why it did not

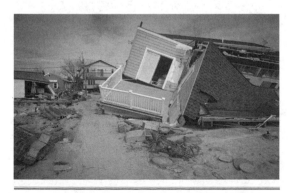

Courtesy of FEMA. U.S. Navy photo by Chief Mass Communication Specialist Ryan J. Courtade/Released

work. Throughout the questioning, collaboration with the community is key as its input is valuable in the development and design of any future disaster management phases.

Public Health Nursing and Emergency Management

It is important that the APRN and the RN be involved in all phases of emergency management. Public health nurses (PHN) know the community in which they work and can supply information that is accurate and pertinent regarding the population they serve. They can assist with the risk assessment and provide information regarding vulnerable populations, including the elderly or physically challenged. The PHN will know the community leaders both informal and formal, police officers, and firefighters and as a result be able to serve as a facilitator between and among all of these individuals and community agencies. Participating in this way, the PHN can contribute to mitigating the adverse outcomes and improving resource sharing. The PHN works to protect the public by being a leader and a dynamic participant in the community while collaborating with the community. The PHN provides care that protects and serves the public by providing physical, psychological, emotional, spiritual, and social support (Londrigan, 2012). More specifically, PHNs are able to carry out best practices that are population based such as "... rapid needs assessments of communities impacted by the incident, population-based triage, mass dispensing of preventive or curative therapies, community education, providing care or managing shelters for displaced populations, and, of course, provision of ongoing continuity in essential public health services" (Association of Public Health Nurses Public Health Preparedness Committee, 2013, p. 4). Ultimately, PHNs work within their communities to improve outcomes through better communication facilitated by collaborative work on issues and by strategizing with the community on the process of implementing population-based best practices. The PHN encourages information sharing and communication between community members. Communication and the exchange of information and resources is an essential goal of emergency management and can help to improve outcomes. This is clearly identified in the position paper *The Role of the Public Health Nurses in Disaster Preparedness, Response, and Recovery* which states, "No single discipline, agency, organization, or jurisdiction can or should claim sole responsibility for the complex array of challenges associated with the disaster, whether caused by nature, humans, or some combination of both" (Association of Public Health Nurses Public Health Preparedness Committee, 2013, p. 4).

During the management of the actual disaster, the RN and APRN schooled in disaster management should have the ability to manage mass casualties. Managing mass casualties includes the capacity to recognize victims' injuries and triage according to the resources available to maximize the capacity for victim recovery and minimize poor outcomes for the individual, their family, the population being affected by the disaster, and communities. Prompt adaptive care saves lives, decreases further injuries, and improves overall recovery (American Nurses Association [ANA], 2016). The ANA stresses the importance of the RN being prepared to respond to a disaster and legal and ethical issues in managing a disaster. There is also the matter of a nurse's preparation and knowledge of emergency preparedness. There is an essential difference between the premise of battlefield medicine and the underlying ethics that the RN must deal with making decisions about how to triage patients and resources. The ANA recommends that the ethical and legal standards of care be maintained in responding to a disaster, suggesting that the federal government protect healthcare providers and other medical team members when responding to a crisis (ANA, 2016). The ANA is part of the workgroup for the Institute of Medicine's (IOM) *Report on Guidance for Establishing Crisis Standards of Care for Use in Disaster Situations* (2009). The guidelines discuss the ethical and legal issues, the significance of standards of care, and the importance of community engagement. The guidelines also stress the importance of a trained and ready medical workforce (IOM, 2009). The ANA has links to websites for RNs to receive training for disaster preparedness. It also provides links for individuals wanting to volunteer and be part of a larger effort. It is the obligation of every healthcare provider to have a working knowledge of the phases of emergency management and possess the knowledge of how to engage before and when a disaster occurs in order to protect and serve the public adequately.

Despite work in the areas of disaster response and education, policies, procedures, and protocols that have been put into place to prepare nurses for these emergencies, efforts have been "episodic and difficult to sustain" (Veenema et al., 2016, p. 11). To address issues in preparing a strong nursing workforce, these authors identified recommendations in nursing practice, education, policy, and research. For example, nurse educators should be examining ways in which they can include disaster management within their courses, as well as develop nursing competencies during disasters that can be included in the American Association of Colleges of Nursing (AACN) *Essentials of Nursing* and the National League for Nursing (NLN) *Guidelines for Nursing*. Further recommendations address volunteerism, interprofessional and intersectorial community-based collaboration (Veenema et al., 2016).

Protecting the Public in a Disaster

In October 2011, the Presidential Policy Directive 8 (PPD-8) was released. The PPD-8 is the first document issued that addresses preparedness goals for the United States (Homeland Security Website, 2015). The directives propelled by recent outcomes seen in the disasters of Hurricanes Katrina and Rita have changed the perspective in emergency preparedness.

The PPD-8 goals along with the shifts in FEMA principles require a broader, community-based approach (Biedrzycki & Kolton, 2012). If the community is not involved, it weakens the preparedness response, or it may make it ineffectual. The plan recommended by the PPD-8 and FEMA recognizes the importance of community involvement. The Centers for Disease Control and Prevention (CDC) in its Strategic Plan (2011) also supports the PPD-8 goals for all stakeholders to be involved in planning, implementation, and evaluation. Efforts are underway to change the view of what preparation means within a cultural context. If the population at risk is prepared and has participated in the preparation for the emergency, it will improve recovery from the event (Lippmann, 2011). Emergency preparedness is the sum of behaviors involved in how an individual, community, or population responds to a disaster, whether it is manmade or natural (Lippmann, 2011, p. 71). Being prepared for the event of a catastrophe is inextricably linked to an individual's interpretation and worldview of disasters. Response and preparation to a disaster are determined within a social context, and preparedness needs to occur within a context that is understandable to the culture of the individuals affected by the emergency.

To help move the locus of control for disaster preparedness, New York State's (NYS) Office of Public Health has created pods as a means of shifting emergency preparedness responsibilities to the communities. This state office has guidance for municipalities on organizing and creating pods for their communities as well as how to provide training for volunteers (University at Albany School of Public Health, 2016). Pods have as their members registered nurses, pharmacists, physicians, and community leaders who are engaged at a local level, recognize the needs of the neighborhood, and can identify needed resources to prepare better for future catastrophes. The teams can receive training through the ANA and FEMA in disaster preparedness programs that are free to the public. The teams also consist of volunteers and local government officials. These groups and

their members may not be incident commanders at the time of the crisis, but they can better inform the commander to assist with preparations, mitigation, response, and recovery. The teams also have protocols to help with surge capacity for hospitals and facilities within their pods. They allow pharmacists to dispense medications in times of crisis and have registered nurses provide triage as well as emergency care. The NYS Department of Disaster Preparedness has an HMP for each locality. The plans are tracked by the state to determine whether the project is ready for implementation within the county or city. These programs help shift the level of responsibility for emergency planning from the federal and state levels to a local level with state and federal support.

Preparedness from a Social and Cultural Context

Healthy People 2020 examines the social determinants of health that may affect an individual, family, population, or community's ability to recover from an emergency. The lack of resources, understanding the availability of services in a disaster, living in areas more vulnerable, and possible mistrust of government agencies may all influence the community's resilience. Individuals in organizations working with these communities need to be culturally competent and socially aware when dealing with vulnerable populations. Poverty as a social determinant affects the ability of a community to recover from a disaster event. Biedrycki and Koltun (2012) discuss the importance of identifying the social determinants of health for a community to better formulate the support needed to recover from a disaster. The failure to integrate these known deficiencies have led to poor outcomes for the poorest and most vulnerable. Social determinants to be considered that contribute to poverty include social attitudes and norms, quality of schools and education, social disorder, crime, and violence, in addition to access to transportation and emerging technologies (Biedrzycki & Koltun, 2012; *Healthy People 2020*, nd.). Another issue to be considered in this context is how the community views a natural disaster. It is important to address the cultural context and the issues related not only to preparedness but also to how disasters are perceived by the affected community. For some Hispanic and Native American cultures, there is a belief that natural disasters are acts of God, and they may not want to prepare for the catastrophe. Included in the cultural aspects are the language barriers specific to each population. This can affect the community's ability to seek help when needed. All these factors affect the community's ability and willingness to respond to a catastrophe. Considering all socioeconomic and cultural factors is imperative if disaster management strategies and processes are to facilitate resiliency.

Resilience

Resilience is the ability of an organization, city, or town to recover and ease the effects of a disaster or event, with the least amount of disruption and within the shortest amount of time (Hemond & Robert, 2012). Resilience is a relatively new concept and is the future of what preparedness will entail. Resilience is the adaptability of an organization (Hemond & Robert, 2012). Appropriate response and planning will both save lives and cost during and after the event. In the conceptualization of resilience, there are physical, behavioral, and social aspects (Paton & Johnston, 2006). The physical aspects involve the actual place or the environment in which the individual, family, and population exist—the community. Behavioral aspects include the interaction of the leadership, the organization, and the people within and around the community that can help to increase resilience (Nirupama, Popper, & Quirke, 2015). The social aspects include the social determinants of health previously discussed. Resilience helps build personal and community preparedness through community commitment, coordination of services, and training for all partners from individual,

local, state, and federal agencies (Plough et al., 2013). Resiliency is also the community's ability to recover once the event has occurred. This concept broadens the approach and invites new stakeholders to the table. The inclusion of the community members in emergency management can improve preparedness and increase resilience. The issues of failure to be aware of and integrated into these known physical, behavioral, and social aspects may facilitate deficiencies in disaster management, leading to poor outcomes for the poorest and most vulnerable populations (Biedrycki & Koltun, 2012). You cannot discuss resilience without including the social determinants of health that affect the outcome and may delay recovery.

One method to increase resilience is through building coalitions (Truglio-Londrigan, 2017; Walsh, Craddock, Gully, Straus-Riggs, & Schor, 2015). Alliances provide the opportunity for healthcare institutions and workforce to come together with public and private sector agencies to develop a plan that will assist with disaster preparedness response. If all stakeholders are at the table, there is a better buy-in from individuals within the community (Truglio-Londrigan, 2017; Walsh et al., 2015). Better communication, sharing education, and training, as well as staff and resources will help build trust among Health Care Coalition (HCC) members. The value of these organizations lies in their ability to help identify and respond to the poor health outcomes among members of the communities in a catastrophe. Resources such as access to services and health care should be made available for those of more impoverished circumstances; establishing resources will lead to a quicker recovery time and increased resilience. A decrease in postdisaster needs will lead to improved financial outcomes. Access to services pre-event will reduce aftermath morbidity and mortality. Examining the vulnerabilities of the environment in which individuals live is important in determining the people and the community's ability to recover and the potential for resilience (Nirupama, Popper, & Quirke, 2015).

Individual resilience is also necessary to promote improved outcomes and help with the stressors of dealing with a catastrophic event. As studied by the Army, resilience is of particular importance for medical staff because of the operating tempo that has occurred since 9/11 with Operation Iraqi Freedom (OIF) and Operation Enduring Freedom (OEF). Fatigue after exposure to repeated traumatic events can lead to compromise of the individual's emotional, physical, cognitive, and social well-being (Adams, Camarillo, Lewis, & McNish, 2010). Adams et al. (2010) discusses how there are key components to maintaining a healthy level of resilience. An individual must be able to manage their health, problem solve, increase their self-esteem, and find positive outcomes in difficult situations to maintain their ability to cope and their level of resilience (Adams et al., 2010). Offering classes that increase the mind–body connection such as guided imagery, breathing techniques, and journaling are all methods that help to maintain the medical provider's resilience when dealing with stressful situations. Although many of these exercises were found to be beneficial in the population studied, it would be difficult to generalize to the population as a whole (Adams et al., 2010). If simple needs such as food and water are not met, it will be difficult for the individual to focus on the process of meditation or any other mind–body experience. This information may be useful, however, when working with other medical personnel who are dealing with tragic events such as mass shootings.

Surge Capacity

In preparation for a catastrophe, surge capacity is anticipated within the hospital setting. Emergency departments have plans in place to manage disasters when they occur. *Medical Surge Capacity* (MSC) is the evaluation and care of a significantly increased number of patients beyond the typical capability of the establishment (ANA Website, 2012). The ANA and the Agency for Healthcare Research and Quality (AHRQ) recommend that hospital facilities use the resources available to them before sending patients to other facilities. Participating in exercises with response

teams of civilian and governmental agencies as well as community members helps to anticipate surge capacity as well as improving response times for the population at risk. Evidence supports emergency exercises improve outcomes during the actual event (Kellman et al., 2011). Having individuals as patients during these exercise helps with the anticipatory needs and makes hospitals and facilities with decontamination zones aware of the materials needed and how long they could sustain the care related to these occurrences. Hospitals must be mindful of the need for more bed availability. Facilities should have a plan in place to increase the number of providers involved and a call system in place to aid in response times. The exercises are timed to measure response. Tabletop exercises can also be done so that there is less expenditure of resources and an ability to determine the impact that surge capacity has to save lives.

Part of the anticipatory need is knowing the vulnerable members of the community. Individual leaders and community members need to participate in these exercises because of their intimate knowledge of the community. If there are vulnerable elderly persons who may not be able to mobilize as efficiently, the community members would be the only ones mindful of these issues. Awareness of the language barriers and cultural background will improve the community's response time and anticipatory planning. Preplanning, exercising, and community involvement are all elements affecting resiliency and surge capacity. All of these circumstances influence the ability of individuals and communities to not only be ready for the disaster but also reduce recovery time.

Hurricane Irene: Resilience in a Vermont Community—Pittsfield, Vermont— Case Study 1

On August 28, 2011, Hurricane Irene struck Vermont and its infrastructure hard. Vermont is a state of many small roads and isolated small towns that are near creeks and small rivers. These places are nestled in the Green Mountains, and all Vermonters are proud of their independent, small town atmosphere. Hurricane Irene hit the small Vermont town of Pittsfield. Pittsfield, Vermont, is a tiny town of 546 people. The township was affected by the rains of Irene on August 28th, and it washed out the only bridge in this municipality. In just 12 minutes, the water level rose two feet. Entire houses were swept away in a matter of minutes. Individuals were left with only the clothes on their back and their animals. On the day of the storm, shortly before the bridge washed away, the power went out. Pittsfield was not only cut off physically from the rest of the state, but they were also cut off from communication. Pittsfield had their emergency management coordinator, who had thought he would never have to deal with such devastation, but within hours of Irene passing, he had coordinated a town hall meeting to discuss the damages and the need to pool resources. The village established a medical clinic with personnel from the village to help sustain them while they waited for assistance. Supplies from the local store were used to feed members of the community together on the town green.

For mitigation of the disaster before the hurricane, the village had prepared by having the highway superintendent dig trenches alongside the road to help divert the water, but there was too much, and it came too quickly (Greenhill, 2011). By the second day after the disaster, the National Guard was able to use helicopters to make drops of food and water. The community members assisted their neighbors. They loaded their all-terrain vehicles (ATVs) with provisions and brought them to the remote regions where individuals were isolated (Greenhill, 2011).

Analysis of the Community of Pittsfield from a Resiliency and Social Determinants Perspective

The community of Pittsfield had resiliency and the ability to respond and recover from the disaster when it occurred. Although there was a large degree of devastation, the community was able to work together to improve outcomes and alleviate the problems they faced. Looking at this population from the perspective of their social determinants, it may help to explain their level of resilience. The ability of the townspeople to coordinate efforts before and during the storm as well as after served to decrease the recovery time and help sustain them while waiting for more definitive care. Social determinants may also have influenced the ability of the small hamlet to recover. The average income for the town was over $50,000 for a family of four. An average income across the United States is $50,000, but it is well above the poverty level for a family of four. According to the Department of Health and Human Services, the federal poverty level for 2016 for a family of four was $24,300. Over 80% of the population of Pittsfield has a high school education or better, and of those, over 40% have a bachelor's degree. Over 97% of the population is white, and less than 2% of the population is unemployed (Onboard Informatics, Citi-Data.Com, 2016). The individuals of this town had resources, a stronger healthier economy, and a livelihood before the disaster; therefore, they were able to recover and display a high degree of resilience. They were able to mitigate circumstances that were barriers to recovery by using resources available to them. This town is an example of how using resilience is critical for disaster preparedness and helps on the road to recovery.

Violence and Mass Shootings—A Disaster of Our Own Making—Case Study 2

According to the Federal Bureau of Investigation (FBI), statistics on homicides in the United States have continued to decline; however, mass shootings have risen sharply since 2007. From 2000 to 2006, the average mass shooting crime rate was 6.4%, and from 2007 to 2014, it has increased to 16.4% (FBI Crime Statistics Website, 2014). According to the most recent data on mass casualties and active shooter incidents from the FBI, there were 160 incidents of active shooters and 1,063 deaths or injuries occurred from 2000 to 2013 (FBI Crime Statistics, 2014). Not included in these statistics is one of the most recent mass shootings on U.S. soil in Florida in June 2016. A gunman opened fire on a gay Orlando nightclub, killing 49 people. Mass shootings are an increasing public health issue. Also not included in these statistics is the shooting of nine individuals in the Emanuel African Methodist Episcopal Church in Charleston, the San Bernardino shooting of 14 people in 2015, or the military shooting in Tennessee in 2015 of five people. The victims are men, women, and children of all races and ages. The distinction for some is that they are hate crimes, such as the most recent in Orlando and the church killings. Some are inspired by the Jihadist movement, such as the victims in the San Bernardino attack. Violence is also directed by white extremist groups, such as the attack on the Sikh temple in 2012 in which six people were killed. These shootings are described by some as a manmade epidemic and need to be addressed from a social, moral, and medical point of view. Regardless of the motive behind the shootings, medical personnel as well as communities need to be ready to respond to these emergencies (New America International Securities, nd).

These events require preparation similar to disaster management response. If there is a warning of an event, or if there is intelligence that alerts of a mass shooting, agencies need to do credible threat assessments (Vernon, 2010). Many times there is no warning, and the incidents vary based on the shooter's agenda. Although there has been much discussion about the failure of the mental health system, studies have shown that less than 5% of shootings between 2000 and 2010 were perpetrated by persons with mental illness (Metzl & Macleish, 2015). Although much of gun violence is said to relate to the mentally ill, this has not been supported by the evidence. There are cases related to the mass shooting, however, such as the Newtown shooting, that supports the theory of failure of the mental health system. The shooter was diagnosed posthumously as having schizophrenia.

As with any disaster, there needs to be discussion about mitigation of these mass shootings and pre-incident planning. Law enforcement trains and supports rapid deployment teams. They have animals that are trained to find wounded under rubble. College campuses and military facilities now demand that their security teams take active shooter training. First responders need to be prepared to handle and respond to the trauma they may be faced with at the scene. Facing the trauma at the incident may mean developing not only the medical skills but building individual resilience to deal with the aftermath of these traumatic event. Hospitals as well as fire departments and emergency medical system (EMS) have to have deployment and surge capacity plans in place for mass casualty management. These agencies must have training opportunities together, and some of these exercises can be a simulations. Incident command centers (ICC) need to be set up, usually outside or near the mass shooting. The incident commander (IC) should be someone with intimate knowledge of the area and the agencies and community involved. Hospitals need to have trauma-trained personnel. Having APRNs and RNs with emergency management and leadership skills will be critical in decreasing morbidity and mortality during very stressful conditions.

The IOM (2013) in its report on firearms and violence recognizes that a public health approach may help in addressing the issue of gun violence from a prevention point of view (IOM Report, 2013). The IOM report states that firearm violence should be put in a public health context and thought of as a contagion (IOM, 2013, p. 16). The significance of the morbidity and the mortality makes it a serious population-based public health problem.

Emergency preparedness is an expanding field in public health. It has become necessary to prepare ahead for the changes that are occurring in our climate as well as our uncertain social environment. The cycle for disaster management is constant and overlapping. Mitigation is an important part of the cycle, and it overlaps the other parts of the cycle of readiness. It is important to decrease the time to recovery by increasing individual and community resilience. Improving outcomes can be accomplished through addressing and mitigating the social determinants of health in the communities. As the largest number of healthcare providers, nursing stands at the forefront as leaders to improve outcomes for communities during and after disasters, whether manmade or natural.

Conclusion

The cycle of disaster management is ongoing, and the steps overlap. Mitigation is intermittent within the cycle and occurs at all steps within the cycle. The focus is changing from disaster preparedness to an emphasis on resilience. Economic losses and loss of life can be diminished by developing systems that address the social determinants of health before the catastrophe. Emergency management will involve all stakeholders and integrate knowledge regarding the culture of the unique groups to create successful plans (Lippmann, 2011). The IOM Report on the *Future of Nursing* (2010) emphasizes that nurses need to practice to the full extent of their education and licensure. Nurses are the largest workforce in the United States, and hence the role of the RN, PHN, and APRN is vital to preparing for and mitigating the effects of a disaster (Spain, Clements, DeRanieri, & Holt, 2012). All nurses can be an educational resource for the community, to educate them on increasing their individual preparedness. The PHN is population based and can take a leadership role, assess the needs of the community, and facilitate communication between agencies. Many times they are the respected healthcare provider and can be approached by different members of the community. The role of APRN, as leader and collaborator during a disaster, supports this recommendation. All nurses need to make the public aware of how to manage in the wake of a natural disaster or disease outbreak. All nurses must be aware of the sanitation conditions and the latest evidence-based practice (EBP) to provide appropriate care to the people within the communities. The APRN and RN working within hospitals need to keep their critical care skills up to date to provide the most effective care possible during a disaster. Nurses must stand willing to participate in teams and provide care wherever needed at the time of the disaster, whether it is manmade or natural. They need to take part in exercises to determine areas of weakness and be the voice of those who may not have a voice within the communities in which they live and work.

Additional Resources

Emergency Nurse Association at: https://www.ena.org/practice-research/Practice/Safety/Emergency Prepared/Pages/FederalLinks.aspx

FEMA—National Response Framework at: https://www.fema.gov/media-library/assets/documents/32230?id=7371

FEMA Emergency Management at: http://www.fema.gov/training

International Federation of Red Cross and Red Crescent Society at: http://www.ifrc.org/en/what-we-do /disaster-management/about-disasters/what-is-a-disaster/

Public Health Foundation at: http://www.phf.org/programs/TRAIN/Pages/default.aspx

CDC Office of Public Health Preparedness Response at: http://www.cdc.gov/phpr/perlc.htm

American Red Cross at: http://www.redcross.org/what-we-do/international-services/disaster-preparedness

ASPCA Disaster Preparedness at: http://www.aspca.org/pet-care/general-pet-care/disaster-preparedness

National Center for Disaster Preparedness at: http://ncdp.columbia.edu/

Ready—Prepare, Plan, Stay Informed at: https://www.ready.gov/

DERA—The International Association for Preparedness and Response at: http://www.disasters.org/

ANA Disaster Preparedness Response at: http://www.nursingworld.org/disasterpreparedness

Healthy People 2020 Disaster Preparedness at: https://www.healthypeople.gov/2020/topics-objectives /topic/preparedness.FBI Active

Shooter Incidents at: https://www.fbi.gov/news/stories/fbi-releases-study-on-active-shooter-incidents

APA Report on Gun Violence in America at: http://www.apa.org/pubs/info/reports/gun-violence-report.pdf

CDC Emergency Preparedness and Response at: https://emergency.cdc.gov/

References

Adams, S., Camarillo, C., Lewis, S., & McNish, N. (2010). Resiliency training for medical professionals. *U.S. Army Medical Department Journal, 48.*

American Nurses Association. (2016). *Disaster preparedness and response.* Retrieved from http://www.nursingworld.org/MainMenuCategories /WorkplaceSafety/DPR

American Psychiatric Association (2013). *Report on gun violence in America.* Retrieved from http://www .apa.org/pubs/info/reports/gun-violence-report.pdf

Association of Public Health Nurses/Public Health Preparedness Committee. (2013). *The role of the public health nurse in disaster preparedness, response, and recovery: A position paper.* Retrieved from www.achne.org/files/public/APHN_RoleOf PHNinDisasterPRR_FINALJan14.pdf

Biedrzycki, P. A., & Koltun, R. (2012). Integration of social determinants of community preparedness and resiliency in the 21st-century emergency management planning. *Homeland Security Affairs, 8*(14), 1–5.

Burkle, F. M. (2006). Population-based triage management in response to surge capacity requirements during a large-scale bioevent disaster. *Academic Emergency Medicine, 13,* 1118–1129.

Centers for Disease Control and Prevention. (2011). *A national strategic plan for public health preparedness.* Retrieved from http://www.upmc-cbn.org /report_archive/pdfs/CDC-Natl-Strategic-Plan.pdf

Danna, D., & Bennett, M. (2013). Providing culturally competent care during disasters: Strategies for nurses. *The Journal of Continuing Education in Nursing, 44*(4), 151–152. doi:http://dx.doi.org /10.3928/00220124-20130327-13

DeLa'O, C. M., Kashuk, J., Rodriguez, A., Zipf, J., & Dumire, R. D. (2014). The geriatric trauma institute: Reducing the increasing burden of senior trauma care. *The American Journal of Surgery, 208*(6), 988–994. doi:http://dx.doi.org/10.1016/ j.amjsurg.2014.08.00

Department of Homeland Security. (2015). *Presidential Policy Directive/PPD-8: National Preparedness.* Retrieved from https://www.dhs.gov/presidential -policy-directive-8-national-preparedness

Federal Bureau of Investigation. (2014). *Active shooter incidents.* Retrieved from https://www .fbi.gov/news/stories/fbi-releases-study-on -active-shooter-incidents

Federal Emergency Management Agency. (2016). *The disaster declaration process.* Retrieved from https://www.fema.gov/disaster-declaration-process

Greenhill, J. (2011). *National Guard helps Vermont recover after hurricane.* Lanham, MD: Federal Information & News Dispatch, Inc. Retrieved from http://library .sage.edu:2048/login?url=http://search.proquest .com/docview/7332?accountid=13645

Healthy People 2020. (nd.) *Disaster Preparedness.* Retrieved from https://www.healthypeople .gov/2020/topics-objectives/topic/preparedness

Hémond, Y., & Robert, B. (2012). Preparedness: The state of the art and future prospects. *Disaster Prevention and Management: An International Journal, 21*(4), 404–417. doi:10.1108/09653561211256125

International Federation of Red Cross and Red Crescent Societies. (2015). *What is a disaster?* Retrieved from http://www.ifrc.org/en/what -we-do/disaster-management/about-disasters /what-is-a-disaster/

Institute of Medicine. (2009). *Report on guidance for establishing crisis standards of care for use in disaster situations*. Washington, *DC*: The National Academy Press.

Institute of Medicine. (2010). *The future of nursing leading the change advancing health*. Washington, DC: The National Academy Press.

Institute of Medicine & National Research Council. (2013). *Priorities for research to reduce the threat of firearm related violence*. Washington, DC: The National Academies Press.

Jakeway, C., LaRosa, G., Cary, A., & Schoenfisch, S. (2008). The role of the public health nurses in emergency preparedness and response: A position paper of the Association of State and Territorial Directors of Nursing. *Public Health Nursing, 25*(4), 353–361.

Jackman, A. M., & Beruvides, M. G. (2013). Approaches to disaster management–examining the implications of hazards, emergencies, and disasters. In J. Tiefenbacher (Ed.), *Hazard mitigation planning in the United States: historical perspectives, cultural influences, and current challenges* (pp. 55–79). Zagreb, Croatia: INTECH Publishing. doi:10.5772/54209

Leifer, S. L., & Glass, L. K. (2008). Planning for mass disaster in the 1950s. *Nursing Research, 57*(4), 237–244.

Lippmann, A. L. (2011). Disaster preparedness in vulnerable communities. *International Law and Policy Review 1*(1), 69–96.

Londrigan, M. (2012, January). Protecting the public nursing call to action. In S. Freidman (President), *Summit on Resilience, Securing our Future through Public-Private Partnerships*. Summit conducted at a meeting at Pace University, New York, NY.

Mann Wall, B., & Keeling, A. (2011). Historical highlights in disaster nursing. In M. Truglio-Londrigan & S. B. Lewenson (Eds.), *Public health nursing: Practicing population based care* (pp. 353–367). Burlington, MA: Jones & Bartlett Learning.

Maxwell, C., Miller, R. S., Dietrich, M. S., Mion, L. C., & Minnick, A. (2015). The aging of America: A comprehensive look at over 25,000 geriatric trauma admissions to U.S. hospitals. *The American Surgeon, 81*(6), 630–636. Retrieved from http://library.sage.edu:2048/login?url=http://search.proquest.com/docview/1692920025?accountid=13645

Metzl, J. M., & MacLeish, K. T. (2015). Mental illness, mass shootings, and the politics of American firearms. *American journal of public health, 105*(2), 240. Retrieved from http://library.sage.edu:2048/login?url=http://search.proquest.com/docview/1646330605?accountid=13645

New America International Securities. (n.d.). *Deadly attacks since 911*. Retrieved from http://securitydata.newamerica.net/extremists/deadly-attacks.html

New York State Homeland Security and Emergency Services. (2014). *Disaster recovery hazard mitigation planning*. Retrieved from http://www.dhses.ny.gov/recovery/mitigation/planning.cfm

Nirupama, N., Popper, T., & Quirke, A. (2015). Role of social resilience in mitigating disasters. *International Journal of Disaster Resilience in the Built Environment, 6*(3), 363.

Office of Disease Prevention and Health Promotion. (2014). Healthy People 2020. *Social Determinants of Health*. Retrieved from: https://www.healthypeople.gov/2020/topics-objectives/topic/social-determinants-of-health

Onboard Informatics, Citi-Data.com. (2016). *Pittsfield, Vermont*. Retrieved from http://www.city-data.com/city//Pittsfield-Vermont.html

Plough, A., Fielding, J. E., Chandra, A., Williams, M., Eisenman, D., Wells, K. B., . . . Magana, A. (2013). Building community disaster resilience: perspectives from a large urban county department of public health. *American Journal of Public Health, 103*(7), 1190–1197. Retrieved from http://search.proquest.com/docview/1399923993?accountid=13645

Spain, K. M., Clements, P. T., DeRanieri, J. T., & Holt, K. (2012). When disaster happens: Emergency preparedness for nurse practitioners. *The Journal for Nurse Practitioners, 8*(1), 38–44. doi:http://dx.doi.org/10.1016/j.nurpra.2011.07.024

Truglio-Londrigan, M., & Lewenson, S. B. (2011). What is public health and public health Nursing. In M. Truglio-Londrigan & S. B. Lewenson (Eds.), *Public health nursing: Practicing population based care* (pp. 1–19). Burlington, MA: Jones & Bartlett Learning.

Truglio-Londrigan, M. (2017). Coalitions, partnerships, and shared decision-making: A primary health care perspective. In S. B. Lewenson & M. Truglio-Londrigan (Eds.), *Practicing primary health care in nursing: Caring for populations* (pp. 89–108). Burlington, MA: Jones & Bartlett Learning.

U.S. Department of Health and Human Services. (2016). *Federal Poverty Guidelines for 2016.* Retrieved from http://adsd.nv.gov/uploaded Files/agingnvgov/content/Programs/Grant /fedpoverty.pdf

University of Albany School of Public Health. (2016). *New York State Department of Health POD training.* Retrieved from http://www.albany.edu/sph/22536 .php

Veenema, T. G., Griffin, A., Gable, A. R., MacIntyre, L., Simons, N., Couig, M. P., . . . Larson, E. (2016). Nurses as leaders in disaster preparedness and response—A call to action. *Journal of Nursing Scholarship, 48*(2), 1–14.

Vernon, A. (2010). Mass-shooting incidents: Planning and response. *Fire Engineering, 163*(9), Special section p. 14.

Wald, L. D. (1917). The visiting nurse in public health work. Speech delivered at the Chapter for Red Cross Junior League Board. Lillian Wald Papers. Writings & Speeches, Nurses & Nursing, Reel 25, Box 37, Folder 3, pp. 1–4. New York Public Library, Humanities and Social Sciences Library, Manuscripts and Archives Division, New York, NY.

Walsh, L., Craddock, H., Gulley, K., Strauss-Riggs, K., & Schor, K. W. (2015). Building health care system capacity to respond to disasters: Successes and challenges of disaster preparedness health care coalitions. *Prehospital Disaster Medicine, 30*(2), 112–122. doi:10.1017/s1049023X14001459

World Health Organization. (2016). *Humanitarian health actions definitions: Emergencies.* Retrieved from http://www.who.int/hac/about/definitions/en/

For a full suite of assignments and additional learning activities, use the access code located in the front of your book to visit this exclusive website: **http://go.jblearning.com/londrigan.** If you do not have an access code, you can obtain one at the site.

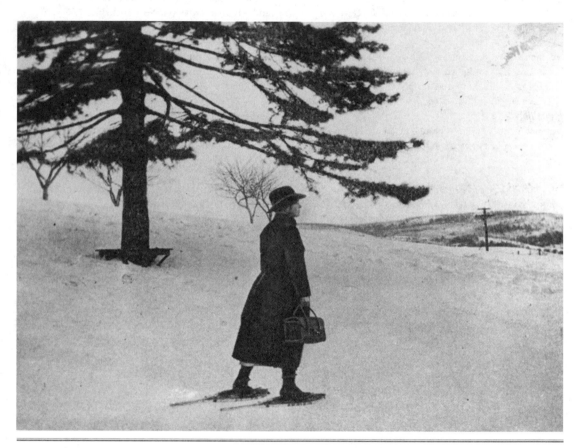

Courtesy of American Red Cross.

CHAPTER 19

Environment and Health

Hollie Shaner-McRae

Since 1904 the anti-tuberculosis movement in this country has grown rapidly. Although it is preeminently a disease of poverty and will never be successfully combated without dealing with its underlying economic causes – bad housing, bad workshops, undernourishment, etc. – the most immediate attack lies in education in personal hygiene, and for this the nurse with her ability to apply scientific truth to the problems of daily life, has been found invaluable. (Wald, 1918, p. 6)

LEARNING OBJECTIVES

At the completion of this chapter, the reader will be able to:

- Discuss the relevance of the environment to health.
- Examine the physical determinants of health, including but not limited to air, water, and soil quality.
- Describe the importance of the built environment as a potential facilitator affecting the health of the public.
- Explore the role of public health nursing practice in environmental health.
- Explore the mid-range model/theory— Environmentally Responsible Clinical Practice Model (ERCPM)—as a guide for practice.

KEY TERMS

- ❑ Bioaccumulation
- ❑ Biocapacity
- ❑ Built environment
- ❑ Determinant of health
- ❑ Ecological footprint
- ❑ Environmental health
- ❑ Environmental regulations
- ❑ Food desert
- ❑ Physical determinant of health
- ❑ Precautionary principle

Introduction

Over time, it has become more and more evident that environmental health is inextricably linked to human health, so much so that the environment is considered one of the **determinants of health** (U.S. Department of Health and Human Services, [USDHHS], 2016a). Furthermore, the environment, at times referred to as a **physical determinant**, is the context within which people "live, learn, play, work, and age" (USDHHS, 2016b, para. 1), thus potentially affecting health and life. The Science & Environmental Health Network (SEHN) blog page on ecological medicine notes,

> The health of Earth's ecosystem is the foundation of all health. Human impact in the form of population pressure, resource abuse, economic self-interest, and inappropriate technologies is rapidly degrading the environment. This impact, in turn, is creating new patterns of human and ecosystem poverty and disease. The tension among ecosystem health, public health, and individual health is reaching a breaking point at the beginning of the Twenty-First Century. (2016a, para. 2)

The purpose of this chapter, therefore, is twofold: 1) to describe environmental health and to discuss how it relates to the health of populations and 2) discuss the role of the nurse in environmental health.

What Is Environmental Health?

The National Environmental Health Association (NEHA) defines **environmental health** as follows:

> the science and practice of preventing human injury and illness and promoting well-being by identifying and evaluating environmental sources and hazardous agents and limiting exposures to hazardous physical, chemical, and biological agents in air, water, soil, food, and other environmental media or settings that may adversely affect human health. (NEHA, 2013, para. 1)

Environmental health professionals and others working in the health field, therefore, focus on topics such as air and water quality, food safety, healthy homes, climate change, vectors and pests, preparedness, and health tracking, all of which affect and are affected by the environment within which we live (NEHA, 2016, para. 1). This thought is supported by the American Public Health Association (APHA), who also identifies that environmental health considers not only how people affect the environment negatively and positively, but also how the environment may affect the people negatively or positively (APHA, 2016a & b). Considering this information, it is clear that when healthcare providers—a term that includes nurses—consider the environment in their practice, they need to question and assess how the environment affects the individual, family, community, and population health (APHA, 2016a & b).

There are certain concepts that more specifically portray the co-relationship between the environment and the people living within that environment. For example, the terms **biocapacity** and **ecological footprint** are useful concepts to understand when one wishes to assess how healthy the environment is, which then will ultimately affect the health of the people. Simply put, "On the supply side, biocapacity represents the planet's biologically productive land areas, including our forests, pastures, cropland, and fisheries. These areas, especially if left unharvested, can also absorb much of the waste we generate, especially our carbon emissions." On the demand side, there is the ecological footprint which considers how "human activities consume resources and produce waste" or "humanity's demand on nature" (Global Footprint Network, 2016, para. 1–2). On a high level, having an understanding of the ecological footprint concept and how it applies to the physical environment, human, and ecological health and even our healthcare delivery systems can prepare nurses to make decisions from a more informed basis and be advocates for judicious use of resources. Another useful concept to understand is that of **bioaccumulation**. This concept explains what happens within the food web or food chain system when chemicals or other pollutants are concentrated within living organisms and then transferred and concentrated as things move up the food chain. For example, consider a pollutant found in water. The pollutant is absorbed by the plankton. The small fish then eat the plankton and take on the cumulative pollutants from the plankton over their lifetime. The larger fish consume the smaller fish and take on even more pollution as they are now absorbing the pollutant from the plankton concentrated within the small fish, as well as the small fish's own concentration of pollutants. Next, consider that a bird consumes many large fish and is taking on all the pollutants now concentrated in each fish's body. Next, humans catch and eat the fish or the bird, taking on all the pollutants that have accumulated, which reflects all the pollutants absorbed starting with the plankton (National Wildlife Federation, 2016).

The totality of environmental health is complex and exists on a multiplicity of levels. Strategies to ensure a healthy environment are varied and many. One strategy to ensure and assure a healthy environment that will sustain a healthy population is the development and implementation of policies, regulations, and laws at the national, state, and local levels. This also includes organizational policy. When considering the environment, regulations are developed and implemented as a way to assure and ensure the people that the environment, within which they live, is being protected from harmful agents that may affect their health and safety. **Environmental regulations**, such as the Clean Air Act, Clean Water Act, and the Resource Conservation and Recovery Act (RCRA), were established in the United States to assure and ensure the protection of water, air quality, and lands. Specifically, the RCRA was initiated to assure and ensure that waste by-products of all types, such as solid waste, biohazard waste, and hazardous chemical wastes,

were managed safely and responsibly. Public policy is made with the best available information at the time. Thus, it is very much possible that some policy and regulatory decisions are made with incomplete, uncertain, or evolving health data. There are also other influences such a lobbyists, for specific industries, who have influence on the shaping of policy. Thus, as health and science research puts forth new findings, existing regulatory frameworks designed to protect the environment and health sometimes become insufficient and outdated. Given that reality, in 1998, a group of healthcare professionals across multiple disciplines came together and met at Johnson Foundation headquarters. During the meeting, an agreement was reached about public health and decision-making in environmental health. The outcome was an agreement known as the Wingspread statement on the **Precautionary Principle**. The statement provides guidance on how to make decisions when there is uncertainty about existing data. It suggested that when an activity raises threats of harm to human health or the environment, precautionary measures should be taken, even if some cause-and-effect relationships are not fully established scientifically. In this context, the proponent of an activity, rather than the public, should bear the burden of proof. The process of applying the precautionary principle must be transparent, open, informed, and democratic, and it must include all potentially affected parties. It must also involve an examination of the full range of alternatives, including no action (SEHN, 2016b, para. 2). When used as a lens and considered as part of governmental and industrial decision-making, the precautionary principle can serve as a long-term protective measure for humankind.

Taking a Closer Look at the Environment

Earlier in this chapter, a definition was offered on environmental health. Within this definition and section, several topic areas were introduced for consideration. An example of these topic areas included air and water quality. Taking a closer look at these areas to demonstrate the relationship that exists between the environment and the health of the people will illustrate the importance of being diligent with regard to the assessment of environmental issues and strategies to address these issues, whether a nurse is working in acute care or a public health nurse working in the community. Specific topic areas that will be addressed include air quality, water quality, toxic substances, and waste, as well as the overall environmental context.

Air Quality

Air is invisible, and the true measures of air quality are not detectable by the human eye. This is not always the case, however, if one considers that smoke from a campfire or a burn barrel is visible and is readily experienced as a respiratory irritant. There are, however, other examples of invisible irritants in the air that are harmful. For example, ozone, particulate levels, and carbon monoxide gas are invisible and are not detectable visually or by smell but are harmful. To gain a better understanding of lung physiology and impacts from air pollutants, visit the National Institute for Environmental Health and Safety website's reference at http://www.niehs.nih.gov/health/topics/conditions/lung-disease/index.cfm.

There has been greater public awareness about clean air as it relates to human health over the last 40 years. Laws and policy changes have emerged that are based on the growing body of scientific evidence linking air quality to human health. Ironic as it sounds, it was less than 30 years ago (the early 1980s) that hospitalized patients and their families were allowed to smoke cigarettes, pipes, and cigars in their hospital rooms, thus transforming the healing environment to a place of secondhand smoke and exposure to carcinogens for all of those around them. At that time, smoking was rampant in restaurants, bars, bowling alleys, offices; on airplanes, trains, and buses; at conferences; and in doctors' offices. Anyone could smoke anytime, anywhere without regard for the impact they were having on others. Asking someone to extinguish their cigarette, cigar, or pipe was almost a cultural taboo. Air pollution associated

with transportation and resulting traffic emissions is significant and contributes to diminished respiratory health and poor health in general (Centers for Disease Control & Prevention [CDC], 2009, para. 1). This information has spurred the U.S. Environmental Protection Agency (USEPA) to develop policy and law directed to assure and ensure clean air. For example, the U.S. Environmental Protection Agency developed the Clean School Bus Program as a way to mitigate the issue of bus emissions and facilitate the elimination of air pollution from school buses to which children and others in school settings are exposed.

As air quality diminishes, people with health conditions such as asthma and chronic obstructive lung disease seek health care more frequently. Exacerbations can be triggered by poor outdoor or indoor air quality or both. Exposure to ozone, smoke, and particulates can be particularly problematic. People who work in specific occupations can have greater exposure to poor air quality. A population most affected by this are firefighters (IAFF, Fire Fighters, 2016). It is well documented that exposure to air pollution and particulates can create increased risk for cardiovascular disease, lung cancer, sudden infant death syndrome, and compromised respiratory health in children (CDC, 2016). Research continues to demonstrate that where there are elevations in the concentration of fine particles in the air, there may be a transient increase in the risk of myocardial infarction, and this risk may linger for hours to days after exposure (Peters, Dockery, Muller, & Mittleman, 2001). The influence of air quality on our health is now a more mainstream topic with daily reports (pollen count, ozone, and particulates) available through all forms of media. Geographic regions with high humidity and poor air quality are cited as particularly challenging for individuals who have underlying respiratory health conditions.

Surface and Ground Water Quality

The impacts of poor water quality on health can be profound. Water pollution can come in various forms. Biological contamination of water occurs from a variety of biological or microbial contaminants. These include bacteria, viruses, protozoan, and parasites. As you become familiar with water pollution in general and the impacts on human and ecological health, consider the categories of water contamination, which include chemical, biological, radiological, and physical contamination. According to the *Healthy People 2020* report, "Poor water quality can lead to gastrointestinal illness and a range of other conditions, including neurological problems and cancer. Some chemicals in and around homes and workplaces can contribute to acute poisonings and other toxic effects" (2016c, para. 5). A recent example of the importance of water quality is that of Flint, Michigan, who made national news with its high lead levels in the drinking water, resulting in negative health outcomes. While the media offers many versions of this tragic story, journalist Michael Moore, a Flint, Michigan, native, offers a unique perspective, and that can be viewed at http://michaelmoore.com/10FactsOnFlint/. And, more recently there have been reports of lead in school water supplies in Newark, New Jersey (McGeehan, 2016) and the Bronx, New York (Small & Kapp, 2017). Furthermore, nurses must be diligent in the political arena when it comes to policy changes pertaining to the environment.

It is not uncommon to learn about similar discoveries of contaminated water supplies in other communities. An interesting case study is unfolding in Bennington, Vermont, where perfluorooctanoic acid (PFOA) was discovered in drinking water impacting nearly 100 families, and the same chemical is in the drinking water in nearby Pownal, impacting 450 families. This situation demonstrates how water contamination can happen and the challenges associated with persistent toxic chemicals in the environment (Markowitz, 2016). In communities that get their drinking water from either public sources or underground wells, ongoing monitoring and testing of water quality is needed from the source. The PFOA case study below offers an in-depth look at how contaminants that migrated from a community chemical plant years ago can show up and adversely impact humans decades later. As you visit the web links listed for you, always reflect upon nurses and their role. At the completion of your readings, work together and consider the question posted at the end of the case study. **Box 19-1** is a case study exercise that may be completed either alone or in teams. Take time to access each of the links, read the information, and answer the questions after all of the steps are completed.

Now, for a totally different perspective on community drinking water and water quality, consider

---

Box 19-1 Perfluorooctanoic Acid (PFOA)—Case Study Exercise

Perfluorooctanoic Acid (PFOA) Case Study

Carry out the following activities:

1. Read the legislative report at the link provided on the case at: http://dec.vermont.gov/sites/dec/files/documents/PFOASummaryForLegislatorsvFINAL3.25.16.pdf
2. Read the Vermont Department of Environmental Conservation website for ongoing PFOA advisory information and health updates at: http://dec.vermont.gov/commissioners-office/pfoa
3. Read U.S. Environmental Protection Agency general information about drinking water contaminants at: https://www.epa.gov/ccl/types-drinking-water-contaminants
4. Read Vermont Department of Health specific information about PFOA at: http://healthvermont.gov/enviro/pfoa.aspx
5. Read the article by Markowitz at http://vtdigger.org/2016/04/05/deb-markowitz-environmental-laws-that-leave-a-lasting-legacy/.
6. Once you have completed these activities, answer the questions listed for you:

(continues)

Box 19-1 *(continued)*

Questions: What is PFOA? What happened in the case study exercise posted for you above? What would you do as a public health nurse to prepare yourself to best serve the community around this issue? Consider what a public health nurse working in that community might be thinking about. How would the PFOA contaminated water potentially impact the health of people in the community? What would a public health nurse need to know to correctly address questions from the community? Where would you go to find out the latest information? How might you use social media to share information with the people living in the community and other health colleagues? What outreach and partnership efforts might you develop to optimize the health and well-being of the community around such issues? Take the intervention wheel outlined in your intervention chapters in this book. How may you apply these interventions to this specific case study?

Figure 19-1 Photo of Water Collection System in Bermuda. Water is piped from roof tiles to cistern below building.

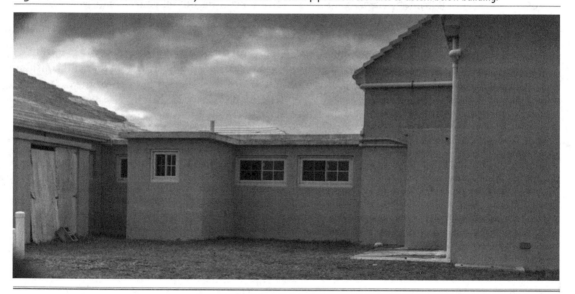

Personal collection from Bermuda, 2016, Hollie Shaner–McRae.

---

the world's island nations, those surrounded by ocean water, that have little if any fresh drinking water available. In Bermuda, for example, nearly all fresh drinking water is captured from rain falling on rooftops (Government of Bermuda, 2016). According to the Consulate General of the United States at Hamilton, Bermuda website (nd), Bermuda relies on rainfall to provide its source of water, and homes have rainwater collection systems, as seen in **Figure 19-1**. Some homes do have a combination of rainwater for cooking and drinking and piped or delivered water for showers, toilets, and laundries. In Bermuda, collected water is stored in cisterns beneath dwellings.

The Government of Bermuda's website on Bermuda water and sewerage offers "Tips for Keeping your Drinking Water Clean" (see **Box 19-2**) as a means to offer helpful information to the people of Bermuda.

One final example of the importance of safe drinking water will be mentioned here. It was

---

Box 19-2 Tips for Keeping Your Drinking Water Clean

Your roof catchment system is your main source for clean drinking water. To maintain your home drinking water quality:

- Keep your roof clean and painted;
- Before cleaning, block the drain pipes so that nothing enters the tank;
- Check your tank levels regularly, at least once a month;
- Clean your tank at least once every five years;
- Trim overhanging trees to prevent leaves from falling onto your roof and entering your tank;
- Disinfect water using ¼ cup of household bleach to every 1,000 gallons of water. To determine the capacity of your tank, in gallons, multiply the tank length × tank width × tank depth × 6.25; and
- When purchasing water, remember only buy enough to take your tank to about half, always leave enough space for rainwater collection

Reproduced from Government of Bermuda. (2016). *Bermuda water and sewage*. Retrieved from https://www.gov.bm/bermuda-water-and-sewage

---

once thought purchasing drinking water distributed in plastic bottles was safe. This is now under increased scrutiny due to concerns about chemical plasticizer, BPA (bisphenol A). While some industry-sponsored sources dismiss the concerns related to BPA, scientists continue to pose questions. For additional information, please read physician and public health activist Ted Schettler's testimony on BPA to the Maryland General Assembly in support of House Bill 33 at http://sehn.org/testimony-on-bpa/. Furthermore, the U.S. EPA has been addressing BPA under the Toxic Substances Control Act (TSCA) through the BPA action plan, which also may be viewed at https://www.epa.gov/assessing-and-managing-chemicals-under-tsca/bisphenol-bpa-action-plan. Ongoing exposure to BPA

through a myriad of sources, including the plasticizer used to make most bottled water plastic containers, provides microdoses of an endocrine disrupting manmade chemical. The U.S. Food and Drug Administration (FDA) has also weighed in on BPA. This information may be seen at http://www.fda.gov/forconsumers/consumerupdates/ucm297954.htm#1, and they continue to study it. The National Institute of Environmental Health Sciences (NIEHS) has also commented on the potential risks and harm from exposure to BPA. This information is posted by the NIEHS may be seen at http://www.niehs.nih.gov/health/topics/agents/sya-bpa/. The CDC does offer guidelines on bottled water; however, their focus is more on how the water is disinfected and the key issues about which immunosuppressed individuals need to be knowledgeable. They do not, however, explore the question of toxins that might leach into the water from the packaging. Information from the CDC may be viewed at http://www.cdc.gov/healthywater/drinking/bottled/. Not only is there a health concern, but the use of these water bottles has also been now shown to have a negative effect on the health of the environment. The *Story of Bottled Water* video explores bottled water with a fresh lens. This story may be viewed at https://www.youtube.com/watch?v=Se12y9hSOM0.

Is bottled water in plastic containers safe? The answer depends on analysis of the evidence, the sources of the evidence, and one's personal threshold for exposure to risk. If one has concerns about the biological purity of drinking water, knowing the source, methods of purification, and evidence of ongoing monitoring instills confidence that the water is safe to drink. If one has concerns about the chemical purity of the drinking water, then consideration to the packaging of the water (type of bottle/container) is worthy of exploration. For anyone informed on the emerging science of endocrine disruptors their impact on the developing fetus, and on the likelihood of latent impacts triggering future adverse health conditions, BPA is likely a concern. Noticing that BPA has become a chemical of international concern, as recently as 2015, the European Food Safety Authority established a working group to review BPA and immune system safety. For further information please view https://www.efsa.europa.eu/en/press/news/160426a.

Public health nurses have the skills to look at an issue and pose questions from multiple perspectives, synthesize the available evidence, and provide education and advocacy for those in their care. It is also key to recognize that as data evolves and is published, advice, perspective, and guidance will also likely shift.

Toxic Substances and Waste

Toxic substances and waste are related to the environment. A person can be exposed to toxic substances through the air they breathe, the water they drink, or their home or workplace environments. The PFOA case study and the discussion about BPA in drinking water are examples of exposure to toxic substances through drinking water. Eating fish contaminated with mercury is another example of exposure to toxic substance through food intake. Examples of exposure to toxic substances in the workplace setting include the workers who work in factories where flavored popcorn is made and thus experienced exposure to flavorings-related lung disease (The National Institute for Occupational Safety and Health, 2016) and the story of the Radium Girls from the early 1900s who suffered from radiation poisoning after exposure to radium paint in a watch factory (Fry, 1998).

Waste generated from all settings needs to go someplace, either down the drain or in the trash. How the waste is managed can impact the health of anyone in contact with it along the way, depending on the type of waste and how it is transported and disposed. Consider the following. There is solid waste, which includes general garbage or trash, and there is recyclable waste, which includes cardboard, paper, plastics, metals, glass, electronics, and durable goods. Biohazard waste includes used syringes, needles, and blood-soaked and contaminated items. Hazardous waste includes chemicals and some pharmaceuticals. Radioactive waste includes radioactive pharmaceuticals and radioactive waste from other sources. In addition, there is construction waste, industrial waste, and other types of waste by-products. The transport and disposal of each waste stream has its own set of challenges. Some waste is sent to landfills and buried. Other waste is sent to incinerators and burned, thus being transformed in the process and emitting another set of airborne by-products, which become global persistent pollutants. Some waste is autoclaved to kill the biological hazard and then either buried or incinerated. Other waste is sent for processing to be recycled and transformed. For example, some plastic scrap is bundled, then unbundled, washed, disinfected and heated, and morphed into a form of small plastic pellets that are then used to create new plastic products. The location of waste-processing facilities, either incinerators, landfills, or recycling plants, are disproportionally located in low-income neighborhoods in the United States and abroad (Fine Maron, 2013). **Box 19-3** offers you a variety of YouTube videos that demonstrate examples of exposure to toxic substances that you may be interested in viewing.

Box 19-3 Video Examples of Exposure to Toxic Substances

1. **What happens during a small mercury spill: from a sphygmomanometer**
   https://www.youtube.com/watch?v=lpZF88fqrl8
2. **Electronic Waste— in China—exposure to mercury and lead**
   https://www.youtube.com/watch?v=ZHTWRYXy2gE
3. **Life in trash—Delhi rag pickers**
   https://www.youtube.com/watch?v=-2TskTnE05w
4. **E-Waste Hell**
   https://www.youtube.com/watch?v=dd_ZttK3PuM

Test Your Knowledge

Can you describe the ways individuals and community members are exposed to toxic substances as a result of a substance spilling or once a substance becomes a waste?

Healthy Homes/Communities and the Environmental Context

The physical home environment can impact health. In order to assess the impact, one needs to consider the systems within the home. What is the source of heat? Forced hot air, baseboard heat, or wood stove? Has the home been tested to ensure radon is not present? What is the source of energy fueling the cookstove? Gas or electric? Is there a fireplace in the home? Is there mold and mildew evident in the bathrooms or basement? What are the finishes in the home? Is there formica or pressboard paneling? Furnishings or carpeting made with an off-gassing formaldehyde? Are there adequate ventilation systems in place for the clothes dryer and cookstove? What products are used to clean the home? Are they bleach based, or are they aerosolized containers? Is there a tobacco/cigar or marijuana smoker residing in the home? What hobbies do the home occupants have? Do they use toxic chemicals as part of their hobby such as glues, adhesives, cleaning chemicals, metals, welding materials, or pesticides? What is the temperature of the hot water coming out of the tap? Is it safe for elders and children? Where is the home located? Is it on a busy street, near highways, or on a country road? What is the noise level within the home? Is it near a noisy highway, airport, or factory? Are pesticides used in the home (ant traps, roach traps, wasp sprays, or rat poison)? Is the home a single-family home, a duplex, an apartment, a condominium, a mobile home, or something more rustic such as housing found in parts of the developing world? Homes come in all shapes and sizes; some are owned, and some are rented. The attributes of a person's home constitutes the physical environment where people spend a great deal of their time. Homes that promote health have clean air, water, and systems in place to manage waste. Thought needs to be given to substances brought into the home and how the home is maintained to prevent degradation that can impact health. The individual, family, and population residing within a community make use of schools, parks, greenways, and the transportation systems, all of which are a part of the greater community and built environment discussed below. Carrying

out home and community assessments will alert the provider and the public health nurse in the identification of environmental issues that need to be addressed.

The Centers for Disease Control and Prevention has a Division of Community Health (DCH). DCH is focused on health from a population basis and is focused on promoting healthy lifestyles and preventing chronic disease. Examples of community health efforts include physical education classes for children to increase their physical activity each day, increasing the number of interprofessional teams in health care to help patients manage chronic diseases, promoting healthy foods and beverage options in public schools and workplaces, and protecting people from exposure to second-hand smoke in indoor and outdoor spaces. From an environmental health perspective, the neighborhood community where one resides can be a favorable environment or less than favorable. For example, the **built environment** is an element of environmental health and is defined by the CDC as including

> all of the physical parts of where we live and work (e.g., homes, buildings, streets, open spaces, and infrastructure). The built environment influences a person's level of physical activity. For example, inaccessible or nonexistent sidewalks and bicycle or walking paths contribute to sedentary habits. (2011, para. 1)

As such, there is an association between the built environment and health conditions (CDC, 2015). Therefore, how communities plan and build their environment is of great importance. The infrastructure of the current public health system in the United States is designed to promote health and prevent disease and is documented in the literature. From an environmental health perspective, it is also useful to consider the environmental infrastructure—the built environment—in a community and explore how the built environment impacts health. Examples of this would be access to sidewalks, access to a transit system, access to a park system, access to fresh fruits and vegetables, either through the location of facilities within the community or access to transportation that leads to a facility. An example of community infrastructure that impacts physical, social, and psychological health is the Hudson River Park in Manhattan. This infrastructure part of the built environment supports health on so many levels. Click on the link to view the park, and see how many things you can identify that would be considered physical infrastructure that support health: https://www .hudsonriverpark.org/explore-the-park. Part of the built environment is access to healthy foods; however, there are many locations in the United States where access to healthy foods is limited. According to the American Nutrition Association (2015) **food deserts** are defined as "parts of the country vapid of fresh fruit, vegetables, and other healthful whole foods, usually found in impoverished areas. This is largely due to a lack of grocery stores, farmers' markets, and healthy food providers" (para. 1). Furthermore, many urban areas of the United States are littered with small community-based stores such as local delicatessens, bodegas, and quickie marts where processed foods high in sugar and unhealthy fats are in surplus (depending on the community). At the end of this chapter, there is a web quest box. This box contains additional information for you to search out on both the built environment and food deserts in the United States.

Environmental Health and the Role of the Nurse

Health of the environment on so many levels is inextricably linked to the health of those residing within it. From a nursing perspective, regardless of the field of nursing practice, there are environmental factors that are influencing the health of the population. A perfect example of this may be asthma and COPD related to poor air quality; or obesity related to limited access to healthy food and environments that prevent physical activity, such as walking; or neurological deficits related to lead exposure in drinking water. Whether you work in acute care, home care, or some other organization, take a moment and reflect on other examples based on where you practice and the population for which you care.

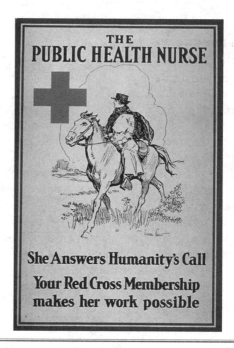

Courtesy of American Red Cross

One of the major components of the Public Health Nursing Assessment Tool in this book is the observation that the public health nurse engages in concerning the totality of the environment. Along with these observations are considerations about how these environmental conditions affect health. According to the World Health Organization (2016), "Environmental risk factors, such as air, water and soil pollution, chemical exposures, climate change, and ultraviolet radiation, contribute to more than 100 diseases and injuries" (para. 1). By reducing and eliminating these risk factors "nearly a quarter of the global burden of disease can be prevented" (WHO, 2016, para. 2). According to the USDHHS (2016d, para. 4), there are six themes that public health nurses and all providers must be aware of when considering environmental health, all of which have already been discussed in this chapter. These six themes include outdoor air quality, surface and ground water, toxic substances and hazardous waste, homes and communities, infrastructure and surveillance, and the health of the global environment. According to Shaner-McRae, and Jas (2007), "There is a direct connection between nursing actions and the health of the environment in health care agencies" (np). The questions that nurses must raise for themselves are "What are these nursing actions?" and "What is environmentally responsible clinical practice?" The answers to these questions rest in the Environmentally Responsible Clinical Practice Model (ERCPM). This model is a map that can guide nurses in their decision-making and actions within their practice. Simply put, the ERCPM is a way of practicing nursing in any setting that takes into account the environmental impacts of the care being delivered, and the nurse chooses actions that protect the environment. It starts with self-awareness that leads nurses to alter their attitudes, resulting in a change in behavior toward choices about conservation. This conservation is about clinical resources and involves water use, supplies, and those continual disposal questions about discarding or recycling: "Discard it as trash, or discard it as biohazard waste?" ERCPM can be something as simple as a disposal decision; for example, it could be about how to discard chemotherapy waste, syringes, or other sharps either in the home or in an acute care setting or it can be more complicated such as researching and ordering the most environmentally preferable finishes for a new hospital wing. It can be collaborating with the materials management leader to ensure that healthcare product purchasing contracts stipulate the procurement of the most environmentally responsible products. It can be more personal decisions, such as the mode of transportation taken for getting to work. Knowing that nearly a pound of air pollution is created for each mile driven in a single passenger automobile, which has deleterious impacts on the environment, the nurse would explore alternatives transportation modes such as walking to work, bicycling to work, carpooling, or public transportation. Every action one takes as a professional nurse and as a citizen has an impact. The energy used to light the workplace, power the elevators (for vertical transport), and heat and cool the indoor environment has an environmental impact. Any option the nurse can make to mitigate negative environmental impact is useful. Using the stairs instead of the elevator, turning off the lights when not

in the office, dimming the lights on the clinical unit, and other similar intentional actions are examples of expressing the environmentally responsible clinical practice model. As citizens, nurses can also advocate for policies that support clean air, clean water, healthy food, exercise, paid time off, physical education for children, healthy workplaces that feature access to light, and support public transportation. Nurses can volunteer to serve on committees and community boards to ensure there are recycling programs; access to safe, well-lit, and maintained stairways; no-smoking policies; and no-idling policies, making sure that buses and trucks cannot idle their engines. Nurses can educate themselves and obtain credentials to be qualified to serve as leaders in organizations that design, deliver, influence, or impact public policy issues.

Shaner-McRae, and Jas (2007) further expound on this in the publication *Environmentally Safe Health Care Agencies: Nursing's Responsibility, Nightingales' Legacy.* For details, please visit http://www.nursingworld.org/MainMenuCategories /ANAMarketplace/ANAPeriodicals/OJIN/Tableof Contents/Volume122007/No2May07/Environmentally SafeHealthCareAgencies.html.

Conclusion

Environmental health knowledge and the application of this knowledge are elements of the nursing practice domain. This domain of nursing practice traces back to Florence Nightingale and her 1859 publication *Notes on Nursing: What it is and what it is not.* In her writings, Florence addressed air quality, water quality, ventilation, the health of houses, cleanliness, and light. She detailed nursing's role in attaining these as integral to creating a healing environment for patients. Fast forward to 2017. There are so many things contemporary nurses can do under the realm of environmental health to contribute to the well-being of populations. This chapter explores the current and future issues related to the environment, the one that Nightingale knew so influenced the health of the community and required the vigilance of not only public health nurses but all nurses (Nightingale, 1949/1893).

Additional Resources

Science and Environmental Health Network (SEHN) at: http://sehn.org/ecological-medicine/

National Environmental Health Association (NEHA) at: http://www.neha.org./

Summary of Clean Air Act at: https://www.epa.gov/laws-regulations/summary-clean-air-act

Summary of Clean Water Act at: Retrieved from: https://www.epa.gov/laws-regulations/summary-clean-water-act

Summary of Resource Conservation and Recovery Act at: https://www.epa.gov/laws-regulations/summary-resource-conservation-and-recovery-act

Healthy People 2020 Environmental Quality at: https://www.healthypeople.gov/2020/leading-health-indicators/2020-lhi-topics/Environmental-Quality

Center for Disease Control Division of Community Health at: https://www.cdc.gov/nccdphp/dch/

Prevention Institute—The Built Environment and Health: 11 Profiles of Neighborhood Transformation at: http://www.preventioninstitute.org/index.php?option=com_jlibrary&view=article&id=114&Itemid=127

Robert Wood Johnson Foundation—Built Environment and Health at: http://www.rwjf.org/en/our-focus-areas/topics/built-environment-and-health.html

Food Empowerment Project at: http://www.foodispower.org/food-deserts/

Feeding America—Hunger and Poverty Facts and Statistics at: http://www.feedingamerica.org/hunger-in-america/impact-of-hunger/hunger-and-poverty/hunger-and-poverty-fact-sheet.html?gclid=Cj0KEQjwxLC9BRDb1dP8o7Op68IBEiQAwWggQCPJdF8_wZv0xmW0DIIy_Nh5NEf56ZhqT_JuW9iwm6kaAs2T8P8HAQ

References

American Nutrition Association. (2015). *USDA defines food deserts.* Retrieved from http://americannutritionassociation.org/newsletter/usda-defines-food-deserts

American Public Health Association. (2016a). *Building and understanding of environmental health.* Retrieved from https://www.apha.org/topics-and-issues/environmental-health/understanding-environmental-health

American Public Health Association. (2016b). Environmental health. Retrieved from https://www.apha.org/topics-and-issues/environmental-health?gclid=CjwKEAjwtLO7BRDax4-I4_6G71USJAA6FjN1MuZVAYFJsJoIOYU2HdLraLDHxyErjpeqgYQ1uJ-28BoCDR7w_wcB

Centers for Disease Control and Prevention. (2009). *Respiratory health & air pollution.* Retrieved from https://www.cdc.gov/healthyplaces/healthtopics/airpollution.htm

Centers for Disease Control and Prevention. (2011). *Impact of the built environment on health.* Retrieved from www.cdc.gov/nceh/publications/factsheets/ImpactoftheBuiltEnvironmentonHealth.pdf

Centers for Disease Control and Prevention. (2015). *CDC's built environment and health initiative.* Retrieved from http://www.cdc.gov/nceh/information/built_environment.htm

Centers for Disease Control and Prevention. (2016). Health effects of secondhand smoke. Retrieved from http://www.cdc.gov/tobacco/data_statistics/fact_sheets/secondhand_smoke/health_effects/

Consulate General of the United States, Hamilton, Bermuda. (nd). *Drinking water.* Retrieved from http://hamilton.usconsulate.gov/essentials.html

Fine, D. M. (2013). *Toxic waste sites take toll on millions in poor nations.* Retrieved from http://www.scientificamerican.com/article/toxic-waste-sites-take-toll-millions-poor-nations/

Fry, S. A. (1998). U.S. radium dial workers: An epidemiological classic. *Radiation Research, Supplement: Madame Curie's Discovery of Radium (1898): A Commemoration by Women in Radiation Sciences, 150*(5), S21–S29.

Global Footprint Network. (2016). *Footprint basics.* Retrieved from http://www.footprintnetwork.org/en/index.php/GFN/page/footprint_basics_overview/

Government of Bermuda. (2016). *Bermuda water and sewage.* Retrieved from https://www.gov.bm/bermuda-water-and-sewage

IAFF Fire Fighters. (2016). Healthy, safety & medicine. Retrieved from http://www.iaff.org/hs/resi/lung_disease_in_fire_fighters.htm

Markowitz, D. (2016). *Deb Markowitz: Environmental laws that leave a lasting legacy.* Retrieved from http://vtdigger.org/2016/04/05/deb-markowitz-environmental-laws-that-leave-a-lasting-legacy/

McGeehan, P. (2016). *New York Times: Drinking water in Newark schools known to have lead problem at least 6 years ago.* Retrieved from https://www.nytimes.com/2016/04/09/nyregion/drinking-water-in-newark-schools-known-to-have-lead-problem-at-least-6-years-ago.html?_r=0

National Environmental Health Association. (2013). *Definitions of environmental health.* Retrieved from http://www.neha.org/about-neha/definitions-environmental-health

National Environmental Health Association. (2016). *Environmental health topics.* Retrieved from http://www.neha.org/eh-topics

National Institute for Occupational Safety and Health. (2016). *Flavoring-related lung disease.* Retrieved from https://www.cdc.gov/niosh/topics/flavorings/

National Wildlife Federation. (2016). *Food webs and bioaccumulation.* Retrieved from https://www.nwf.org/Wildlife/Wildlife-Conservation/Food-Webs.aspx

Nightingale, F. (1893/1949). Sick nursing and health nursing. In I. A. Hampton. (Ed.), *Nursing of the Sick-1893,* pp. 24–43. New York, NY: McGraw-Hill Book Company.

Peters, A., Dockery, D. W., Muller, J. E., & Mittleman, M. A. (2001). Increased particulate air pollution and the triggering of myocardial infarction. *Circulation.* doi:http://dx.doi.org/10.1161/01.CIR.103.23.2810

Science & Environmental Health Network. (2016a). *Ecological medicine.* Retrieved from http://sehn.org/ecological-medicine/

Science & Environmental Health Network. (2016b). *Precautionary principle.* Retrieved from http://www.sehn.org/precaution.html

Shaner-McRae, H., & Jas, V. (2007). Environmentally responsible health care agencies: Nursing's responsibility, Nightingale's legacy. *Online Journal of Issues in Nursing. 12*(2). Retrieved from http://www.nursingworld.org/MainMenuCategories/ANAMarketplace/ANAPeriodicals/OJIN/TableofContents/Volume122007/No2May07/EnvironmentallySafeHealthCareAgencies.html

Small, E. & Kapp, T. (2017). *Lead levels in Bronx school's water 16 times higher than in Flint, Michigan.* Retrieved from https://www.dnainfo.com/new-york/20170206/morrisania/elevated-lead-levels-ps-41-is-158

U.S. Department of Health and Human Services. (2016a). *Determinants of health.* Retrieved from https://www.healthypeople.gov/2020/about/foundation-health-measures/Determinants-of-Health

U.S. Department of Health and Human Services. (2016b). *Social factors.* Retrieved from https://www.healthypeople.gov/2020/about/foundation-health-measures/Determinants-of-Health#social

U.S. Department of Health and Human Services. (2016c). *Environmental quality.* Retrieved from https://www.healthypeople.gov/2020/leading-health-indicators/2020-lhi-topics/Environmental-Quality

U.S. Department of Health and Human Services. (2016d). *Environmental health.* Retrieved from https://www.healthypeople.gov/2020/topics-objectives/topic/environmental-health

U.S. Environmental Protection Agency. (2016). *Clean school bus.* Retrieved from https://www.epa.gov/cleandiesel/clean-school-bus#you-can-do

Wald, L. D. (1918, December 11). Visiting nursing. Written for the Foreign Bureau. Lillian Wald Papers. Writings & Speeches, Nurses & Nursing II, Reel 25, Box 37, Folder 4, pp. 1–9. New York Public Library, Humanities and Social Sciences Library, Manuscripts and Archives Division, New York, NY.

Wikipedia. (2016). *Radium girls.* Retrieved from https://en.wikipedia.org/wiki/Radium_Girls

World Health Organization. (2016). *Environmental health.* Retrieved from http://www.who.int/topics/environmental_health/en/

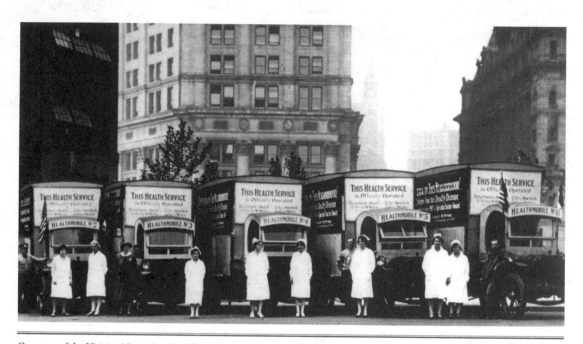

Courtesy of the Visiting Nurse Service of New York.

CHAPTER 20

Epilogue: Nursing and Primary Health Care

Marie Truglio-Londrigan
Joanne Singleton
Sandra B. Lewenson

. . . we have been comrades in work trying to think in a broad way about nurses' opportunities and obligations which translated into the service that is now so generally understood as public health nursing is the democratizing of the nurses' service. What our message was and still is . . . namely, that the age-old woman's profession of nursing has assumed new social values with the changing conditions and the development of social self-consciousness particularly among women, and that the time has come for adjusting the nurses and the profession to meet community—social needs in a large way. (Wald, 1918, p. 2)

LEARNING OBJECTIVES

At the completion of this chapter, the reader will be able to

- Discuss the difference between primary health care and primary care.
- Describe how the Declaration of Alma-Ata influenced primary health care.
- Debate the challenges to the delivery of primary health care.

KEY TERMS

- ❑ Cultural authority
- ❑ Declaration of Alma-Ata
- ❑ Primary care
- ❑ Primary health care
- ❑ Social legitimacy

When the authors of this book began to contemplate what type of content would be presented within its pages, it was clear that the focus would be on the public and how healthcare providers may work together, with the public, in the achievement of one primary goal: access to care and health for all Americans. The areas to be discussed would be the science of public health as well as the types of interventions that are necessary for the attainment of our goal. The implementation of these interventions in a collaborative way with the public, however, is not enough. What we still need, as a nation, is to shift our view of the world so that we first acknowledge a broader healthcare model that includes multiple professionals engaged in the securing of better health outcomes for all people. This means moving our agenda away from a paternalistic, medical model that has dominated much of the 20th- and early-21st-centuries healthcare policies and practices to one that embraces a more holistic approach to health care. All nurses, and especially public health nurses, are at the forefront of providing leadership toward such an approach. We believe that this public health book may provide the knowledge, stamina, and courage to accomplish this goal.

When President Barack Obama signed the Patient Protection and Affordable Care Act (PPACA) in 2010, the possibilities of what may be for our healthcare system shifted. For some, the imbalance is still overwhelming; for others, there is still excitement. Even with a new administration in Washington beginning, some of the essential ideas of the PPACA may endure, although this is yet to be determined. What we do know is that the PPACA is not just about physician-provided medical care to individual patients (Deville & Novick, 2011). Rather, there is a demonstrable commitment to disease prevention, wellness, and population-based work dedicated to social justice and the elimination of health inequities (Mohammed, Stevens, Ezeonwu, & Cooke, 2017). As we know, these elements loom large in the philosophy of primary health care and have permeated the chapters throughout this book. The authors of this

book and of this chapter embrace this shift and believe that this book offers a path toward achieving comprehensive **primary health care**, a path that Sambala, Sapsed, and Mkandawire (2010) have noted as having the ability to ". . . unlock barriers to healthcare services and contribute greatly to determining collective health through the promotion of universal basic health services" (p. 181). This chapter also reflects our ideas about primary health care that evolved further following the completion of the book, *Primary Health Care: Practicing Population Based Care* in 2017. An outcome of both, the new book and the revision of this public health book helped shape this final chapter where we reconsider primary health care in light of the broader meaning of this term. We invite the reader to consider all aspects of public health and primary health care in relationship with public health nursing's role in making this shift and to continually expand their thinking to include the overall notion of primary health care.

The Declaration of Alma-Ata

In 1978, the saying "Health for All" was coined by the World Health Organization (WHO), and the idea of primary health care was derived as the means of achieving this goal. So strong was this belief that at the International Conference on Primary Health Care (1978), the **Declaration of Alma-Ata** expressed a call to action by all governments and world communities to promote and to protect all people. This Declaration contains 10 principal points, the 6th and 7th of which speak specifically to the idea of primary health care. The entire Declaration may be viewed in **Box 20-1**.

A careful review of this document informs the reader of the view of the world and by extension the view of those who authored the Declaration of Alma Ata who placed this vision into words. **Box 20-2** provides an overview of this view of the world and health.

This view of the world and health care reflects specific principles or values that guide decision-making

---

Box 20-1 Declaration of Alma-Ata

Declaration of Alma-Ata International Conference on Primary Health Care, Alma-Ata, USSR, September 6–12, 1978

The International Conference on Primary Health Care, meeting in Alma-Ata this twelfth day of September in the year Nineteen hundred and seventy-eight, expressing the need for urgent action by all governments, all health and development workers, and the world community to protect and promote the health of all the people of the world, hereby makes the following

Declaration:

I

The Conference strongly reaffirms that health, which is a state of complete physical, mental and social well-being, and not merely the absence of disease or infirmity, is a fundamental human right and that the attainment of the highest possible level of health is a most important world-wide social goal whose realization requires the action of many other social and economic sectors in addition to the health sector.

II

The existing gross inequality in the health status of the people particularly between developed and developing countries as well as within countries is politically, socially and economically unacceptable and is, therefore, of common concern to all countries.

III

Economic and social development, based on a New International Economic Order, is of basic importance to the fullest attainment of health for all and to the reduction of the gap between the health status of the developing and developed countries. The promotion and protection of the health of the people is essential to sustained economic and social development and contributes to a better quality of life and to world peace.

IV

The people have the right and duty to participate individually and collectively in the planning and implementation of their health care.

V

Governments have a responsibility for the health of their people which can be fulfilled only by the provision of adequate health and social measures. A main social target of governments, international organizations and the whole world community in the coming decades should be the attainment by all peoples of the world by the year 2000 of a level of health that will permit them to lead a socially and economically productive life. Primary health care is the key to attaining this target as part of development in the spirit of social justice.

VI

Primary health care is essential health care based on practical, scientifically sound and socially acceptable methods and technology made universally accessible to individuals and families in the community through their full participation and at a cost that the community and country can afford to maintain at every stage of their development in the spirit of self-reliance and self-determination. It forms an integral part both of the country's health system, of which it is the central function and main focus, and of the overall social and economic development of the community. It is the first level of contact of individuals, the family and community with the national health system bringing health care as close as possible to where people live and work, and constitutes the first element of a continuing health care process.

(continues)

Box 20-1 *(continued)*

VII

Primary health care:

1. reflects and evolves from the economic conditions and sociocultural and political characteristics of the country and its communities and is based on the application of the relevant results of social, bio-medical and health services research and public health experience;

2. addresses the main health problems in the community, providing promotive, preventive, curative and rehabilitative services accordingly;

3. includes at least: education concerning prevailing health problems and the methods of preventing and controlling them; promotion of food supply and proper nutrition; an adequate supply of safe water and basic sanitation; maternal and child health care, including family planning; immunization against the major infectious diseases; prevention and control of locally endemic diseases; appropriate treatment of common diseases and injuries; and provision of essential drugs;

4. involves, in addition to the health sector, all related sectors and aspects of national and community development, in particular agriculture, animal husbandry, food, industry, education, housing, public works, communications and other sectors; and demands the coordinated efforts of all those sectors;

5. requires and promotes maximum community and individual self-reliance and participation in the planning, organization, operation and control of primary health care, making fullest use of local, national and other available resources; and to this end develops through appropriate education the ability of communities to participate;

6. should be sustained by integrated, functional and mutually supportive referral systems, leading to the progressive improvement of comprehensive health care for all, and giving priority to those most in need;

7. relies, at local and referral levels, on health workers, including physicians, nurses, midwives, auxil-iaries and community workers as applicable, as well as traditional practitioners as needed, suitably trained socially and technically to work as a health team and to respond to the expressed health needs of the community.

VIII

All governments should formulate national policies, strategies and plans of action to launch and sustain primary health care as part of a comprehensive national health system and in coordination with other sectors. To this end, it will be necessary to exercise political will, to mobilize the country's resources and to use available external resources rationally.

IX

All countries should cooperate in a spirit of partnership and service to ensure primary health care for all people since the attainment of health by people in any one country directly concerns and benefits every other country. In this context the joint WHO/UNICEF report on primary health care constitutes a solid basis for the further development and operation of primary health care throughout the world.

X

An acceptable level of health for all the people of the world by the year 2000 can be attained through a fuller and better use of the world's resources, a considerable part of which is now spent on armaments and military conflicts. A genuine policy of independence, peace, détente and disarmament could and should release additional resources that could well be devoted to peaceful aims and in particular to the accelera-tion of social and economic development of which primary health care, as an essential part, should be allotted its proper share.

Box 20-1 *(continued)*

The International Conference on Primary Health Care calls for urgent and effective national and international action to develop and implement primary health care throughout the world and particularly in developing countries in a spirit of technical cooperation and in keeping with a New International Economic Order. It urges governments, WHO and UNICEF, and other international organizations, as well as multilateral and bilateral agencies, nongovernmental organizations, funding agencies, all health workers and the whole world community to support national and international commitment to primary health care and to channel increased technical and financial support to it, particularly in developing countries.

The Conference calls on all the aforementioned to collaborate in introducing, developing and maintaining primary health care in accordance with the spirit and content of this Declaration.

Reproduced from World Health Organization. (1978). Declaration of Alma-Ata. Retrieved from www.euro.who.int/__data/assets/pdf_file/0009/113877/E93944.pdf. Copyright 1978, World Health Organization.

Box 20-2 Worldview in Primary Health Care

- Universal health care that is accessible to all which is reflective of all aspects of personal, family, population, and environmental health.
- Universal healthcare building from the economic, sociocultural, and political characteristics of the nation, state, and local communities.
- Universal health care that is community driven through the co-participation of community participants working collectively in shared decisions.
- Universal health care that represents a systematic processes with focused attention on use of best evidence and technology.
- Universal health care made possible through the enhancement of available resources and through intersectoral work and community collaboration.

---

and collective action to assure and ensure access, quality, and equity of care delivery throughout the healthcare delivery system. Furthermore, the Declaration of the Alma-Ata specifically describes primary health care as essential to the achievement of accessible health by all its citizens.

Primary Health Care

As previously mentioned, the sixth and the seventh principal points speak specifically about primary health care. The Alma-Ata Declaration of 1978 formally defined primary health care as:

essential health care based on practical, scientifically sound, and socially acceptable methods and technology made universally accessible to individuals and families in the community through their full participation and at a cost that the community and country can afford to maintain at every stage of their development in the spirit of self-reliance and self-determination. It forms an integral part both of the country's health system, of which it is the central function and main focus, and of the overall social and economic development of the community. It is the first level of contact of individuals, the family, and community with the *national health system bringing health care as close as possible to where people live and work, and constitutes the first element of a continuing health care process.* (WHO, 1978, para. 6)*

The Declaration of the Alma-Ata is very specific when it comes to primary health care and highlights several principles that guide action:

- Reflects the culture of the nation and its people; therefore, the development of health initiatives takes place with the people and where the people are. In this way, these health initiatives will be culturally sensitive and appropriate, thus making them congruent with the people and their ideas, values, and beliefs.
- Addresses all areas of health, including health promotion, disease prevention, and curative care, including the availability and accessibility of needed medications and immunizations as well as rehabilitation. In this way, primary health care is seen as a philosophy and a way to practice that is inclusive of all contexts, not just one of community.
- Includes education toward the attainment of health as well as essentials for public health, such as clean water, sanitation, and nutrition. Education must reflect cultural ideas, values, and beliefs as well as focus on educational strategies that are congruent with the population and their needs. The education of primary health care includes the level of formal educational attainment by the people as well as specific education concerning what knowledge and skills are needed to make healthy decision choices.
- Involves more than healthcare practitioners and is inclusive of multiple sectors of the community and thus multiple partners.
- Requires maximum participation and partnering with individuals, families, communities, and

populations. This partnering may be a challenge, but it reflects a true working relationship where all individuals are considered essential and all voices are heard—where all people assume responsibility in shared decision-making in the development of health initiatives and the movement toward stated goals.

Primary health care is comprehensive health care, comprehensive in its breadth and depth. Primary health care is guided by the overriding principle that health is a basic human right that requires the action of many, but it also recognizes that there are inequities that are unacceptable and should be a concern to all. The Declaration acknowledges that health for all has sociopolitical and economic implications that ultimately must address social determinants of health (Scott, Crawford-Browne, & Sanders, 2016). Furthermore, the Declaration is clear that the people need to be active participants in the attainment of this health, both individually and collectively, at the local and community level with intersectoral involvement (Scott, Crawford-Browne, & Sanders, 2016). Additionally, not only are people key to the attainment of health, but governments also must work together with its people to formulate policies that will facilitate and sustain health through primary health care. In fact, there is evidence that suggests community participation and the mobilization of the people bridges the gap between the community and the healthcare system because of the already established connections and trust within the community (Cheng, Wahidi, Vasi, & Samuel, 2015) resulting in positive health outcomes (Bath & Wakerman, 2015). Sambala, Sapsed, and Mkandawire (2010) further this discussion as they stress how primary health care is capable of delivering services to deal with the resiliency of global public health issues (p. 181). They identify that the ability to deliver these services is due to the fact that primary health care has "sophisticated and organized infrastructure, theories, and political principles, with which to deal adequately with the issues of inequity, inequality, and social injustice . . ." (p. 181). Lewenson and Truglio-Londrigan (2017)

---

* Reproduced from World Health Organization. (1978). Declaration of Alma-Ata. Retrieved from www.euro .who.int/__data/assets/pdf_file/0009/113877/E93944.pdf. Copyright 1978, World Health Organization.

explain that "the concepts embedded in the philosophy of primary health care—shared decision-making, collaboration, social justice, community orientation, access for all citizens, and equity of services—may also permeate primary care, public health, and population-based care, depending on how they are operationalized" (p. xiii). These ideas allow nurses, especially public health nurses, to think about how to implement the broad ideas inherent in primary health care.

Take a few minutes, and as a group critically examine the Declaration of Alma-Ata provided for you in Box 20-1, specifically points VI and VII. Think about the type of care you have seen rendered in your past clinical experiences. Identify one specific care initiative and answer the following questions:

- In what way is the care initiative reflective of the Declaration of Alma-Ata and primary health care?
- In what way is the care initiative effective or ineffective?
- Can you take one of your clinical experiences and shape and shift it so that it is reflective of the worldview and practices of primary health care?

Evolution of Primary Health Care

It has been almost 40 years since the introduction of the Declaration of Alma-Ata, and many have questioned how far we have come as a nation and globally. Although it is true there have been changes and improvements with water access, sanitation, and antenatal care, there have been other areas where progress has not been as obvious. For example, health and the attainment of health have been unequal across countries, and the identification of inequalities within countries is noted (WHO, 2008). Presently, the United States faces inequities and disparities in many identified areas. These areas include infant mortality rates; life expectancy and rates of disease within specific populations; elevated risk factors in certain populations such as smoking rates, access to care, nutrition, and physical activity;

and in the social determinants of health, including poverty, inadequate housing, and unsafe working conditions (Association of State and Territorial Health Officials [ASTHO], 2016).

Why the Struggle?

Although it is clear that there has been progress in the area of primary health care, there are still challenges ahead. In the U.S. healthcare system, primary care appear to be a driving force. We still hold on to a system that focuses on a biomedical model, specialization, and curative care with an emphasis on disease along with technology, short-term results, and fragmentation of service delivery (WHO, 2007). Part of the struggle with embracing primary health care is that despite the term, it still creates confusion for some. Gordon and Plamping (1996) initially discussed the lack of a shared understanding of primary health care and indicated that one of the reasons for this is that hospital care is much more visible and demonstrative, and primary health care is much more abstract and complex. For example, consider some of the points that are made in the definition of primary health care. When the definition describes culture and the importance of culture, what does this mean? Are we really culturally and socially astute? Do we really conduct cultural assessments and understand the communities and people we are working with? When we develop community health initiatives, are they really culturally congruent and developed with the people in the community? When we develop these initiatives, whose community are we referring? Is it the community as defined by the people, or is it a community defined by the involved agencies, administrators, large hospitals, or some other external group (Wayland & Crowder, 2002)? When we speak about community participation, what do we mean by this? Do we really understand the importance of this type of participation or the complexity of the process? Do we understand how to initiate partnerships and coalitions and sustain those partnerships? What about communication and shared decision-making in these partnerships? Are we ready to live in a world where we share and facilitate the empowerment of the people? The purpose of these questions is to illustrate the complexity of primary health care and to also demonstrate that the principles and values inherent within this view of the world may not be embraced by all.

The purpose of the extensive list of questions is to bring to light the principles and values that are important to consider when building a healthcare system that embraces primary health care. These values, concepts, and ideas "serve as standards for how we understand ourselves and the world around us, and we often use them as a basis for our decisions and actions" (Heard, 1990, p. 1). In American culture, certain values may be more dominant than others at varying points in time. Beauchamp (1985) noted that in the United States the dominant language of politics is that of individualism, whereas the community is considered secondary. Individualism is rooted deeply in our historical consciousness. Individualism focuses on "the human condition as it exists apart from others and serves to promote ideas of personal freedom, self-improvement, privacy, achievement, independence, detachments, and self-interest" (Heard, 1990, p. 3). The second value, known as community, sets forth a view of people "within the context of human relationships. It concentrates on qualities that people have through their associations with others such as intimacy, benevolence, fellowship, belonging, dependence, social involvement, and the public good" (Heard, 1990, p. 3). To further explain this, contemplate the term of *access and equity*, which is so essential for primary health care. If we speak of access and equity of services, we must also ensure education, social, and economic justice for all. From what values do these emanate? When one considers this question, some will select the value of community, especially because that particular value speaks to the public good. Given the emphasis on the value of individualism within the American culture, it may explain why individuals who lean toward the values of individualism may have difficulty understanding and ultimately welcoming the idea of primary health care.

Analyzing the two values of individualism and community, we can see the tension that exists between them because they both are present in our American culture. This does not mean that a transformation in our social consciousness is impossible. What it does mean is that there needs to be a willingness to listen and be open to the idea of primary health care for there to be a shift in our view of the world and health care that will lead to a cultural transformation in our ideas. Remember that with this cultural shifting of ideas and values there is an opportunity for acceptance of primary health care, which will lead to a restructuring of policies and redistribution of care and services. Heggenhougen (1984) noted primary health care will "ultimately lead to a reduction in the greater benefit for the few to the greater benefit for the many" (p. 217). How do you suppose this is received by the few? According to Cueto (2004), there is increasing resistance among some professionals because "they fear losing privileges, prestige, and power" (p. 1872). Our present healthcare system is steeped in our own American culture, with certain values being stronger than others. Taking this into account, any alteration in our view of the world and health care will require a shift toward seeing that health for all citizens is a fundamental right that can take place only with the restructuring of our healthcare system (Mohammed et al., 2017; Nickitas, 2017). Political process and the political parties that govern and develop policies, as witnessed in the 2016 Presidential election, brings change in the way the government responds to the health needs of populations—including such examples as changes in environmental regulations and in the proposed repeal of the Affordable Care Act.

Primary Health Care Includes Primary Care

A final point to be made about the struggle for primary health care refers to the confusion that exists between it and the term **primary care**. They are not one and the same, although the similarities in their names may cause individuals to believe that they are. "Primary care is often used interchangeably with primary medical care as its focus is on clinical services provided predominantly by [general practitioners], as well as by practice nurses, primary/community health care nurses, early childhood nurses, and community pharmacists" (The University of New South Wales, 2010, para. 3). According to a report of the National Primary Health Care Conference of 2004, primary care

> *deals mainly with the prevention and treatment of sickness.... Primary care may involve immunization, preventative advice (stop smoking, get some exercise), diagnosis and treatment of illness, but it stops short of a comprehensive, intersectional approach to producing or enhancing health. Perhaps most importantly, primary care is focused on individuals and families, but not the community as the unit of intervention.* (Edwards et al., 2004, p. 4)

Primary care serves the necessary purpose of treating the patient on the basis of a model that "involves a single service or intermittent management of a person's specific illness or disease condition in a service that is typically contained to a time—limited appointment, with or without follow-up and monitoring or an expectation of provider—client interaction beyond that visit" (Keleher, 2001, p. 59). Hence, in the United States, primary care "remains a medical model" (Murray, 2011, p. 3). This primary care has served us well, and because of this accomplishment of our medical care system, physicians have achieved **cultural authority** that has also lead to the establishment of **social legitimacy** (De Ville & Novick, 2011, p. 106), making it difficult to shift our views that may be more in line with primary health care. Lewenson and Truglio-Londrigan (2017) define primary care in part as a point-of-care service model that fits within the primary health care paradigm (p. xii). Primary health care then broadly incorporates the various models of care using a population-based focus and a public health mind-set.

Primary care refers to a way of practicing between the practitioner and the individual or family. It may include a population-based focus or not, but the focus of the relationship is more one-to-one, whether with a physician, a nurse practitioner, or a physician's assistant. These practitioners address the efforts of accomplishing what the Robert Woods Johnson Foundation calls a "culture of health" (Hassmiller, 2017) by addressing the individuals or families in front of them. This culture stresses the importance for primary care providers to have an awareness that the person/family sitting in front of them must return to his or her or its home and communities. They must build and integrate into their practice an understanding of where their patients live, learn, work, and play and how this influences the choices their patients/families make (Hassmiller, 2017; Robert Wood Johnson Foundation, 2015). This broadening of the philosophical framework presents them with a vision of people who are participants in their care and in shared decisions that pertain to their care (Truglio-Londrigan, 2017). Furthermore, providers must broaden their views in a way that includes an awareness of intersectoral and interprofessional collaborative practice building primary health care initiatives with the people in the communities. As this shift takes place, cultural authority and social legitimacy too will shift from a biomedical model to one of collaboration, but who are these others that we need to practice with? We know the people living within the communities, but do we know who the professionals and other disciplines are? Do they know and understand nursing, and do they reach out to us? Alternatively, do we reach out to them? Who are the individuals they work with? What are the issues they face on a daily basis? Is there synergy between and among these professionals and disciplines? Can we inform one another? Can we collaborate with one another to build this culture of health?

Colleagues from varying professions and disciplines were invited to participate in the development of this chapter. These individuals were informed that this book provides the historical context, skills, and knowledge that public health nurses need to know for their practice. And, to foster an understanding of other professionals and disciplines in the hope that this enhanced understanding will facilitate collaboration. The ability to engage in collaborative work, using primary health care approaches, starts with an introduction to one another and a dialogue that broadens one's view of the world, one's place in the world, and the relationships one has with others. To this end, the authors of this chapter asked individuals outside of nursing what they did in their practice, who they worked with, and issues that they face daily. Some even went so

far as identifying the need to connect with nurses to "get the job done." The purpose of this portion of this chapter is to begin a conversation where we start the necessary dialogue leading to action and ultimately change. **Box 20-3** is the introduction that will heighten our awareness of these professionals and disciplines. As public health nurses build their practices within a primary health care philosophical frame of reference, these are some of the questions that they (and other healthcare providers) must attend.

Box 20-3 Interprofessional, Interdisciplinary, and Intersectoral Practice

Example 1:

Screening Children for Developmental Delays

Karen S. Edwards, MD, MPH,
Professor, School of Health Sciences and Practice, New York Medical College;
Vice President for Education, Training and Research,
Westchester Institute for Human Development.

I am educated both as a general pediatrician and in public health. My career has included being a general pediatrician working with children with special healthcare needs and their families and being a faculty member providing interprofessional and interdisciplinary education for future health professionals who work with children with disabilities and in providing leadership to improve outcomes. From my perspective, care to this vulnerable population must be carried out through collaborative work with many professional disciplines, with participation from the individuals and families.

Screening children for developmental delay is an important responsibility shared by public health providers and healthcare systems to ensure early identification of developmental delays and appropriate referral for evaluation and timely intervention. In light of very strong evidence that prompt initiation of early intervention for children with delay impacts positively on child outcomes, it is imperative that all primary care providers screen regularly for developmental delays according to recommended schedules, using proven screening tools, and make appropriate referrals when screening reveals a possible developmental issue.[1] A recent nationwide survey revealed that, by parental report, only 30.8% of children aged 12 months to 5 years who had at least one healthcare visit in the past 12 months received standardized developmental and behavioral screening conducted during the visit.[2] Although this represents an increase over the same survey conducted 4 years previously, it falls far short of expectations. Primary care professionals may thus benefit from easy access to evidence and materials that support timely screening.

Parents have an important role in noticing possible developmental issues and bringing them to the attention of their child's primary care provider. Parents can be supported in this role through parent education that can be delivered by the multitude of professionals. The "Learn the Signs. Act Early" campaign of the federal Centers for Disease Control and Prevention (https://www.cdc.gov/ncbddd/actearly/) provides high-quality, evidence-based print materials and web-based tools for parents and professionals to support their roles in early recognition, screening, and referral concerning developmental delays. Materials

Box 20-3 *(continued)*

available at the site include videos and checklists describing developmental milestones expected at each age; detailed information for professionals concerning screening schedules and screening tools; public service announcements and videos concerning the importance of early identification of developmental delays; and a large collection of free print materials that can be ordered.

[1]Council on Children with Disabilities; Section on Developmental Behavioral Pediatrics; Bright Futures Steering Committee; Medical Home Initiatives for Children With Special Needs Project Advisory Committee. (2006). Identifying infants and young children with developmental disorders in the medical home: An algorithm for developmental surveillance and screening. *Pediatrics, 118*(1), 405–420.

[2]National Survey of Children's Health. NSCH 2011/12. Data query from the Child and Adolescent Health Measurement Initiative, Data Resource Center for Child and Adolescent Health website. Retrieved from *www.childhealthdata.org*

Example 2:

The Challenge of Staying Home with the Double Jeopardy: Minor-to-Moderate Cognitive Impairment and Fall Risk*

Jane Bear-Lehman, PhD, OTR/L, FAOTA
Professor and Chair
College of Health Professions
Pace University, New York, NY
New York College of Dentistry

There are limited health services research and evidence-based programming focused on elderly fall prevention despite high fall-related morbidity and mortality. Moreover, persons with minor-to-moderate dementia living in the community have an increased risk of falls.

A multidisciplinary collaborative representing public health, sociology, occupational therapy, neurology, and rehabilitative medicine adapted an evidence-based fall prevention program (PROFET) for delivery to community-dwelling elderly, newly diagnosed with mild-to-moderate dementia, who had not experienced a fall-related injury. Program participants were enrolled through the Pearl I—New York University, Barlow Center for Memory Evaluation and Treatment. The elder participants in this collaborative effort were diagnosed with mild-to-moderate dementia. In addition, there was evidence of intrinsic risk factors indicative of poor functionality such as decreased cognition, slowed gait, decreased balance, decreased grip strength, and increased polypharmacy. Similarly, these elders also demonstrated evidence of increased extrinsic risk factors, which included hazards in the home environment with challenged navigation and transitioning in sitting and rising from bed, chairs within the home, and need for increased safety in their living space, including the need for assistive devices in the bathroom and kitchen, all of which were identified through a comprehensive clinical assessment and home visit. An individualized fall risk reduction protocol was developed for each elder participant (N = 7). Data were collected on the short-term (6 to 12 months) impact of the program on reduction in fall risk factors, fear of falling, and falls experienced.

In conclusion, even though the process was complicated given the new diagnosis of dementia, the outcomes of this research revealed that the overall design was feasible and, more importantly, that the window for learning new skills to prevent falls is longer than originally thought, as our cohort of seven were able to remain in their residences when we contacted them up to one year after diagnosis of mild-to-moderate dementia. Three of the seven reported a noninjurious fall, and all seven were stable in their mild-to-moderate impaired cognitive status.

(continues)

Box 20-3 (continued)

The outcomes also revealed that the first year or two post diagnosis is opportune for learning a traditional fall prevention program, allowing for successful participation in occupational and physical therapy to improve upon body strength, learn exercises, and for the development of an important and safe walking program, all of which is not part of the usual and customary intervention among those with the diagnosis of mild-to-moderate dementia.

Our clinical education programs need to expand the reach of fall prevention efforts to include at-risk clinical populations, such as community residents with mild-to-moderate dementia, to substantially reduce healthcare costs and sustain health and functioning for patients and their care providers.

It is recommended that the clinical education program for healthcare providers recognize the benefit of a home assessment to improve safety in the home and assist in lifestyle planning for the patient and the family and to promote safety while still capable of learning new skills. It is advised that the home assessment take place soon after but not at the time of initial diagnosis of mild-or-moderate dementia. It is also important to provide an opportunity for the individual to participate in a fall prevention program while learning new motor skills is still possible. It is also important for healthcare providers to identify ways to facilitate collaboration between and among the involved professionals and to be familiar with other community support resources that the families need in order to attend to the pressing challenges of early diagnosis of mild-to-moderate dementia.

*This work is supported by a grant from the National Institutes of Health/National Center for Research Resources through New York University's Clinical and Translational Institute (CTSI). "C-PROFET: Piloting an Early Intervention Fall Prevention Program for Community-Dwelling Elderly with Dementia," 1UL1RR029893, Jane Bear-Lehman, PhD, Victoria H. Raveis, PhD, James Galvin, MD, Valery Lanyi, MD, 2013-2015.

Example 3:

Collaboration in Mental Health and Confidentiality

Margaret Fitzgerald, J. D.
Associate Professor
Criminal Justice and Security
Dyson College of Arts and Sciences
Pace University
Pleasantville, NY

Individuals and families experiencing stressful situations and/or mental health issues often seek help from multiple agencies and multiple professionals. It is not unusual for more than one agency or professional to respond to and provide assistance to these individuals in crisis and address the multiple issues that arise. The problem that occurs because of the rules of confidentiality is that these agencies and multiple professionals may not know that other mental health organizations or professionals are involved. Consequentially, there are often conflicting approaches to the treatments given to this vulnerable population. This is not helpful and could even cause more distress and oftentimes leads to additional issues.

Healthcare professionals have sought solutions to address this issue. One such example involved a group of healthcare workers from varying professions who sought to relieve the situation by carrying out collaborative monthly joint meetings. At these meetings, the client was referred to by name, and a comprehensive clinical plan was drawn up for the month with input from all organizations and professions and at times the client. The concept of confidentially was addressed as it was waived by the clients before they could be treated. This program was very successful as there was a decrease in disruptive behavior over the year.

Box 20-3 *(continued)*

Example 4:

Public Policy and Populations: Are We Safeguarding the Vulnerable

Paul Londrigan, MA
Adjunct Professor, Political Science
Dyson College of Arts and Sciences
Pace University
Pleasantville, NY

At first glance, the fields of political theory and that of nursing seem to be strange bedfellows. What could political theorists, a group criticized by some for building castles in the sky, possibly have to offer health-care providers and nurses whom, as I understand it, base many of their interventions on evidenced-based practice? More than the reader of this book would probably guess at first blush. By virtue of the fact that public health nursing focuses on populations rather than atomistic individuals, the seemingly disparate fields of nursing, public policy, and political theory can be stitched together. The thread that does the stitching is governmentality, a concept developed by the French social theorist Michel Foucault.[1] Governmentality operates as a form of power that, much like public policy and public health nursing, addresses the population. The objective of this form of power is to intervene in the population and foster the birth rate, mortality rate, and literacy rate while simultaneously attempting to tame contingency.

What the reader should realize, as Foucault eventually did, is that governmentality as a form of power is not always altruistic, nor is it value neutral. The underlying suggestion is that the idea of a population may not always be a homogeneous unit. Populations can be disaggregated into different groups such as the elderly, the young, the mentally incompetent, the delinquent, and the deviant. By virtue of this disaggregation, some groups may be purposefully cast out of a population or treated prejudicially for political purposes. This raises the question who gets excluded from public health policies by virtue of their exclusion from the population? Anecdotally, if one were to survey the totality of public health policy in the United States or the broader world, one would surely find that some public health policy systematically favors some segments of a population while imposing serious hardships on others. In sum, if it is the objective of public health providers to safeguard access to healthcare services for all members of society, it is crucial to be attentive to public policy and the powers behind policies' creation. This leads me to wonder what the outcomes would be if political scientists and the profession of nursing work together more closely to benefit populations?

[1] Foucault, M. (2005). *The hermeneutics of the subject: Lectures at the Collège De France 1981–1982.* New York, NY: Picador.

Example 5

Safeguarding the Safety of Older Adults

Christopher A. Pariso, BS
Criminal Justice Technical Operations Coordinator
University of New Haven
Center for Analytics
New Haven, CT

In caring for an elderly population, there are many factors to consider in one's quest to maintain health and safety. The elderly are often vulnerable targets for identity theft, financial fraud, and physical abuse,

(continues)

Box 20-3 *(continued)*

as evidenced by data that can be pulled from large data sets. These acts are a concern for law enforcement personnel. This vulnerability may stem from a variety of factors, including a lack of understanding of modern technology, reduced social support and availability of networks, and in some cases diminished mental capacity and cognitive functions. The nature of the fraud itself can take many forms, but there are common factors in each that can be seen.

Scammers targeting the elderly will most commonly seek three things: a direct payment or money transfer; credit card or bank account numbers; and personally identifying information, such as Social Security numbers. Fraudulent emails and phone calls, such as claiming to be an IRS agent demanding payment for past taxes, are one tactic used to gain this information. Similar ploys might be used by a scammer going door to door pretending to be a utility worker or a city official. In some cases, the exploitation of the elderly could come from someone in regular contact with the elder, such as an in-home helper or meal delivery person. Cash, credit cards, valuables, or documents with sensitive information frequently are left in the open on kitchen tables, for example, making the elderly easy targets for opportunistic theft.

In order to prevent the elderly from falling victim to these scams and to implement safety measures, there must first be awareness that such scams exist. Education and resources provided by law enforcement varies from city to city. Some locations do offer seminars and reading materials detailing the common sources of fraud. Police departments in some locations have also partnered with banks and other private businesses to provide educational seminars to raise awareness. The possibilities of partnering with nursing are endless from an education perspective to practice perspectives for the expressed purpose of providing the elderly and their families with the necessary knowledge to protect themselves. Working together with this vulnerable population has the potential to turn the cards on those who would prey on those considered vulnerable.

Example 6

Incorporating an Oral Health Screening Tool as a Component of a Community Outreach Screening Visits for Frail Older Adults—The Importance of Collaborative Practice

Rima B. Sehl, DDS, MPA
Associate Professor and Director of Health Promotion
Department of Cardiology and Comprehensive Care
New York University College of Dentistry, New York, New York

Improving the ability of a complex healthcare system to respond to the increasing oral health needs of the vulnerable frail older adults—as essential health care—is extremely challenging. Untreated oral diseases do not resolve when left untreated and can profoundly impact quality of life of individuals. The existing model of dental practice has limited the delivery of oral health care in nontraditional settings and the dentist in making home visits. Community-dwelling frail elderly are more often unable to access oral health care in the traditional office setting. The interrelationship of oral and general health provides a strong rationale for interprofessional partnership and collaboration between nursing and dentistry in order to respond to the oral health needs of frail older adults living in the community. Community outreach and screening are interventions that lead to early detection and early treatment of diseases including oral diseases. Incorporating an oral health screening tool as a component of a community outreach or screening visit will allow a community or public health nurse (a nondental healthcare professional) to identify elderly with dental problems and refer them for the needed care. This interprofessional collaborative model will require the development of a system to ensure access to oral health care for diagnosis, treatment, and follow-up, and mechanisms to address the gap in oral health education and training of nondental professionals.

Box 20-3 *(continued)*

Reflection Upon the Words of Our Colleagues

Reading the words of our colleagues from the various professions and disciplines, it becomes evident that all are working with vulnerable populations from older adults to children to those with issues in mental health. All seem to be faced with issues that plague the particular vulnerable population and are either conducting research to identify strategies to eliminate the issue or developing initiatives using evidence-based practice or espousing the need to advocate in the form of collaborating on policy as an intervention to support and empower the vulnerable toward self-efficacy and self-reliance. Furthermore, the establishment of strong interprofessional and interdisciplinary teams across sectors may facilitate strong knowledge networks that facilitate the generation of information and adoption of that information, which may ultimately lead to policy and planning (Armstrong & Kendall, 2010). The point the authors of this chapter wanted to make is that there are others—professionals, disciplines, and other stakeholders working in varying sectors—who we as nurses can partner and collaborate with, thus providing the necessary synergy toward change. We need to understand these professionals, but at the same time, we need to educate them as to what nurses do and what nurses bring to health care. Take the time to read each of the examples. Work in teams, and ask yourselves the following questions:

1. As a profession, how can we work collaboratively with this profession or discipline to achieve health for this particular population?
2. What are the processes that we would need to incorporate in this collaborative to assure and ensure a systematic approach?
3. What types of primary health care programs can we develop collaboratively?
4. Are there any programs already being implemented, inclusive of nursing, with evidence to suggest positive outcomes?
5. How may we engage the targeted population so that they are working with a team?

Finally, consider the specific questions listed below in relation to the specific example in this box.

Example 1: Considering the information presented in this example, what role can nurses play when working with this specific population?

Example 2: This describes an initiative where there is a collaborative, and nursing is not involved. Is there a place for nursing at this table? If yes, what is that place? How can nursing gain access to this table?

Example 3: What are some of the benefits of working in teams with patients and their families?

Example 4: This describes public policy as a public health intervention designed to protect the public. However, the author describes concerns that populations may still be treated prejudicially whereby public policy may not recognize them and their needs. Reflect upon this example. What do you see in your clinical arena? Are there populations that are left behind?

Example 5: Do you see a way and a means to partner with your local law enforcement to develop safety programs for the elderly in your local communities? What role do you see the elderly play in the development and implementation of these safety initiatives?

Example 6: Do you see a role for nursing in the essential health service of dental care? What is that role? Be creative and develop an initiative that addresses this issue. Who would you invite to be a member of the initiative?

The Teaching of a Philosophy

This book focuses on population-based care and public health nursing for educational purposes. It also includes the ideas of primary health care throughout, showing the relationship between and among the concepts that fit within the larger primary health care paradigm. Nursing has at times practiced according to the principles of primary health care, and yet many in nursing are not familiar or practice under this broad philosophical approach. The authors of this book recognized a paucity of scholarship and educational resources, placing nursing within the primary health care paradigm (Lewenson & Truglio-Londrigan, 2017). Furthermore, the authors of this book also recognized that the teaching of these concepts was challenging and forced faculty to draw on scholarship outside of nursing that often omitted nursing from their work, thus adding to the invisibility that nurses and the profession often experience. These reflections led us to question how we teach primary health care that includes the ideas of intersectoral and interprofessional collaboration. The answer to this question was to publish another book in 2017 titled, *Practicing Primary Health Care in Nursing: Caring for Populations*. Placing nursing within the broader discussion of primary health care facilitates our ability to develop curricula and teach nursing students using the ideas of primary health care.

According to Cueto (2004), one of the struggles of medicine in the acceptance and the application of primary health care is in the fact that "there is no steady effort to reorganize medical education around primary health care" (p. 1872). Can the same be true for nursing education? We believe that by placing the ideas of primary health care squarely within the chapters of this book, we can begin to see a steady effort to teach nurses and change our educational practices.

In learning any health profession, acquisition of knowledge and skills toward competency is essential to practice. Providing knowledge and skills requires a dedicated focus to include this content in the curriculum, including didactic and clinical experiences. With this experience, however, comes a greater responsibility to understand the many social determinants of health that impact those we care for in the world of primary care and make the connection with primary health care. In preparing students for the health disciplines, differentiating primary care and primary health care is imperative to addressing and meeting the needs of the nation's health. Helping students understand this difference will allow them, when they are ready, to have their aha! moment and embrace the larger context of practice. An education about primary care without primary health care is an incomplete education.

The second chapter of this book, written by Sandra B. Lewenson, is titled *Public Health Nursing in the United States: A History*. Reading this chapter informs us that nurses, particularly in public health nursing, have been practicing primary health care all along. As you read this chapter, point out the areas to which the Declaration of Alma-Ata refers. **Box 20-4** provides a more detailed example.

Conclusion

History provides us with important lessons from those who came before. How did the conduct of these nurses emulate the principles of public health nursing and primary health care? Perhaps it is our professional heritage that facilitates our acceptance of these three words and a willingness to embrace all that primary health care has to offer. In fact, if one considers the 17 intervention strategies, these in and of themselves demonstrate the methods that nurses in general may use to practice primary health care. Furthermore, this chapter allows us to consider and articulate the connections between primary health care and the public health nursing interventions that we, as a profession, have always performed and will continue to perform. We in the profession of nursing are poised to meet the challenges in the recent Institute of Medicine report, *The Future of Nursing* (2011), specifically key message number three, which states, "Nurses should be full partners, with physicians and other health professionals, in redesigning health care in the United States" (p. 4) as well as Robert Wood Johnson's (2015) *Charting Nursing's Future*.

Box 20-4 Primary Health Care and Public Health Nursing: An Example From History

The noted early-20th-century public health nursing leader, Lillian D. Wald, believed in primary health care, even though the term itself was not yet used. Wald contributed to the health of populations living in urban centers as well as in rural communities. Not content to provide access to health care just to those living in New York City, Wald believed that those living in rural communities throughout the United States deserved the same kind of care. Wald's visionary leadership led to the establishment of the Red Cross Rural Nursing Service, which opened in 1912 and continued, under different names, until the middle of the 20th century. Wald saw the American Red Cross as a viable organization that could expand its wartime activities into peacetime initiatives that would bring public health nursing services into rural communities. Wald sought support from philanthropists, governmental officials, and nursing leaders to create a structure that supported public health nursing efforts in rural, isolated communities.

Each nurse who met the requirements for joining the American Red Cross and had a minimum of 4 months' additional training as a public health nurse in rural communities could serve in this new capacity. These nurses would go into communities and work with various organizations within these communities, such as school boards, boards of health, or women's clubs, to bring health education, vaccinations, and other primary health care-type activities to the populations living within the communities. One of the later directors of this rural public health nursing service, Elizabeth Fox (1932), described the growth of this service throughout the first half of the 1900s as follows: "One by one, to the southern mountains, to mining camps, to farming counties, to small towns, to an industrial village, went Red Cross nurses, often the first to undertake rural work in a given state, and with them went a constant stream of wise advice and encouragement" (p. 173). These nurses provided bedside nursing when needed, set up well-baby clinics in rural settings, brought nursing into schools and industrial settings, arranged classes for mothers in home hygiene and care of the sick, and educated populations about how to stay healthy. Fox (1921) saw Red Cross public health nurses as the trailblazers; they tried to "fill the gaps in the health organization of the country and to blaze the trail in the unreached areas" (p. 108). Between 1912 and 1947, there were over "3,109 public health nursing services in about 1,800 counties under the sponsorship of some 2,100 chapters—a notable contribution to the health of America and an influence on many other agencies" (Kernodle, 1949, p. 469).

Adapted from: Lewenson, S. (2015). Town and country nursing: Community participation and nurse recruitment. In J. C. Kirchgessner & A. W. Keeling (Eds.), Nursing rural America: Perspectives from the early 20th century (pp. 1–19). New York, NY: Springer Publishing Company.

Additional Resources

United Nations Sustainable Development Goals at: http://www.un.org/sustainabledevelopment/sustainable-development-goals/

World Health Organization Millennium Development Goals at: http://www.who.int/topics/millennium_development_goals/en/

Millennium Project Historic Site at: http://www.unmillenniumproject.org/index.htm

World Health Organization—Primary Health Care at: http://www.who.int/topics/primary_health_care/en/

> **World Health Organization—Primary Health Care The Bulletin Series at:** http://www.who.int/topics /primary_health_care/en/
>
> **Primary Health Care Performance Initiative at:** http://phcperformanceinitiative.org/
>
> **Video Primary Health care at:** https://www.youtube.com/watch?v=JrEguvyCsV8
>
> **Mary Bassett—Why Your Doctor Should Care about Social Justice at:** https://www.ted.com/talks /mary_bassett_why_your_doctor_should_care_about_social_justice?language=en

References

Armstrong, K., & Kendall, E. (2010). Translating knowledge into practice and policy: The role of knowledge networks in primary health care. *Health Information Management Journal, 39*(2), 9–17.

Association of State and Territorial Health Officials. (2016). *Policy and position statements.* Retrieved from http://www.astho.org/Policy-and -Position-Statements/Policy-Statement-on -Achieving-Optimal-Health-for-All/

Bath, J., & Wakerman, J. (2015). Impact of community participation in primary health care: What is the evidence? *Australian Journal of Primary Health, 21*(1), 2–8.

Beauchamp, D. E. (1985). Community: The neglected tradition of public health. *Hastings Center Report, 15*(6), 28–36.

Ceng, I-H., Wahidi, S., Vasi, S., & Samuel, S. (2015). Importance of community engagement in primary health care: The case of Afghan refugees. *Australian Journal of Primary Health, 21*(3), 262–267.

Cueto, M. (2004). The origins of primary health care and selective primary health care. *American Journal of Public Health, 94*(11), 1864–1873.

DeVille, K., & Novick, L. (2011). Swimming upstream? Patient Protection and Affordable Care Act and the cultural ascendancy of public health. *Journal of Public Health Management and Practice, 17*(2), 102–109.

Dock, L., & Stewart, I. M. (1938). *A short history of nursing* (4th ed.). New York, NY: G. P. Putnam's Sons.

Edwards, J., Hicks, S., O'Neill, M., Corby, L., Kulkarni, L., Wiktorowicz, B., & Cooper, J. (2004). *A thousand points of light? Moving forward on primary health care.* A synthesis of key themes and ideas from the National Primary Health Care Conference, Winnipeg, Manitoba. Retrieved from http://www .eicp.ca/en/resources/pdfs/PHC_Conference _Synthesis_Report.pdf

Feinsilver, J. (1993). *Healing the masses: Cuban health politics at home and abroad.* Berkeley: University of California Press.

Gordon, E., & Plamping, D. (1996). Primary health care: Its characteristics and potential. In E. Gordon & J. Hadley (Eds.), *Extending primary care: Polyclinics, resource centers, hospitals-at-home* (pp. 1–15). Oxford, UK: Radcliffe.

Hassmiller, S. B. (2017). Nursing's role in building a culture of health. In. S. B. Lewenson & M. Truglio-Londrigan (Eds.), *Practicing primary health care in nursing: Caring for populations* (pp. 33–60). Burlington, MA: Jones & Bartlett Learning.

Heard, G. C. (1990). *Basic values and ethical decision: An examination of individualism and community in American society.* Malabar, FL: Robert E. Krieger Publishing.

Heggenhougen, H. (1993). PHC and anthropology: Challenges and opportunities (Review of the book *Anthropology and primary health care*). *Culture, Medicine and Psychiatry, 17*(2), 281–289.

Heggenhougen, H. K. (1984). Will primary health care efforts be allowed to succeed? *Social Sciences and Medicine, 19*(3), 217–224.

Institute of Medicine. (2011). *The future of nursing: Leading change, and advancing health.* Washington, DC: National Academies Press.

Keleher, H. (2001). Why primary health care offers a more comprehensive approach for tackling health inequities than primary care. *Australian Journal of Primary Health, 7*(2), 57–61.

Kernodle, P. B. (1949). *The Red Cross nurse in action 1882–1948*. New York, NY: Harper and Brothers.

Lewenson, S. B., & Truglio-Londrigan, M. (2017). Preface. In S. B. Lewenson & M. Truglio-Londrigan (Eds.), *Practicing primary health care in nursing: Caring for populations* (pp. xi–xix). Burlington, MA: Jones & Bartlett Learning.

Lewenson, S. (2015). *Town and country nursing: Community participation and nurse recruitment*. In J. C. Kirchgessner & A. W. Keeling (Eds.), Nursing rural America: Perspectives from the early 20th century (pp. 1–19). NewYork, NY: Springer Publishing Company.

Mohammed, S., Stevens, C. A., Ezeonwu, M., & Cooke, C. L. (2017). Social justice, nursing advocacy, and health inequities: A primary health care perspective. In S. B. Lewenson & M. Truglio-Londrigan (Eds.), *Practicing primary health care in nursing: Caring for populations* (pp. 61–74). Burlington, MA: Jones & Bartlett Learning.

Murray, L. R. (2011). Public health and primary care: Transforming the U.S. health system. *The Nation's Health, 41*(3), 1–35.

Nickitas, D. (2017). The economics of caring for populations: A primary health care perspective. In. S. B. Lewenson & M. Truglio-Londrigan (Eds.), *Practicing primary health care in nursing: Caring for populations* (pp. 75–87). Burlington, MA: Jones & Bartlett Learning.

Rifkin, S., & Walt, G. (1986). Why health improves: Defining the issues concerning comprehensive primary health care. *Social Science Medicine, 23*(6), 559–566.

Robert Wood Johnson Foundation. (2015). The value of nursing in building a culture of health (Part 1): Reaching beyond traditional care settings to promote health where people live, learn, and play. *Charting Nursing's Future*. Retrieved from http://www.rwjf.org/en/library/research/2015/04/the-value-of-nursing-in-building-a-culture-of-health-part-1-.html

Sambala, E. Z., Sapsed, S., & Mkandawire, M. L. (2010). Role of primary health care in ensuring access to medicines. *Croatian Medical Journal, 51*(3), 181–190.

Scott, V., Crawford-Browne, S., & Sanders, D. (2016). Critiquing the response to the Ebola epidemic through primary health care approach. *BMC Public Health, 16,* 410. doi:10.1186/s12889-016-3071-4

Truglio-Londrigan, M. (2017). Coalitions, partnerships, and shared decision-making: A primary health care perspective. In S. B. Lewenson & M. Truglio-Londrigan (Eds.), *Practicing primary health care in nursing: Caring for populations* (pp. 89–108). Burlington, MA: Jones & Bartlett Learning.

The University of New South Wales. (2010). *Primary Health Care Connect*. Retrieved from http://www.-phcconnect.unsw.edu.au/

Wald, L. D. (1918, May 1). Address to graduates of Johns Hopkins Hospital. Lillian Wald Papers. Reel 25, 1918, pp. 1–12. New York City Public Library. New York, NY.

Wayland, C., & Crowder, J. (2002). Disparate views of community primary health care: Understanding how perceptions influence success. *Medical Anthropology Quarterly, 16*(2), 230–247.

Whiteford, L., & Branch, L. (2008). *Primary health care in Cuba: The other revolution*. Lanham, MD: Rowman & Littlefield.

World Health Organization. (1978). *Declaration of Alma-Ata*. Retrieved from www.euro.who.int/__data/assets/pdf_file/0009/113877/E93944.pdf

World Health Organization. (2008). *The world health report 2008: Primary health care now more than ever*. Geneva, Switzerland: Author.

World Health Organization. (2011). *The bulletin series: Primary health care 30 years on*. Retrieved from http://www.who.int/bulletin/primary_health_care_series/en/

For a full suite of assignments and additional learning activities, use the access code located in the front of your book to visit this exclusive website: **http://go.jblearning.com/londrigan.** If you do not have an access code, you can obtain one at the site.

Glossary

advocacy: Acting on someone's behalf with the intention to ultimately build the capacity of the individual, family, community, or system so that they may ultimately support their own cause.

Affordable Care Act (ACA): Signed by President Barack Obama in March 2010, this federal statute is intended to reform U.S. health care and provides for multiple healthcare changes and benefits.

agent: That which causes or contributes to a health problem or condition. The agent may be infectious, chemical, or physical, and it is one of the parts of the epidemiological triangle.

age-specific rate: Provides information about a disease for a particular age group.

American Red Cross: The lead emergency response agency in United States, founded by Clara Barton in 1881.

analytic assessment: The process of identifying appropriate data and information sources.

analytical epidemiology: Illustrates the causal relationship between a risk factor and a specific disease or health condition. It seeks to answer the questions how and why with regard to the cause of a disease and the effects.

assessment: The process of gathering data from a wide variety of sources and critically analyzing the data to identify strengths and weaknesses and to prioritize the weaknesses.

Association of Community Health Nursing Educators (ACHNE): A nursing organization that provides a meeting ground for those committed to excellence in community and public health nursing education, research, and practice.

assure: Public health providers assure individuals, families, communities, and populations about health matters by verbally providing information and relieving any concerns they may have about issues they are facing.

assurance: Requires that public health agencies provide needed services and that the services are guaranteed for those unable to afford them.

attack rate: The incidence of a disease in a particular population over a period of time. This is important for the study of a single disease outbreak or epidemic during a short time period.

bioaccumulation: The accumulation of substances, such as pesticides or other chemicals in an organism. It occurs when an organism absorbs a possibly toxic substance at a rate faster than at which the substance is lost by catabolism or excretion.

biocapacity: The capacity of a given biologically productive area to generate an ongoing supply of renewable resources and to absorb its spillover waste.

Black Death: The second recorded pandemic of the disease known as the bubonic plague swept across Europe from Central Asia in the 14th century, causing millions of deaths and devastating entire villages.

built environment: An element of environmental health and is defined by the CDC as including all of the physical parts of where we live and work (e.g., homes, buildings, streets, open spaces, and infrastructure).

case finding: Actions and activities that help the healthcare professional locate individuals and families with identified risk factors and/or active disease and connect them with resources.

case management: Activities and actions that facilitate the seamlessness of a system's operation, thereby enhancing the capacity of the system. A system functioning at maximum capacity enhances the coordination and provision of services that optimize self-care of an individual and family.

chain of infection: Description of how an infectious disease results from the interaction between and among the agent, host, and environment. Transmission, direct or indirect, of an infectious agent takes place after the agent leaves its reservoir (host) by a portal of exit, such as the mouth when coughing. The agent then enters the susceptible host via a portal of entry, such as a skin wound, to infect the susceptible host.

coalition building: Promotes and develops partnerships among agencies and organizations for a common purpose. The coalition, via the partnership, serves to bring about change as all members work together toward the common vision and solve problems or enhance an already existing healthcare initiative.

collaboration: The working together of two or more individuals or organizations to achieve a common goal.

collective action: Refers to groups of people who organize social or political activities in order to address a shared need.

community-engaged learning: Provides students hands-on, real-life experiences while benefitting the community and its health.

community health nurse: Any nurse who works in the community setting and focuses on the health of the community.

community organizing: Activities that bring together various community groups with a common goal and mobilize resources in the identified community to develop, implement, and evaluate the outcome of their initiative as they work collectively.

community partnership: A community partner may be, but is not limited to, the following: local, state, national, international, public, community-based, private and academic organization.

consultation: Interactive problem solving with a community, system, family, or individual that generates optimal and optional solutions to issues.

core functions of public health: Assessment, policy development, and assurance. Each of the functions requires a specific set of skills to ensure that the 10 essential services that fall under the three core functions are accomplished.

counseling: An interpersonal relationship between a health professional and a community, system, family, or individual, with the intention to increase self-care and coping.

crude rates: Measure of the experience of an entire population in a specific area with the certain disease or condition being investigated.

cultural authority: Dictates specific behaviors and expectations within a group or society of respect and acceptance that confers authority, dominance, and influence for a particular idea, value, or belief over another.

culturally competent care: A healthcare provider's set of attitudes and behaviors that takes into account a client's or population's cultural beliefs, values, health practices, and ways of behaving in social interactions, which may differ widely from the expectations of the healthcare provider.

culture: The lifeways, folkways, rituals, taboos, and practices of a group of people who share symbols, values, and patterns of behavior.

data: Discrete elements or entities that are objective and that have not been interpreted.

database: A system or structure that allows for data to be stored in an organized way so that it may be easily accessed.

data mining: Discerning patterns and relationships from large aggregate data sources.

Declaration of Alma-Ata: Introduced in the 1978 World Health conference, which initiated the goal of primary health care for all.

delegation: Direct care tasks a registered professional nurse carries out under the authority of another healthcare practitioner as permitted by law. Delegation also includes any direct care tasks a registered professional nurse entrusts to other appropriate personnel to perform while still being responsible for that task.

descriptive epidemiology: The extent of an outbreak in terms of who gets the disease, where the disease occurs, and when the disease occurred. It is concerned with the acquisition of information about the occurrence of states of health, such as characteristics of person, place, and time. Descriptive epidemiology is essential for the description of the characteristics of disease occurrence and in the development of a hypothesis.

determinants of health: One of the four foundational health measures that serve as an indicator of progress toward achieving the goals of *Healthy People 2020*.

developmental and life-course perspective: The early life experiences of an individual that contribute to his or her susceptibility to disease later in life.

directly observed therapy: Administering or observing a patient as he or she self-administers prescribed medication to ensure that adherence and compliance with treatment are achieved.

disaster: A sudden, devastating occurrence within a community that demands a nursing and medical response.

discrimination: The process by which people are treated differently because they are members of a particular group. Particular isms such as racism (bias against racial and ethnic groups), sexism (bias against women), ageism (bias against elders), heterosexism (bias against gays and lesbians), ableism (bias against disabled), and classism (bias against people of lower economic class) are forms of discrimination.

disease and health event investigation: The systematic collection and analysis of data about a threat to a population that ascertains the source of the threat, identifies cases and others at risk, determines strategic measures for action, and evaluates outcomes.

disparities: One of the four foundational health measures that serve as an indicator of progress toward achieving the goals of *Healthy People 2020*.

district nurse: A mid-19th-century English term that refers to a nurse whose main focus was caring for the sick poor in their homes.

ecological footprint: The impact of a person or a community on the environment, expressed as the amount of land required to sustain the person's or the community's use of natural resources.

economic policy: Set of rules or laws mandated by government to maintain financial growth and tax revenues, often influenced by political beliefs as well as the policies of parties.

education: One of the social determinants of health.

effectiveness: The degree to which we are sure that the intervention we are proposing will achieve our stated goal.

electronic health record: Individual and population health information that is collected and stored in a digital format with the potential of being shared across health settings.

emergency preparedness: Completion of the steps and actions to prepare for unexpected emergency situations and to be able to deal with the emergency as it is taking place, as well as in its aftermath.

ensure: Public health providers ensure and guarantee the achievement of health through the development of specific policy and laws using collaborative efforts.

environment: A factor that is considered extrinsic, which has an effect on the agent and the opportunity for exposure. It is one of the parts of the epidemiological triangle.

environmental health: The branch of public health that is concerned with all aspects of the natural and built environment that may affect human health.

environmental regulations: Laws, rules, and requirements that generally cover two things: pollution control (regulating how much pollution a facility releases) and conservation management (maintaining the health of ecosystems).

epidemic: Occurs when new cases of a particular disease, in a particular population, in a given time period is greater than expected.

epidemiological triad: The traditional model of infectious disease causation. The triad has three components: the agent, the host, and the environment.

epidemiology: The scientific discipline that studies the distribution and the determinants of diseases and injuries in human populations.

Essentials of Baccalaureate Nursing Education: Publication that identifies the framework for designing and assessing professional practice nursing education programs.

essentials of public health: The 10 essential public health services include responsibilities of local public health systems as well as strategies necessary for building a healthy, integrated public health system capable of facilitating the health of the public.

ethical issues: Ethics includes actions by the nurse that promote compassion, respect, justice and dignity of the individual, family, community, and population. From a technological perspective ethical issues therefore would include confidentiality, accurate data entry and analysis, and cybersecurity for electronic health records.

ethnocentrism: The interpretation of the world according to the norms of one's own culture.

evidence-based medicine: The application of research evidence as the best evidence to guide decision making. The term was first developed and used by medical professionals and was noted to be the new way of medical practice.

evidence-based practice: A systematic framework for decision making that uses the best available evidence in conjunction with the professional's expertise and the client's values and preferences to guide problem solving about how to best approach a situation.

food deserts: Parts of the country where fresh fruit, vegetables, and other healthful whole foods are scarce.

general health status: One of the four foundational health measures that serve as an indicator of progress toward achieving the goals of *Healthy People 2020*.

healthcare access: Helping people obtain appropriate healthcare resources in order to improve or maintain their health.

healthcare cost: Cost of goods and services directly related to the care of individuals, families, communities, and populations.

health disparities: Gaps in health care related to the existence and the quality of health care for individuals, families, populations, communities, and systems.

health inequity: Health inequities are noted differences in the health of different populations.

health literacy: The degree to which individuals have the capacity to obtain, process, and understand basic health information and services needed to make appropriate health decisions.

health promotion: A primary level of prevention that includes strategies and behaviors that an individual engages in to enhance health. These strategies are not focused on any one particular disease but rather focus on the individual, family, or population's overall health and optimal level of wellness.

health-related quality of life: One of the four foundational health measures that serve as an indicator of progress toward achieving the goals of *Healthy People 2020*.

health teaching: The communication of knowledge, facts, ideas, and skills that change competencies, attitudes, values, beliefs, behaviors, and practices of individuals, families, communities, and systems.

Healthy People 2010: A comprehensive, nationwide health promotion and disease prevention agenda that serves as a road map for improving the health of all people in the United States.

Healthy People 2020: A collaborative process that will build from the goals and objectives set forth in *Healthy People 2010*.

HIV: Human immunodeficiency virus, which is the cause of acquired immune deficiency syndrome (AIDS).

home care nurse: A nurse who provides care to individuals and families across the health continuum within their homes.

host: Individual affected by intrinsic factors and environmental exposure, susceptibility, and/or response to a causative agent. It is one part of the epidemiological triangle.

incidence rates: The number of new cases of a specified disease reported during a given time interval.

income: One of the social determinants of health.

income inequality: Describes where wealth is concentrated and who controls the wealth in society. Income inequality measures the degree of income variation in a population.

index case: The start of any investigation, which begins with an event, such as disease, that presents in an individual.

infection control: A discipline concerned with the prevention of infection within a healthcare setting and/or the factors and steps that need to be taken in the event of an infection to eliminate and control its spread.

influence: The ability to persuade an individual or group.

informatics: An academic field that is concerned with the application of information science and technology to public health practice and research.

information: Data that are interpreted, organized, and structured.

information technology: The study, development, and implementation of computer-based technology that the healthcare professional can use to access information; identify information for best practice; and apply technology in educational initiatives, communication, and in the support of research.

Institute of Medicine (IOM) Reports for Nursing Education: Publication based on the series of IOM reports aimed at improving the safety and overall quality of health care in the United States that addresses areas of interest to nurse educators in preparing students in public health.

interprofessional education: When students from two or more professions learn together during their professional education with the objective of cultivating collaborative practice for providing patient-centered care.

Intervention Wheel: Developed at the Minnesota Department of Health, the intervention wheel model depicts 17 intervention strategies applied to three levels of practice, which public health nurses can use across various practice settings.

investigation: The search for health data, using skills for assessing individuals, families/groups, and populations, and skills in informatics to access information regarding a particular need.

knowledge: Information that is synthesized so that relationships are identified and formalized.

least infringement: An acknowledgment of the importance of being mindful of individual and minority interests.

life course model: A model that suggests that the socioeconomic position of the family during childhood affects the child's health status, educational choices, and occupational choices in the future.

maintaining health: Engagement in activities that sustain an individual's present level of health.

Minnesota Department of Health Population-Based Public Health Nursing Practice Intervention Wheel Strategies: An organizing framework public health nurses use to guide their practice.

monitoring: Observation of a population, specific group(s), or individuals while continuously making adjustments to what is occurring.

morbidity rate: The rate of illness, injury, or disability in a population (i.e., the number of people ill during a time period divided by the number of people in the total population).

mortality: A measure of the frequency of occurrence of death in a defined population during a specified interval.

multilevel analysis: An analysis necessary to understand all of the factors that contribute to disease. In a multilevel analysis, all factors are examined on an individual level and on an environmental level, such as a neighborhood, community, city, state, and so forth.

national health initiative: Plans intended to inform, enhance, and guide public health efforts across a nation.

necessity: Something that is required or indispensable.

network: A type of collaboration that usually involves informal or formal relationships where there is cooperation and coordination among partners.

nursing history: Examining the social, political, and economic context in which nursing evolved over time.

nursing informatics: The integration of nursing science, computer science, and information science to manage and communicate data, information, knowledge, and wisdom in nursing practice.

Nursing's Social Policy Statement: A document that focuses on the relationship between the profession of nursing and society in general. The statement focuses on the care and health of society and how the profession and individual nurses develop and meet the challenge of providing care with social justice in mind through political and legislative action.

occupation: A job or profession. One of the social determinants of health.

outreach: The process of locating individuals, families, and/or populations of interest for the purpose of information dissemination and/or provision of service.

pandemic: An epidemic that spreads to a larger populations beyond to several countries or continents.

participant observation: A technique in which the nurse makes careful observations of specific processes, actions, or communications while providing care as a participant in the activity.

personal health record: The personal record related to a patient and the information pertaining to that patient.

physical determinant of health: The context within which the individual, family, or population resides including where they live, work, and play.

policy development and enforcement: Actions and activities that place health issues on decision makers' agendas, acquire a plan of resolution, and determine needed resources. Policy development results in laws, rules, regulations, ordinances, and policies. Policy enforcement compels others to comply with the laws, rules, regulations, ordinances, and policies created in conjunction with policy development.

politics: The process of collective decision making performed by a group of people involved with government, religion, corporate, or academic issues.

population: A group of individuals who share specific characteristics such as social, physical, cultural, economic, or environmental characteristics.

population-focused care: Application of intervention wheel strategies that will access and provide care to a specific population.

population perspective: Viewpoint that suggests that an individual's risk for health problems cannot be isolated from the community in which he or she resides or from the population or society to which he or she belongs.

precautionary principle: Provides guidance on how to make decisions when there is uncertainty about existing data. It suggested that when an activity raises threats of harm to human health or the environment, precautionary measures should be taken, even if some cause-and-effect relationships are not fully established scientifically.

preexposure prophylaxis: A prevention strategy for individuals who are HIV negative to prevent new infections.

preparedness: The ability to engage in an effective response to a disaster or other emergency.

prevalence rates: A measure of the number of people in a given population who have a specific existing condition at a given point in time.

prevention/preventing disease: Engaging in an action or initiating an intervention to prevent the occurrence of a disease or an event.

primary care: Treatment of the patient based on a model of intermittent management of a person's specific condition, generally contained to a time-limited appointment, with or without follow-up, monitoring, or evaluation. Provider–client interaction beyond this visit may or may not take place.

primary health care: Bringing health care that is universally accessible to the people via their full participation.

primary prevention: Actions taken to prevent disease and/or injury and require strategies including health promotion and specific protection.

proportionality: The quality of corresponding in size or amount to something else.

public health: Both a science and an art that ensures the public's health by engaging in interventions that promote health and prevent disease, prolonging life through organized community efforts.

public health ethics: Involves a systematic approach to clarify, prioritize, and justify possible courses of public health based on ethical principles, values, and beliefs of stakeholders, and scientific and other information.

public health informatics: The systematic application of information, computer science, and technology to public health practice and learning.

public health nurse: A term coined by Lillian Wald in the early 20th century that describes the work of the visiting nurse who cares for the sick at home and provides health promotion and disease prevention measures in the community. The work of the public health nurse is population focused and takes place on three practice levels: individual/family, community, and system.

Public health nurse education: Specific educational knowledge, competencies, and skills, with focus on public health and the delivering care to populations.

public justification: Any intervention needs to be justified to the public. The justification needs to be provided in terms that are consistent with the values and the discourses of the community.

public policy: Encompasses the choices that a government makes regarding goals and priorities and the way it allocates resources to attain those goals.

Quad Council: Comprised of ACHNE, the Association of State and Territorial Directors of Nursing (ASTDN), APHA public health nursing section, and the American Nurses Association's Congress on Nursing Practice and Economics (ANA) to address priorities for public health nursing education, practice, leadership, and research and to be the voice for public health nursing.

quarantine: The isolation of a contagious individual from the remainder of the population.

racism: Prejudice, discrimination, or antagonism directed against someone of a different race based on the belief that one's own race is superior.

rate: The primary measurement used to describe the occurrence of a health problem. It is a measure of the frequency of a health-related event in a specific population within a given period of time. A rate consists of a numerator and a denominator and calculated by dividing the number of conditions or events by time, and multiplying by a base multiple of 10.

referral and follow-up: Actions and activities that serve to assist individuals, families, and/or populations by connecting them to needed services for possible treatments and other resources, including follow-up to identify outcomes.

regional health information exchanges: Organizations established to electronically collect and organize a core set of data from multiple organizations within a community or region.

resilience: The ability of an organization, city, or town to recover and ease the effects of a disaster or event with the least amount of disruption and within the shortest amount of time.

risk: The probability that an event will occur within a specific time period.

risk reduction: Completion of specific strategies designed to reduce risk or the probability that an event will occur.

ritual: An act often associated with key life events. It may enhance joy, as in the case of celebratory traditions such as weddings and holidays; provide a sense of comfort, as in the case of death and dying; or promote a gracious lifestyle, as exemplified by table manners and the offering of food to guests.

screening: A strategy of the Intervention Wheel that serves to identify individuals with disease who are asymptomatic or those individuals with health risk factors.

secondary prevention: Strategies that facilitate early detection of disease, thus resulting in early diagnosis, early treatment, and prevention of spread to others and long-term disability. An example of secondary prevention would be screening.

service learning: A hands-on approach to education where community service, instruction, and reflection serve as a meaningful learning experience.

social capital: Social resources such as parks, medical facilities, schools, and economic investments that are needed to ensure that communities have the resources to maintain health.

social context: A guiding concept of social epidemiology. The social context of behavior addresses individual behavioral risk factors such as smoking and drinking and examines these behaviors in a larger social context, or examines the social influences or conditions that contribute to specific behaviors.

social epidemiology: The study of epidemiology that deals with social distribution and social determinants of health and disease. Social epidemiology makes the case that social determinants of health, which consist of socioeconomic status (income, occupation, and education), socioeconomic position, and discrimination, can influence health outcomes.

social determinants of health: The situations in which people are born, live, work, and play that affect living conditions and ultimately health.

social justice: Justice as it is considered and applied to every aspect of society and to every member of society.

social legitimacy: Popular acceptance of a prevailing idea, value, or belief.

social marketing: Actions and activities that operationalize social marketing principles and the application of appropriate technology for program design with the expressed purpose of influencing the knowledge, attitudes, values, beliefs, behaviors, and practices of a population of interest.

social policy: Guidelines for the creation of positive living conditions for the people's welfare, such as in regard to housing, education, and health.

socioeconomic position: Determined by an individual's socioeconomic status. How much money an individual has, his or her educational attainment, and his or her occupation have a bearing on and reflect the individual's socioeconomic position, or standing in society.

socioeconomic status: Consists of family income, educational level, and occupation.

Spanish Influenza: An epidemic of 1918–1919 (caused by the virus H1N1) that developed toward the end of World War I and was estimated to have caused a global mortality of between 50 and 100 million.

specific protection: Considered in the primary level of prevention, it focuses on a particular disease and/or injury and the prevention of those situations before they take form by stopping the causal event. Examples of these actions include immunizations, environmental sanitation, and nutrition.

state-sanctioned control measures: Government-implemented measures to control the spread of a disease. During the Black Death, Italian city-states were at particular risk. These states were the first to introduce systematic measures to protect their populations from plague.

stereotyping: To generalize to all members of a group.

surge capacity: A measurable representation of the ability to manage a sudden influx of patients.

surveillance: The monitoring of health events and the facilitation of the ongoing systematic collection, analysis, interpretation, and evaluation of data for the purpose of planning, implementing, and evaluating public health initiatives.

teaching–learning strategy: Method of education to meet the needs of and enhance the learning of a specific individual, family, community, population, or system.

telehealth: The use of technology to deliver health care, health information, or health education at a distance.

tertiary prevention: Strategies that stop a disease from progressing and prevent further disability. An example of tertiary prevention is rehabilitation and education on maximum use of an individual's capabilities, thus supporting his or her human capital.

the 5 A's: A framework for the healthcare practitioner to use when working with populations at the individual/family, community, and systems levels of practice to assess how well the population can gain entry into needed resources and use those resources with ultimate positive outcomes.

tobacco use: The leading preventable cause of premature death in the United States. The majority of tobacco users smoke cigarettes, with a smaller number smoking cigars and pipes. Smokeless tobacco is the smallest user group, which includes snuff and chewing tobacco. Passive smoking is a process where nonsmokers inhale smoke.

visiting nurse: A term used interchangeably, at one time in the United States, with district nurse. This term also refers to the educated nurse who provides care for the sick public in their homes.

vulnerable populations: A group of individuals who are at greater risk than other populations and who also share specific characteristics such as social, physical, cultural, economic, or environmental characteristics.

xenophobia: The conscious fear of foreigners.

Index

Note: Boxes, figures, and tables are indicated by b, f, and t following the page number.